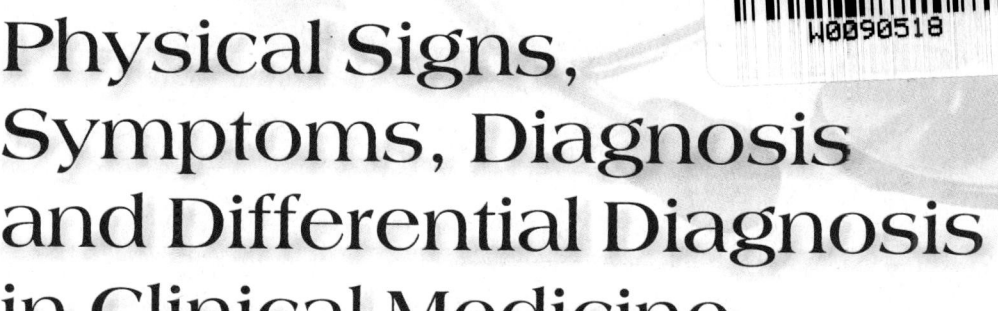
Physical Signs, Symptoms, Diagnosis and Differential Diagnosis in Clinical Medicine

Physical Signs, Symptoms, Diagnosis and Differential Diagnosis in Clinical Medicine

S N Chugh
MD, MNAMS, FICP, FIACM, FICN, FISC, FIMSA
Ex-Senior Professor of Medicine
Pt BD Sharma PG Institute of Medical Sciences
and
Ex-Pro Vice Chancellor
Pt BD Sharma University of Health Sciences
Rohtak, Haryana

Ashima
MBBS (Gold Medalist), MD
ex-senior resident, GB Pant Hospital
New Delhi

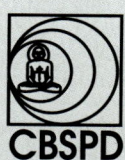

CBSPD

CBS Publishers & Distributors Pvt Ltd

New Delhi • Bengaluru • Chennai • Kochi • Kolkata • Lucknow • Mumbai
Hyderabad • Jharkhand • Nagpur • Patna • Pune • Uttarakhand

Disclaimer

Science and technology are constantly changing fields. New research and experience broaden the scope of information and knowledge. The authors have tried their best in giving information available to them while preparing the material for this book. Although all efforts have been made to ensure optimum accuracy of the material, yet it is quite possible some errors might have been left uncorrected. The publisher, the printer and the authors will not be held responsible for any inadvertent errors or inaccuracies.

Physical Signs, Symptoms Diagnosis and Differential Diagnosis in Clinical Medicine

ISBN: 978-93-86478-17-7

Copyright © Authors and Publisher

First Edition: 2017

Reprint: 2025

All rights reserved. No part of this book may be reproduced or transmitted in any form or by any means, electronic or mechanical, including photocopying, recording, or any information storage and retrieval system without permission, in writing, from the authors and the publisher.

Published by Satish Kumar Jain and produced by Varun Jain for

CBS Publishers & Distributors Pvt Ltd

4819/XI Prahlad Street, 24 Ansari Road, Daryaganj, New Delhi 110 002, India
Ph: 011-23266838, 23289259   Website: www.cbspd.com
                                 e-mail: delhi@cbspd.com

Corporate Office: 204 FIE, Industrial Area, Patparganj, Delhi 110 092, India
Ph: 011-49344934   Fax: 011-49344935   e-mail: publishing@cbspd.com; publicity@cbspd.com

Branches

- **Bengaluru:** Seema House 2975, 17th Cross, K.R. Road, Banasankari 2nd Stage, Bengaluru 560 070, Karnataka, India
  Ph: +91-80-26771678/79   Fax: +91-80-26771680   e-mail: bangalore@cbspd.com

- **Chennai:** 18/8B, Subbaraya Street, Shenoy Nagar, Chennai 600 030, Tamil Nadu, India
  Ph: +91-44-42032115, 26681266   e-mail: chennai@cbspd.com

- **Kochi:** 42/1325, 1326, Power House Road, Opposite KSEB, Power House, Ernakulum 682 018, Kochi, Kerala, India
  Ph: +91-484-4059061–65   Fax: +91-484-4059065   e-mail: kochi@cbspd.com

- **Kolkata:** 147, Hind Ceramics Compound, 1st Floor, Nilgunj Road, Belghoria, Kolkata 700 056, West Bengal, India
  Ph: +91-33-25330055/56   e-mail: kolkata@cbspd.com

- **Lucknow:** Basement, Khushuma Complex, 7 Meerabai Marg (behind Jawahar Bhawan), Lucknow 226 001, UP, India
  Ph: +91-522-4000032   e-mail: tiwari.lucknow@cbspd.com

- **Mumbai:** PWD Shed, Gala No. 25/26, Ramchandra Bhatt Marg, Next JJ Hospital, Gate No. 2, Opp. Union Bank of India, Noorbaug Mumbai 400 009, Maharashtra, India
  Ph: +91-22-66661880/89   e-mail: mumbai@cbspd.com

Representatives

- **Hyderabad** 0-9885175004   • **Jharkhand** 0-9811541605   • **Nagpur** 0-8692091830
- **Patna** 0-9334159340   • **Pune** 0-9664372571   • **Uttarakhand** 0-9716462459

Printed at: Nutech Print Services, Faridabad, Haryana, India

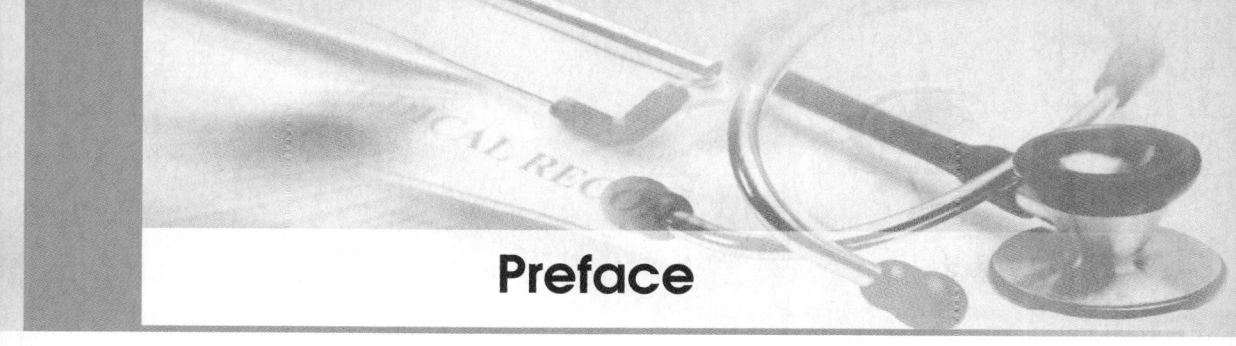

Preface

It gives us immense pleasure to introduce the first edition of our book entitled *Physical Signs, Symptoms, Diagnosis and Differential Diagnosis in Clinical Medicine* to medical students and physicians. In the present era of high profile sets of investigations, the physical signs occupy the back seat. Physicians rely more on investigations than the physical signs forgetting that they are clues to diagnosis. Investigations are planned based on provisional diagnosis/differential diagnosis. Mind thinks about what you see, therefore, we should not forget the significance of physical signs.

A student/physician after taking the detailed history, analysing the symptoms, interprets the physical signs and comes to some physical diagnosis. After critical analysis of the signs, he/she narrows down the differential diagnosis and then plan the investigations. Missing or misinterpretation of physician signs can point to erroneous diagnosis. Therefore, we have introduced this book for picking up correct clinical signs and interpret them correctly to give correct provisional diagnosis/differential diagnosis.

The book has been written on the request of our students and younger teachers, so as to apprise the students, about the clinical significance of physical symptoms and signs. A large number of books are available on clinical examinations but some lack in substance while others lack in the analysis of symptoms/signs clues to diagnosis/differential diagnosis. This book gives you detailed analysis of symptoms pertaining to various systems, their analysis and the detailed physical signs to highlight the diagnosis and differential diagnosis. At the end of each unit, brief synopsis of various diseases/conditions is provided for viva voce at the bedside.

We think this book will cater the need of the students and physicians and they would like it for making prompt spot provisional diagnosis.

We are thankful to CBS Publishers who have provided me the opportunity to introduce this book and we are happy that they have brought a colourful edition of this book.

SN Chugh
Ashima Chugh

Contents

Preface v

UNIT I
General Physical Examination 1

General Physical Examination	1
Head (Cranium)	4
The Eye Examination	6
Examination of Ear, Nose, Throat	8
The Neck	17
Regional lymphadenopathy	18
The Breast and Axillae	20
The Extremities	20

UNIT II
Examination of Respiratory System 29

Respiratory System	29
Symptoms related to Upper Respiratory Tract and their Analysis	29
Symptoms of Lower Respiratory Tract and their Analysis	31
History	36
General Physical Examination of Respiratory System	36
Examination of Upper Respiratory System	39
Examination of Lower Respiratory System (Chest examination)	41
Adventitious/Added Sounds	54
Examination of the Posterior Chest	58
Differential Diagnosis	59
Brief Synopsis of Common Respiratory Diseases	59

UNIT III
Cardiovascular System 71

Symptoms and their Analysis	71
The History	77
General Physical Examination	78
Systemic Examination of Cardiovascular System	89
Differential Diagnosis of Murmurs	101
I. Ejection Systolic (ES) or Midsystolic Murmur	102
II. Pansystolic Murmurs	104
Diastolic Murmurs	105
Continuous Murmurs	107
Physical Signs of Different Cardiovascular Conditions	108
Peripheral Vascular System	115
Examination	116
Brief Synopsis of Peripheral Vascular Disease	120
The Venous System	122
Brief Synopsis of Venous Disorders	122

UNIT IV
The Urogenital System and Sexually Transmitted Diseases 127

I. Common Urinary Symptoms and their Analysis	127
II. Symptoms of Sexually Transmitted Diseases (STDs)	133
The History	133
Examination—General Physical and Urogenital System (Abdomen Examination)	135
Examination of The Male Genitalia	139
The Scrotum and its Contents	141
Differential Diagnosis of a Scrotal Swelling	143
Examination of Female Genitalia	143
Brief Synopsis of Common Renal Disorders	146
Brief Synopsis of Genital Diseases and Hernia	149

UNIT V
Nervous System 153

Common Symptoms and their Analysis	153
History	161
Examination—General Physical	162

Physical Signs, Symptoms, Diagnosis and Differential Diagnosis

Systemic Neurological Examination	170
Mental Status/Higher Mental Functions	170
Speech and Language	172
Examination of Cranial Nerves	176
The Motor System Examination	203
Testing for the Cerebellar Functions	222
Gait	225
The Sensory System	234
Nerve lesion (Entrapment Neuropathy)	242
Autonomic Nervous System (ANS)	243
Nervous System at a Glance	246
Brief synopsis of the Neurological Disorders	247
Epilepsies	252
Polyneuropathies	252
Postinfective Polyneuropathy (Guillain-Barré syndrome)	253
Myasthenia Gravis	254
Multiple Sclerosis	254
Syringomyelia	255
Motor Neuron Disease (MND)	255
Paraplegia	256

UNIT VI
Gastrointestinal and Hepatobiliary Systems — 257

Symptoms of Gastrointestinal System	257
Symptoms of Hepatobiliary System	268
History	271
Examination—General Physical and Systemic (Abdominal examination)	271
Examination of Inguinal Region	292
The Back of Abdomen	292
Examination of the Anus, Rectum and Prostate	292
Examination of Abdominal Lump/Mass	294
Brief synopsis of common GI Tract Hepatobiliary Disorders	299

UNIT VII
Examination of Breasts and Axillae — 313

Common Symptoms Related to Breast	313
Examination of Breasts	316
Brief Synopsis of Breast Diseases	319

UNIT VIII
Haematological Disorders — 321

Pattern of Haematological Disorders	321
History	331
Examination of a Patient with Haematological Disorder	332
Systemic Examination	337
Brief Synopsis of Common Blood Disorders	337
Laboratory Diagnosis of Hematological Disorders	342

UNIT IX
Endocrine Disorders — 347

Symptoms of Endocrine System	347
History	348
General Physical Examination (GPE)	349
Systemic Examination	357
Brief Synopsis of Endocrinal Disorders	357

UNIT X
Examination of Musculoskeletal and Locomotor System — 371

Major Symptoms of Rheumatic Diseases	371
History	376
Examination of Locomotor System	377
Examination of Individual Joints	380
Examination of the Spinal Column	385
Examination of Limb Joints	389
Brief synopsis of Rheumatological disorders	401

UNIT XI
Dermatological Disorders — 407

Symptoms of Skin Disorders and thier Analysis	407
History	408
Examination—General	410
Examination of Nails	419
Examination of Hair	420
Brief synopsis of Common Skin disorders	420

UNIT XII
Vitals and the Unconscious Patient — 427

Symptom Unconsciousness	427
History	428
Examination—General Physical	429
Systemic Examination	433
Other Systems Examination	438
Brief Synopsis of Different Comas	438
Index	445

Unit I

General Physical Examination

- Symptoms and their Analysis
- History
- Examination (Physical Signs and Systemic Signs)
- Diagnosis and Differential Diagnosis
- Brief Synopsis of lymphadenopathy and oedema

GENERAL PHYSICAL EXAMINATION

1. GENERAL OBSERVATIONS
- Abnormal facial appearance/symmetry
- Abnormal gait, posture, movements
- Abnormal sound/breath
- Abnormal swelling/nutrition
- Change in colour of skin and mucous membrane
- Abnormal height and weight.

SIGNS

Facial Expression

☞ *Look at the face for appearance and expression*

- Mask-like expressionless face suggests depression, parkinsonism and hypothyroidism.
- Agitated face indicates hypomania.
- Swollen face indicates periorbital oedema (nephrotic/nephritic syndrome, cirrhosis, hypothyroidism, CHF, hypoproteinemia, etc.).
- A staring look (frightening face) suggests Graves' disease.
- Moon-facies with red-cheeks suggest Cushing's syndrome.
- Mongoloid face (small, flat face, upward slanting eyes, depressed nose, protruded tongue resembling idiotic face) indicates Down's syndrome (trisomy).

Special types of facies are:
i. Leonine face is seen in leprosy (*see* Fig. 11.31).
ii. Congenital syphilitic face consisting of Hutchinson's teeth, saddle nose and keratitis is seen in congenital syphilis.
iii. Mitral facies (malar flush) is characteristic of mitral stenosis.
iv. Cyanotic (bluish) face is characteristic of cyanotic heart disease, SVC obstruction, COPD, etc.

- Elfin facies (wide mouth, large lower lips, pointed chin, widely spaced teeth, widely set eyes and protruding ears) are seen in supravalvular aortic stenosis.
- Hypertelorism (eyes are set apart due to epicanthal folds) is seen in congenital heart disease.
- Thalassemic face (frontal bossing, prominent cheeks) is seen in thalassemic patients.

☞ *Look at the complexion, i.e. dark/fair/abnormal*
- Normal complexion of most of Indians is dark/fair.
- Abnormal complexion such as pallor indicates anaemia and cherry-red complexion is due to polycythaemia/carboxyhaemoglobinaemia.

(Read the abnormal skin colour in dermatology)

☞ *Observe state of clothing and hydration*
- Shabby dress and soiling of underwear indicate dementia.
- Excessive clothing indicates cold intolerance in hypothyroidism or drug addiction (to hide the scar mark) or a patient suffering from skin disease.

☞ *Observe state of consciousness*
- Read it under unit of examination of unconscious patient.

Physical Signs, Symptoms, Diagnosis and Differential Diagnosis

☞ Observe abnormal gait/posture/movement (read them also in unit on nervous system examination).

Typical postures observed during general physical examination are:
- Patients of cor pulmonale (COPD), pericardial effusions and CHF adopt a peculiar **sitting posture on the bed** with arms resting on the table and legs hanging down (**orthopnoeic posture**).
- Patient with abdominal colic tosses in the bed or may have hot water bottle on the abdomen.
- Patients with emphysema may puff out his/her cheeks (*purse lip breathing*) while sitting in bed.
- **Stooped posture** while standing is seen in parkinsonism.
- **Hemiplegic posture:** There is a characteristic limb asymmetry displaying adduction of upper limb with flexion at elbow and pronation and flexion of the wrist. The lower limb is hyperextended.
- **Lordotic posture** (sway-back posture) is seen in pseudohypertrophic muscular dystrophy.
- **Normal decubitus posture** in bed is dorsal recumbent (patient lies flat on the back) or normal supine posture. **Lateral decubitus posture** whether right lateral or left lateral is adopted in respiratory diseases (pleural effusion, empyema, pneumothorax), cardiovascular diseases (cardiomegaly), meningitis, appendicitis, etc. In meningitis, patient adopts **coiled up decubitus (curled up) posture**.
- **Decubitus posture of thromboangiitis obliterans** is a sitting up posture with legs hanging down and the head resting on knees even during sleep. This relieves agonising pain in the lower limbs.
- **Kneeling posture (Prayer's posture)** is adopted to relieve orthopnoea in patients with CHF, pericardial effusion, mediastinal tumour. This is similar to orthopnoeic posture described above.
- **Squatting posture (knee-chest position)** is seen in children with Fallot's tetralogy (congenital cyanotic heart disease). This posture provides resistance against right to left shunt, allows more blood to flow for oxygenation into the lungs to relieve cyanosis.
- **Prone posture:** It may be habitual in certain persons, but common in tuberculosis of the spine, acute gastroenteritis.
- **Astasia abasia:** A hysterical patient may at times not be able to stand (ataxic) but is able to walk and move the legs in bed.

☞ Observe the built/body habitus/constitution

The normal average body built is called **normosthenic**
- **Asthenic of hyposthenic built** is thin long under developed body with long neck, flat chest, slender fingers.
- **Hypersthenic built** is short, broad stout built with short neck, muscular chest and large stubby fingers.

☞ Observe the stature and measure upper and lower segments (body proportions)

The **stature** means sum total of upper segment (top of head to pubis symphysis) and lower segment (pubis symphysis to soles of feet). The **span** is the distance between the tips of the middle fingers of the two hands with the arms stretched out and held horizontally.

> *Note.* Normally the span and stature are more or less equal and so are the upper and lower segments, the abnormality arises when either there is premature or delayed epiphyseal fusion.

- **In premature epiphyseal fusion** (precocious puberty) the stature is greater than the arm span and upper segment is greater than lower.
- **In delayed epiphyseal fusion** there is tall stature and arm span is greater than stature (height) and upper segment is greater than lower segment; for example in Marfan's syndrome, homocysteinuria, Klinefelter's syndrome, constitutional, and enuchoidism.
- **Tall stature** means height more than 97 percentile of the normal population. The *causes* of tall stature are given in Box 1.1. Gigantism is generalised tall stature due to excess of growth hormone with normal body proportions. Kallmann's syndrome is another cause of tall stature with normal body proportion and hypogonadism.

Box 1.1 Causes of Tall Stature

I. Congenital
- A normal variant
- Cerebral gigantism (abnormally tall individual with pointed chin, prominent forehead and hypertelorism)
- Marfan's syndrome
- Homocysteinuria
- Klinefelter's syndrome

II. Endocrinal causes
- Hyperthyroidism
- Precocious puberty
- Pituitary gigantism
- Kallmann's syndrome

- **Short stature or dwarfism** means decrease in height more than expected in normal person.

General Physical Examination

A child more than 2.5 SD below the mean for chronological, age, growth velocity below 5th percentile on the growth velocity curve is called **short stature**.

> Dwarfism means height below 3rd percentile of normal population of same age and sex.

The **causes** include:
1. **Hereditary** (genetic or primary)
2. **Endocrine dwarfism,** e.g. cretinism or hypothyroidism, Fröhlich's syndrome, pituitary dwarfism (infantilism), Turner syndrome (45X0), Noonan syndrome, polyostotic fibrosa cystica (Albright syndrome), Laurence-Moon-Biedl syndrome.
3. **Skeletal dwarfism,** e.g. cerebral dwarfism achondroplasia, osteogenesis imperfecta, spondyloepiphyseal dysplasia (tarda or congenita). It is short limbs and short trunk type of dwarfism.
4. **Storage diseases,** e.g. mucopolysaccharidoses (Hurler's syndrome, Hunter's syndrome, etc.)
5. **Systemic dwarfism,** i.e. systemic diseases leading to dwarfism include renal rickets, congenital heart diseases, coeliac disease, diabetes type I.
6. **Metabolic diseases,** e.g. von Gierke's disease (glycogen storage disease).
7. **Infective causes,** i.e. syphilis (congenital).

Note. Chromosomal, endocrinal, metabolic, nutritional and psychological abnormalities produce proportionate dwarfism.

☞ Look for status of nutrition

The state of nutrition depends mainly on the distribution of adipose tissue or fat in the body. On the basis of weight and height, BMI is calculated, and on the basis of weight vis à vis, BMI, the individuals are classified as *normal, overweight* and *underweight* as follows:

I. **Mild undernutrition** (body weight reduction from 90 to 80% of International Standard and BMI reduced from 20 to 18 kg/m²).
II. **Moderate undernutrition** (weight reduction from 80 to 71% and BMI reduction from 18 to 16 kg/m²).
III. **Severe malnutrition** (weight reduction below 70% and BMI reduced below 16 kg/m²).

The **overweight** and **obesity** on the basis of BMI (WHO) are graded as follows:
- Normal   13–25 kg/m²
- Overweight   < 30 (26–29) kg/m²
- Obesity   ≥ 30 (30–39) kg/m²
- Morbid obesity   ≥ 40 kg/m²

Waist/Hip Ratio

☞ Measure the waist (between costal margins and iliac crests and hip (at greater trochanter) and calculate the ratio.

- Normal waist/hip ratio is < 0.8
- Waist/hip ratio > 0.9 indicate central obesity

☞ Decide whether person is overweight, obese or underweight

Obesity may be mild, moderate and severe. Types of obesity depend on the distribution of fat and may be of diagnostic value, i.e.
1. Generalised obesity is either an alimentary or exogenous obesity (excessive intake of food).
2. Central or truncal obesity is common in Cushing's syndrome and hypothyroidism
3. Girdle type obesity involving hips, buttocks and abdomen is due to pituitary or hypothalamic in origin.
4. The trochanteric type involving the hips only is usually a hypogonadal obesity.
5. Localised obesity where large deposits of fat are more or less confined to neck region is seen in beer drinkers or alcoholics called *cervical lipomatosis*.

The **causes** of overweight/obesity include positive energy balance due to hereditary (genetic), hypothalamic, psychological (food faddism), physical inactivity and drugs (steroids, oral contraceptives, insulin, etc.).
Obesity can be endocrinal, i.e. Cushing syndrome, adiposogenital syndrome, hypothyroidism, Prader-Willi syndrome, Fröhlich's syndrome, Laurence-Moon-Biedl syndrome, polycystic ovarian syndrome, hypogonadism, menopausal syndrome, and idiopathic.

Underweight is due to malnutrition such as protein energy malnutrition resulting in oedema (*kwashiorkor*) and total calories malnutrition, i.e. *marasmus* resulting in thin lean person, thyrotoxicosis, type I DM, coeliac disease, tuberculosis, malabsorption, HIV infection, malignancy, anorexia nervosa, Addison's disease and depression.

☞ Assess the nutritional status by muscle bulk, subcutaneous fat and sign and symptoms of nutrients and vitamins deficiency.

☞ Assess the tone of muscles and measure muscle bulk (left arm circumference).

Toneless muscles (flabby muscles and decreased muscle mass indicate decreased nutrition. Normal left mid-upper arm circumference in males is 25.5 cm and in females 23 cm).

☞ Measure triceps skin fold thickness of the left mid-arm by Lange's or Herpenden's calipers
- Normal average adult triceps skin fold thickness is as follows:
  Males   12.5 mm
  Females   16 mm

Reduced skin fold thickness indicates malnutrition.

☞ Assess fat distribution, i.e. localised/generalised.

- Localised deposition of fat results in lipomas (Fig. 1.1).
- Localised lipoatrophy is seen after insulin injection (insulin lipoatrophy).
- Truncal deposition of fat and camel hump is seen in Cushing's syndrome.
- Xanthomas are lipid nodules present in subcutaneous tissue along the tendons of muscles, are associated with hyperlipidaemia.

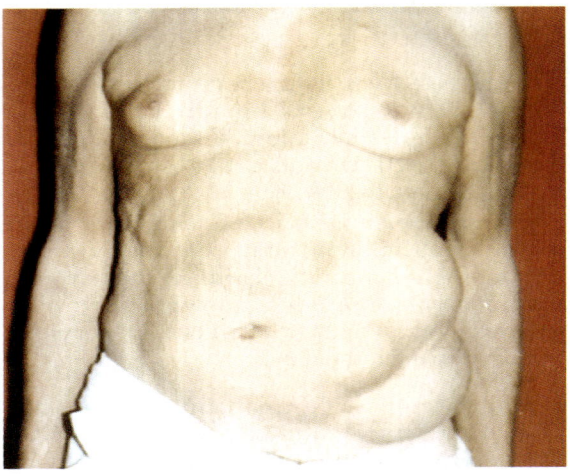

Fig. 1.1: Multiple abdominal wall lipomas. Note the multiple swellings.

State of Hydration

☞ Assess hydration state by skin elasticity, intraocular tension, BP, moistness of tongue, JVP and weight.

Dryness of tongue and mouth, soft sunken eyeballs (reduced intraocular tension), loss of skin elasticity, low BP and JVP and loss of weight suggest dehydration (volume depletion).

Odour/Smell

☞ Is there any foul smell from breath?

Foul breath is called *halitosis*. The **causes** are:
Foul breath may be due to bad orodental hygiene, stomatitis, atrophic rhinitis, follicular tonsillitis, sinusitis, bronchiectasis, lung abscess, ingestion of substances like onion, garlic and excessive fermentation in the stomach due to neoplasm.

Typical foul breath
- *Alcoholic breath* in alcoholic intoxication, is easily recognised.
- *Fruity odour* (acetone smell) occurs in diabetic ketoacidosis, starvation, metabolic acidosis.
- *Urinous or ammoniacal smell*. It occurs in uraemia.
- *Musty sweety odour* or *ammoniacal odour (fetor hepaticus)* occurs in liver cell failure.
- *Pungent garlic odour* is typical of poisoning by OP compounds, aluminium, phosphide and arsenic.
- *Very offensive fecal breath* occurs in gastrocolic fistula.

HEAD (CRANIUM)

☞ *Measure the skull circumference and note any abnormality*

The average skull circumference measured circumferentially along the lines drawn horizontally backward from supraorbital ridges to the occipital protuberance is 13 inches at birth, 18 inches at 1 year, 20 inches at age 7 and 21 inches at age 15 years and 22 inches in adult.

- The skull may be unduly large called *macrocephaly*.
- The *microcephaly* (small skull) may be due to cerebral agenesis, toxoplasmosis, cytomegalic inclusion disease.
- The macrocephaly may be due to hydrocephalus (Fig. 1.2) or megalencephaly, Paget's disease (the skull becomes larger and larger in adult life requiring larger and larger sizes of hats), acromegaly (large head and face with prominent supraorbital ridges) or gargoylism. In achondroplasia head appears to be larger due to short stature (dwarfism).
- The head circumference is larger than normal in Paget's disease. Face is small and legs are bowed.

☞ *Look at the shape of skull*

Abnormal shapes of the skull are:
  i. **Oxycephaly** (tower skull). It results from early closure of coronal and sagittal sutures

resulting in decrease in A-P as well as vertical diameter of skull giving the head an elongated shape with pointed vertex. It is familial.

ii. **Acrocephaly** (high pointed head with broad base) is less common. It is associated with syndactyly of hands and feet. It is seen in craniofacial dysostosis.

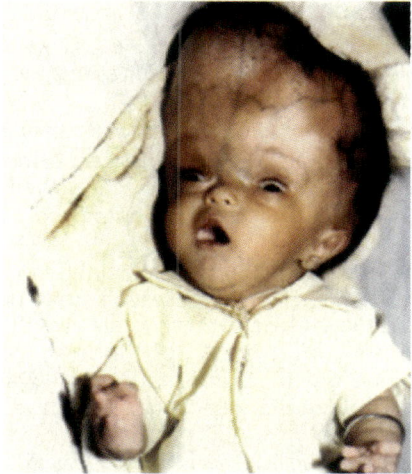

Fig. 1.2: Macrocephaly (hydrocephalus with 'sun setting' sign).

iii. **Dolicocephaly**. Narrow bifrontal transverse diameter constitutes narrow forehead, is seen in Edward's syndrome (a trisomy).
iv. **Rachitic (boxy) head**. There is bossing of head (prominent frontal and parietal bones) with square shape head or oblong head.
v. **Brachycephaly**. There is bicoronal synostosis with loss of supraorbital contour on both sides. The head assumes a spherical shape.
vi. **Platybasia (basilar invagination)**. As the name suggests, there is upward displacement (invagination) of basilar portion of occipital bone with reduction in the size of posterior fossa. The deformity is congenital and associated with fusion of two or more cervical vertebrae (*Klippel-Feil syndrome*) or stenosis of foramen magnum. Basilar impression may be acquired in osteogenesis imperfecta, rickets, osteomalacia and Paget's disease.
vii. **Craniotabes (softening of skull)**. Soft skull with egg-shell crackling on palpation (craniotabes) is early sign of rickets, disappears before the end of first year.
viii. **Other abnormalities** such as lumps or tumours (meningocoele, Fig. 1.3), metastastes, neuroma and aneurysm may also produce localised swelling.

☞ *Look and palpate the anterior and posterior fontanelles*

- Normally anterior fontanelle closes at 16 months, posterior at 6 weeks and cranial sutures at 6 months.
- Sunken or depressed frontanelles suggest *dehydration or marasmus*; while bulging frontanelles suggest *raised intracranial pressure* (meningitis, hydrocephalus, subarachnoid haemorrhage).
- Premature closure of the sutures indicates craniostenosis, while delayed closure is seen in hydrocephalus, cretinism and congenital syphilis.

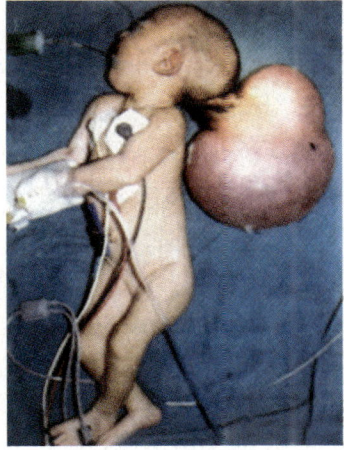

Fig. 1.3: Localised bulge due to encephalocoele.

THE SCALP

☞ *Examine the skull for dandruff (seborrhoeic dermatitis) or any abnormality of hair*

- **Bull dog scalp** (thick corrugated scalp with thick skin and subcutaneous tissue) is seen in acromegaly.
- **Syphilic mop** (excessive growth of hair over the head) is seen in congenital syphilis.
- **Greying of hair** is physiological (after age of 40 years), but may be familial or due to mental stress and ischaemic heart disease, atherosclerosis, prenicious anaemia or progeria (premature senility).

HEAD MOVEMENTS

☞ *Note any movements or fixation of the head*

- Normally head movements may occur in old age, in certain families, in alcoholics and may be habitual spasms (tics).

- Abnormally, they may be seen in paralytic agitans or parkinsonism (a slow coarse head rotatory or head nodding or shaking of the head movements), severe AR (head nodding with each heartbeat), chorea (jerky or variable movements of head).
- Titubation is a phenomenon of irregular oscillations of the head and neck while standing. It occurs in multiple sclerosis, cerebellar disease and in Friedreich's ataxia.
- **Head fixation (lack of normal head movements)** indicates cervical rigidity, is seen in meningitis, tetanus, cervical spine disease (trauma, spondylosis), cervical lymphadenitis, torticollis, retropharyngeal abscess, strychnine poisoning.

THE FOREHEAD

☞ Look at the forehead for prominence, wrinkling and local lesions

- Prominence of forehead with prominent supraorbital ridges indicates *acromegaly*.
- *Frontal bossing* is seen in thalassaemia, hydrocephalus.
- Absence of bilateral wrinkling over the forehead indicates Graves' disease (Joffroy's sign).
- Bilateral wrinkled forehead suggests anxiety, psychoneurosis old age or bilateral ptosis.
- Loss of unilateral wrinkling indicates Bell's palsy (7th cranial nerve palsy).
- Local lesions, i.e. skin eruptions may occur in acne, chickenpox, measles, local skin diseases.
- Nodules over the forehead may be due to cyst, tumour, etc.

THE TEMPLE

☞ Palpate the temple for tenderness and pulsation of temporal artery.

- Tender, painful and irregular temporal arteries in old persons indicate *temporal arteritis*. The lingual and jaw claudication is characteristic of this condition
- Thickened, palpable temporal arteries suggest *atherosclerosis*.

THE EYE EXAMINATION

☞ Look at the eyes for expression/behaviour

- Dull and apathetic eye expression indicates a psychiatric disorder or hypothyroidism.
- Shiny, bright and staring eyes indicate Graves' disease

- Patients with ocular pain or photophobia wear dark glasses.
- Patient having diplopia may close one eye
- Patient with hemianopia may bump into objects on the blind side.
- Patients with central loss of vision cannot make eye to eye contact.

The Eyelids

Note the position of the lid in relation to eyeball. Inspect the palpebral fissure, oedema of the lids, xanthelasma and redness of eyes

Pull down the lower lid while patient looks up

To evert the upper lid, ask the patient to look down, grasp the eyelashes, press gently on the upper border of tarsal plate with a tip and swing the lashes up.

- Palpebral fissure is *wide* in facial nerve palsy, parkinsonism, Graves' disease; *narrow* in ptosis, Horner's syndrome, myasthenia gravis, etc.
- Xanthelasma (small lipid laden swelling) appears on the inner canthus in diabetes, hyperlipidaemia, nephrotic syndrome, hypothyroidism.
- Oedema of the lids (periorbital oedema) may be due to nephrotic syndrome, hypothyroidism, angioneurotic oedema, CHF, cirrhosis, SVC obstruction, cavernous sinus thrombosis.
- Redness of eyelids is due to blepharitis, Weil's disease.
- Stye is an infected follicle or a small abscess over the upper or lower lid, is commonly seen in diabetics.
- Mikulicz's syndrome consisting of enlargement of lacrimal glands (bilateral swelling over upper eyelids) and parotid glands (bilateral swelling over the angles of the jaw) is an autoimmune disorder.
- Chalazion is a growing tumour or cyst of meibomian gland in the eyelid.
- Dacrocystitis is inflammation and swelling at the inner canthus of the eye.
- Tophi containing urate crystals can be seen over the eyelids in gout.
- Ectropion (eversion of the free edge of eyelid) may occur due to old age, facial paralysis or scarring of the lids following burns.
- Entropion (rolling in or inversion of the eyelid) may be due to spasm of orbicularis oculi or due to scarring.
- Lid-lag, lid retraction, infrequent blinking, lagophthalmos, etc. are signs of Graves' disease (read unit on examination of endocrine system).
- Frequent blinking is seen as habitual spasms (tics), in nervousness, local eye irritation.
- Tremors of lids occur in parkinsonism.

The Eyeballs

☞ *Look at the eyeballs for prominence or retraction and for other abnormalities*

- Prominence of the eyeball is due to exophthalmos or proptosis (read exophthalmos on examination of endocrine disorders).
- Enophthalmos (sunken eyeballs) are seen in dehydration, Horner's syndrome.
- Microphthalmia is seen in Patau's syndrome.
- Panophthalmitis is infection of eyeball with loss of vision.

Note: Read nervous system examination for cranial nerves innervating the eyes.
Read conjugate deviation and Doll eye's movements in examination of unconscious patient.

The Conjunctiva

☞ *Examine the conjunctivae for inflammation, ulceration, haemorrhage, spots and scar*

- Bright red conjunctivae indicate conjunctivitis due to any cause.
- Petechial conjunctival haemorrhage occurs in SABE, leukaemias, aplastic anaemia; while subconjunctival haemorrhage occurs in hypertensive patients, following bouts of whooping cough, during convulsion, fracture of base of skull. Pterygium is a fold of membrane that extends from outer part of bulbar conjunctiva to the cornea, seen in old persons.
- Bitot's spots are white glistening plaques (spots) of desquamated epithelium found over conjunctiva in vitamin A deficiency (Fig. 1.4).

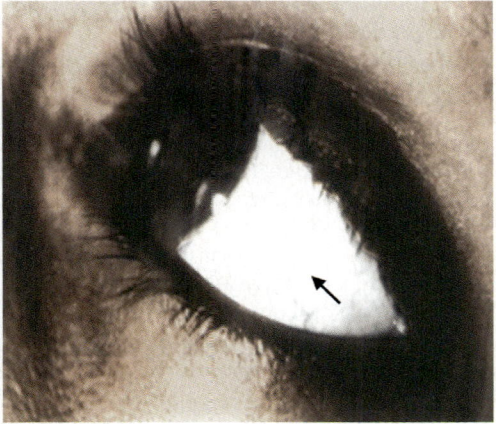

Fig. 1.4: Bitot's spots. Note the white glistening spots (←) at the sclera near the lateral angle of the eye.

The Sclera

☞ *Examine sclera for colour, vascularity, inflammation, etc.*

- Sclera is yellow in jaundice, red in scleritis or episcleritis (extra-articular manifestation of collagen vascular disorder).
- Blue sclera occurs in osteogenesis imperfecta, Marfan's syndrome, Ehlers-Danlos syndrome and trisomy 18.
- Dark grey or lead coloured sclera is seen in argyria, after use of silver salts for long time.
- Pearly white sclera is seen in idiopathic hypochromic anaemia.
- Scleral pigmentation occurs in alkaptonuria.

The Cornea

☞ *Examine the cornea for opacity, scar, ulcer, abrasion, etc. Look at the lens for opacity.*

- *Clouding of cornea* occurs due to corneal oedema, herpes simplex infection, acute glaucoma.
- *Corneal abrasions* can occur following chemical burns (alkali or acid burns), arcus senilis.
- *Corneal arcus.* It is ill defined greyish white crescent or circle just within outer margin of the cornea. It is due to lipid infiltration and is a degenerative condition due to old age. A clear zone of iris from the limbus distinguishes it from Kayser-Fleischer ring. It sometimes may be associated with hyperlipoproteinaemia.
- *Kayser-Fleischer ring* (Fig. 1.5) It is a golden brown pigmentary ring around the cornea just internal to the limbus. It is sometimes visible to the naked eye but confirmation of the ring is done by slit-lamp examination. It is diagnostic of Wilson's disease.
- *Corneal opacities.* Presence of corneal opacities or old scars indicates old injuries, ulcers, inflammation or gonococcal ophthalmia.
- *Opacification of cornea* is seen in Hurler's syndrome while corneal calcification indicates long standing hypercalcaemia (hyperparathyroidism), most commonly seen when serum phosphate levels are raised.
- *Interstital keratitis* due to cellular infiltration of deeper layers of cornea with other sphilitic stigmatas (Hutchinson's teeth and saddle nose) suggest congenital syphilis while *exposure keratitis* is seen in exophthalmos or in Bell's palsy or 5th nerve paralysis causing loss of corneal sensation.

- *Keratomalacia* is opaque, cloudy, glossy cornea due to Vit. A deficiency, it is associated with night blindness, dry and shrunken conjunctivae (xerosis or xerophthalmia).
- *Phlyctenular keratitis* (small greyish or yellowish nodules over the cornea) may appear in debilitated children and patients with tuberculosis.
- *Corneal ulcer* (a localised erosion or loss of substance of cornea) is due to trauma, tuberculosis, malignancy, hypopyon and following herpes zoster ophthalmicus.
- *Keratoconjuctivitis sicca* means dry cornea and conjunctivae, is seen in Sjögren's syndrome.

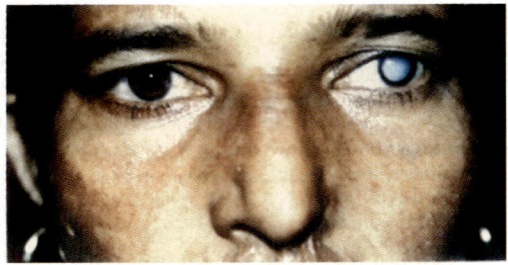

Fig. 1.6: Cataract (lens opacity) of left eye.

The Pupil
The examination of the pupil has been discussed in neurology (cranial nerve examination).

The Fundus
Examination of ocular fundus has been discussed in neurology.

Movements of the Eyeballs
Read neurology—cranial nerve examination.

EXAMINATION OF EAR, NOSE, THROAT
Read it under upper respiratory system also.

The Ears
☞ Examine the ears for congenital malformations, nodules, discharge, shape and size, pulsations, local lesions. Palpate them for tenderness.

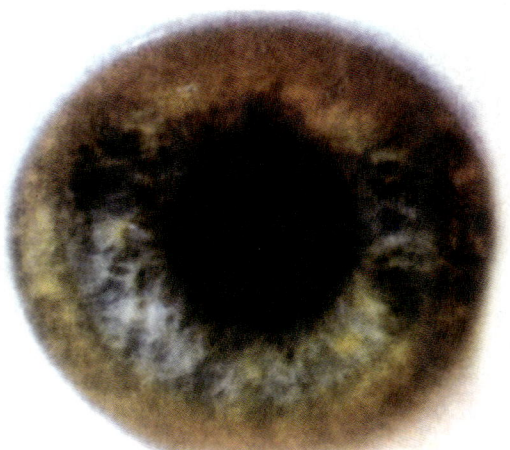

Fig. 1.5: A Kayser-Fleischer ring. It is seen in Wilson's disease.

The Iris
Normally iris is black in colour and has a central hole called pupil.

☞ Look at the iris for discolouration, inflammation, etc.
- *Discolouration of iris (heterochromia)* indicates intraocular disease or albinism.
- *Muddy sclera* with a small pupil with ciliary congestion indicates iritis, a manifestation, rheumatoid arthritis, connective tissue diseases or sarcoidosis.

The Lens
The normal lens is not visible on inspection.

☞ Examine the lens with torch for whiteness, displacement
- *Ectopia lentis* (displaced lens) is seen on slit-lamp examination in Marfan's syndrome.
- *Advanced cataract* (chalky white lens) is seen in the central hole of cornea (Fig. 1.6).

- *Unduly large prominent protuding ears* may be seen in Marfan's syndrome.
- *Small ear lobe with angular overlapping helix* is seen in Down's syndrome.
- *Cauliflower ears* (grossly deformed, thickened, flexible ears) are common in wrestles (Fig. 1.7). They are due to repeated injuries to the ears.
- *Buddhas ears* (elongated, hanging ears) are seen in leprosy. There may be thickening of the ears.
- *Low set ears* (draw a line from the outer canthus of the eye to the ear on the same side. If one-third of the pinna is above this line, it suggests low set ears) are seen in Edward's syndrome, Patau's syndrome, and Noonan syndrome.
- *Hairy ears* in a neonate may be associated with maternal diabetes mellitus.
- *Tophi* over ear indicate gouty arthritis.
- *Bluish-black discolouration of ears* occurs due to cyanosis, frostbite, haematoma, ochronosis, angiomatous tumour.
- *Local lesions,* i.e. boils, furuncles, herpetic vesicles, sebaceous cyst, haematoma, lupus, etc. are not uncommon.

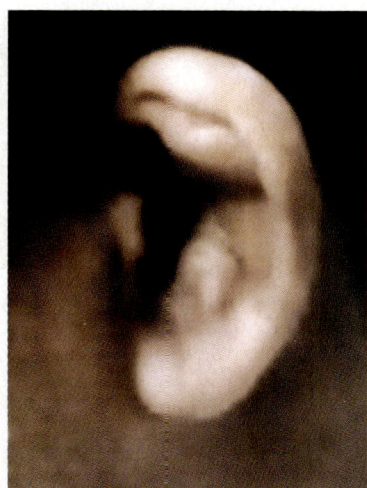

Fig. 1.7: Cauliflower ears due to repeated trauma in a wrestler.

- *Ear lobe pulsations* can be felt in severe AR, thyrotoxicosis, TR, coarctation of aorta.
- *Ear discharge* suggests an ear infection.
- *Ear tenderness* may be due to lesion of external auditory meatus, mastoiditis, mumps, parotitis, etc.
- *Prominent crease over ear lobule* is associated with increased incidence of IHD.

The Nose

The symptoms pertaining to nose have been discussed in respiratory system.

☞ *Examine the nose for symmetry or any deformity*

- **Saddle shape nose** results from either bony destruction (syphilis) or cartilage destruction (tuberculosis, leprosy, trauma, septal haematoma or septal abscess, Wegener's granulomatosis, polychondritis, etc.)
- **Broad nose** may be due to hypertelorism, bony tumour, chronic sinus infection, myxoedema.
- **A bulbous nose** with coarse, pitted and flushed skin (*Rhinophyma*) is common in old age with acne rosacea.
- **Breaked nose** is seen in Werner's syndrome and progeria.
- **Chronic redness of nose or its tip** may be due to chronic alcoholism (alcoholic stigmata), acne rosacea, SLE, liver cirrhosis, polycythaemia.
- A **plum-colour appearance of nose** is seen in lupus pernio.
- **Lupus pernio** (a violaceous infiltrated plaques) over the nose is pathognomonic of sarcoidosis.
- **Boil or furuncle** may produce acute redness.

- **Active alae nasi** (excessive working of alae nasi) are seen in pneumonia, COPD, laryngeal obstruction.
- **Nasal regurgitation of fluid** on drinking suggests bulbar palsy, cleft palate (refer to Fig. 1.14) or perforated syphilitic palate.

☞ *Test for patency of the nose for nasal obstruction*

- Read respiratory system for its causes and analysis.

☞ *Inspect the inside of the nose with speculum. Look at the nasal mucosa and note its colour, swelling, bleeding or exudate*

- Mucosa is red in rhinitis due to any cause.
- Crusting of the mucosa is seen in atrophic rhinitis.

☞ *Look at the nasal septum for deviation or perforation*

- Read the cause of deflected nasal septum in respiratory disease unit.
- Black eschars may be seen in nasal cavity.

☞ *Look inside the nose for bleeding spots*

- Read the causes of bleeding nose (epistaxis) under symptoms of respiratory disease unit.

THE MOUTH

The examination of the mouth is carried out in sitting position either on bed or on a chair with the help of a torch and a tongue depression (spatula).

☞ *Look at the lips for inflammation, ulcer, nodule, granuloma, pigmentation, telangiectasia, cysts, etc. (Table 1.1).*

TABLE 1.1: Abnormalities of the Lips as a Clue to Diagnosis	
Abnormality	*Causes/Diagnoses*
• Cleft lip/hare lip	A congenital abnormality
• Blue lips	Cyanosis due to any cause
• Pale lips	Anaemia
• Swollen/oedematous lips	Angioedema, acute nephritic or nephrotic syndrome, traumatic biting, epileptic fit, insect bite, abscess, carbuncle, cancer oris or corrosive poison
• Lip hypertrophy (large lips)	Myxoedema, acromegaly, cretinism, common in some African tribes
• Thin lips	Racial or familial
• Parched lip (dry erythematous lips)	Typhoid fever, dehydration
• Parted lips with open mouth	Nasopharyngeal obstruction (adenoids), dyspnoea associated with poor nasal airway, fascio-scapulo-humeral dystrophy,

Contd.

Abnormality	Causes/Diagnosis
Contd.	scleroderma, mongolism, cretinism, idiocy, bulbar palsy, stomatitis, mouth breathing, parkinsonism
• Frothing of lips	Acute pulmonary oedema, epileptic fit, rabies, hemiplegia, Bell's palsy
• Cracks/fissuring of angles of lips (angular cheilitis)	Trauma, local infection, anaemia, stomatitis, vitamin B complex deficiency, diabetes
• Chancre (painless sore) with regional lymphadenopathy	Primary syphilis
• Telangiectasia of lips	Hereditary telangiectasia, CREST syndrome (calcinosis cutis, Raynaud's phenomenon, esophageal dysfunction, scterodactyly and telangiectasia)
• Pursed lips	COPD
• Fish mouth	Obesity with Cushing's syndrome
Mobility of mouth (opening/closing) clue to diagnosis	
• Inability to open the mouth (jaw muscle spasms) or pain during opening	Tetanus, temporomandibular arthritis (RA), ankylosis of temporomandibular joint, Vth nerve palsy, local pain (mumps, quinsy, trichinosis, Mikulicz's syndrome)
• Inability to close the mouth	Drugs (metochlopramide) subluxation of temporo-mandibular joint or its hypermobility (hypermobility syndrome)
Smiles as clue to diagnosis	
• Transverse smile	Facial myopathy
• Sneering smile	Myasthenia
• Fixed or suppressed smile	Scleroderma, Wilson's disease
• Unilateral smile	Bell's palsy
• Sardonic smile (risus sardonicus)	Tetanus
• Excessive smile	Mania
• Absent smiling	Melancholia
• Slow sluggish smile	Parkinsonism

- **Desquamation of lips** is common in cold weather.
- **Vesicles over the lips** with crusts are seen in herpes simplex labialis (*see* Fig. 11.25).
- **Recurrent cheilitis** with small blisters and exfoliation (a premalignant condition) is seen in fishermen and farmers exposed to sunlight.
- **An indolent ulcer** on the lower lip with indurated margin may suggest epithelioma (cancer) of the lip.
- **A granuloma** (soft red raspberry-like) on the lips occur due to trauma.
- **Circumoral pigmentation** extending to lips occurs in Peutz-Jeghers syndrome (polyposis syndrome).
- **Aphthous ulceration** (small painful ulcers with a white or yellow base and a red halo of hyperaemia) is seen in ulcerative colitis, Crohn's syndrome, Behçet's syndrome, coeliac disease. Commonly, it is idiopathic in origin (Fig. 1.8).

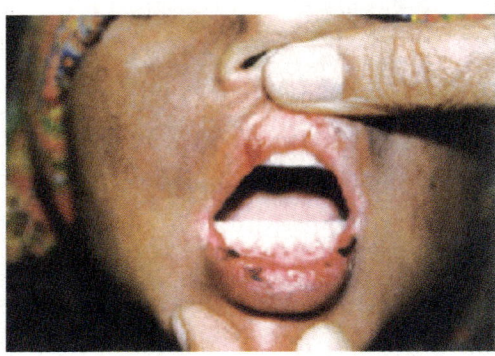

Fig. 1.8: Aphthous ulceration. Note the superficial ulcers on inner aspects of both lips with hyperaemia. The ulcers have whitish base.

☞ *Look at the teeth for decay (caries), discolouration, shape, erosion, etc.*

- **Dental caries** is visible as chalky white area in the enamel surface of the teeth.
- **Tartar deposits** (brown deposits) occur on incisors and canine teeth in smokers.
- **Reddish brown discolouration** of teeth may be seen in chewers of betel nuts.
- **Staining of permanent and deciduous teeth** in the form of yellow-grey bands is seen in children (< 8 years) treated with tetracyclines.
- **Furrowed or striated teeth** (transverse grooves on teeth) may occur during fevers, rickets.
- Children of expectant mothers are also at risk of **staining** after 14 weeks of pregnancy if treated with tetracyclines.
- The **teeth may be pitted or mottled** yellow-brown (*Maldon teeth*) in fluorosis (Fig. 1.9).
- **Peg-shaped teeth** may be seen in ectodermal dysplasia.
- **Dentonogenesis imperfecta** (teeth are translucent, dentine is malformed, rapid attrition and discolouration) may occur in osteogenesis imperfecta.

- **Premature loss of decidual teeth** is most common in hypophosphatasia.
- **Projecting teeth** may be congenital, familial or due to acromegaly.
- **Tumour arising** in association with teeth is dentigerous cyst, odontomas, epithelial tumour.

Abnormal shapes of the teeth are:
- **Notching of incisors** is common in nail biters or who hold hair clips between their teeth.
- **Notched, separated and peg-shaped upper incisors** are seen in congenital syphilis (*Hutchinson's teeth*).
- The two central upper incisors are sometimes lost in *leprosy*.
- **Teeth are poorly developed** in *juvenile hypothyroidism*.
- **Eruption of teeth** may be delayed and transverse ridging is sometimes seen in *scurvy* and *rickets*.
- **Enlargement of lower jaw (prognathism)** in acromegaly leads to alteration of biting line so that lower teeth may close outside the upper ones. The teeth are widely spaced.
- **Attrition of teeth.** Teeth are worn down by repetitive use in old persons leading to the recession of gums—called *attrition*. This process leads to apparent increase in the length of teeth.
- **Acid erosion of incisors** in children may be a sign of gastro-oesophageal reflux disease (GERD).
- **Serrated/dentated teeth** with serrated biting edges are due to malnutrition.

THE GUM

☞ Now look at the gums for recession (attrition) inflammation, plaques, bleeding, hypertrophy and ulceration.

- Normally, healthy gums (gingivae) are pink and adhere firmly and closely to the teeth.
- **Attrition of teeth and recession of gums.** There is recession of the gums from the teeth in old age so that the teeth appear longer and are prone to infection.
- **Gingivitis** is inflammation of the gums producing red and swollen gums.
- **Acute herpetic gingivostomatitis** due to herpes simplex virus producing small vesicles on the lips and gums is common among infants and children.
- **Acute necrotising ulcerative gingivitis (Vincent's infection) and periodontitis is caused by fusiform bacteria.**
- Spirochaetes produces **painful tender gums which bleed on pressure.** There is associated foul breath (**halitosis**). In chronic gingivitis teeth may become loose.
- **Bleeding gums** (spontaneous or on brushing) may be seen in scurvy, thrombocytopenia, leukaemia, bleeding diathesis.
- Pus coming out on squeezing the gum indicates pyorrhoea. Necrosis or sloughing of the gums may occur in neutropenia, malnutrition, severe gingivitis, Vincent's angina, vit. deficiencies.
- **Firm, hypertrophied gums** are seen in sarcoidosis, phenytoin therapy (Fig. 1.9) use of cyclosporine, nifedipine, amlodipine and also seen myelomonocytic leukaemia.
- **Soft, haemorrhagic gums** are seen in scurvy.
- **Spongy, hypertrophied and haemorrhagic gums** are seen in thrombocytopenic purpura and acute leukaemia.
- **Gum atrophy** can occur following acute gingivitis, Vincent's angina, wasting disease and old age.
- **Spongy and haemorrhagic gums** occur in cyanotic congenital heart disease.
- **A punctate/stippled blue line on gums** is seen in chronic lead poisoning (lead line); bismuth and mercury poisoning (uncommon).
- **A reticulated whitish pattern** is typically seen in lichen planus.
- **Violet colour tumours of the gums** indicate Kaposi's sarcoma.

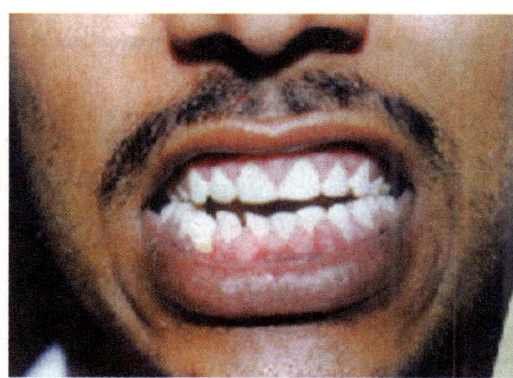

Fig. 1.9: Gum hypertrophy. Note the firm hypertrophied gums due to phenytoin toxicity (uncommon).

THE TONGUE

☞ Ask the patient to protrude out the tongue. Examine the tongue for (i) asymmetry, (ii) size, (iii) fasciculation or tremors, (iv) colour, (v) moistness, (vi) fur, and (vii) atrophy/hypertrophy

Size. The various abnormalities of the *size of tongue* are:

- *Macroglossia* is produced by tumour, angioedema, cretinism, acromegaly, amyloidosis, Down's syndrome, Hurler's syndrome, insect bite.
- *Microglossia* (small tongue) is seen in dehydration (shrivelled tongue), malnutrition, atrophic glossitis, XII nerve paralysis, typhus (parrot tongue), facial hemiatrophy, pseudobulbar palsy and Simmond's disease.

Congenital abnormalities of the tongue are:
- *Fissured tongue* (deep fissures over the tongue) is a congenital abnormality.
- *Geographic tongue* in which circular flattened atrophied filiform papillae are interspersed with zig-zag lines of hypertrophied filiform papillae producing a geographic map over the tongue. It is a congenital of abnormality seen in children.
- *Tongue tie* (a congenital abnormality) produces inability to protrude the tongue due to short frenulum.

Colour. *Is tongue pale, red or discoloured?*
Normal tongue is greyish red in colour
- *Pale tongue* is due to anaemia, leukoplakia
- *Curdy white tongue* is due to furring (bad oral dental hygiene or candidiasis)
- *Purple or bluish red tongue* is due to polycythaemia
- *Red-fiery tongue (raspberry tongue)* is seen in scarlet fever, niacin deficiency, acute glossitis, ingestion of berries and red sweets, pan chewers.
- *Magenta coloured tongue* is seen in ariboflavinosis, Vit B_{12} deficiency.
- *A orange red tongue* is seen in polyarteritis nodose and after antibiotic therapy.
- *Blue tongue* indicates cyanosis
- *Black tongue* (Fig. 1.10) indicates fungal infections (chromogens), antibiotic therapy (penicillin), iron and bismuth ingestion or tobacco-chewing.

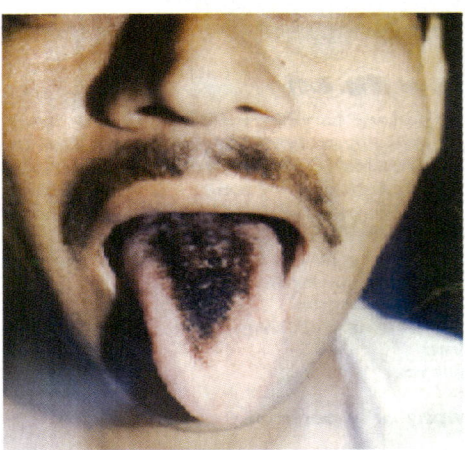

Fig. 1.10: Black tongue in tobacco chewers.

Fur (coating): *Is there any furring or coating of the tongue?* The fur consists of epithelial cells, debris, food residue and microorganisms.
- *Black-furred tongue* is seen in fungal (acetinomycosis) infection or chromogens and following antibiotics.
- *White furring* is due to bad orodental hygiene.
- *Curdy white furring* suggests candidiasis.
- *White mucous patches* over the tongue are seen in chronic leukoplakia (Fig. 1.11), a precancerous condition.

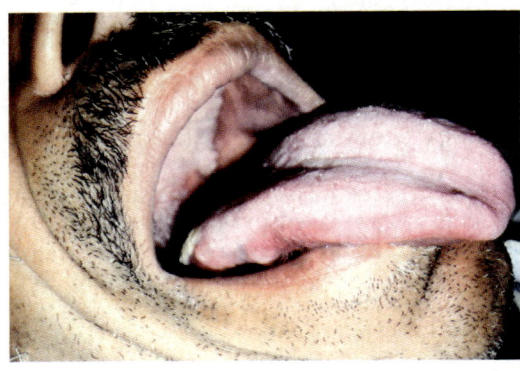

Fig. 1.11: Leukoplakia of the tongue. Note the white smooth patches with firm margins on the side of the tongue.

- *Hairy furring with mucous patches* called hairy leukoplakia suggests HIV infection.
- *Excessive furring* is seen in mouth breathers, smokers, milk drinkers, gastritis or dyspepsia, constipation, alcoholism, fevers, acute exanthematous infection, cirrhosis of liver.
- *Unilateral furring* is seen in unilateral paralysis of the tongue.
- A *dry thick brown furring* is seen in uraemia or acute liver cell failure.

The papillae: *Look at the papillae. Are they atrophied or hypertrophied (stand out prominently)?*
- *Bald tongue* (generalised atrophy of the papillae) is seen in iron deficiency anaemia, coeliac disease, pellagra, malnutrition, malabsorption.
- *Rhomboid tongue* (Lozenge-shape areas of loss of papillae with fissuring) is geographical variation, hence, of no consequence.
- *Strawberry tongue* (bright red papillae standing out of thick white fur) is seen in scarlet fever, toxic shock syndrome and Kawasaki disease.

Moistness of tongue. *Is the tongue dry or moist?*
Normal tongue in health is moist. The **causes** of dry tongue are:
- Mouth breathers, smokers.
- Dehydration, prolonged fevers

- Xerosis (Vit. A deficiency)
- Anticholinergics
- Sjögren's syndrome
- Uraemia, coma due to any cause
- Hyperventilation (anxiety state)

Pigmentation. *Is the tongue pigmented?* Normally tongue is not pigmented but in tropics it is not uncommon to see patches of pigmentation. They are not of any significance.
- *Dark brown patches of pigmentation* over the tongue may be seen in Addison's disease (*see* Fig. 9.18), Nelson's syndrome, cachexia of malignancy, Peutz-Jeghers syndrome, malabsorption.
- *Bright red patches* are seen in glossitis due to any cause.

Tongue movements. *Look at the resting tongue inside the mouth for tremors*
- *A tremulous tongue* may be noted in paralytic agitans, parkinsonism (post-encephalitic) delirium tremens, anxiety, thyrotoxicosis.
- *Fasciculations of the tongue* may occur in XII cranial nerve palsy, wasting diseases, motor neuron disease.
- *Spastic or rigid tongue* is seen in pseudobulbar palsy. Clonic spasms (tongue displaying sudden jerks) are seen in chorea, habit spasms, epilepsy, GPI, stuttering.
- *Immobile tongue.* Ask the patient to move the tongue inside the mouth. Paretic or immobile tongue is seen in bulbar palsy, amyotrophic lateral sclerosis, malignancy of tongue.
- *Permanently protruded tongue* (tongue remains permanently protruded out of the mouth), is seen in prognathism, macroglossia, mongolism, idiocy.
- *Deviation of the tongue* occurs due to XII cranial nerve palsy, malignant infiltration of the tongue, facial nerve palsy.
- *Lizard/reptile tongue*: The protruded tongue is withdrawn back with lizard or reptile speed in rheumatic chorea.

In XII nerve palsy, the tongue is atrophic, motionless and exhibits fasciculations.

Ulcer: *Look at the tongue for an ulcer (S)*
- Ulcer on the tongue may be single or multiple. A single ulcer may be carcinomatous (Fig. 1.11, 1.12), tuberculosis, syphilis, dental trauma. Multiple ulcers may be aphthous or dyspeptic ulcers, ulcerative stomatitis, Vincent's disease, secondary syphilis, herpes, pemphigus, eczema and vitamin B-complex deficiency.
- Recurrent ulceration is commonly aphthous but may be due to agranulocytosis, leukaemia, skin diseases (lichen planus, pemphigus, erythema multiforme, Stevens-Johnson syndrome, SLE and Behçet's syndrome).
- *A carcinomatous ulcer* is single, hard, indurated, irregular deep ulcer on the side of the tongue (Fig. 1.12) with regional neck lymphadenopathy. It is painless.

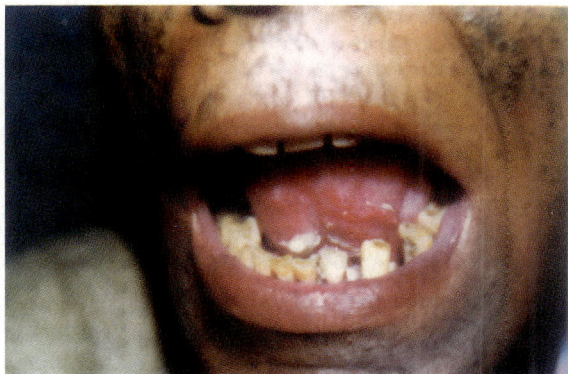

Fig. 1.12: Carcinoma of the tongue. Note the irregular growth with ulceration.

- *A tubercular ulcer* is usually present at the tip of the tongue with sloughed granulomatous base and *undermined margins*. It is painful but not hard.
- *A syphilitic ulcer* may be single (primary chancre or a gumma) or multiple (secondary syphilis) but are rarely seen now-a-days. They are superficial ulcers, scattered all over the tongue, painful with greyish base and punched out appearance associated with shotty lymphadenopathy of neck.
- *Dental ulcer* is located opposite to jagged or broken tooth on the margin of the tongue.
- *A frenulum ulcer* is seen on the frenulum of tongue in whooping cough.
  - *Mucosal neuromas* on tongue may be seen in multiple endocrine neoplasia (MEN II syndrome).
  - *Secondary deposits* on the tongue are rare but can occur in medullary carcinoma of thyroid.

THE ORAL MUCOSA/BUCCAL MUCOSA

☞ Look at the oral mucosa for inflammation, lesion, pigmentation, petechial haemorrhage, mucous patches, etc.

a. **Red oral lesions**
   i. *Red, swollen, tender buccal mucosa* indicates stomatitis which may be catarrhal (due to poor oral hygiene, debility, infection and use of broad spectrum antibiotics) or

aphthous (aphthous ulceration) or *ulceromembranous* (Vincent's angina) or may be due to *thrush* (Candida infection), *denture induced* (ill-fitted denture) or *erythematous nodular* (Kaposi sarcoma, Fig. 1.13), erythroplasia (carcinoma).
  ii. *Widespread red oral mucosa* is seen with *candida infection*, avitaminosis, Vit. B. deficiency, pellagra, riboflavin deficiency, irradiation, mucositis, lichen planus, polycythaemia.
  iii. *Localised red patches* (erythroplakia) involving the tongue, buccal mucosa, floor of the mouth indicate malignancy.

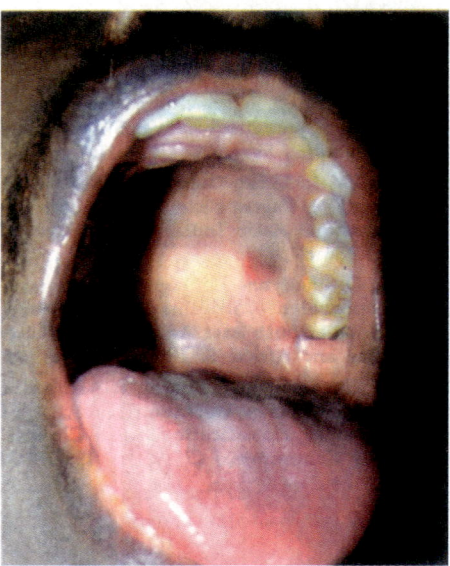

Fig. 1.13: Kaposi's sarcoma on the left side of the hard palate as red nodule in a patient with HIV infection.

  b. *White oral lesions*
    i. *White oral lesions* may be due to lichen planus, burns (chemicals), hairy leukoplakia (HIV), neoplasia, cheek biting and can be idiopathic.
    ii. *Koplik's spots* (small bluish-white spots on an erythematous base) on buccal mucosa occur in measles.
  c. *Cobblestone appearance of the mucosa* may be seen in Crohn's disease.
  d. *Petechial haemorrhages on buccal mucosa* are seen in purpura, hemorrhagic diseases, endocarditis, rubella, SLE and scurvy.
  e. *Mucous patches* (snail track painless ulcers) are seen in secondary syphilis; while painful ulcers can occur due to trauma, stomatitis, trigeminal, herpes zoster, infectious mononucleosis, hand-foot-mouth disease, blood dyscrasias (leukaemia, neutropaenia).
  f. *Lichenoid eruptions* may occur due to amalgams, drugs, hepatititis C infection or graft-versus-host disease.
  g. *Submucosal fibrosis* (fibrous band formation) with stiffening of mucosa resulting in restriction of chewing movements, occurs in pan (betel) chewers.

THE PALATE

☞ *Observe the palate for the following defects*

1. **Cleft palate** (a median symmetrical defect of congenital origin is shown in Fig. 1.14). It can lead to regurgitation of food and drink.

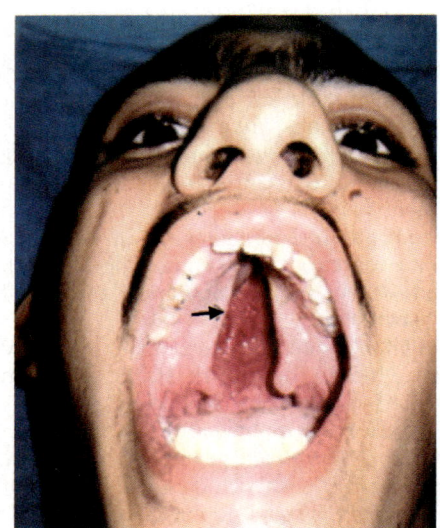

Fig. 1.14: Cleft palate.

2. **High arch (dome-shaped) palate.** It may be seen as a congenital abnormality associated with congenital heart disease or due to Marfan's syndrome. Trisomy syndrome, Turner's syndrome.
3. **Perforation of palate.** It may be seen in syphilis, tuberculosis, actinomycosis, diphtheria and trauma.
4. **Reddened and oedematous palate** is seen in obstructive sleep apnoea due to heavy snoring.
5. **Anaesthesia of palate** occurs in trigeminal nerve paralysis.
6. **Paralysis of soft palate** either unilateral or bilateral is seen in bulbar and pseudobulbar palsy, post-diphtheric paralysis.
7. **Vesicles over palate** are seen in herpes simplex or zoster infection, chickenpox.

8. **Ulcers over palate** occur due to stomatitits (read causes of buccal ulcers), syphilis, malignancy, deficiency diseases or blood dyscrasias.
9. **Tumour** (soft, nodule) suggests malignancy, while hard nodule indicates exostosis, chondroma.
10. **Pigmentation:** Palatal pigmentation may be seen in Addison's disease and Peutz-Jeghers syndrome.

THE FLOOR OF THE MOUTH

- On upturning the tongue, certain structures, i.e. frenulum linguae, sublingual ridge and Whartson's papilla are normally seen.
☞ *Note any cyst/swelling in the floor of the mouth*
- A *retention cyst* of a mucous gland (ranula), an *obstructive cyst* of salivary gland or *a congenital inclusion cyst* or a *sublingual dermoid cyst* can occur.

THE FAUCIAL TONSILS

☞ *Look at the tonsils in tonsillar fossa for enlargement, abscess and infection*
- **Acute tonsillitis** is an inflammation of tonsils leading to their enlargement, odynophagia and cough. It may be *bacterial* (common) or *secondary* to acute exanthem like measles or scarlet fever. Repeated attacks of acute tonsillitis lead to *chronic tonsillitis* with follicular hyperplasia and exudation of pus on pressing the tonsillar bed. There may be regional lymphadenopathy.
- **Quinsy (peritonsillar abscess)** is localised collection of pus adjacent to or outside the tonsil leading to pain during deglutition, enteric fever with rigors and cervical lymphadenitis.
- **Faucial diphtheria**. It is characterised by greyish or yellowish white membrane over the tonsils which bleed on scrapping.
- Infectious mononucleosis is characterised by **cheesy white exudate confined to tonsils**.

THE FACE, CHEEKS AND JAWS

The Face. The facial appearance and their abnormalities have already been discussed under general observations.

☞ *Note the following types of facies which form an important clue to the diagnosis (Table 1.2)*

☞ *Look at the face for eruptions, scales, skin lesions, telangiectasia*
- *Angry red crusted eruptions* on the cheeks suggest atopic dermatitis.
- *Greasy scales* over nasolabial folds, eyebrows and ears indicate *seborrhoeic dermatitis*.

TABLE 1.2 : Face as an Index to the Diagnosis

Description of face	Diagnosis and type of face
Pale and puffy face with swollen eyelids and dull expression. The skin is dry, thick with loss of hair on the lateral third of the eyeball	Hypothyroidism (*myxoedema face*)
Large oblong face with protruding lower jaw (prognathism), coarse features, large nose, thick lip and large tongue, wide teeth and prominent eyebrows and cheeks	Acromegaly (*acromegalic face*)
Round, flushed *plethoric face* with acne and hirsutism	Cushing syndrome (*moon-face*)
Frightening face with prominent eyeballs, staring look, excessive sweating (moist face)	Hyperthyroidism (*Exophthalmos face*)
The *premature face*, skin shallow and pale, with wrinkles and furrows and absence of facial hair	Hypognadism (*eunuchoid face*)
An immobile, fixed, *expressionless* face	Parkinsonism (*mask-like face*)
Asymmetric and depressed face with drooling of saliva from an angle of the mouth with frequent use of handkerchief to wipe it out	C.V.A. hemiplegic or apoplectic face
Inequality or asymmetry of face due to muscle wasting on one side of face with wide palpebral fissure, deviation of angle of the mouth	Bell's palsy, congenital hemiatrophy of face (*asymmetrical face*)
Bilateral ptosis (narrow palpebral fissure), open mouth, noticeable sneering smile towards the end of the day (evening)	Myasthenia gravis (*myasthenic face*)
Facial muscles and eye muscles atrophy leading to opening of mouth, dropping of lids or transverse smile and difficulty in closure of the eyes and dysphagia	Oculopharyngeal myopathy (*myopathic face*)
'*Hound dog*' *face* with frontal baldness, atrophy of masseters, temporalis and sternomastoids	Myotonic dystrophy or paramyotonia
Rounded face with prominence over the angle of the jaws (bilateral parotid enlargement)	Mumps (*parotid face*)
Saddle nose, rhagades, Hutchinson's teeth (*syphilitic face*)	Congenital syphilis
Spasm of the facial muscles with retraction of the angles of the mouth producing a characteristic sardonic smile (*sardonic face*)	Risus sardonicus in tetanus
Bluish face, lips, nose, ear with congestion and oedema increasing on stooping	Cyanotic heart disease Superior vena cava (SVC) obstruction (*cyanotic face*)

Contd.

Contd.	
Description of face	**Diagnosis and type of face**
Malar flush (mitral facies)	Mitral stenosis
Leonine face (read facial appearance in the beginning)	Leprosy
Elfin-like face (read facial appearance)	Supravalvular aortic stenosis
Puffy, swollen, pale face with baggy eyeballs and narrow palpebral fissure (*nephrotic face*)	Nephrotic/nephritic syndrome
Mongoloid face (read facial appearance)	Down's syndrome (Fig. 1.15)
Macrocephaly, bushy eyebrows, thickened stiff lip, nares and face, depressed nasal bridge, wide bony ridge in the middle of face	Hurler's syndrome or mucopoly-saccharidosis (gargoyle-like face)
Macrosomia with sunken cheeks, hypoplasia of malar bones and mandible	Mandibulofacial dysostosis
Atrophy of the facial muscles, muscles of mastication and atrophy of neck muscles	Myotonic muscular dystropy (hatchet face)
Multiple pitted scars like rain drops over the face (*scarred face*)	Healed lesions of small pox (pox-face)
Short narrow face (forehead) with small mouth, short palpebral fissures, micrognathia (small mandible)	A trisomy called Edward syndrome (pinched face)
Red nose (tip), earlobules, flushed face, sunken cheeks, shiny eyeballs, eyes icteric and congested. (*cirrhotic face*)	cirrhosis of liver
Thalassemic face (read facial appearance)	Thalassaemia

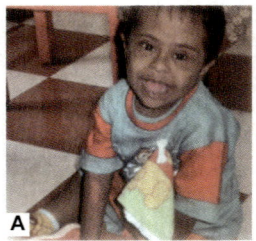 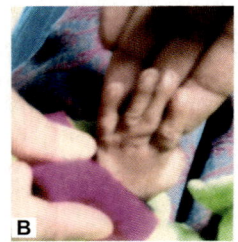

Figs 1.15A and B: (A) Mongoloid face in Down's syndrome; (B) Clinodactyly (hypoplasia of middle phalanx of little finger resulting in incurving of it).

- *Moisted crusted lesions* can occur due to *rosacea*.
- *Scaly silvery white lesion* over face can be due to *psoriasis*.
- The skin over the face and cheek is common site for acute *pustular lesions, boils, lupus vulgaris* and *acne* (read dermatology).

- *Photosensitive erythrodermic facial eruption* is due to SLE, while chronic patches of erythema, scaling, telangiectasia with keratotic plugs in the hair follicles indicate *discoid lupus*.
- *Tightening of smooth facial skin* (skin cannot be lifted off the face) with improper smile and closure of the mouth (partially open mouth called *tobacco pouch mouth*) suggests *scleroderma*.
- *Violaceous hue* with oedema of facial expression indicates *dermatomyositis*.
- *Telangiectasia* of face, lips, eyebrows, mucous membrane of nose, mouth may be seen in *Osler-Weber-Rendu-syndrome* (hemorrhagic telangiectasia) while spider angiomata and telangiectasia of cheek occur *in cirrhosis of liver*.

☞ **Look at the colour of face**
- *Facial pallor* may be familial but commonly occurs due to severe anaemia due to any cause.
- *Flushed face* (cutaneous vasodilatation) may be *physiological* (weather-bitten, cold climate, high altitude), or *pathological* (alcoholism, polycythemia, carcinoid syndrome, mastocytosis, menopause (hot flushes), phaeochromocytomas, drug-induced, e.g. nifedipine, calcitonin, nicotinic acid, anaphylaxis or anaphylactoid reactions, etc).
- *Facial erythema* suggests dermatomyositis, SLE, ENL (erythema nodosum leprum—a reaction in leprosy).
- *Depigmentation of face* occurs in leucoderma, albinism.
- *Excessive pigmentation* could be racial, idiopathic, melanosis due to any cause (read causes of hyperpigmentation in *section on dermatology*).
- *Facial sweating*, i.e. generalised sweating indicates hyperhydrosis due to phaeochromocytoma, thyrotoxicosis, idiopathic, etc. while localised sweating occurs in trigeminal neuralgia. Asymmetrical gustatory sweating limited to face, head and neck on one side after eating indicates misdirected regeneration of lingual nerve in facial nerve palsy.

☞ **Look for any involuntary movements of face**
- *Tics* involving the face are habitual spasms causing blepharospasms, frequent blinking, grimacing of face.
- *Facial spasms*, e.g. unilateral occur in Bell's palsy, trigeminal neuralgia, chorea while bilaterally occur in tetanus, meningitis, encephalitis, etc. Facial spasms may be tonic or clonic.
- *Facial grimace* may occur due to dystonia, phenothiazine toxicity.
- *Facial myoclonus* is seen in encephalitis lethargica.

THE NECK

The neck is examined in a good light with the patient comfortably sitted on the bed/couch facing the examiner. Neck is examined in the following order.

Inspection

☞ *Inspect the neck for position, size, shape, symmetry, abnormal movements, swelling of thyroid, engorgement of veins and pulsations.*

- **Congenital abnormalities** in the neck include cysts (*thyroglossal cyst*), vascular malformations, i.e. hemangioma, lymphangioma.
- **A thin long neck** is common in hyposthenic individuals and in patients with wasting diseases, emaciation and cachexia.
- **A short and broad neck (bull neck)** is seen in hyperasthenic and obese individuals and Klippel-Feil syndrome.
- **A camel hump/buffallo hump** is due to central obesity in Cushing's syndrome.
- **Webbing of the neck** is seen in ovarian dysgenesis, Turner's syndrome, Klippel-Feil syndrome and Ulrich-Noonan syndrome.
- **Head retraction (hyperextension of neck)** due to spasm/rigidity of neck muscles (*neck rigidity*) is seen in meningitis, meningism, encephalitis, tetanus, strychnine poisoning, subarachnoid haemorrhage, cervical spine injury (fracture, dislocation).
- **Torticollis (wry neck)** is an abnormal deviation with rotation of the head to one side, may be encountered in myofibrositis due to chill or trauma, secondary to caries of spine, drug reaction, could be congenital or hysterical.
- **Abnormal movements of the neck** include torticollis (clonic jerking of head with rotation), head nodding (nodding spasm/*salaam* spasm), habit spasms, and also seen in hysteria, chorea, parkinsonism, encephalitis, aortic regurgitation (*de Musset's sign*).

☞ *After surveying the neck from front, the head is slightly extended and rotated to each side in turn in order to define sternomastoid muscles and the anterior and posterior triangles on either side.*

- **Weak neck muscles** produce flexion of neck, prevent extension and even the normal upright position of neck. This may occur in myotonic muscular dystrophy, polymyositis.
- **Backward tilting of head (swan-neck)** is due to atrophy or paralysis of one or both sternomastoids either as a congenital abnormality or due to XI cranial nerve paralysis.
- **Atrophy of sternomastoid** is an invariable finding in dystrophic myotonia and poliomyelitis.
- **Cervical oedema** is subcutaneous oedema either due to thrombosis of superior vena cava or infection and inflammation of cervical veins. It can be a part of generalised anasarca.
- **Subcutaneous emphysema** over the chest may extend into the neck producing crepitus.
- **Lipomatosis** (multiple lipomas) over the neck is a common finding in alcoholics and beer drinkers.
- **Pachydermatocoele** (*elephantiasis neuromatosa*) is due to neurofibromatosis characterised by hypertrophy of skin and subcutaneous tissue.
- **Cellulitis of neck** produces red painful brawny swelling of neck, occurs due to septicaemia.
- **Scrofuloderma** (involvement of skin due to rupture of a lymph node) can be seen in tubercular lymphadenopathy.
- **Dancing carotids** are a sign of aortic regurgitation or wide pulse pressure due to high cardiac output of any other cause (anaemia, thyrotoxicosis, etc.)
- **Tumours** such as lipoma, carotid body tumour, lymphoma, secondaries deposits, etc. are not uncommon in the region of the neck.
- **Jugular venous pulse and pressure (JVP).** Read it in unit on cardiovascular system.

Palpation

Palpation is carried out from the front, side and the back of neck for palpation of a mass (tumour) or masses (lymph nodes), thyroid gland, trachea and blood vessels. Active and passive movements, neck stiffness and wasting of neck muscles are also noted.

- Palpation is also done for local tenderness and signs of inflammation and deformities of the spine.
- **Palpation of trachea.** It is discussed in the unit on respiratory sytem.
- **Thyroid gland** (inspection and palpation of thyroid gland is discussed in the unit on endocrine system examination).
- **Tumour.** The mass in the neck is palpated and described for its *size, shape, adherence, tenderness, mobility* and *surface*.

Tumours in the region of the neck are multiple lipomas, lymph node, secondaries, etc.

- **Pulsations:** *Pulsations over the carotids are felt.* Weak pulsations indicate carotid artery stenosis (a cause of CVA) while dancing carotids are seen and felt in aortic regurgitation.
- **Neck stiffness.** It is elicited by passively flexing the neck with both hands. The causes of neck stiffness are discussed in inspection.
- **Wasting of muscles of neck.** The muscles are palpated for tone and movements (read testing for the XI cranial nerve in neurology).

- **Neck movements.** The various neck movements and their significance are discussed in the unit on rheumatology.

Auscultation

☞ *Auscultate the thyroid for bruit (Graves' disease) and other blood vessels such as carotids for bruit (carotid artery stenosis in a case with CVA).*

Lymph Nodes (Read Unit VIII also)

☞ *Examine the lymph nodes in the neck for number, size, site, consistency, discrete or matted, mobility, tenderness, fluctuation, condition of the surrounding skin and draining area.*

The various groups of lymph nodes to be examined in the neck are given in Fig. 1.16.

☞ *Examine from behind the submental, tonsillar, submandibular, supraclavicular, preauricular and deep cervical nodes.*

- For palpation of these lymph nodes, read the Clinical Methods in Medicine by Prof SN Chugh.

☞ *Significant lymphadenopathy means*

- Soft, flat lymph nodes of < 1 cm size anywhere in the body are usually benign and require follow-up.
- Inguinal lymph nodes of more than 2 cm size are abnormal, need evaluation.

Lymph node size of 1 × 1 cm is significant and to be evaluated.
Abnormal lymphadenopathy (size > 1 cm in neck and more than 2 cm in groin).

- Soft, non-tender, matted nodes (attached to each other) suggest tubercular lymphadenitis. Matting occurs due to periadenitis. Discharge, sinus or scar of previous suppuration of untreated cases may be present.
- **Tender node** resulting from acute stretching of the capsule signifies inflammatory or infective pathology.
- **Lymphangitis** means superficial lymphatic vessels appear as red streaks running between the nodes and sites of original infection, occurs due to filarial lymphangitis, bacterial or infective lymphangitis.
- **Fixity or immobility of lymph nodes** indicates inflammatory or malignant pathology. On the other hand, mobile, discrete non-tender lymph nodes indicate lymphoma.
- **Fluctuation of a lymph nodes** suggests pus forming conditions like abscess, sepsis or tuberculosis.
- **Consistency.** Firm and rubbery (elastic) lymph nodes suggest lymphoma. Hard, non-tender fixed nodes which progressively enlarge suggest malignancy.
- **Bubo.** It is an inflammatory swelling of one or more lymph nodes in the inguinal region suggesting plague. Masses of lymph nodes may suppurate and drain pus, e.g. chancroid, lymphogranuloma venereum.

REGIONAL LYMPHADENOPATHY

Cervical Lymphadenopathy (Fig. 1.16)

Causes
- Upper respiratory tract infection.
- Viral illness (infectious mononucleosis)
- Oral or dental lesions
- Secondaries from primary head, neck, breast, lung and thyroid malignancy.
- Lymphoma and leukaemias
- A part and parcel of generalised lymphadenopathy.

Examination
Scalene node: Node is present deep to sternomastoid muscle on the scalenus anticus muscle.
  Method of palpation: Finger is dipped through the clavicular head of sternomastoid behind the clavicle.
  Significance: Secondary involvement of the lymph nodes due to bronchial carcinoma.

Jugulodigastric node: Most commonly enlarged lymph node, indicates URTI and tonsillitis.
  Palpate it just posterior to the angle of the mandible.
  Examine the posterior triangle of the neck up to the back for posterior auricular and occipital lymph nodes (scalp infection).

Waldeyer's ring: Waldeyer's ring constitutes a group of lymphatic structures, which surround the opening of digestive and respiratory tracts.

External Waldeyer's ring consists of the following groups of lymph nodes, i.e.
- Occipital (posteriorly) nodes
- Posterior auricular (behind the ear)
- Pre-auricular (front of the ear)
- Jugular and tonsillar
- Submandibular
- Sub-mental (anteriorly)

Significance: Waldeyer's ring adenopathy occurs with local disease or as a part of generalised lymphadenopathy especially in patients with non-Hodgkin's lymphoma.

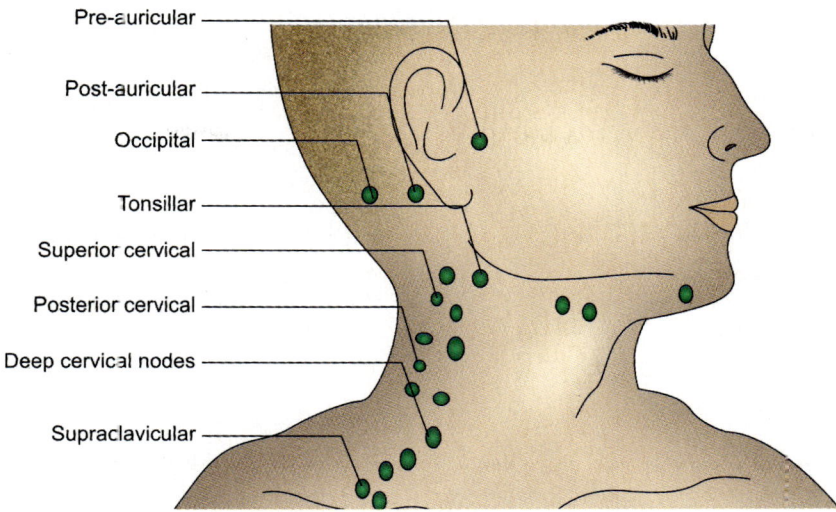

Fig. 1.16: Groups of lymph nodes in the neck.

Virchow's node (Troisier's sign): Enlargement of left supraclavicular node occurs due to metastatic lesion from GIT or testicular malignancy.

Axillary Lymphadenopathy
Causes
a. Infection or injury to the ipsilateral upper limb
b. Breast and chest wall disease
c. Lymphoma
d. Part of generalised lymphadenopathy.

Method of examination
Examiner sitting in front of the patient supports the patient's upper limb with his own arm on the side to be examined.
   Finger tips are inserted into the axillary pit (right finger tip for left axilla and *vice versa*) and anterior, posterior and medial walls are palpated in turn.

Epitrochlear Nodes
Causes of enlargement
- Infection and inflammation of ipsilateral hand
- Secondary syphilis
- Non-Hodgkin's lymphoma

Method of examination
Patient's elbow is partially flexed and grasped by the examiner's hand (right hand for right epitrochlear node and *vice versa*) while patient's wrist is supported by the examiner's non-examining hand. Feel the epitrochlear node with the thumb.

Inguinal and popliteal lymph nodes (read examination of feet and legs).

INGUINAL LYMPHADENOPATHY (Read examination of lower limbs in this unit)

GENERALISED LYMPHADENOPATHY (Read it also in Unit on Haematology)

Definition: Enlargement of three or more non-contiguous areas of lymph nodes is called generalised lymphadenopathy.

Causes
Infection
- Viral infection
- Infectious mononucleosis
- HIV infection
- Disseminated tuberculosis, histoplasmosis, etc.

Immunologic
- Rheumatoid arthritis
- SLE
- Sjögren's syndrome

Malignancies
- Hodgkin's and non-Hodgkin's lymphoma
- CLL (chronic lymphatic leukaemia)
- ALL (acute lymphoid leukaemia)

Storage diseases
- Gaucher's disease
- Niemann-Pick disease

Endocrine disorders
Graves' disease

Drug-induced
For example, phenytoin sodium, carbamazepine, allopurinol.

THE BREAST AND AXILLAE
Read it under a separater unit

THE EXTREMITIES

THE HANDS

☞ *Examine the hand for moistness, size, shape, temperature, colour, creases, deposits, and abnormal movements.*

- **Dryness of hands** is seen in dermatitis, wasting diseases, myxoedema, dehydration, Vit. A deficiency, icthyosis or xeroderma. The '**sweaty palms**' indicate hyperthyroidism, nervousness, neurocirculatory asthenia, shock or hypotension, hypoglycaemia and vasovagal syndrome.
- **Palms of hands are pale** in anaemia, shock, hypothyroidism, oedema; **while they are pink** in polycythaemia, CO poisoning, carcinoid syndrome, **blue** in cyanosis, **yellow** in **jaundice** and carotenemia, xanthomatosis and **bright red** in palmar erythema due to cirrhosis of liver, rheumotoid arhritis or vasculitis, shoulder hand syndrome, pregnancy, thyrotoxicosis.
- **Alteration in the colour (pigmentation and depigmentation) of the palm** may be seen in exanthematous fevers (due to eruptions) i.e. rubella, measles, scarlet fever, pellegra (pigmentation), Addison's disease (pigmentation of creases of palm), hemachromatosis (blackening of palms), local skin conditions, Raynaud's phenomenon (tricolour response) and leucoderma and albinism (depigmentation).
- **Cold hands** (Washerman hands) occur due to vasoconstriction, can be seen due to cold hypersensitivity, Raynaud's phenomenon, scorpion sting.
- **Palmar xanthomas** occur in hypothyroidism, diabetes mellitus, familial hyperlipidaema, biliary cirrhosis and nephrotic syndrome.
- **Single palmar crease** is seen in Down's syndrome (Fig. 1.17).
- *Hyperkeratosis of palms* may be seen in maid servants, psoriasis, scleroderma due to toxic effect of drugs.

Handshake

☞ *Ask the patient to shake the hand with you.*

Handshake is a diagnostic clue to the following diseases:
- Violent handshake suggests mania
- Subdued handshake is characteristic of melancholia.
- Interrupted handshake (sudden withdrawl of hand) is seen in schizophrenia.
- Handshake with persistent grip (slow relaxation) suggests myotonia dystrophica.
- Tremulous handshake is felt in parkinsonism.

Handwriting

☞ *Ask the patient to write*
- *Inability to write is motor agraphia* due to CNS diseases. *Inability to write* also can occur due to peripheral nerve lesion, spasticity of hand muscles, wasting of small muscles (motor neuron disease), painful joint conditions or bone injuries/deformities. Cramps may occur during writing are called *muscle cramps*.
- *Abnormal handwriting* occur in schizophrenia, chorea, thyrotoxicosis and general paralysis of insane (GPI). In hepatic encephalopathy, there is bizarre handwriting.

Abnormal Movements

The abnormal movements that involve the fingers are; choreiform movements, clonic movements, Writer's cramp, carpopedal spasms (Fig. 1.18) of tetany, jacksonian fits and epileptiform convulsion.

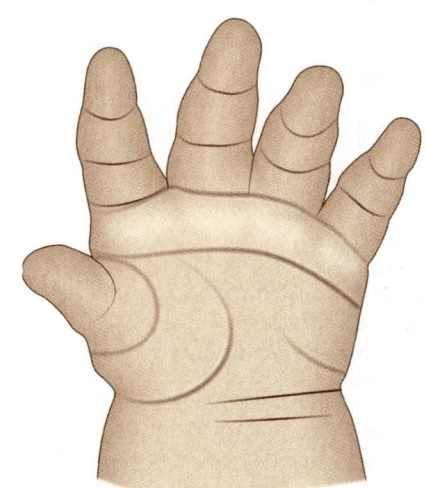

Fig. 1.17: Down syndrome (note single palmar crease).

General Physical Examination

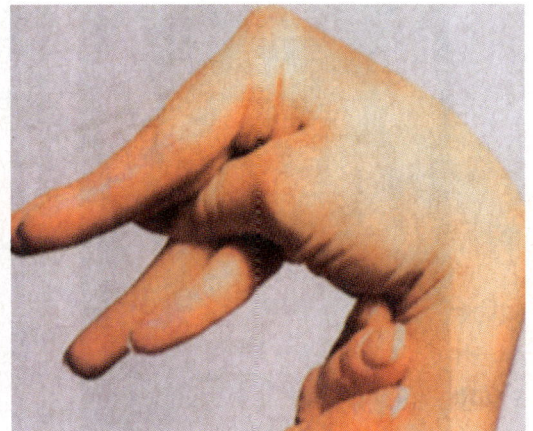

Fig. 1.18: D'accoucheur hand (also called obstetric hand). Note the spontaneous carpopedal spasm producing flexion of the thumb and adduction and apposition of fingers.

Deformities/Contractures/Abnormal Hands and Fingers (Box 1.2)

☞ Examine the hands (Box 1.2) and fingers for deformities, contractures, shape and size or any other abnormalities (Table 1.3).

Box 1.2 Hand as a Diagnostic Tool

Morphological feature	Diagnosis
Flexed posture of hand and arm	Hemiplegia
Large hands and palms	Gigantism, Marfan's syndrome
Trident hand (short hand) with divergent fingers like spokes	Achondroplasia
Short spade-like hands	Acromegaly (see Fig. 9.16)
Wrist drop	Radial nerve palsy, lead neuropathy, other peripheral neuropathies
Ulnar deviation of hand	Rheumatoid arthritis (see Fig. 10.10)
Main De'accoucheur or obstetric hand	Tetany (Fig. 1.18)
Square hand	Nodular OA
Deformity	Trauma, rheumatoid arthritis
Claw hand (main en griffe)	Paralysis of interossei and lumbricals
Prayer's hand: Inability to approximate the palmar surface of hands and finger (Fig. 1.19)	Diabetic cheiroarthropathy

Oedema of hands	May be part of generalised oedema, may be due to local venous or lymphatic obstruction or disuse in hemiplegia
Mongoloid hand (short thick hands with curving of little fingers and a single simian (transverse) line or palms	Down's syndrome (mongolism), Fig. 1.16
Broad, short, stubby, stout fingers	Acromegaly (see Fig. 9.16), pseudo-hypoparathyroidism
Fingerised thumb	ASD
Short metacarpals, i.e. bradydactyly (short fingers)	Down's syndrome, Turner's syndrome
Pseudoclubbing	Trauma, leprosy, hyperparathyroidism, occupational
Thyroid acropatchy (pseudoclubbing due to subperiosteal new bone formation)	Graves' disease

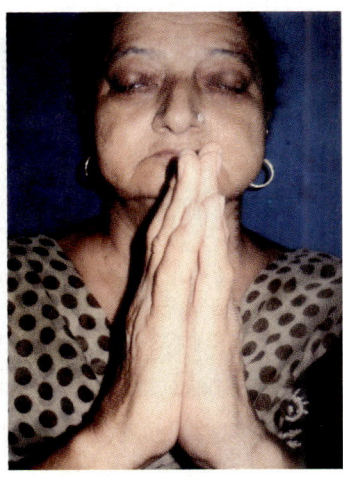

Fig. 1.19: Prayer's hand in a patient with rheumatoid arthritis.

TABLE 1.3: Fingers as Clue to Diagnosis

Description of finger	Cause
• Arachnodactyly (long, slender fingers—Fig. 1.20)	• Marfan's syndrome, Kallmann's syndrome (hypogonadotrophic hypogonadism), homocystinuria
• Polydactyly (an extra finger, 6th finger—Fig. 1.21A)	• Laurence-Moon-Biedl syndrome, congenital heart disease, Turner syndrome

Contd.   *Contd.*

Contd.

Description of finger	Cause
• *Syndactyly* (united or jointed fingers—Fig. 1.21B)	• Poland's syndrome, congenital heart disease
• *Sclerodactyly* (tight skin over phalanges—Fig. 1.22B)	• Scleroderma
• *Clinodactyly* (an incurving of the little finger)	• Down's or Hurler's syndrome
• *Clubbing* of the fingers	• Read the description and causes under respiratory and cardiovascular system

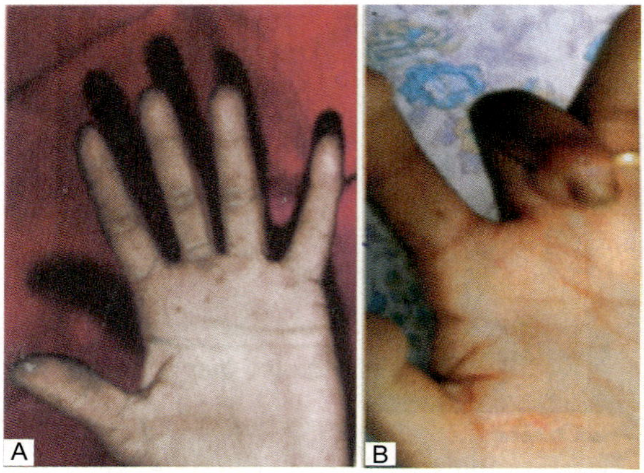

The Nails

Growth of nails is slowed by acute illness and ischaemia. It is increased in psoriasis. Injury is the commonest cause of nail deformity. Some important changes in the nails are depicted and discussed in the unit on dematology.

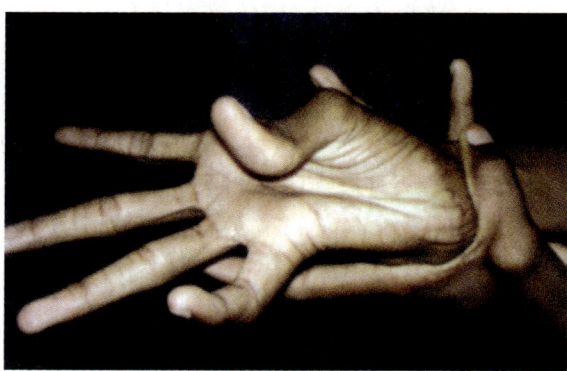

Fig. 1.20: *Arachnodactyly*: Long slender fingers with wrist sign positive.

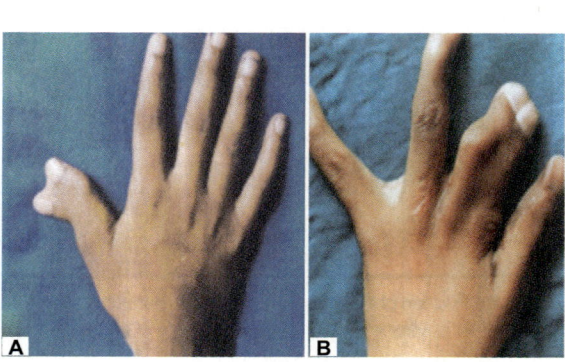

Figs 1.21A and B: Deformities of fingers. (A) Polydactyly (an extra thumb); (B) Syndactyly.

Figs 1.22A and B: (A) Pigmentation of hands and creases of the palms in pellagra; (B) Sclerodactyly.

Nail Folds

Examination of the nail folds should accompany examination of nails but here they are described separately.

Paronychia or whitlow refers to inflamed, bolstered and swollen nail folds. The *causes* are:
- Poor peripheral circulation
- Persons involved in wet-work
- Diabetes
- Persons overenthusiastic in manicuring their cuticles.

Vascularity and Pulsations

☞ *Examine the nails for vascularity and pulsation*

- **Arteritis** may cause small necrotic lesions and digital infarcts at the base of the nail and on the pulps, is seen in endocarditis, SLE and connective tissue disorders (scleroderma), PAN cryoglobulinaemia, RA.
- **Capillary pulsations** are seen by putting the tip of a pintorch under the pulp. They are characteristically seen in aortic incompetence.
- **Raynaud's phenomenon (blanched fingers and gangrenous fingers):** Read peripheral vascular examination.
- **Venous abnormalities** are seldom seen, but the linear marks or phlebitis caused by intravenous injection of drugs in addicts ('mainliners') are characteristics.
- **Absent pulsation** (radial or digital) is seen in embolisation to small vessels.
- **Dactylitis.** Acute tender swelling of a finger due to trauma and inflammation is seen in infection (tuberculosis), sarcoidosis and sickle cell anaemia.

Swellings

☞ Look for any swelling. The different swellings and their significance have been discussed in unit on rheumatology.

THE FEET AND THE LEGS

The examination of feet is done by *inspection* and *palpation*. The examination of feet is just similar to examination of hands.

Inspection

☞ Look at the feet for the following

1. **Morphology**, e.g. *pes cavus* or *pes planus*. Pes cavus (Fig. 1.23) is a fixed deformity where both feet are more or less symmetrically high-arched which can be demonstrated by observing the arch

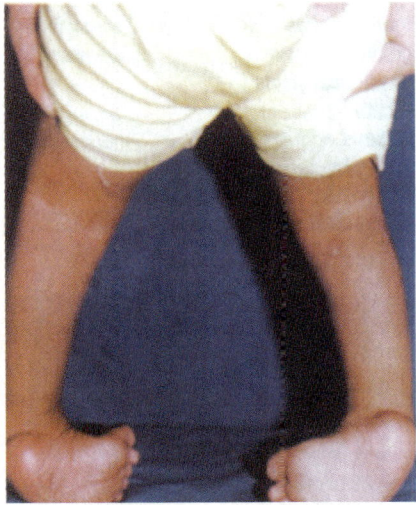

Fig. 1.24: Talipes equinus varus—a congenital abnormality of the feet.

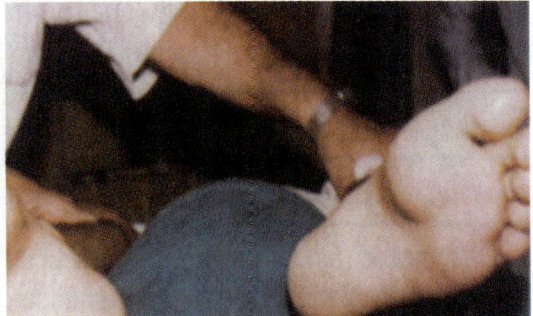

Fig. 1.23: Pes cavus. Note the high arching of both the feet leading to hollowness of soles.

of foot when patient stands on the floor (there is exaggeration of the longitudinal arch in *pes cavus*) or by taking a foot-print on a white paper after painting the foot with some colour or after immersion of the feet in water and asking the patient to walk barefooted.

The *pes cavus* (*claw foot*) results from wasting of small muscles (interossei and lumbricals) of foot due to poliomyelitis, spina bifida, Friedreich's ataxia, syringomyelia, peroneal muscle atrophy (Charcot-Marie-Tooth disease), familial peripheral neuropathies (Refsum's disease) and may be idiopathic.

Talipes equinus varus (Fig. 1.24) is a congenital abnormality seen in infants/children. There may be supernumerary toe or underdeveloped toes (Fig. 1.25).

2. **Posture**

☞ Look at the posture of feet

- Plantar flexion of the foot occurs in hemiplegia, which may be associated with extension and adduction of lower limb.

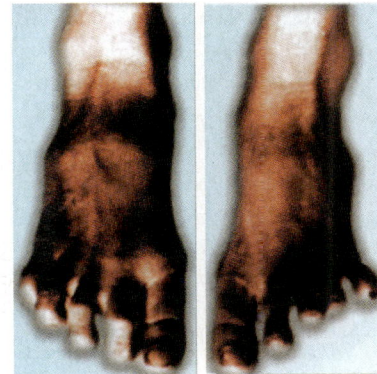

Fig. 1.25: Underdeveloped and maldeveloped toes of left foot.

- Foot drop is seen in sciatic or common peroneal nerve palsy or peripheral neuropathies.

3. **Size**

☞ Look at the size of feet

- Feet are large and broad in acromegaly. There is increase in the size of the shoes. Oedema feet also causes increase in feet dimensions.

4. **Colour**

☞ Look at the feet for any colour change

- By and large changes in the colour of the skin of the feet are similar to those of the skin in general (*read changes in skin colour*).
- The *trophic changes* (varicose ulcer, black-staining) at or around the ankle are seen in varicosity of

veins or venous insufficiency (Fig. 1.26). There is central pallor with atrophy and erythematous borders of plaques seen in necrobiosis lipoidica diabeticorum (*see* Fig. 9.2).

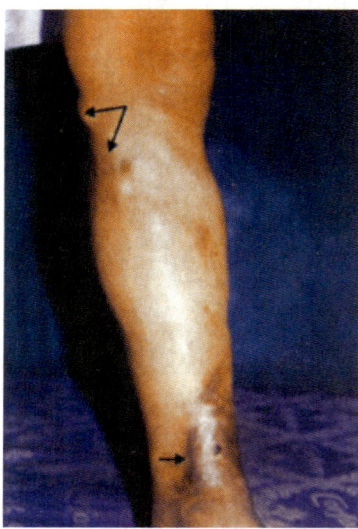

Fig. 1.26: Varicose veins (←↓) with varicose ulcer (→). Note the brown pigmentation around the ankle (→).

5. Temperature
☞ *Note the temperature of the feet*
- The feet are warm or cold similar to hands (read examination of temperature of hands).
- The toes become cold, red and then blue due to chilblain (cold injury) (Fig. 1.27) producing pain due to vasospasm.

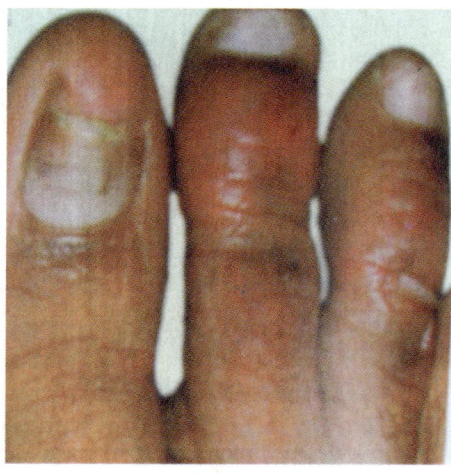

Fig. 1.27: Chilblain. Note the red erythematous plaques over the toes due to cold injury.

6. Vessels and pulsations
☞ *Note the condition of veins and their pulsations.*
- Veins stand out prominently over the calf and the ankle in varicosity and venous thrombosis.
- Pulsations may be absent in embolisation to the vessels or arteritis due to occlusive arterial disease (*pulseless disease* or *Takayasu's arteritis*, *Buerger's disease*).
- Digital gangrene may occur due to arterial obstruction (diabetes, Buerger's disease, occlusive arterial disease) leading of amputation of a digit (Fig. 1.28).
- Vasculitis (palpable purpura, urticarial rashes, maculopapular eruptions) may be seen in SLE, infections and may be due to drugs.

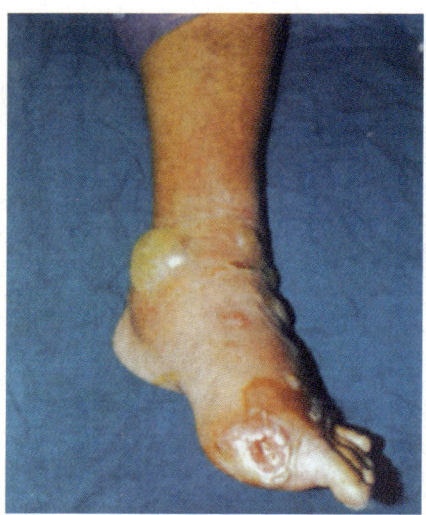

Fig. 1.28: Diabetic foot. There is blistering of the skin with amputation of left big toe. There is impending gangrene of other toes digit.

- Erythromelalgia is a vasomotor disturbance of extremities producing redness due to vasodilatation exaggerated by standing, exertion and heat.
- Acrocyanosis is bluish discolouration of feet/hands associated with coldness and sweating while chillblain produce red plaques over toes due to cold injury (Fig. 1.24).
- Varicose veins (dilated, prominent superficial veins (Fig. 1.25), venous thrombosis/deep vein thrombosis can occur during prolonged bed rest, during surgery/fracture, trauma, CHF, malignancy and puerperium.

7. Joints
☞ *Look at the small joints of feet for swelling and deformity*

- *Arthritis* may involve small joints of the foot in rheumatoid arthritis and psoriasis. The ankle may be involved in osteoarthritis. Swelling of ankle may be due to trauma or bleeding into joints (hemarthrosis) in coagulation disorder, e.g. haemophilia.
- Painful swelling of joints of big toe is seen in gout, (podagra).
- *Neuropathic joint* (*Charcot joint*) commonly involves the knee, hip and ankle producing painless huge swelling of the joint with presence of loose bodies in the joint. Crepitus may be felt over the joint. The joint becomes hypermobile.

8. Inguinal Nodes

Palpate

☞ *Palpate horizontal nodes just below the inguinal ligament and vertical nodes along the saphenous vein.*

Causes of inguinal lymphadenopathy
- Infection (tuberculosis, plague), trauma to the lower extremities
- Sexually transmitted diseases
- Lymphomas
- Metastatic cancer from primary in the rectum, genitalia and lower extremities.
 Part and Parcel of Generalised Lymphadenopathy

Popliteal Lymph Nodes

☞ *Palpate deeply into the popliteal fossa with both hands with the knee partially flexed.*

Causes of enlargement of popliteal nodes
- Knee joint disease.
- Infection and trauma to the lower limb.
- All causes of generalised lymphadenopathy.

9. Trophic ulcers
☞ *Look for trophic changes, i.e. ulcer over pressure points*
- They may be seen in neuropathy commonly in diabetic neuropathy at pressure points, i.e. sacrum (Fig. 1.29), heel and pad of great toe. In diabetic foot, there is vasculopathy, infection and dermopathy, and there may be loss of digit(s).

10. Abnormalities of feet and toes (Read Unit on Rheumatology)

11. Oedema (Fig. 1.30)
☞ *Look at the feet for oedema*
- Oedema means collection of fluid in the interstitial tissue as a result of either increased hydrostatic pressure (e.g. CVS disease) or reduced oncotic

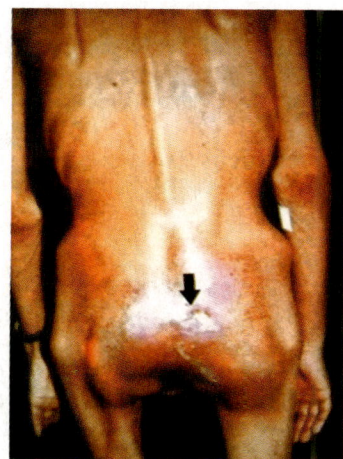

Fig. 1.29: Pressure sores over the sacrum (↓) and iliac crest formed in a patient who was lying in an unconscious state for a long period.

pressure (e.g. hypoproteinaemic states) or due to increased capillary permeability or local venous or lymphatic obstruction.

Usually oedema is demonstrated by the presence of a pit by applying firm pressure over subcutaneous tissue over an area against the hard surface usually the bone.

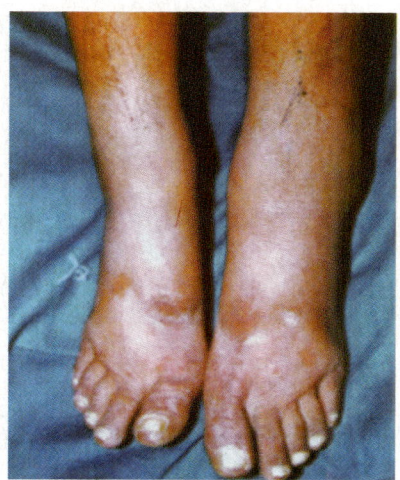

Fig. 1.30: Oedema of feet and legs.

Testing for Dependent Oedema

1. Ankle Oedema (Fig. 1.30)
- The swelling of feet is apparent and complained by the patient. It is checked by applying firm pressure with the right thumb (e.g. till the nail blanches) for at least 5–10 sec not exceeding

30 seconds at the ankle above the medial malleolus, lower end of tibia or upper part of shin bone and then the pressure is released. Presence of a **pit** staying for >30 seconds indicates pitting oedema.
- The extent of oedema is assessed by spread over the tibia; in the mid-thigh, in sacral area and abdominal wall.

2. Sacral Oedema

It is demonstrated by putting pressure with the right thumb over the subcutaneous tissue in sacral area while the patient is lying prone or on one side. Presence of a **pit** indicates oedema **(Fig. 1.31)**. Otherwise also, pitting of sacral area may be seen in oedematous patients confined to bed for prolonged period.

3. Abdominal Wall Oedema (Parietal Oedema)
- Oedema of abdominal wall or thigh can be demonstrated by pressing the chest piece of the stethoscope or the tips of the fingers of right hand and looking for the **pit**.
- It can also be demonstrated by pinching the skin between the thumb and index finger for 15 to 20 seconds and then released. Presence of **pits** at the site of pressure indicate oedema.

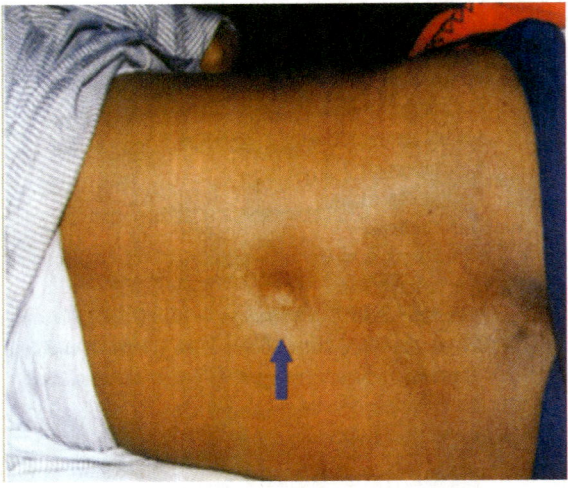

Fig. 1.31: Oedema over the back near or at sacral area. Pressure over the skin and subcutaneous tissue with the thumb against the vertebral column left behind a pit (↑).

Types

Oedema may be **pitting** or **non-pitting**. **Pitting oedema** is due to collection of fluid into the subcutaneous tissue while **nonpitting oedema** is due to infiltration of subcutaneous tissue by any other substance than fluid, i.e. lymph, myxomatous tissue, thickening and hypertrophy of subcutaneous tissue.

A. Pitting Oedema

1. **Generalised oedema.** It is present throughout the body; is due to disorders of heart, kidney, liver, gut, etc. It can also be nutritional or idiopathic. It may be associated with ascites or hydrothorax.
2. **Localised oedema.** It involves a part of the body, is due to venous or lymphatic obstruction, allergy or inflammation. It is unilateral.
3. **Postural oedema.** It may occur due to prolonged standing, old age, hemiplegia but is unimportant.
4. **Unilateral oedema.** Cyclical oedema may be unilateral.

B. Nonpitting Oedema

Occurs in lymphatic obstruction, i.e. lymphoedema **(Fig. 1.31)** or myxoedema.

Distribution of Oedema

When oedema is due to fluid retention, then its distribution is governed by gravity. This is the reason that oedema first appears in dependent parts such as legs, back of thighs and sacral region in the semirecumbent position. If the patient lies flat, it may involve face and hands; for example oedema due to renal disease appears first on the face early in the morning just getting up from the bed, then subsequently gets distributed over the legs when patient is ambulatory.

Causes (Table 1.4)

Pathogenesis of Generalised Oedema

It is also called *anasarca*

1. **Increased hydrostatic pressure** resulting in transudation of fluid from intravascular to interstitial compartment leading to oedema. The causes are given in **Table 1.4**.
2. **Reduced oncotic pressure.** The oncotic pressure depends on the plasma proteins. The conditions associated with hypoproteinaemia result in oedema as a result reduced oncotic pressure (for causes read the **Table 1.4**).
3. **Renin-angiotensin system.** Stimulation of renin-angiotensin-aldosterone system (cirrhosis and renal diseases) results in retention of sodium and H_2O and may contribute to oedema.
    Primary or secondary hyperaldosteronism in patients with hepatic cirrhosis and nephrotic syndrome cause oedema.
4. **Release of ADH.** Reduction in effective fluid volume results in release of ADH to conserve water.

TABLE 1.4: Causes of Oedema

1. Pitting oedema

(A) Increased hydrostatic pressure
- Congestive heart failure or cor pulmonale
- Pericardial effusion
- Constrictive pericarditis
- Budd-Chiari syndrome

(B) Reduced oncotic pressure
- Cirrhosis of liver
- Nephrotic syndrome
- Hypoproteinaemia (nutritional, malabsorption, protein losing enteropathy)

(C) Increased vascular permeability/vasodilatation
- Beriberi
- Epidemic dropsy
- Drugs, e.g. nifedipine/amlodipine

(D) Retention of salt and H_2O
- Cushing syndrome or corticosteroids use
- Oral contraceptives (e.g. oestrogen)
- Liquorice

(E) Venous obstruction

2. Nonpitting oedema
- *Myxoedema*. It may become pitting if CHF is superadded over myxoedema.
- *Lymphatic oedema*, e.g. filariasis or lymph node removal (Fig. 1.32). It is recurrent and intractable oedema in lymphogranuloma venereum, radiation, malignancy, congenital abnormality
- *Angioneurotic oedema*
- *Scleroderma* (painless oedematous induration)

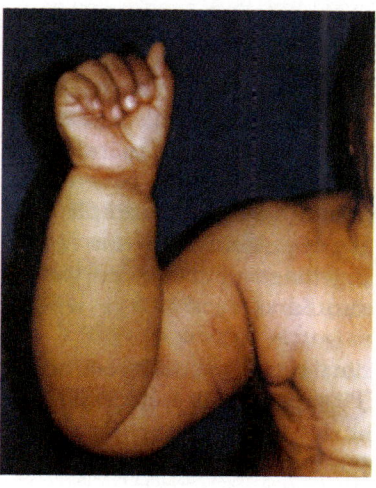

Fig. 1.32: Unilateral lymphoedema. Note the huge swelling, thickening and induration of skin of upper extremity. The lymphoedema occurred due to removal of lymph nodes during surgery for carcinoma of the breast. Note the scar of mastectomy.

5. **Stimulation of anti-natriuretic hormone or peptide (ANP).** In CHF, there is stimulation of anti-natriuretic hormone from the distended right atrium which inhibits salt loss and conserves Na^+ and H_2O.

Differential Diagnosis of Oedema

The characteristic features of oedema due to various causes/conditions are given in Table 1.5.

TABLE 1.5: Differential Diagnosis of Oedema

Cirrhotic	Renal	Cardiac	Angioneurotic	Lymphoedema	Venous oedema
• Pitting oedema appears on the legs with ascites	• Oedema starts first on the face (puffiness of face) then on the legs. It is pitting type	• Oedema appears first on legs then on face. It is pitting type	• It is solid or non-pitting oedema	• Oedema is soft in early stage, becomes indurated, hard and non-pitting	• Soft pitting ankle or leg oedema
• Signs or stigmatas of chronic liver disease may be present	• Oedema is usually noticed in the morning	• Patient will be dyspnoeic, may have tachypnoea and tachycardia	• Results from hypersensitivity, involves eyelids, tongue, lips, face, etc.	• Mostly unilateral, may be bilateral	• Prominent vein and skin thickening may be present
• Signs of portal hypertension, e.g. caput medusae, ascites, fetor hepaticus and splenomegaly may be present	• Ascites is common	• Raised JVP, cyanosis, cirrhotic faeces	• It is acute in onset	• Skin thickening present	• Ulceration and pigmentation over leg, ankle and foot common

Contd.

Contd.

Cirrhotic	Renal	Cardiac	Angioneurotic	Lymphoedema	Venous oedema
• Past history of jaundice or hepatitis or hematemesis • Signs of liver cell failure, i.e. palmar erythema, gynaecomastia, loss of axillary and pubic hair, parotid enlargement, Dupuytren's contractures, flapping tremors, bleeding tendencies, white nails, etc. may be present	• Sacral oedema in nonambulatory patients • Evidence or history of a renal disease in the past	• Tender hepato-megaly • Signs of RVH may be present	• Associated with itching • Congenital variety due to C1 esterase deficiency	• Oedema involves legs, feet, toes, and scrotum • Caused by lymphatic obstruction due to tumour, fibrosis, inflammation, radiation and lymph node removal	• Usually unilateral, occasionally bilateral • Caused by venous obstruction or vulvular incompetence of the deep veins
• USG will show sunken or enlarged liver with disturbed echotexture and increased portal vein diameter (>13 cm) and splenomegaly	• Urine shows massive albumi-nuria	• Evidence of a cardiac disease, e.g. cardio-megaly, 3rd heart sound, murmurs, etc.	• May become life-threatening emergency if glottis is involved	• Congenital variety is due to hypoplasia of lymph vessels, (*Milroy's disease*)	• It commonly occurs during pregnancy, postpartum period due to hyper-coagulable state
	• Other features of hypopro-teinaemia and hyper-cholesterolaemia may be present	• Ascites may also be present		• Oedema is intractable and recurrent	

Unit II

Examination of Respiratory System

- Symptoms and their Analysis
- History
- Examination (General Physical and Systemic Signs)
- Diagnosis and Differential Diagnosis of Lung Lesions and Acute Dyspnoea
- Brief Synopsis of Common Respiratory Diseases

RESPIRATORY SYSTEM

It consists of
- **Upper respiratory system** consisting of nose, nasopharynx, pharynx, larynx and trachea.
- **Lower respiratory system** consisting of bronchi, lungs and pleura.

Symptoms and Signs

Symptoms of upper respiratory tract	Symptoms of lower respiratory tract
• **Nose and nasopharynx,** e.g. nasal discharge, nasal obstruction, sneezing, epistaxis, headache	• **Bronchi and lungs,** e.g. cough, expectoration, haemoptysis, tightness of chest, dyspnoea, orthopnoea, wheezes and apnoea
• **Pharynx,** e.g. sore throat, fever, dry cough, dysphagia	• **Pleura,** e.g. pleural pain, pleural effusion (dyspnoea on exertion), crackpot sounds in chest (hydropneumothorax), acute dyspnoea (pneumothorax)
• **Larynx,** e.g. hoarseness, cough, stridor, pain throat	
• **Trachea,** e.g. pain, hoarseness, cough, dyspnoea, stridor	• **Diaphragm,** e.g. hiccups, shoulder pain

SYMPTOMS RELATED TO UPPER RESPIRATORY TRACT

1. NASAL OBSTRUCTION

It is often associated with local discomfort, nasal discharge, and causes difficulty in breathing, may lead to mouth breathing and dryness of the mouth, persistent sore throat and snoring. Acute nasal obstruction may be due to trauma or to deviated nasal septum. *Vasomotor rhinitis* or *seasonal allergic rhinitis* is the common cause of nasal blockage. Long standing nasal obstruction suggests either deflected *nasal septum* or a *nasal polyp*. Nasal obstruction may be *unilateral* or *bilateral*.

2. NASAL DISCHARGE/RUNNING NOSE

It is a common symptom of acute inflammation or infection of the nose, may be *watery* (*nasal catarrh*), *mucoid*, *purulent* or *blood-stained*. The discharge is often bilateral but may be unilateral. A unilateral blood-stained discharge with nasal obstruction indicates nasal or sinus malignancy.

3. EPISTAXIS

Epistaxis means bleeding from the nose, can occur due to nasal and extranasal causes. The causes of epistaxis are given in Box 2.1.

Symptom Analysis

Q. Ask about the age.
- Foreign body, diphtheria or adenoids are common causes in children. Epistaxis in adults follows trauma, hypertension and bleeding disorder.

Q. History of trauma.
- Local trauma by finger or by injury can lead to epistaxis. Minimal trauma can precipitate epistaxis in bleeding/coagulation disorders.

Q. Is it recurrent or episodic?
- Episodes of epistaxis occur in uncontrolled HT and ITP.

Box 2.1 Causes of Epistaxis

1. **Nasal diseases**
   - Rhinitis
   - Tumours
   - Diphtheria
   - Trauma
   - Sinusitis
2. **Haematological disorders**
   (i) *Due to platelet (bleeding) disorders*
      - Leukaemia
      - Idiopathic thrombocytopenic purpura (ITP)
      - Aplastic anaemia
      - von Willebrand's disease
      - Glanzmann's disease
   (ii) *Coagulation disorders*
      - Haemophilia
      - Afibrogenaemia/hypofibrogenaemia
   (iii) *Miscellaneous*
      - Hypersplenism (pancytopenia)
3. **Systemic disorders**
   (i) *Infection*
      - Typhoid, malaria, measles, high fever, influenza
   (ii) *Hypertension*
   (iii) *High altitude*
   (iv) *Collagen vascular diseases*

Q. **What is quantity of blood loss?**
   - Small blood loss indicates local cause.
   - Profuse bleeding indicates HT or bleeding disorder.

Q. **History of high grade fever.**
   - Typhoid, influenza, infectious mononucleosis indicate vascular phenomenon as a cause of haemoptysis.

Q. **Family history.**
   - Positive family history suggests hemorragic disease/diathesis.

4. NASAL PAIN

Nasal pain is an uncommon symptom, occurs during acute severe infection of the nose or may be secondary to infiltration of the anterior maxillary nerves as they pass along the nasal floor and lateral nasal wall.

Persistent localised pain centred over a sinus suggests sinus infection. Tenderness can be elicited over the involved sinus.

Pain of trigeminal neuralgia or migraine may be referred to nose.

5. SNEEZING

It is deep inspiration followed by forceful uncontrollable expiration through nose associated with a characteristic sound. It is a protective expulsive reflex initiated by irritation of nasal airways. It helps to clear the nasal passages off irritants, noxious substances/gas/particles.

Causes
   i. Excessive, sneezing is associated with vasomotor rhinitis, nasal polyp or allergic rhinitis or deviated nasal sputum.
   ii. Influenza, whooping cough
   iii. **Drugs:** Salicylates, opium, iodides can produce it.
   iv. Psychogenic, e.g. neurosis, hysteria.

6. SORE THROAT

The mouth being an open cavity and tonsils being the policemen of the throat are predisposed to irritation and infection leading to sore throat. Sore throat due to tonsillitis or pharyngitis is associated with fever, chills and in children, dysphagia. There may be formation of an abscess at different sites such as peritonsillar area (*quinsy or peritonsillar abscess*), or retropharyngeal space (*retropharyngeal abscess* presenting as a bulge on posterior pharyngeal wall) or parapharyngeal area (e.g. *parapharyngeal abscess* presenting as a swelling around the angle of the mandible). *A grey membrane* over the tonsils is formed in *diphtheria*.

Symptom Analysis
Ask about the following
- Ask about irritation in throat, pain, fever, chills and rigor
- Ask about difficulty in swelling or painful swallowing (odynophagia)
- Ask about any associated rash (i.e. rubella, herpes zoster, glandular fever)
- Ask about swelling in the neck (grandular fever)
- Ask about tachycardia, mouth breathing, tachypnoea (diphtheria).

7. STRIDOR

It is noisy breathing mainly during inspiration produced by partial obstruction of larynx or trachea or main bronchi. It is usually associated with dysphonia. It is distinguishable from wheezing by different quality and pitch of the note or sound.

Causes
- Foreign body impaction, acute tracheobronchitis, epiglottitis, diphtheria, adenoid enlargement, angioedema, retrosternal goitre can produce laryngeal stridor.
- Tracheal stridor is due to tracheal stenosis and tetany.

8. DYSPHONIA (HOARSENESS)

The hoarseness of voice results from involvement of vocal cord either locally or its paralysis due to damage to recurrent laryngeal nerve or the main trunk of the vagus. The hoarseness may be *acute* (irritation or inflammation of the cord) or *chronic* (nodule, papilloma or polyp of the cord). The *causes* of hoarseness are:

A. Local
  i. *Acute*, e.g. smoke inhalation, exposure to dust
  ii. *Chronic*
   - Laryngeal oedema (chronic laryngitis)
   - A vocal cord nodule (hyperkeratosis)
   - Papilloma of the cord
   - Foreign body, a polyp, carcinoma of larynx.

B. Neurological
  i. *Recurrent laryngeal nerve palsy*
   - Thyroid disorders, e.g. neoplasia, thyroid surgery
   - Neoplasia of oesophagus
   - Neoplasia of apex of the lung (*Pancoast tumour*)
   - Aortic aneurysm
   - A left atrial hypertrophy in mitral stenosis.
  ii. *Involvement of main trunk of vagus*
   - Jugular bulb involvement
   - Infiltrative nasopharyngeal carcinoma/bronchial carcinoma.

C. Systemic illness
   - Myxoedema, angioneurotic oedema.

Symptom Analysis
- Ask about the hoarseness if present, whether acute or chronic.
- Ask about neurological and systemic diseases known to cause hoarseness.

9. DYSPHAGIA

It means difficulty in swallowing. Pain during swallowing is called *odynophagia*.

Causes
  i. Squamous cell carcinoma of oropharynx
  ii. A pharyngeal pouch—a diverticulum between two parts of inferior constrictor muscles.
  iii. Involvement of hypopharynx by inflammation, webs (pharyngeal web-post-cricoid web), stricture and tumours.

The other causes of dysphagia are discussed under GI tract symptoms.

Symptom Analysis
Read GI tract symptoms.

10. LUMP IN THE NECK (LYMPHADENOPATHY)

Certain deep cervical lymph nodes may get enlarged and palpable in the neck due to diseases of the pharynx. The most commonly enlarged lymph node is *jugulodiagastric* which becomes enlarged in upper respiratory tract infection especially tonsillitis, pharyngitis and in neoplasm of the pharynx.

Symptom Analysis
- Ask about history of lump(s) in the neck
- Ask about sore throat, tonsillitis if neck swelling present.

SYMPTOMS OF LOWER RESPIRATORY TRACT

1. COUGH

It is defensive mechanism that helps to keep the respiratory tract clear and protects it against the entry of foreign material from outside.

Cough is defined as violent expiratory effort to clear the tracheobronchial secretion and is produced by rise in intra-bronchial or intratracheal pressure against closed glottis. With opening of the glottis, the pressure is released with throwing of secretions out of trachea with production of sound of cough. The cough is the most common symptom of respiratory disease. It may be *dry* or *productive*. It is produced by stimulation of the sensory nerves of the respiratory mucosa by inflammatory, mechanical, chemical and thermal stimuli. Rarely, it may arise due to irritation or stimulation of the pleura during the aspiration of a pleural effusion/empyema.

Symptom Analysis
Ask about

Q. **What is onset of cough, acute or chronic?**
  - *Acute paroxysmal cough* indicates asthma, foreign body in the larynx or bronchus, or irritation due to inhalation of gases.
  - Continuous cough indicates malignancy lung.
  - Chronic cough (> 2 years) indicates COPD.

Q. **What is the nature/type of cough?**
  - Read Table 2.1

Q. **Is cough dry or productive?**
  - *A persistent dry cough* is associated with pulmonary tuberculosis, URI, sinus infection, pharyngitis, tracheitis.
  - *Productive cough* indicates COPD, lung abscess, bronchiectasis, tuberculosis, asthma.

Q. Is cough spasmodic?
- *Cough associated with wheezing* (spasmodic) occurs in whooping cough, asthma, bronchitis, pulmonary oedema.

Q. Is it intermittent or episodic?
- Episodes of cough and sputum indicate asthma or bronchitis.

Q. Is it painful or distressing?
- Laryngitis, tracheitis, pneumonia or pleurisy produce painful coughing.

Q. What is its relation to posture, time and meal?
- Cough aggravated by lying posture indicates lung abscess, bronchiectasis, pulmonary oedema.
- Nocturnal cough relieved by sitting indicates LVF; morning cough indicates lung abscess and bronchiectasis.
- Cough increased by swallowing indicates broncho-oesophageal fistula.

TABLE 2.1: Characteristics of Cough in Diseases of the Bronchi and small Airways

Disease/Cause	Characteristics of cough
Bronchitis	Dry or productive, worse in the morning
Asthma	Dry or productive, worse at night
Bronchial carcinoma	Persistent, dry usually with haemoptysis
Pneumonia	Initially dry, later productive with or without blood tinge. It is associated with chest pain
Pulmonary embolism	Dry, hacking cough with pleuritic chest pain in patients with DVT
Bronchiectasis	Productive, copious in amount, postural relationship (change in posture induces sputum production), more in the morning, may be blood stained
Pulmonary oedema	Productive with pink frothy sputum, often at night, associated dyspnoea, orthopnoea, PND, crackles and wheezes
Interstitial lung disease	Dry, irritant and distressing cough associated with dyspnoea.

Q. What are associated features?
- *Bovine cough with hoarseness* of voice indicates laryngitis, vocal cord paralysis.
- *Dysphagia associated with cough* indicates mediastinal compression.
- *Persistent cough producing syncope* indicates chronic airway obstruction, or mediastinal compression.
- *Cough with strider* indicates laryngeal or tracheal obstruction.

2. SPUTUM (EXPECTORATION)

The abnormal tracheobronchial secretion is called *sputum*.

Symptom Analysis

If history of sputum production is positive, then:

Ask about the following

Q. Ask about the quantity of sputum, i.e. small or large.
- A large amount of sputum occurs in *bronchiectasis, bronchitis, lung abscess* or a *cavity*.
- Small amount is seen in *asthma*, COPD and *interstitial lung diseases*.

Q. What is the character of sputum?
- The four main types of sputum include *serous, mucoid, mucopurulent* or *purulent* and *rusty*. (Table 2.2) The specimen of sputum may be inspected for nature wherever possible.

Q. What is the colour of sputum, i.e. white, yellow or green, pinkish, brown (rusty)?
- *Mucoid* (white) sputum is more viscous than *purulent* (yellow) sputum, hence, is more difficult to expectorate. It is seen in bronchitis.
- *Mucoid purulent* (yellowish white) sputum occurs in pneumonia and asthma.
- *Purulent* (yellow) sputum is seen in bronchiectasis, lung abscess.
- *Rusty sputum* is seen in pneumococcal pneumonia.
- Pinkish or red sputum indicates haemoptysis.

TABLE 2.2: Sputum Characteristics and their Causes

Type	Character/Nature	Cause
Serous	Clear, watery, frothy, may be pink	Acute pulmonary oedema; Bronchoalveolar carcinoma
Mucoid	Clear, grey, white, may be frothy or black (soot)	Chronic bronchitis; COPD; Bronchial asthma; Asthmatic bronchitis
Mucopurulent or purulent	Yellow, green, brown	All types of bacterial broncho-pulmonary infections; Pulmonary eosinophilia
Rusty	Rusty, golden yellow	Pneumococcal pneumonia

Q. Is sputum foetid (foul smelling)?
- The sputum is foul tasting/smelling (foetid) in *bronchiectasis, lung abscess* or *anaerobic (bacteroides) infection of the lung*.

Q. Is there any postural relation of sputum?
- Postural variation in cough and sputum is characteristic of *lung abscess, a cavity* and *bronchiectasis*.

Q. Is there any diurnal variation of sputum?
- Cough and sputum are more in the morning than evening in *lung abscess, a cavity full of secretion* and *bronchiectasis*.

Q. Is sputum blood stained?
- Read haemoptysis.

3. HAEMOPTYSIS

The coughing up blood in the sputum is called *haemoptysis*. It may be in the form of drops or streaking of the sputum (*pneumonia*) or may be frank blood in the sputum (lung cancer). It may be recurrent or may be just an occasional episode. Although, most patients know whether blood has been coughed up or vomited, yet haemoptysis is occasionally confused with haematemesis. The distinguishing features between the two are listed in Box 2.2.

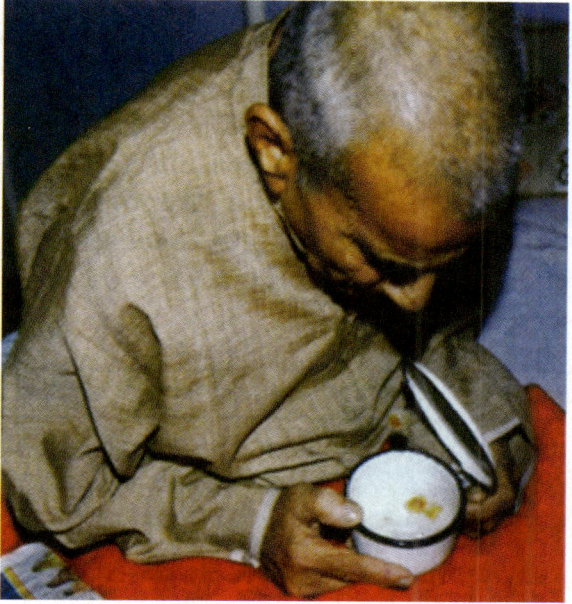

Fig. 2.1: Haemoptysis. Note the red colouration of the sputum.

Box 2.2	Differentiation Between Haematemesis and Haemoptysis
Haemoptysis	*Haematemesis*
• Cough present	• Nausea, vomiting present
• Blood in the sputum (Fig. 2.1)	• Blood in the vomitus containing food particles
• The prodromal symptom is either irritation of throat or cough	• The prodrome is either nausea, retching or abdominal discomfort
• Blood is bright red or frothy	• Blood is magenta-coloured or brownish-black due to formation of acid haematin
• Blood in sputum is alkaline in reaction (taste)	• Reaction of blood is acidic (taste)
• It is mixed with sputum	• It is mixed with food particles

Causes
1. Pulmonary infection
2. Bronchial carcinoma
3. Tuberculosis
4. Bronchiectasis
5. Lung abscess
6. Bronchitis (acute or chronic)
7. Mitral stenosis
8. Bronchial adenoma
9. Secondaries in the lungs
10. Laryngeal tumour
11. Connective tissue diseases
12. Goodpasture's syndrome
13. Blood dyscrasias and anticoagulation
14. Chest trauma
15. Iatrogenic, e.g. after bronchoscopy or biopsy (trans-bronchial or trans-thoracic).

Symptom Analysis

Q. Ask about age.
- The haemoptysis in *childhood* occurs due to tuberculosis, mitral stenosis, pneumonia and bronchiectasis.
- In *adults*, common causes include tuberculosis, mitral stenosis, lung cancer, lung abscess, COPD.

Q. History of trauma.
- Gunshot wound, lung trauma, fracture of ribs can lead to hemoptysis.

Q. Ask about the quantity, i.e. small or large.
- *Mild haemoptysis* with steaking of the sputum occurs in pneumonia, pulmonary infarct.
- *Profuse haemoptysis* occurs in mitral stenosis, bronchiectasis, tuberculosis, bronchogenic carcinoma.

Q. Is it associated with pain chest?
- Haemoptysis with pain chest occurs in diseases involving the lung and pleura, i.e. pulmonary infarct, pneumonia, lung abscess, lung cancer, etc.

Q. What are associated features?
- Associated fever, chills, rigors indicate pneumonia.
- Associated weight loss, anorexia, cachexia indicate malignancy.
- Associated low grade fever with evening rise of temperature, sweating, anorexia indicate pulmonary tuberculosis.

Q. Is there a family history?
- Relatives of patient with tuberculosis may give positive family history of haemoptysis.

Q. Is haemoptysis frank or associated with sputum?
- *Frank haemoptysis* occurs in bronchial adenoma, bronchial carcinoma, pulmonary infarct, tuberculosis.
- *Sputum with haemoptysis* occurs in lung abscess, bronchiectasis, tuberculosis.

Q. Is haemoptysis recurrent?
- Recurrent haemoptysis indicates adenoma/carcinoma of bronchus, lung infarction, mitral valve disease.

4. DYSPNOEA

Dyspnoea is defined as awareness of breathing, may be due to cardiac or respiratory disease, but sometimes it may occur as a result of disorders of other systems e.g. diabetic ketoacidosis, anaemia, thyrotoxicosis.

The **causes** of dyspnoea due to respiratory diseases (*respiratory dyspnoea*) are:
- Bronchial asthma
- COPD
- Bronchial carcinoma
- Pneumonia
- Interstitial lung disease
- Tension pneumothorax
- Large pleural effusion
- Pulmonary embolism
- Lobar collapse
- Laryngeal oedema (anaphylaxis)

ORTHOPNOEA AND PND (PAROXYSMAL NOCTURNAL DYSPNOEA)

Read it under cardiovasuclar system. The orthopnoea and PND in respiratory diseases are uncommon, occur in COPD.

Dyspnoea Analysis

If dyspnoea is complained of, then:

Ask about the following

Q. Mode of onset, duration and progression.
- *Respiratory dyspnoea* may be of *acute or sudden onset* (pulmonary oedema, pulmonary embolism, pneumothorax) or *slow insidious onset* (chronic cor pulmonale, interstitial lung disease, COPD), may be *continuous* and *progressive* (diffuse interstitial lung disease, occupational diseases) or *intermittent/episodic* (asthma).
- Dyspnoea of years duration with progression indicates COPD, pulmonary fibrosis, chest wall deformities.

Q. Is dyspnoea related to posture?
- Dyspnoea in sitting position which gets relieved on lying down indicates the possibility of left atrial myxoma, ball valve thrombus or orthostatic hypertension.
- Breathlessness on lying down indicates LVF, COPD, diaphragmatic paralysis.

Q. What are aggravating and relieving factors?
- Diurnal variation of dyspnoea is characteristic of bronchiectasis, lung abscess.
- Dyspnoea which improves at weekend or on holidays (rest) suggests occupational asthma or extrinsic allergic alveolitis.
- Some diseases such as asthma may be provoked by coughing or laughing or exertion or following exposure to allergans/ irritants.
- *Nocturnal dyspnoea* which may awaken the patient from sleep is a typical feature of nocturnal asthma, pulmonary oedema and COPD. *Orthopnoea and paroxysmal nocturanal dyspnoea* (PND) may be seen in heart failure and severe COPD and such patients may have to sleep in the sitting position propped up by pillows.

Q. What are associated symptoms?
- *Fever* indicates infection of lung or pleura.
- The symptoms associated with dyspnoea include cough, wheeze, sputum, haemoptysis and chest pain. Their significance has been discussed.
- Palpitation, fatigue and oedema legs indicate cor pulmonale or anaemia.

Q. What is severity of dyspnoea?
- Though grading systems exist to assess the cardiac and respiratory disabilities (NYHA classification) but simple questions like breathlessness on daily activities may

provide an effective functional assessment of the severity of dyspnoea.
- Grading of dyspnoea (read CVS)

Q. Does apnoea occur in between dyspnoea?
Apnoea is defined as cessation of breathing, can occur in following conditions:
- Voluntarily holding of breath for sometimes.
- Cheyne-Stokes breathing in which apnoea alternates with hyperventilation.
- *Sleep apnoea syndrome* (read from the textbook).

WHEEZING

Wheezing is defined as whistling or musical sounds produced in the chest. It is due to narrowing of the bronchi as a result of mucus plugging or bronchoconstriction. Many patients may become so accustomed to wheeze that they cease to be aware of its presence.

Causes
1. Asthma
2. COPD, chronic bronchitis
3. Acute pulmonary oedema (LVF)
4. High altitude pulmonary odema
5. Anaphylaxis
6. Inhalation of gases/fumes
7. Carcinoid syndrome, mastocytosis.

Symptom Analysis

Ask about the following

Q. Onset, i.e. acute or chronic.
- Acute wheezing occurs in asthma, anaphylaxis, acute LVF, carcinoid syndrome.
- Chronic wheezing indicates COPD, chronic bronchitis, bronchiostenosis (adenoma, carcinoma bronchus).

Q. Is wheezing intermittent or episodic?
- *Episodic wheezing* indicates asthma
- *Continuous wheezing* indicates COPD.

Q. Is wheezing associated with dyspnoea or cough?
- *Wheezing and dyspnoea* occur in all respiratory diseases with bronchial involvement and CHF (cor pulmonale).
- *Cough with wheezing* is due to asthma, bronchitis, COPD, bronchial obstruction, irritant fumes/gases.

5. CHEST PAIN AS RESPIRATORY SYMPTOM

Any type of pain in the chest is called *chest pain* which may arise from the pain sensitive structures around the chest (skin, muscles, nerves), chest wall (bone/cartilage) and inside the chest (pleura and lungs). The chest pain due to cardiovascular diseases has seen dealt in CVS. Localisation of chest pain helps in making the clinical diagnosis. In general, pain originating from the lungs, pleura or chest wall tends to be **peripheral**; while pain arising from the centrally situated structures, i.e. heart, aorta, trachea, mediastinum, oesophagus is **central**.

The **causes** of chest pain depending on the location are given in Table 2.3. Pain from other organs may also get referred to the chest (referred pain). It can also be psychogenic.

Symptom Analysis

Q. What is the site of pain? Is it central or peripheral?
- *Central or retrosternal chest pain* (Table 2.3) due to repeated coughing is seen in tracheobronchitis or chronic bronchitis/COPD.
- *Central chest discomfort/heaviness* is felt in mediastinal compression due to mass lesion, i.e. a tumour or lymph node enlargement (Table 2.3) or spontaneous pneumothorax.

TABLE 2.3: Respiratory Causes of Chest Pain

Central (retrosternal)	Peripheral
Mediastinal causes	**Pleural involvement**
• Compression due to tumour, mass lesion	• Pulmonary infarct (small peripheral vessel)
• Mediastinitis	• Pneumonia
• Tracheitis	• Pneumothorax
• Thoracic outlet syndrome	• Tuberculosis
Rheumatological causes	• Malignancy
• Costochondritis (Teitz syndrome)	• Connective tissue disorders
Pulmonary Causes	**Musculoskeletal chest wall pain**
• Tracheobronchitis	• Rib injury/fracture
• Chronic bronchitis	• Intercostal muscle injury
• COPD	• Direct invasion of chest wall by tumour or metastases
• Spontaneous pneumothorax	
	• Epidemic myalgia (Coxsackie B infection)
	• Spinal nerve root involvement in Pott's disease (tuberculosis of spine) or vertebral disease or prolapsed disc
	• Post-herpetic neuralgia

- *Peripheral respiratory chest pain* is due to involvement of lung and pleura, i.e. pneummia, pulmonary infarction, tuberculosis, malignancy lung.

Q. Does pain worsen on coughing, sneezing or breathing?
- Unilateral sharp, stabbing chest pain which is made worse by coughing and breathing, is characteristic of pleuritis or chest wall disease (myalgia, fibromyalgia, rib fracture).
- Sometimes, a patient of pleuritis may hold breath or take shallow respiration due to pain.

Q. Is pain chest intermittent or continuous?
- Intermittent pain is pleuritic while continuous, dull, localised pain indicate mass lesion (Table 2.4).

TABLE 2.4: Differences between Pain of Mass Lesion and Pleural Pain

Mass lesion pain	Pleural pain
Localised, retrosternal	Diffuse, side of chest
Dull, central pain	Sharp, stabbing peripheral pain
No relation to respiration	Increases with respiration
Persistent, continuous	Intermittent
No pleural rub	Pleural rub may be heard

Q. What is the nature and severity of pain?
- Constant dull or sharp persistent pain is felt in malignant lung tumours. It is neither related to coughing nor breathing.
- A typical chest pain with no localisaion or relation to coughing or breathing is characteristic of anxiety neurosis. These patients have anxious look.

HISTORY

Present History
Describe the complaints, e.g. cough, sputum, dyspnoea, chest pain, haemoptysis, etc. in chronological orders with *mode of onset, duration, progression of symptoms, aggravating* and *relieving factors, associated symptoms* with treatment being taken.

Past History
- Ask about the past history of tuberculosis, asthma, rhinitis, childhood measles and whooping cough, chest injury and recurrent chest infections.
- Ask about history of epilepsy (convulsions), surgery and prolonged immobilisation (fracture).

Family History
- Ask about family history of asthma, cystic fibrosis (bronchiectasis), eczema, hay fever and tuberculosis.
- Familial alpha-1 antitrypsin deficiency can lead to emphysema, ciliary dyskinesia and bronchietasis (*Kartagener syndrome*).

Personal and Occupational History
Ask about
- History of smoking and alcohol intake.
- History of past and present occupation. *Occupational asthma is known to occur in workers exposed to allergens such as isocyanates (varnishes, soldering and electronic industry), animal and insects allergen (laboratories), platinum salts (metal refirning industry) and allergens from flour and grains (flour mills, farmer, grain handlers).*
- *Certain extrinsic allergic disorders occur due to prolonged exposure to allergens in environment such as farmer's lung (exposure to moudly hay), bird fancier's lung (handling pigeons), malt worker's lung (germinating barley) humidifier fever (contaminated air-conditioners), cheese workers lung (mouldy cheese) and maple bark stipper's lung (bark from maple) occur due to fungal antigen allergen.*
- *Similarly workers in coal mining, silica, asbestos industries are prone to develope occupational lung disease.*

Drug History
Ask about full drug history, i.e. drugs taken in the past or being taken. Ask about the history of drug intake available on the counter.
- ACE inhibitor therapy provokes recent onset cough.
- Beta blockers can precipitate asthma.
- Antimitotic, e.g. methotrexate, bleomycin can cause pulmonary fibrosis.
- Nitrofurantoin therapy can result in intestinal pulmonary fibrosis.

EXAMINATION OF RESPIRATORY SYSTEM

Examination of upper respiratory system.
Examination of lower respiratory system.

General Physical Examination (GPE)
General assessment should be made by making the patient resting on a bed inclined at an angle of 45° and supported by pillows. In this unit physical signs related to respiratory system (chest) are discussed.

Examination of Respiratory System

The points to be noted on GPE are:

General appearance, rate and nature of breathing
☞ Note whether patient is comfortable or dyspnoeic at rest (Fig. 2.2). Note the grade of dyspnoea. Also note whether alae nasi or accessory muscles of respiration working.
- Activity of extrarespiratory muscles indicates airflow obstruction.
- Read the grading of dyspnoea in CVS examination.

Physique nutrition, hydration, weight, smell, sound, etc.
☞ Note the form, physique, state of nutrition and hydration. Record the weight.
☞ Note any cough, audible wheeze, stridor and hoarseness. Note any smell in breath.
- Foul smelling breath (halitosis) indicates lung sepsis or bronchiectasis
- Wheeze audible both to the patient and doctor occurs in cardiac and bronchial asthma (read the causes of wheezes).
- Stridor indicates laryngeal/tracheal obstruction.
- Horseness suggests recurrent laryngeal nerve paralysis.

Face
☞ Examine the face, mouth, lips and tongue for anaemia, polycythaemia, central cyanosis.
- Pursed-lip breathing suggests severe COPD (Fig. 2.2). This indicates severe airflow obstruction.
- Oedema and puffiness of face indicate cor pulmonale, secondary amyloidosis due to suppurative lung disease, hypoproteinemia due to massive expectoration.
- Blue lips and tongue (under surface) indicate central cyanosis.
- Anaemia in respiratory disease is due to haemoptysis and nutritional deficiencies.
- Polycythaemia is secondary to COPD (hypoxaemia), respiratory failure.

The Eyes
☞ Examine the eye as it is likely to be involved in many respiratory disorders:
- Phlyctenular keratoconjunctivitis suggests primary tuberculosis.
- Iridocyclitis may be a manifestation of tuberculosis or sarcoidosis.
- Horner's syndrome may occur due to involvement of cervical sympathetic in lung carcinoma or compression by a tubercular lymph node mass.
- Conjunctival chemosis, suffused face, retinal vein dilatation and papilloedema may be seen in type II respiratory failure or superior vena cava obstruction.

The Neck
☞ Examine the neck for the following
- Look excavation of the suprasternal and supraclavicular fossae.

Excavation of the suprasternal and supraclavicular fossae during inspiration occurs in COPD, suggests advanced airflow obstruction.

- Look for carotid pulsations.

Bounding carotid pulsations in respiratory disease are seen in hypoxia and hypercapnia (type II respiratory failure).

- Look for jugular venous pulse and pressure (for this, read CVS examination).

However, raised JVP and distended neck veins indicate right ventricular failure (cor pulmonale) or superior vena cava obstruction. The differences between the two are given in Table 2.5.

☞ Look for lymph node enlargement.

Cervical lymphadenopathy: Palpate for enlargement of lymph nodes in supraclavicular fossa, cervical and axillary regions.

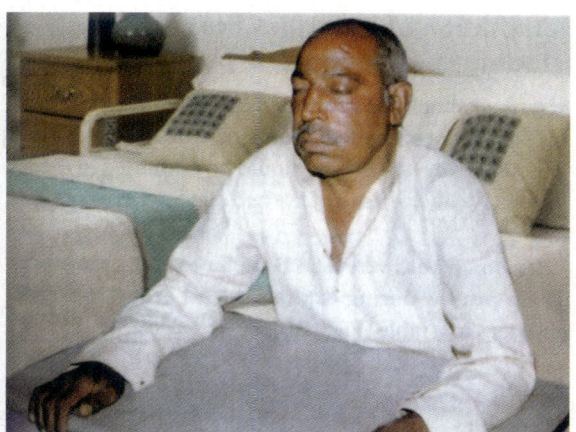

Fig. 2.2: Purse-lip breathing in COPD. Note the sprouting of the lips during inspiration.

TABLE 2.5: Differential Diagnosis of Distended Neck Veins

Right ventricular failure	Superior vena cava obstruction
Distended veins with prominent *v* and *y* collapse	Distended neck veins with absent venous waveforms or pulsations
Swollen face without suffusion or chemosis	The face is swollen, plethoric with conjunctival chemosis
Visible veins on the chest	Prominent veins over the chest
Other associated features of CHF such as cyanosis, pitting peripheral oedema, hepatomegaly and ascites may be present	Associated features such as stridor (due to tracheal obstruction) or dysphagia (oesophageal obstruction) may be present

- The scalene node in particular be examined by dipping the palpating finger behind the clavicle through the clavicular insertion of sternomastoid muscle. The enlarged lymph nodes have a variety of causes (read lymphadenopathy in examination of neck in Unit I on general physical examination) but infection (e.g. tuberculosis) and malignancy (lung cancer) need special mention.

Cervical nodes 1 cm or more in diameter are considered as abnormal, need further evaluation.

☞ *Look for subcutaneous/mediastinal emphysema*
- In *subcutaneous emphysema and mediastinal emphysema*, the air usually escapes into the neck leading to localise or diffuse swelling of neck which gives crackling sensation on palpation.

The Trachea

☞ *Note the position, palpable length above suprasternal notch and 'tracheal tug'.*
- Normally the trachea is either central or slightly to the right. Normally a good length of trachea is palpable in the neck. The method of palpation of trachea has been demonstrated in examination of lower respiratory system (read palpation).

A reduction in palpable length of trachea and tracheal tug indicate severe airflow obstruction.

Extremities

☞ *Examine the hands and feet*
- The hands should be examined for *pallor* (anaemia), *redness* (polycythaemia), cyanosis (CO_2 narcosis), and *clubbing of the fingers*. The feet are examined for *pitting oedema*.

- Cyanosis in respiratory disease is **mixed** type (central as well as peripheral), occurs due to, pneumonia, pneumothorax, massive pulmonary embolism, COPD, severe acute asthma, respiratory failure, diffuse interstitial lung disease and high altitude pulmonary oedema (read the causes of cyanosis as symptoms and signs of CVS).
- Clubbing of the fingers (read symptoms and signs of CVS). In respiratory disease, it occurs in bronchiectasis (Fig. 2.3), lung abscess, bronchogenic carcinoma, COPD, interstitial lung disease, tuberculosis, etc. Clubbing is graded as follows:

Grades of clubbing

Grade I (*normal*): Softening of the nailbed due to hypertrophy of the tissue leading to obliteration of Lovobend's angle, i.e. angle formed between nail-bed and adjacent skin fold (normal < 160°) when both nails of the 4th finger are placed opposite to each other on a bold surface (Fig. 2.3).

Grade II: In addition to grade one there is ballotability and fluctuation of the nailbed (fluctuation sign is positive) due to spongy thickening of the subungual tissue. This is demonstrated by palpating the nailbed with index finger by holding the terminal phalanx between thumb and middle finger. Schamroth's sign is positive, i.e. a lozenge-shaped window is seen when two fingers are held together between the nails of fingers (obliteration of angle with window formation, Fig. 2.3).

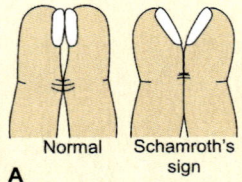
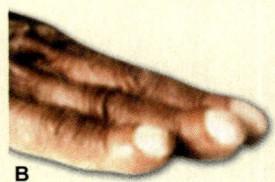

Normal   Schamroth's sign
A   B

Figs. 2.3A and B: (A) Demonstration of Schamroth's sign; (B) Drumstick clubbing in a patient with bronchiectasis. (read the grading of clubbing).

Grade III (bulbous swelling of finger ends): There is bulbous enlargement of ends of the fingers with excessive convex curvature of nails in both planes giving drumstick appearance to the fingers (Fig. 2.3B).

Grade IV (pulmonary osteoarthropathy): In addition to grade III changes, there is involvement of wrists and ankles at times knees, elbow.

- Pitting oedema feet indicate hypoproteinaemia due to massive expectoration or cor pulmonale.

The Skin

☞ *Examine the skin*

- Skin examination as a whole is important for respiratory system. Some of the skin and subcutaneous lesions are associated with respiratory diseases.

- Scar and sinuses are seen in scrofuloderma (tubercular lymphadenitis), erythema nodosum in sarcoidosis, skin metastases occur in lung malignancy, distended veins are seen in SVC obstruction and anastomotic channel in coarctation of aorta.

OTHER FEATURES

☞ *Look for other features*

In a patient of respiratory disease, one should look for:
- *Low grade fever, weight loss* for tuberculosis and cachexia of malignancy.
- *Peripheral signs of right ventricular failure*, e.g. orthopnoea, raised JVP, cyanosis, pitting oedema and hepatomegaly for cor pulmonale.
- *Peripheral signs of II respiratory failure* (CO_2 narcosis) such as flapping tremors (warm extremities, bounding/collapsing pulses).
- *Look for level of consciousness* (response to command and ability to cough).
- *Look for signs of anaemia* (pale conjunctivae, tongue, mucous membrane, nails and palmar creases) and *polycythaemia* (suffused face, cyanosis).

EXAMINATION OF UPPER RESPIRATORY SYSTEM

The Nose and Nasal Sinuses

☞ *Inspect the anterior and inferior surfaces of the nose. Note any asymmetry or deformity of the nose*

- Saddle-shape deformity of the nose may follow destruction of the bony septum from syphilis and the cartilaginous septum following tuberculosis or leprosy, or following trauma, septal haematoma or septal abscess.
- The nasal septum may be depressed in other destructive conditions, e.g. midline granuloma or Wegener's granulomatosis.

- Deviation of the nasal septum is a common deformity visible **(Fig. 2.4)**.

Gentle pressure on the tip of the nose with your thumb will widen the nostrils and now with the help of a penlight or otoscope light, you can have a partial view of each nostril. If tip of the nose is tender, then manipulate the nose more gently and as a little as possible.

- The tip of nose may be red in chronic alcoholics
- Tenderness of the nasal tip or alae suggests local infection such as furunculosis, erysipelas, etc.
- Skin malignancy may involve the skin over the nose.

☞ *Test for the patency of nasal passage*

It may be assessed either by pressing on each ala nasi and occluding the front of each nostril in turn and asking the patient to sniff, or by holding a tongue depressor beneath each nostril and comparing the surface misting of the depressor on the two sides.

Patency of the nasal passage is occluded by a variety of causes as listed under the symptom of nasal obstruction.

☞ *Inspect the inside of the nose* with the help of a biprong nasal speculum and reflected illumination from a head mirror. Look at the nasal mucosa that covers the septum and turbinates. Note its colour, any swelling, bleeding or exudate.

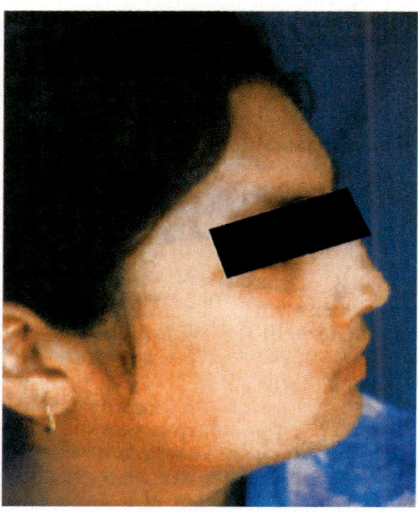

Fig. 2.4: Inspection of the nose: Note the visible deformity of the nasal septum.

- The **atrophic rhinitis or Ozena** is characterised by atrophied mucosa overlaid by foul-smelling dry crusts.
- In *viral rhinitis*, the mucosa is red and swollen; in allergic rhinitis, it may be pale, bluish or red.
- The most common disorders of vestibule (nasal cavity) are **furunculosis** and **vestibulitis**. In the later condition, the vestibule becomes crusted and excoriated as a result of infection usually secondary to repeated trauma from rubbing or cleaning the nose.

☞ *Look at the nasal septum for any area of granulation and septal perforation.*

- **Klebsiella rhinoscleromatis** causes *rhinoscleroma*—a granulomatous disease of upper respiratory tract.
- *Black eschars* in diabetics may be seen in nasal cavity in mucormycosis.
- Fresh blood from the nose may be seen in epistaxis. **Causes of septal perforation** include trauma (nose pricking) surgery and intranasal use of cocaine or amphetamines or inhalation of industrial products, e.g. nickle and chrome.

Note any abnormalities on the lateral wall of the nasal cavity, e.g. hypertrophy of nasal turbinate or a nasal polyp or an ulcer or a mass.

- In *allergic rhinitis*, inferior turbinate is hypertrophied, red and tender.
- *Nasal polyps* are pale, semitranslucent non-tender masses that usually come from the middle meatus.
- *Ulcer* may result from nasal use of cocaine or other drugs, e.g. pituitary preparations and blastomycosis (*Blastomyces dermatitidis*).

☞ *Examine the postnasal space with the help of a small postnasal mirror.* The manoeuvre is best performed with the patient leaning forward, with mouth opened and the tongue firmly depressed with a tongue depressor. A postnasal mirror is warmed over the flame of a spirit lamp and passed into the mouth over the upper surface of the tongue until it lies in the space between the uvula, the tongue, and the faucial pillars.

Note the hypertrophy or any polyp in this space.

The site is common for:
- Carcinoma
- *Antrochoanal polyp*—a benign polyp arising from the nasal septum and protruding through the middle meatus.

- *Hypertrophy of the posterior end of the inferior turbinate* (*mulberry terbinate*).
- ☞ *Palpation for sinus tenderness.* Press on the *frontal sinuses* under the bony brows, avoiding pressure on the eyes. Then press up on the *maxillary sinuses* over the cheeks (Fig. 2.5).

Local tenderness together with pain, fever and rhinorrhoea suggest *acute sinusitis* involving the frontal or maxillary sinuses. Transillumination may be useful for diagnosis. Absence of glow on one or both sides on transillumination suggests either a thickened mucosa or secretion in the sinus involved.

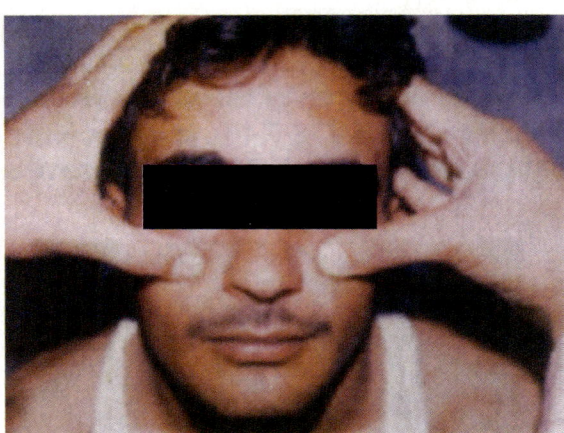

Fig. 2.5: Elicitation of maxillary sinus tenderness.

EXAMINATION OF THROAT

Ask the patient to open the mouth.

☞ *Examine lips, teeth, gums.*

☞ *Examine the tonsils for exudate. Examine oropharynx and floor of the mouth.*

☞ *Finally examine the posterior wall of pharynx for any swelling, vesicles, ulcers or pus.*

- The anterior oropharynx should be examined with a head light or with a head mirror. First check the lips, teeth, and gums, floor of the mouth and opening of submandibular duct and the buccal mucosa.
- The more distal portion of oropharynx and larynx can be inspected only with a laryngeal mirror or fibre-optic laryngoscope.
- A white exudate over the tonsils is seen in glandular fever while yellow punctate follicular exudate is seen in streptococcal tonsillitis. Exudate with membrane formation,

white to green in colour starting from the tonsils and spreading to fauces and pharynx is seen in *diphtheria*. If this condition is suspected, a swab should be taken for bacteriological examination.
- Small lymphatic nodules are normally common on the posterior wall of pharynx.
- In *chickenpox* (*herpes varicella*), there is erythema of pharyngeal wall and buccal mucosa followed by vesicles which progress to round or oval ulcers with a white slough. In *Coxsackie virus infection* (*herpangina*) similar lesions may be present on the pharynx and soft palate.
- In the *common cold* (infection of nose or sinuses) mucus or pus may be visible trickling down the back of the throat. *Peritonsillar abscess* (*quinsy*) and *retropharyngeal abscess* are now-a-days less common.

EXAMINATION OF LOWER RESPIRATORY SYSTEM (CHEST EXAMINATION)

It is described under four heads:
1. *Inspection*: Looking at the chest.
2. *Palpation*: Confirming the findings of inspection.
3. *Percussion*: To define resonant and dull areas on the chest.
4. *Auscultation*: To hear normal and abnormal sounds.

Examination of Anterior and Lateral Chest

☞ Positioning

The patient should be examined in the supine position with arms somewhat abducted. A patient who is having difficulty in breathing on lying down, should be examined in the sitting position or with the head of the bed elevated to a comfortable level.

Persons with severe COPD prefer to sit leaning forward, with lip-pursed during expiration and arms supported on their knees or a table (Fig. 2.2).

☞ Inspection

1. **Shape of the chest.** Observe the following
   - Symmetry
   - Antero-posterior (AP) and transverse diameter
   - Hollowing, flattening or bulging
   - Subcostal angle
   - Position of shoulders and spine.

Normal chest is bilaterally symmetrical with smooth contours and slight recession in infraclavicular regions.

Its transverse diameter is more than the AP diameter, the ratio being 7:5.

The subcostal angle is acute ($<70°$)

The interspaces are oblique; wider anteriorly than posteriorly.

📖 *Abnormalities of chest*

Unilateral prominence of the chest. One side of the chest may become prominent or protuberant in pleural effusion, pneumothorax, tumours, aneurysm and empyema necessitans. *Localised bulge* may occur in aortic aneurysm, pericardial effusion, liver abscess, etc.

Unilateral or localized depression of the chest: Chest may be unilaterally depressed in fibrosis, collapse, thickened pleura and unilateral muscle wasting of chest.

Flat chest: The AP diameter is decreased and chest becomes flat. It is seen in children due to adenoid/lymphoid hypertrophy, rickets and advanced tuberculosis.

2. Respiratory rate and rhythm

Count the respiratory rate and note its rhythm
- The adult respiratory rate is 14–20 min and respiratory rhythm is regular with inspiration longer than expiration.
- The respiratory rate is higher in infance and childhood normally. It increases with excitement, exertion, emotion, fever, diseases of heart and lungs; decreases in respiratory rate (bradypnoea) occurs in narcotic poisoning, hypothyroidism, uraemia, raised ICP and coma.
- The *rhythm* of respiration is normally regular becomes irregular during exertion, emotion and during sleep.
- **Abnormal respiratory patterns are**
  - *Irregular respiratory pattern* may be noted in meningitis, coma, shock or in moribund patients. It may be a pre-terminal event.
  - *Rapid shallow breathing* occurs in restrictive lung disease while *slow breathing* is characteristic of respiratory depression.
  - *Kussmaul's breathing* (deep and slow noisy breathing) is seen in ketoacidosis, uraemia, salicylate poisoning, metabolic acidosis.
  - *Cheyne-Stokes breathing* (periods of hypernoea alternate with periods of apnoea) is seen in LVF, raised intracranial tension, respiratory failure and narcotic poisoning.

- *Biot's (ataxic) breathing* occurs in meningitis and raised intracranial tension.
- *Deep stertorous (noisy) breathing* is seen in deep coma.
- *Ataxic breathing* (irregular rate and rhythm) occurs in medullary lesions.
- *Sighing* (breathing with frequent sobs) *respiration* is seen in hyperventilation and hysterical episode
- *Paradoxical respiration* occurs in flail chest.

Prolongation of respiratory phase. The upper airway obstruction produces stridulous breathing (noisy breathing) with or without prolongation of inspiratory phase.

Lower airway obstruction (below the larynx) produces prolongation of expiratory phase with wheezes/rhonchi. This is seen in asthma, bronchitis, COPD, etc.

3. **Type of breathing movements**
   Note the type of breathing and the presence of any abnormal inspiratory or expiratory movements
   - In majority of the males and some females, the normal breathing is *abdominothoracic* (mainly abdominal).
   - In majortiy of females, the normal breathing is thoracoabdominal (mainly thoracic).

   Abnormal breathing movements are
   i. *Thoracic breathing.* This occurs when diaphragmatic movements are inhibited either by paralysis or by abdominal pain or restricted by raised intra-abdominal pressure caused by ascites, gaseous distension of the bowel, a large ovarian cyst or pregnancy.
   ii. *Abdominal breathing.* It occurs when there is restriction of chest movements either by ankylosing spondylitis or paralysis of intercostals muscles or pleural pain.

4. **Note any deformity of the chest**
   The deformities of the chest are:
   a. *Barrel-shaped chest:* The AP diameter is increased, becomes equal or more than transverse. The subcostal angle is wide (obtuse). The sternum is more arched, spines become unduly concave forwards. The ribs become less oblique. This shape is normal during infancy but abnormally seen in COPD (emphysema).
   b. *Funnel chest (Cobbler's chest, pectus excavatum):* There is hollowing of the sternum which may cause compression of heart and great vessels and may produce murmurs. The normal heart shadow may appear enlarged on chest X-ray (*Pomfret's heart*). This may be either congenital, or an occupational deformity in Cobbler.
   c. *Pigeon chest (Keeled chest, pectus carinatum):* The sternum is displaced anteriorly, increasing the AP diameter and leading to depression on either side of sternum. This is characteristically seen in rickets. Other chest signs of rickets (*rickety rosary*-beading of costochondral junctions, *Harrison's sulcus*—a transverse groove passing outwards from the xiphisternum to the mid-axillary line) may be present.
   d. *Traumatic flail chest:* The side of the chest is depressed due to fracture of multiple ribs (*flail chest*) resulting in paradoxical movement of the thorax, i.e. the injured area moves inwards during inspiration and outwards during expiration.
   e. *Dumb-bell shape chest.* The chest is protuberant anteroposteriorly at its middle and the heart is placed obliquely in it.
   f. *Kyphoscoliosis*: There is backwards bending (kyphosis) due to thoracic convexity and lateral bending (scoliosis) due to lateral and rotatory curvature of thoracic spines. This deformity may be congenital and associated with hereditary ataxias. The asymmetry of the chest may decrease the size of thoracic cage and restrict lung expansion.

5. **Lesion on the chest wall (skin and subcutaneous tissue)**
   Look for *cutaneous* (e.g. eruptions, purpuric spots, bruises, scars, sinuses) *and subcutaneous lesions* (e.g. inflammatory swelling, subcutaneous tumour, nodule, sebaceous cyst, sarcoid nodules, vascular anomalies). These have already been highlighted during general physical examination.

6. **Movements of the chest (expansion of the chest)**
   Observe the chest movements and compare the range of chest movements on the two sides during normal and deep breathing
   - To compare the range of movements in the infraclavicular regions, position the patient supine, shoulders relaxed and symmetrical with the head resting on a pillow and the head and trunk in a straight line. Then ask the patient to take deep steady breaths while inspecting the infraclavicular regions tangentially.
   - Assess lower anterior chest movements by inspecting the patient semirecumbent and breathing deeply.

   Note the intercostal recession or indrawing of the intercostal spaces during movements of the chest. Observe for the prominence and activity of accessory muscles of respiration.

Normally both sides of the chest move uniformly without any indrawing of intercostal spaces. Accessory muscles of respiration are usually not required for act of breathing, hence, are not prominent. The alae nasi are not active.
- When lung compliance is reduced (stiff lung) there will be indrawing of intercostal spaces, i.e. in COPD, fibrosis, lung collapse.
- Alae nasi and accessory muscles of respiration are working actively in airflow obstruction (COPD with or without acute exacerbation).

During the movements of the chest, there is usually expansion of the chest, hence, both are interchangeably used. The **causes of diminished movements or expansion** of the chest are given in Table 2.6.

TABLE 2.6: Causes of Diminished Movement/ Expansion of the Chest

Unilateral diminished movement/expansion	Bilateral diminished movement/expansion
1. Massive collapse of the lung (a foreign body, bronchial adenoma/ carcinoma)	1. Bronchial asthma
	2. COPD
	3. Extrinsic allergic alveolitis
2. Consolidation	4. Bilateral pulmonary fibrosis (idiopathic, drug induced)
3. Consolidation collapse	
4. Fibrosis of the lung	
5. Thickened pleura	5. Guillain-Barré syndrome
6. Pleural effusion	
7. Pneumothorax or hydropneumothorax	6. Respiratory muscle paralysis
8. Diaphragmatic paralysis	7. Poisonings, e.g. narcotics

There can be diminished movements/expansion of the chest in a localized part due to underlying lung or pleural disease such as fibrosis, collapse of the lung, localised pleural effusion, diaphragmatic paralysis.

A good test of the diaphragm movement is to ask the patient to sniff vigorously; patient with diaphragmatic paralysis is unable to do so.

N.B. In normal movements of the chest, the lower parts move first followed by the upper part, but in COPD (emphysema) with barrel-shaped chest, the chest moves as a whole (*en bloc*).
- If the patient is breathless, examine him/her in semirecumbent or sitting position. Note any abnormality of inspiratory or expiratory movement.
  i. Abnormal inspiratory movements produced by contractions of accessory mucles of respiration (sternomastoids, scaleni and trapezii) are seen in patients with gross overdistension of lungs. The intercostal recession or indrawing of the ribs, excavation of supraclavicular fossae and suprasternal notch and widening of the subcostal angle invariable accompany diminished movements in patients with COPD (Fig. 2.6). More violent inspiratory movements are seen in laryngeal or tracheal obstruction.
  ii. Paradoxical movements of chest occur in flail chest (read abnormalities of chest).

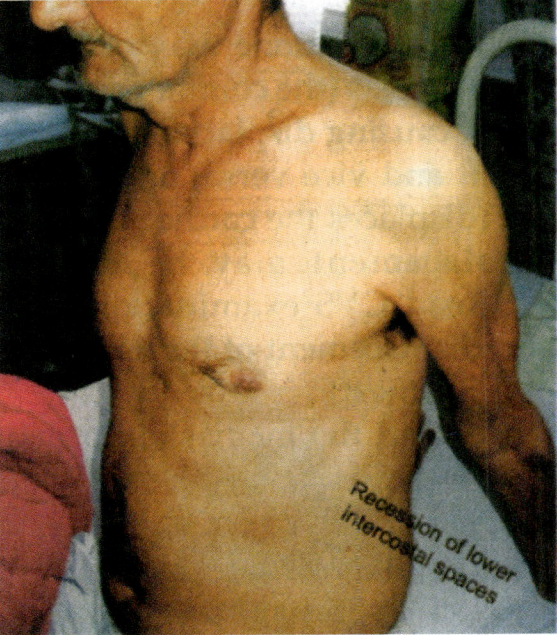

Fig. 2.6: Chronic obstructive pulmonary disease (COPD). Note the barrel-shaped chest, excavation of the supraclavicular fossae, prominence of sternomastoid and recession of intercostal spaces.

  iii. Abnormal expiratory movements are produced by contractions of abdominal muscles and latissimus dorsi. These are observed when either the compliance of the lungs is reduced (e.g. emphysema) or there is severe airway obstruction (bronchitis or bronchial asthma). Such patients prefer to sit upright (Fig. 2.2), gasping on a bed table or the back of a chair. Many patients have purse-lip breathing.

7. The cardiac apex, trachea and mediastinum

Look at the position of the *apex beat* (read CVS examination). Position of the apex beat is decided by position of mediastinum. It may be pulled to same side (lung collapse or fibrosis or thickened pleura or following pneumotectomy) or pushed to opposite side by pleural effusion, pneumothorax.

Inspect the trachea from the front for any deviation from its usual midline position.

- On inspection, sternomastoid muscles become unduly prominent on the side to which trachea has been shifted. This is called *Trail's sign* (Fig. 2.7B). This finding has to be confirmed on palpation.

Look for mediastinal shift
- The position of the mediastinum is decided by the position of the trachea and that of cardiac impulse (apex beat). The mediastinal shift occurs in a variety of diseases given in Box 2.3.

☞ Palpation

Palpation is done to confirm the findings of inspection. In addition, perform tactile vocal fremitus.

i. *Palpate the chest wall for any local swelling or bony prominences, crepitus and tenderness*
   - Fluctuation sign is positive in an abscess on the chest wall.
   - Rickety rosary or scorbutic rosary produce swelling of costochondral junctions. Bony swelling is a hard mass.
   - A *crepitus* (crackling sound) due to presence of air will be felt on palpation of subcutaneous emphysema. A crepitus in the supraclavicular region with a little or no crepitus over the chest wall indicates mediastinal emphysema.
   - Identify the site of *tenderness* so as to find out the cause of pain. The **causes of pain and tenderness** are chest injury, inflammatory myositis, fibromyalgia chest, rib fracture, secondaries in the ribs, herpetic intercostal neuralgia, pleurisy and pericarditis.

ii. *Note the position of cardiac impulse. Palpate the trachea for any deviation*
   - Displacement of cardiac impulse alone may occur in chest deformities such as *scoliosis* (the commoner form, with convexity to the right causing displacement of the cardiac impulse to the left and *vice versa*) and *funnel chest* with central depression (displaces the cardiac impulse to the left). The displacement may be due to cardiovascular causes (read CVS examination) and respiratory causes (read displacement of the apex beat under inspection of anterior chest).

iii. *Palpation of trachea*
   - For any deviation (Fig. 2.7A), place your finger along one side of the trachea with neck slightly flexed to accommodate the finger. Note the space between it and the sternomastoid muscle. Compare it with the other side. Normally, the spaces should be symmetrical and equal. A smaller space on one side than other side indicates shift of trachea to that side.
   - Masses in the neck may shift the trachea to the opposite side.
   - Tracheal deviation may also signify mediastinal shift—an important problem in the thorax.

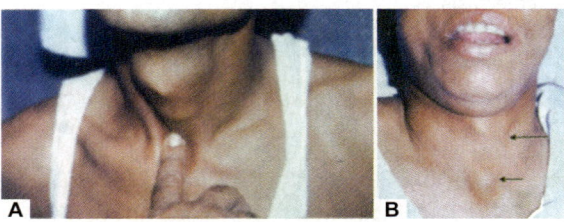

Figs 2.7A and B: (A) Palpation of trachea; (B) Trail's sign. The sternomastoid muscle stands out prominently on the side of the trachea is shifted (left side in this case).

Palpable length of trachea
- On full inspiration, the length of trachea between suprasternal notch and the lower margin of cricoid cartilage is 3 to 4 fingers breadth (2–3 inches), called palpable length of trachea.
- In old age and in hyperinflated lungs, the palpable length of the trachea decreases during expiration. Tracheal descent on inspiration is noticed by placing a fingertip on thyroid cartilage in COPD.

Tracheal tug, i.e. descent of trachea with each heartbeat occurs in severe AR.

iv. *Palpate the intercostal spaces for narrowing or widening*

- Unilateral widening occurs in tumour of the lung or pneumothorax, pleural effusion while unilateral narrowing indicates fibrosis or collapse of the lung on that side or pneumonectomy.
- Bilateral widening indicates COPD (emphysema).

The shift of the trachea and the mediastinum may be due to pull or push. The causes of mediastinal shift have been discussed in Box 2.3.

v. *Assess the other abnormalities seen on inspection*
   - Confirm the findings of inspection by palpation such as skin lesion, pulsations, venous hum or thrill.

Box 2.3	Positions of the Mediastinum in Respiratory Diseases		
Central	**Pulled to the same side**	**Pushed to the opposite side**	
• Bronchitis • Asthma • Pulmonary suppuration, e.g. lung abscess, bronchiectasis • Consolidation • Emphysema • Interstitial fibrosis	• Collapse • Fibrosis • Thickened pleura • Pneumonectomy or lobectomy	• Pleural effusion • Pneumothorax • Hydropneumothorax or pyopneumothorax	

vi. *Measurement of chest expansion*
- The observed expansion of the chest must be confirmed by palpation manually (Figs 2.8A and B) as well as by tape (Fig. 2.9)
  Place your thumbs along a costal margin just below the nipples, your hands along the chest wall laterally. Shift the tips of the thumbs a bit medially so as to approximate them in the centre. Ask the patient to inhale deeply. Observe how far your thumbs diverge as the thorax expands. The distance between the thumbs indicates degree of chest expansion. If one thumb remains closer to the midline, this confirms the diminished expansion on that side (*differential expansion*). This gives you an idea of expansion of each side as well as total chest expansion. Repeat the process on the back.

Measurement of chest expansion by tape (Fig. 2.9): Record with a tape measure the maximum inspiratory/expiratory difference in the lower chest (at the level of nipple in males and 4th or 5th intercostal space in females). This gives you actual total expansion not expansion of each hemithorax.

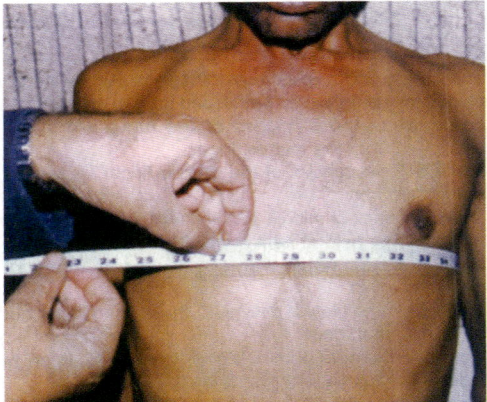

Fig. 2.9: Measurement of expansion of the chest by measuring tape. Encircle the tape around the chest at the level of nipple. Note the reading of the tape during full expiration. Ask the patient to take breath as deep as he can while you let loose the tape. Now note the reading during full inspiration. The difference between the two reading indicates expansion of chest.

Differential expansion (expansion of each hemithorax): One can measure the expansion on each side during full inspiration by the manual method as well as by measurement as described above. This is measured from midsternal line to the level of spine on each side.
- Diminished expansion on one side indicates collapse or fibrosis of the lung on that side.

Palpation of intercostal spaces. In case of abnormal chest, palpate the intercostal spaces with pulp of the fingers on each side at corresponding levels to know any widening or narrowing.

- Narrowing or overcrowding of intercostal spaces on one side occurs in atelectasis, collapse, fibrosis, thickened pleura, pneumonectomy/lobectomy.
- Bilateral narrowing is seen in interstitial lung diseases or bilateral pulmonary fibrosis.

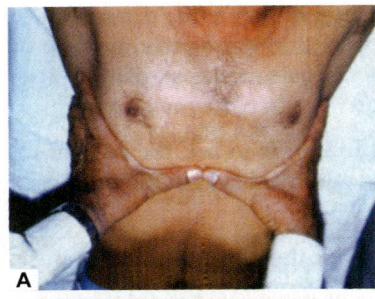

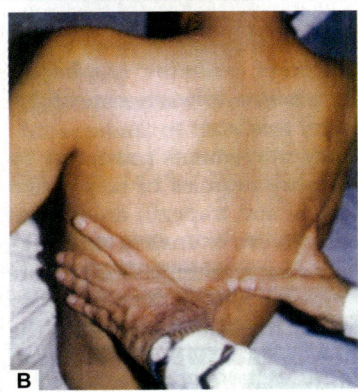

Figs 2.8A and B: Manual measurement of chest expansion on the back. (A) Front of chest; (B) Back of chest.

- Widening of spaces on one side occurs in pleural effusion and pneumothorax, and on both sides in emphysema (COPD).

Assessment of tactile vocal fremitus. Tactile vocal fremitus refers to perception of vibrations transmitted to chest wall from the voice box (*larynx*) via the tracheobronchial tree during the act of phonation (speaking).

During phonation, vibrations produced from the larynx (*voice box*) are transmitted from the larynx to trachea, bronchi, lungs and then to the chest wall and set the chest wall to vibrate. These vibrations may be detected by palpation with the palm of the hand placed flat on the chest, called *tactile vocal fremitus*.

vii. *Perform the vocal fremitus on each side*

Method (Fig. 2.10): Vocal fremitus is performed and compared on both sides of the chest using the ball or ulnar surface of the hand when patient is asked to repeat some words, say, *ninety-nine* or *one-one-one*. The examining hand perceives distinct vibrations.

Points to be noted in tactile vocal fremitus are:
- *Intensity of the sound* perceived, i.e. increased, decreased or absent.
- To determine whether *change in intensity is localized* or *generalized*. This is done by comparing the vocal fremitus in corresponding areas on the two sides of the chest (Fig. 2.10).

Note: Do not include cardiac area for comparison of vocal fremitus on the corresponding area on the other side as it is normally diminished in this area.

Abnormalities of vocal fremitus

The causes of *increased*, *decreased* or *absent tactile vocal fremitus* are listed in Table 2.7.

vii. *Other palpable vibrations*
- Palpate for *crackles, rales, pleural rub* or *wheezes/rhonchi*.

A palpable pleural friction rub: It is a rubbing sound produced due to rubbing of the parietal pleura towards the end of inspiration or during beginning of expiration. It occurs in pleurisy due to any cause, e.g. pleurodynia, consolidation, pulmonary infarction, early pleural effusion. It is felt over the area of pleura involved. It becomes absent with formation of pleural effusion.

Palpable crackles or rales: Coarse crackles or rales are bubbling or gurgling sounds; may become palpable in bronchiectasis and pulmonary fibrosis. They represent bronchi or bronchioles filled with secretions.

Palpable wheeze/rhonchi: Wheeze (a humming or whistling sound), may be audible as well as palpable in bronchial asthma, cardiac asthma, carcinoid syndrome, drug allergy. A palpable persistent rhonchus indicates bronchial adenoma/carcinoma.

viii. *Perform special manoeuvres if required.*

Valsalva and Müller manoeuvres: Normally supraclavicular fossa bulges during Valsalva manoeuvre and refracts during Müller manoeuvre. In carcinoma of the apex of the lung, the supraclavicular fossa does not show any change during these manoeuvres while the normal side exhibits characteristic buldging and retraction. Other diseases that produce similar effect include apical thickened pleura (tuberculosis), fungal infections, radiation and pneumothorax.

☞ Percussion

Percussion of the chest means to set the chest wall and underlying tissues into motions producing audible sounds and palpable vibrations. Percussion note helps you to distinguish whether the chest contains an air (pneumothorax), fluid (pleural effusion) or a solid tumour. It penetrates only about 5–7 cm into the chest, therefore, will not help to detect the deep seated lesions.

Normal areas of resonance and dullness on chest: The regions of the thorax where a resonant percussion note is normally found correspond approximately to the surface marking of the lungs. The heart normally produces an area of dullness to the left of the sternum from the 3rd to 5th spaces (cardiac dullness). Percuss the left lung lateral to it. The liver dullness starts from the 5th intercostal space downwards on the right side.

TABLE 2.7: Abnormalities of Tactile Vocal Fremitus

Increased	Decreased	Absent
• Consolidation	• Bronchial asthma	• Pleural effusion
• A large superficial cavity	• Emphysema	• Pneumothorax
	• Pulmonary fibrosis	• Hydro- or pyopneumothorax
	• Lung collapse with obstructed bronchus	
	• Thickened pleura	

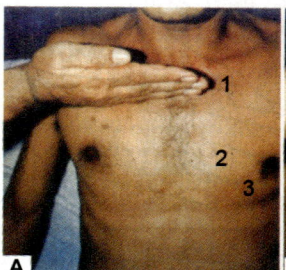
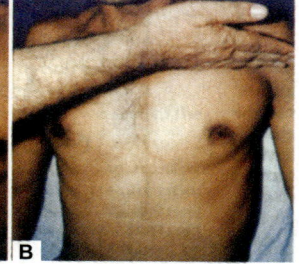

Figs 2.10A and B: Vocal fremitus. (A) Comparison is made on the both sides at corresponding areas (1, 2 and 3) from above downwards toward lower part of chest.

Method: The technique of percussion is illustrated in Fig. 2.11 and Box 2.4.

Box 2.4: The Method of Percussion for Right-handed Doctor/Student (Fig. 2.11)

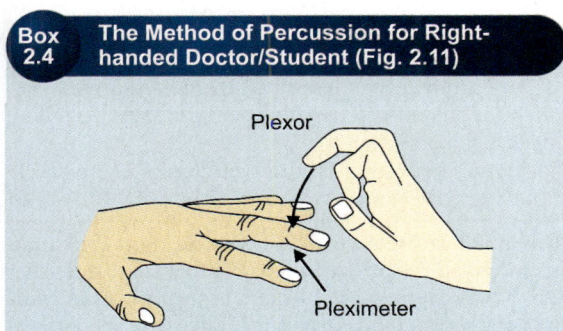

Fig. 2.11: Method to deliver the stroke with plexor (tapping finger) on pleximeter finger (finger that receives stroke). The corresponding areas to be percussed are labelled in Fig. 2.12.

- The middle finger (pleximeter finger) of the left hand is placed on the part to be percussed usually an intercostal space and others fingers of the hand are slightly separated from the middle finger.
- Make a good contact of the middle finger of left hand by pressing the finger firmly into intercostal space.
- Strike the back of middle phalanx with the tip of the right middle finger (plexor) held at right angle. The movement should be at the wrist rather than at elbow so as to produce *hammer effect*.
- With your plexor or tapping finger, deliver the lightest percussion that produces a clear note (Fig. 2.11). For a thick chest wall use heavier percussion. However, if a louder note is needed, apply more pressure with the pleximeter finger.
- As soon as the blow is delivered, the striking finger must be raised off the pleximeter finger each time. The pleximeter finger is moved on identical areas on two sides.
- Compare the note obtained from identical sites on two sides. The area percussed must be more or less equidistant from the two ears of the examiner.
- Map out the area of impaired dullness (excluding cardiac and hepatic) by percussing from a resonant to a dull area but not otherwise.
- In woman, to enhance percussion, gently displace the breast with your left hand while percussing with the right.

Remember the rules of percussion
1. Always percuss from resonant to dull area over one side of the chest. The *vice versa* is not true.
2. Compare the corresponding areas on two sides of the chest simultaneously.

Steps of percussion
While the patient keeps both arms by the side of the chest, percuss the front of the chest in a symmetric fashion from above (apices) to below (bases of the lung). Percuss first one side of the chest and then the other at each level and at similar locations marked in Fig. 2.12. Omit the areas over the scapulae as bone alters the percussion note over the lungs. *Identify and locate the area of any abnormal percussion note.*

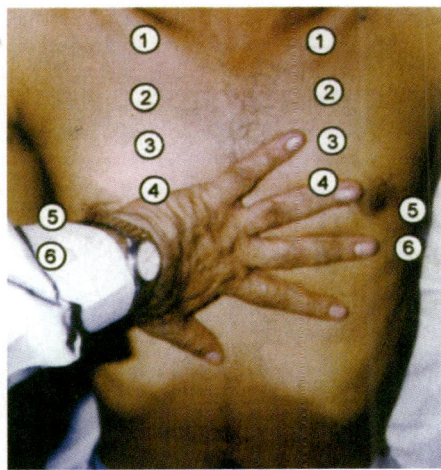

Fig. 2.12: Percussion of the front of the chest. Note the placement of fingers parallel to intercostal spaces. The areas to be percussed are labelled and encircled.

While percussing the lower posterior chest, stand somewhat to the side rather than directly behind the patient. This allows you to place your pleximeter finger more firmly on the chest and makes tapping more effective.

While comparing two areas, use the same percussion technique in both areas. Percuss or strike twice in each locations (Fig. 2.12). *Try to detect differences in percussion notes by comparing one area with another.*

- *Normal lung resonance*: The normal lung resonance is resonant note without any resistance, is due to air containing lungs called vesicular resonance. It varies from case to case and over different areas and bulk of chest.

Remember. Normal lung resonance is replaced by dullness when fluid or solid tissue is interposed between air containing lungs and the chest wall beneath your percussing fingers. For example:

- **Dull note** over consolidation is due to solidification of the lung as the alveoli are filled with fluid and blood cells. Similarly dull note on percussion is elicited over a solid growth (tumour) or collapse (airless alveoli) and fibrosis of the lung.
- **Stony dull note** (a marked resistance to pleximeter finger on percussion) is elicited when either the fluid (pleural effusion) or blood (hemothorax) or pus (empyema) occupies the pleural space.

- **Hyper-resonant note.** Normal lung resonance becomes *hyper-resonant* when either the lungs are hyperinflated (emphysema) or air is present in pleural cavity (pneumothorax).

Learn to identify five percussion notes. You can practice a few of them on yourself. Normal lungs are resonant. The other percussion notes are described in Box 2.5.

Box 2.5 Percussion Note

Type	Detected over
Resonant	Normal lung
Tympanic (drum-like resonance)	Stomach or air-filled hollow viscus, pneumothorax, superficial empty cavity
Hyper-resonant (no resistance during percussion)	Pneumothorax, emphysema, asthma, air-filled large bulla or a thin-walled cavity, eventration of diaphragm
Impaired/dull note (slight resistance felt on percussion)	• Consolidation • Thickened pleura • Collapse • Fibrosis • Solid tumour
Stony dull (mark resistance felt while percussion)	Pleural effusion, empyema

Normal Liver Dullness

Define the normal liver dullness above downwards in midclavicular line and note the intercostal space of dullness.

Remember: The normal liver dullness lies in the right 5th intercostal space in midclavicular line, in the 7th space in anterior axillary line and in the 9th space in scapular line. Abnormalities of liver dullness are:
   i. Liver dullness is pushed up (e.g. 4th intercostal space or above) in midclavicular line in amoebic and pyogenic abscess of the liver, collapse of the lower lobe of the right lung, right hemidiaphragmatic paralysis and eventration of right dome of diaphragm.
   ii. It may be pushed down to 6th space in emphysema and right-sided pneumothorax, pleural effusion and right-sided subphrenic abscess.

Normal Cardiac Dullness

Define cardiac dullness

The normal cardiac dullness is defined in the 3rd and 4th left interspace along the parasternal line and 5th space up to midclavicular line by starting percussion from anterior axillary line (i.e. the lowest cardiac dullness corresponds to the apex beat). While defining the border of the heart, the long axis of the pleximeter finger must be parallel to the expected position of the heart.

Remember
- The cardiac dullness is masked or obliterated in severe obstructive emphysema or left-sided pneumothorax. Area of cardiac dullness may be increased in cardiomegaly and pericardial effusion.
- It may get merged with dullness of left pleural effusion, if fluid is massive.

Normal Traube's area on left side (Fig. 2.13). It is bounded above by lower part of 5th intercostal space (i.e. 6th rib) below by the costal margins on left side and on the left by midaxillary line.

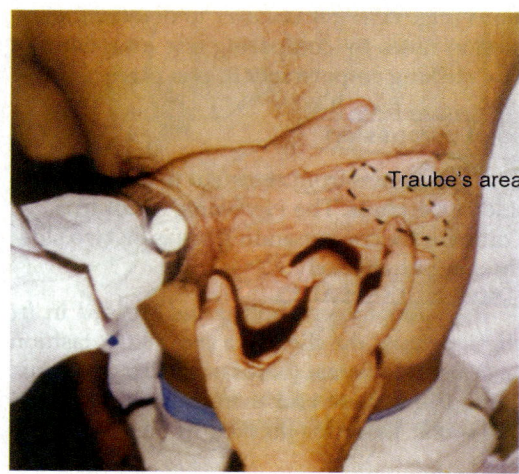

Fig. 2.13: Percussion for the Traube's area.

- *Percuss Traube's area for resonance.*

Percussion note is resonant because normally stomach occupies this area (tympanic note). It becomes dull in left-sided pleural effusion, fluid or solids in the stomach.

Splenic Dullness

- *To define the area of splenic dullness*
  A smaller area of dullness or diminished resonance in the 8th intercostal space in the mid-axillary line left to the Traube's area is attributed to the spleen on that side. In case of splenomegaly, this area as well as Traube's area become dull on percussion.

Identification of descent of diaphragm or diaphragmatic excursion by tidal percussion. First, define the level of diaphragm by percussion on anterior chest in midclavicular level during quiet respiration.

- To *estimate the extent of diaphragmatic excursion*, one has to determine the distance between the level of dullness on full expiration and the level of dullness on full inspiration. Tidal percussion is used for this purpose. This is now-a-days obsolete procedure. The diaphragmatic excursions/movements are better assessed radiologically.

Normal diaphragmatic excursion is 5 to 6 cm. The diaphragmatic excursion is reduced in subpulmonic pleural effusion, atelectasis, diaphragmatic paralysis and liver abscess.

Mediastinal Dullness

The mediastinal percussion normally is confined to the right sternal border and half an inch to left sternal border in 2nd to 4th intercostal space, the dullness extending beyond it indicates mediastinal widening indicating mediastinal tumour/mass. This is elicited by light percussion in lying down position.

Defining the Lower Border of Lung Resonance.

By percussing the bases of lung, normally, during quiet breathing, the lower border of lung resonance corresponds to 6th rib in midclavicular line, 8th rib in midaxillary line and 10th rib in scapular line. It may be slightly lower on left than right side.

- The lower border of the lung resonance is lowered in emphysema and pneumothorax (bases of the lungs are resonant/hyper-resonant), *raised* in lung fibrosis, collapse consolidation, ascites, pleural effusion and abdominal tumour (lung bases are dull).

How to correlate percussion note with anatomy of the lung: When an abnormality on percussion note is due to lung consolidation or collapse, it is usually possible to identify the lobe or lobes involved by reference to the surface marking of the fissures (Fig. 2.14) but unless a lobe is totaly solidified (consolidated), the area over which the percussion note is impaired is often much smaller than would

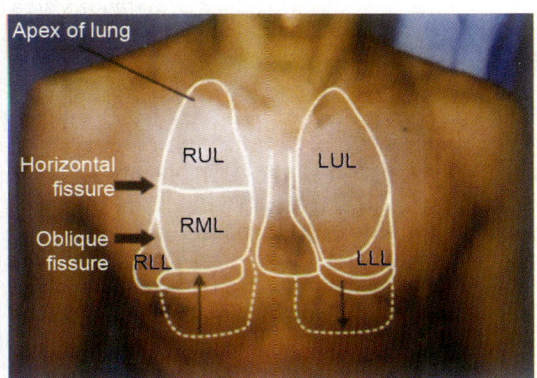

Anterior view (front of chest)

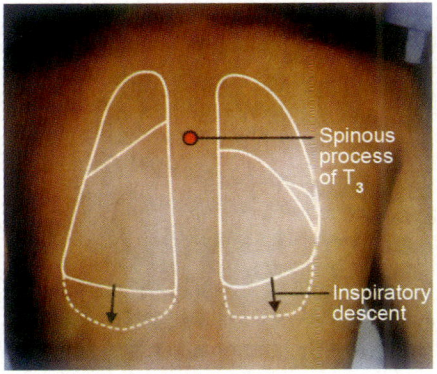

Posterior view (back of chest)

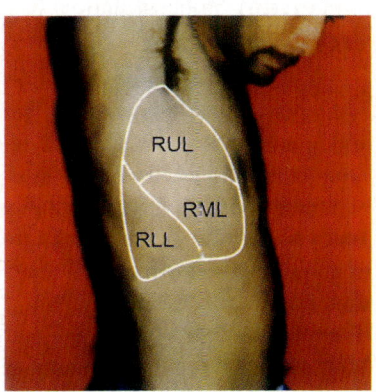

Right lateral

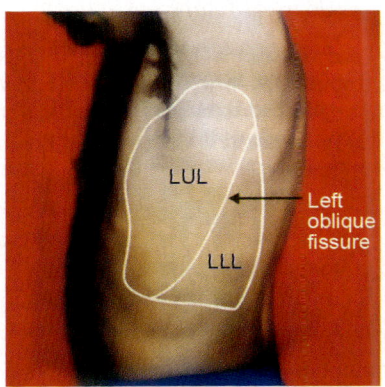

Left lateral

Fig. 2.14: Surface markings of the lungs in different views. Read the division of lungs into lobes by the fissures from the text.

be expected from the surface marking, this is even more striking when a lobe is collapsed.

> Do not rely too much on percussion note alone in localizing the pulmonary or pleural lesion. Percussion combined with auscultation for breath sounds and voice sound are more rewarding.

Remember

> However, small lesions, such as areas of segmental collapse or consolidation and deep-seated lesions may not produce any abnormal physical signs. Even with a larger lesion, the signs may be partly or completely obscured if the lungs are emphysematous. Generalized hyper-resonance on both sides is rarely of diagnostic significance.
> - A small lesion may not cause any change in percussion note.
> - Pleural fluid < 200 ml may not be detected on percussion, needs USG for confirmation.

ABNORMAL PERCUSSION NOTES

Shifting Dullness

The dullness in the pleural effusion does not shift because there is no space for the fluid to shift but there is rising dull (read rising dullness). In case of hydropneumothorax in sitting position, the upper area being occupied by the air is hyper-resonant, while the lower area occupied by free fluid is dull/stony dull. On changing the posture to lying down (supine), this area of dullness shifts along the lower part of the anterior chest as fluid splashes over a wider area by displacing the air. The free air provides the space for fluid to shift. This is called *shifting dullness*. It is a characteristic sign of hydropneumothorax or a large cavity or a cyst containing both air and fluid.

Method: To demonstrate shifting dullness, first define the upper border of dullness on anterior chest by percussing above downwards in upright position. By keeping the pleximeter finger on the dull area, patient is made to lie down; repercuss the same dull area for shift. The dullness shifts down due to shift of fluid. The degree of shift can be defined by now percussing the area further down to find new area of dullness.

Rising Dullness

In moderate pleural effusion, the dullness from the anterior chest rises in the axilla called *rising dullness* comes down to lowest at the spine, thus forming a S-shaped curve called *Ellis curve*. This phenomenon is attributed to *capillary suction*.

Method. To demonstrate rising dullness, define the area of dullness by percussion on the anterior chest wall in supine position. Mark this area. Now percuss the axilla from armpit downwards. Mark the area of dullness. Now percuss the posterior chest wall on the same side above downwards. Mark the area of dullness. Now join all the three areas, this will form a curve called *Ellis curve*, the highest point of which lies in the axilla and lowest point on the posterior chest near the spine.

HORIZONTAL LEVEL OF DULLNESS

To elicit the horizontal fluid level in hydropneumothorax, patient is made to sit comfortably with arms above the head and chest fully exposed.

Percussion is done from above downwards (resonant to dull area) in the front along midclavicular line, lateral chest wall along midaxillary line and back (along scapular line) in the conventional way. During such percussions a point of dullness is reached on the front, lateral chest wall and back where these points are marked with skin pencil. These three points are joined transversely and a horizontal line is drawn encircling the affected chest wall. This is upper border of fluid level.

> *Remember.* The transition between a hyper-resonant note above and a dull note below suggests a upper level of fluid in a case with hydropneumothorax.

Percussion myokymia is noticed during percussion in chronically ill debilitated cachexic patients where a percussion stroke over the front of chest causes a transient twitchings of the muscles (myotatic irritability), more marked on the affected side. This may be seen in an advanced case of pulmonary tuberculosis and malignancy.

Hyper-resonance. A percussion note having pitch in between normal lung resonance and tympany of stomach is taken as *hyper-resonant*. It can normally be elicited over the normal lung tissue when the chest is held in full inspiration. **Pathologically**, it occurs unilaterally in pneumothorax, a large air-containing cavity or air cyst or bullae, or in eventration of the diaphragm and bilaterally in emphysema.

Skodaic resonance. A hyper-resonant note with a boxy quality is elicited just above the level of pleural effusion. This is called *skodaic resonance*.

Kronig's isthmus (apical resonance). A band of lung resonance (*Kronig's isthmus*) 5 to 6 cm in width is present in the lower part of the neck connecting the anterior and posterior aspects of side the chest. It is bounded medially by neck muscles and laterally by shoulder muscles. Its absence on either side indicate apical pulmonary fibrosis while its increased width bilaterally suggest voluminous lungs of emphysema.

Bell tympany: It is high-pitched tympanitic or metallic sound heard over pneumothorax when a silver coin placed flat on the affected side is percussed with a second coin, the metallic sound produced is heard with stethoscope or ear over the opposite chest resembling to the sound of church bell.

Ewart's sign: In a large pericardial effusion, there may be an area of dullness with a patch of bronchial breathing at the angle of left scapula due to compression of the lung called *Ewart's sign*.

Gerhardt's sign: It refers to change in percussion note over an area of chest wall when patient changes recumbent position to sitting or standing position. It is due to lung cavity containing both fluid and air.

Friedreich's sign: When the percussion note over an area of chest wall becomes higher in pitch during forced inspiration than during expiration, it is called *Friedreich's sign*. It is suggestive of a lung cavity, the change of note is due to increased amount of air during inspiration altering the tension of the walls of the cavity.

Cracked-pot resonance is tympanic resonance, can be elicited normally over the chest of an infant during crying and abnormally over a cavity communicating with a bronchus. It is due to sudden expulsion of air from the cavity into the bronchus through the communication.

☞ **Auscultation**

Auscultation of the lungs is done for assessing the airflow through the tracheobronchial tree. It is extremely valuable technique for diagnosing the most of the pulmonary as well as pleural lesions. Auscultation involves:
1. Listening to the sounds generated by breathing called *breath sounds* (whether *vesicular, bronchovesicular* or *bronchial*).
2. *Intensity of breath sound* (increased/diminished). If intensity of breath sound is suspected to be high or bronchial breathing is suspected, then one should listen to the sounds of the patient's spoken or whispered voice (words) so as to decide whether it is *bronchophony, whispering pectoriloquy* or *aegophony*.
3. Listening for any added or adventitious sound such as *crackles (crepitations), rhonchi (wheezes)* and *pleural rub*.

Method of auscultation (Fig. 2.15)
- *Positioning*: The patient should be in the usual lying down or upright position either sitting or

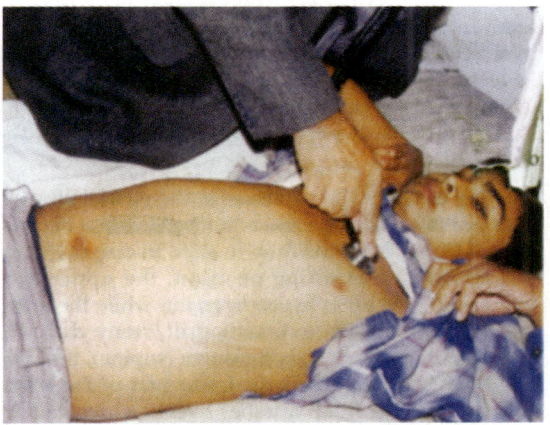

Fig. 2.15: Auscultation of the anterior chest.

standing. Patient should slightly bend forwards during examination of back. In case seriously ill or bed riddened patients, back is examined by tilting the patient first to one side and then to other side. In moribund patient chest piece should be slipped underneath the patient without turning.
- Listen with diaphragm of a stethoscope after explaining the patient to breathe deep as he/she can through an open mouth. You can switch on to hear with the bell of stethoscope if you suspect abnormal sounds being produced by the rubbing of the diaphragm with clothes or hair on the chest itself. Patient should not produce noise by taking deep breaths during examination.
- Pattern of auscultation is similar to percussion, moving from one side to the other and comparing corresponding areas of the lungs (*see* Fig. 2.12).
- If you hear or suspect abnormal sounds, auscultate adjacent areas so as to decide the extent of abnormality.
- Listen to at least one full breath in each location.
- Auscultate in two stages; first to compare the intensity of the breath sounds and then for *vocal resonance*.

Note. Avoid prolonged deep breathing as it may cause giddiness or tetany and also avoid auscultation within 2–3 cm of the midline.

Auscultate anteriorly from above the clavicle down to 6th rib, laterally from the axilla to the 8th rib and posteriorly down to the level of the 11th rib. While listening to the breath sounds:
- Note the quality (rustling, tubular or blowing) and amplitude of inspiration and expiration. Note the intensity of breath sounds.

- Identify if there is a silent gap between inspiration and expiration.
- Is inspiration longer or shorter than expiration? Is expiration prolonged?
- Listen for added (adventitious) sounds.

Always remember
- Intensity (loudness) of breath sounds may decrease when airflow is decreased or when transmission of the sound to the chest is poor. It is increased when bronchus communicates with chest wall, i.e. over a cavity or bronchopleural fistula.
- A gap between inspiration and expiration suggests bronchial breath sounds.
- Normally inspiration is longer than expiration. It becomes equal to expiration in bronchial breathing. Inspiration becomes hollow also.

Auscultation in Special Situations

1. If there is difficulty in distinguishing between *coarse crackles* and *a pleural rub*, repeat auscultation after the patient has been asked to cough forcefully.

Forceful coughing changes the character or intensity of crackles but not of pleural rub.

2. Do not ask the patient with a severe pleuritic pain (consolidation) to take frequent deep breaths or to cough. Test the vocal resonance first, if an area of increased vocal resonance is found, then ask the patient to take one or two deep breaths, and now bronchial breathing will be audible in the same area.
3. When the abnormal breath sounds are heard, define the extent of the area by moving the stethoscope with each breath from the normal to abnormal zone and note the level at which the intensity of breath sounds changes sharply.

BREATH SOUNDS

Breath sounds are produced by passage (rushing) of the turbulent air flow through tracheobronchial tree. The breath sounds have intensity and quality.

Classification and pathogenesis

Breath sounds are classified into three main types, e.g. *vesicular*, *bronchial* and *bronchovesicular*. Normally when person breathes, air enters through the tracheobronchial tree and the breathing remains bronchial in main bronchi, becomes bronchovesicular up to tertiary bronchioles, gets converted into vesicular by alveoli which are heard normally all over the chest. This is called *normal vesicular breathing*.

Normally we have also a normal loud bronchial breathing over trachea. Bronchial breathing occurs when any disease process involves the alveoli (collapse, or consolidation of lung, etc.) because the filtering effect of alveoli is abolished.

The type of breath sound depends on the intensity, pitch and the relative duration of their inspiratory phase and expiratory phase.

Types of Normal Breath Sounds

1. *Vesicular*. It is described above. It is heard all over the chest.
2. *Tracheobronchial*. It is normally heard over the trachea and lower cervical spine on the back. Inspiration is shorter than expiration. There is a pause.
3. *Bronchovesicular (mixed) breathing*. It is heard normally over and around the upper part of sternum and 3rd and 4th dorsal vertebrae. It is intermediate in intesity and inspiration and expiration are equal.

Factors determining transmission of sounds

1. Rate of air flow through the lung under the stethoscope.
   - Lesser the airflow, lesser the intensity heard.
2. Acoustic properties of the lungs and chest wall.
   - Breath sounds become less intense in diseases of alveoli as well thick chest wall.
   - Fluid and air in the pleura are bad conductor of sounds, hence, they are not heard in pleural effusion and pneumothorax.
- The intensity of breath sound may be *normal, reduced or increased* which varies from patient to patient and in different situations (Box 2.6).

Vesicular Breath Sound (Fig. 2.16)

Mechanism of production: It is the sound produced by passage (rushing) of air in and out of the alveoli which filter out or dampen the higher frequency sounds but transmit the lower frequency sounds hence, the breath sounds are quieter and vesicular in type. It is normally heard all over the chest. Its characters are discussed in Fig. 2.16.

Variations. Common variations are:
1. *Diminished vesicular sound*: The causes have already listed in Box 2.6.
2. *Vesicular breath sounds with prolonged expiration* (Fig. 2.16C). This is due to increased airway resistance during expiration either due to spasm or obstruction resulting in prolongation of expiration which becomes equal to inspiration. The **causes** are:

Box 2.6 Intensity of Breath Sounds

Diminished
A. Decreased air entry
- Collapse of a part of lung
- COPD
- Paralysis of respiratory muscles

B. Extensive destruction of the lung, e.g. interstitial fibrosis

C. Poor transmission of breath sounds
- Obesity (thick chest wall)
- Oedematous chest wall
- Thickening of pleura
- Pleural effusion/empyema
- Pneumothorax
- Emphysema

Increased sound
- Thin chest persons
- Consolidation
- A large cavity communicating with bronchus
- Bronchopleural fistula (open pneumothorax)
- At the apex of pleural effusion

Note: When sounds have increased intensity auscultate for bronchophony, whispering, pectoriloquy

Absent breath
- Large pneumothorax (closed)
- Massive pleural effusion
- Collapsed of the lung with obstructed bronchus

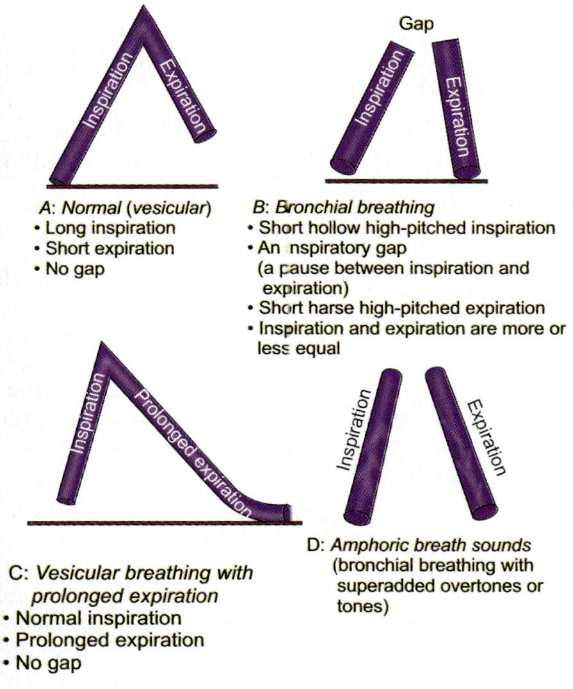

A: Normal (vesicular)
- Long inspiration
- Short expiration
- No gap

B: Bronchial breathing
- Short hollow high-pitched inspiration
- An inspiratory gap (a pause between inspiration and expiration)
- Short harse high-pitched expiration
- Inspiration and expiration are more or less equal

C: Vesicular breathing with prolonged expiration
- Normal inspiration
- Prolonged expiration
- No gap

D: Amphoric breath sounds (bronchial breathing with superadded overtones or tones)

Figs 2.16A to D: Respiratory breath sounds (diagram).

- Bronchial asthma
- Chronic bronchitis and emphysema (COPD)

3. *Harsh vesicular (bronchovesicular).* In this type, intensity of both inspiration and expiration are increased. It is heard in compensatory emphysema.

Abnormal Breath Sounds

Bronchial Breath Sound (Fig. 2.16B)

Mechanism of production. It is the sound produced by passage of the air through larger airways (bronchi and bronchioles). When the lung between these airways and the chest wall becomes airless due to disease the sound from the bronchial tree will be conducted to the chest wall without undergoing the process of filtration by alveoli (i.e. alveolar part of inspiration is cut off resulting in a gap between inspiration and expiration). The causes of bronchial breathing are given in Table 2.8. The characteristics of bronchial sounds are depicted in Fig. 2.16.

> The gap between inspiration and expiration is characteristic of bronchial breathing.

Types of Bronchial Breathing

1. *Tubular (high-pitched, low intensity).* It is a breathing sound produced in large airways resembling the sound produced as you are blowing through a large tube. It is typically heard over pneumonic consolidation. It can also be heard over pulled up trachea on right side in upper lobe fibrosis (*pulled up trachea syndrome*), but will not be heard in axilla. The various causes are given in Table 2.8.

   Transmitted tabular breathing. Sometimes tracheal breath sounds may be transmitted through a mass in the middle or posterior mediastinum over the upper thoracic spine called *D'Espine sign.*

2. *Cavernous (low-pitched, high intensity):* It is produced by a vibrating chamber such as a cavity. The resonance produced is of hollow quality.

3. *Amphoric breathing (high-pitched with overtones):* It is a metallic quality sound resembling sound produced by blowing a narrow-neck wide mouth bottle. There are overtones superimposed on breath sound. The causes include *bronchopleural fistula* and a *large cavity* (Table 2.8).

> *Remember.* The confirmatory sign of bronchial breath sound is increased vocal resonance with whispering pectoriloquy over the area of bronchial breathing.

Causes

The causes of three types of bronchial breathing are tabulated (Table 2.8).

TABLE 2.8: Causes of Bronchial Breath Sounds

High-pitched bronchial sound	Low-pitched bronchial sound
1. *Tubular breathing* • Pneumonic consolidation • Large superficial pulmonary cavity • Collapsed lung lobe surrounded by large bronchi • Above the level of pleural effusion (effusion compresses the lower lung alveoli and brings the patent bronchus of upper lung near the chest) • Malignant lung with patent bronchus • Massive tubercular infiltration • Pulmonary infarct	1. *Cavernous breathing* • Localised areas of pulmonary fibrosis, e.g. chronic pulmonary tuberculosis, chronic suppurative pneumonia (lung abscess), a cavity (empty) and pulled up trachea to one side (pulled trachea syndrome) 2. *Amphoric* (Fig. 2.15D) It is low-pitched bronchial breathing with superadded tones and overtones, or with a metallic tone. The sound resembles the whistling sound produced by blowing air across the mouth of a narrow neck glass bottle. It is produced in; • Bronchopleural fistula (open pneumothorax) • A big thin-walled cavity connected with a narrow patent bronchus

TABLE 2.9: Causes of Increased/decreased/absent Vocal Resonance

Increased	Decreased	Absent
• Consolidation • A cavity communicating with bronchus • Bronchopleural fistula. • At the apex (just above) of pleural effusion posteriorly • Fibrosis of the lung	• Thickened pleura • Emphysema • Interstitial lung disease	• Pleural effusion • Pneumothorax • Collapse of lung due to obstructed bronchus • Empyema

Vocal Resonance

Vocal resonance refers to listening of the vocal sounds (laryngeal vibrations) with the help of stethoscope as the patient repeats some words such as *"ninety-nine, one-one-one"*. Normally, the ear perceives no distinct syllables but a resonant sound, the intensity of which depends on the loudness and depth of the patient's voice and the conductivity of the lungs.

Palpation for vocal fremitus is closely allied to listening for vocal resonance. High-pitched sounds which are not easily palpable can be heard as vocal resonance. The vocal resonance like vocal fremitus has to be compared on each side of the chest. Each point examined on one side must be compared with corresponding point on the other side. Normal vocal resonance gives the impression of sound being produced near the chest piece of stethoscope. If it seems to be produced near the ear than the stethoscope, the resonance is said to be increased. If the intensity of the sound is diminished then it is designated as *decreased vocal resonance*. The causes of increased or decreased vocal resonance are tabulated (Table 2.9). Remember, the causes are more or less same as discussed in tactile vocal fremitus.

Once the vocal resonance is found to be increased hyper-resonance, proceed further to decide whether it is;

1. **Bronchophony.** It is said to be present when spoken sounds are clearly audible but the words are indistinguishable. It conveys the impression that the sound is being produced near the ear piece of stethoscope rather than chest piece. This is heard in consolidation.
2. **Whispering pectoriloquy.** It is much increased vocal resonance where the whispered sound or words are not only clearly and loudly audible but are clearly distinguishable. It conveys the impression that words are being uttered directly into the examiner's ear.
   It is heard in:
   • A cavity communicating with bronchus.
   • A large consolidation where both bronchophony and whispering pectoriloquy are present.
3. **Aegophony.** When the nasal or bleating character is imparted to the spoken sound, it is called *aegophony*.
   It is heart in;
   • Open pneumothorax
   • At the apex of pleural effusion on posterior chest.

ADVENTITIOUS/ADDED SOUNDS

The sounds which are either superimposed or added to the usual breath sounds are called *added or adventitious or extrasounds*. They may arise in the pleura or in the lung.

Extraneous sounds: These are sounds not produced in the lungs and pleura but are produced by external structures and resemble added sounds from which they are to be differentiated. They are:
1. *Sound resembling crackles* may be produced by movement of the stethoscope on hairy skin of the patient. The shaving of chest or wetting of the hair may eliminate these sounds.

Examination of Respiratory System

TABLE 2.10: Differential Diagnosis of Adventitious Sounds (Figs 2.17A to E)

Fig. 2.17	Phase of respiration	Character	Causes
A. Crackles 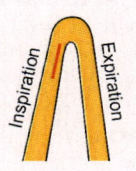	**Fine inspiratory crackles.** They begin in mid-inspiration and continue into late inspiration. They arise from opening up of smaller airways	Profuse, fine and persist from breath to breath. They are heard at the bases of lungs, hence, depend on the gravitational forces of the lungs. They vary with position change over last few hours	They are heard in pneumonia, early congestive heart failure (pulmonary oedema) and interstitial lung disease or lung fibrosis
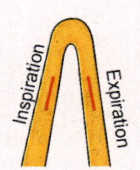	**Early inspiratory crackles.** They are heard in early part of inspiration. Crackles come from large airways	Scanty, coarse in nature	They occur in chronic bronchitis and asthma
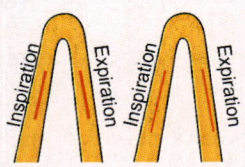	**Coarse inspiratory and expiratory crackles.** They are heard during middle of inspiration and throughout expiration. They arise from secretions within large airways	Coarse clicking, bubbling sounds. They are altered by coughing	Heard in bronchiectasis, a cavity and in lung abscess
B. Wheezes and rhonchi 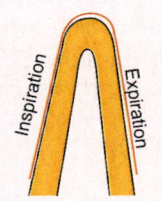	**Wheezes** are high-pitched sounds having hissing or shrilling quality. **Rhonchi** are low-pitched sounds with snoring quality. They are heard either in expiration or in both phases of respiration	Musical sounds produced by air buzzing past the airways. Rhonchi suggest secretions in large airway obstructions	**Causes** include bronchial asthma, bronchitis, COPD, cardiac asthma (LVF), localized obstruction due to malignancy, carcinoid syndrome, anaphylaxis respiratory allergies, inhalation of gases and fumes
C. Pleural rub 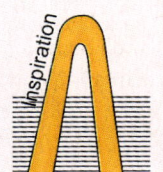	**Pleural rub.** It is heard in both phases of respiration, does not change its character with coughing. It is accentuated by pressure over the chest by stethoscope. Frequently associated with pain and tenderness of chest	• Rubbing or scratching superficial continuous sound • Disappears on holding the breath. Sometimes, it may get transiently eliminated by forced breathing but reappears again during normal or shallow breathing	It occurs in pleuritis due to any cause such as pleurodynia, pulmonary consolidation, pulmonary infarction and following pleural biopsy
D. Mediastinal crunch 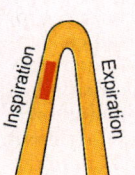	**Mediastinal crunch** has no relation to respiration but is synchronous to heartbeat. Best heard in the left lateral position	Precordial crackling or crunching sound produced by compressing the sternum	It occurs in mediastinal emphysema (pneumomediastinum)
E. Stridor	**Stridor** is a loud inspiratory wheeze or sound produced by closure of glottis	Loud Wheezing sound	It occurs in partial obstruction of trachea (tracheal stridor) or larynx (laryngeal stridor)

2. *Sounds resembling pleural rub* may be produced by movements of the stethoscope on the patient's skin.
   This sound is eliminated by firmly pressing the stethoscope on the chest.
3. *Sounds of muscular contractions* in a shivering patient may produce noisy sound. Change in the position may eliminate the noise.

Types of Adventitious/Added Sounds
I. **Lung sounds**
   1. *Discontinuous*. These are intermittent, non-musical and brief sounds called *crackles or rales*.
   2. *Continuous sounds*: These are musical sounds that persist in most of the respiratory cycle or throughout the cycle (both inspiration and expiration). These include *wheezes* (high-pitched sound) or *rhonchi* (low-pitched) sounds.
II. **Pleural sound**
   - *Pleural rub*. It may be continuous or discontinuous.
III. **Other sounds**

A. Crackles or Rales or Crepitations (Table 2.10 and Fig. 2.17)
These are short, explosive sounds often described as bubbling or clicking noises. They may be heard during inspiration (*fine crackles*) or both during inspiration and expiration (*coarse crackles*).

Pathogenesis
1. *Fine crackles/crepitations*. These are crackling sounds, mimic the artificial sound produced by rolling a few hairs near the ear between thumb and forefinger. They result from tiny explosions when small airways deflated during expiration open during inspiration, thus indicate either exudation or inflammation.
   Causes of fine crackles
   - First stage of pneumonia (lung congestion)
   - Early exudative pulmonary tuberculosis
   - Atelectasis collapse of lung
   - Pulmonary oedema.
2. *Coarse crackles/crepitations*. They result from air bubbles flowing through the secretions in a tightly closed airways, i.e. cavity or dilated bronchi. They are heard during both inspiration and expirations. They are heard over an area of bronchiectasis or a cavity, lung abscess and frequently heard with rhonchi in a case with bronchitis.
3. *Medium crackles*. They are intermediate in loudness and character between fine and coarse crackles, heard in bronchitis, fibrosis due to involvement of small-sized bronchi or bronchioles.

Special Forms of Crackles
1. *Post-tussive crackles/rales*. The crackles which are not heard during normal respiration, but are heard following coughing are called *post-tussive crackles*. They signify that the cavity is filled with secretions which are dislodged during coughing allowing the air to bubble through the fluids/secretions, producing the crackles/rales.
2. *Leathery or sticky rales/crackles*. These are produced by sticky exudate in large airways. They are characteristically heard in bronchiectasis at one or both bases of lung.
3. *Cavernous/amphoric rales/crackles:* These are medium-pitched sounds with echo-like quality, suggest presence of exudate within cavities communicating with bronchi.

B. Wheezes and Rhonchi
These are continuous musical sounds produced by airflow through large airways. They occur due to narrowing of the airways either by spasm or by secretions or by extraneous compression. The causes of wheezes have been enumerated in Table 2.10.

The differences between pleural rub and coarse crackles are tabulated in Table 2.11.

TABLE 2.11: Differences between Pleural Rub and Coarse Crackles

Pleural rub	Coarse crackles
Superficial and loud	Deep, not so loud
Rubbing or scratching continuous sound	Bubbling or clicking interrupted sound
Audible during both phases of respiration	May be inspiratory or inspiratory and expiratory
Usually heard over a smaller area of chest wall	Audible over a wider area or heard diffusely over the chest
Not altered by coughing	May change its character or intensity on coughing
Accentuated by pressing the chest piece of stethoscope firmly over the chest wall	No accentuation
Associated with pain and tenderness	Usually not associated
Caused by rubbing of roughened pleural surfaces	Caused by tiny explosions produced by sudden opening up of smaller airways deflated during expiration or due to air bubbles flowing through secretions

Types of Wheeze

1. *Monophonic:* This a single musical sound arising from of a single bronchus narrowed by a tumour, or extrathoracic obstruction or a foreign body or bronchial stenosis. It may be inspiratory, expiratory or both and does not change its intensity with position.
   Random monophonic wheezes of single note of varying duration, pitch, timing may be scattered all over the chest in patients with asthma and anaphylaxis.
2. *Polyphonic:* These are usually expiratory musical sounds containing several notes of different pitches, can be heard at a distance. Because of expiratory narrowing of airways (asthma, COPD), there can be a large number of wheezes in expiration than inspiration. Multiple polyphonic wheezes are heard in bronchial asthma and chronic bronchitis. These wheezes arise due to dynamic narrowing of the several bronchi by congestion of mucus lining, contraction of smooth muscle and mucus plugging, which get accentuated during expiration.

> Occasionally, in severe asthma and COPD, the patient is no longer able to force enough air through the narrowed bronchi to produce wheezing. The absence of wheezing leads to silent chest. This should not be mistaken for improvement, actually is a bad prognostic sign.

Pleural rub: A continuous rubbing or grating or scratching sound produced by rubbing of roughened surfaces of both parietal and visceral pleura is called *pleural friction/rub.* The common site of pleural rub is axillary region where friction between two pleural surfaces is maximum, but can be heard anywhere over the chest. It differs from crackles (Table 2.11) and pleuropericardial rub (Table 2.12).

Stridor (Fig. 2.10E): It is a loud monophonic wheeze associated with laryngeal spasm or tracheal stenosis (read it as a respiratory symptom). The noise is often inspiratory and expiratory.

TABLE 2.12: Difference between a Pleural Rub and Pleuropericardial Rub

Pleural rub	Pleuropericardial rub
• Associated with phases of respiration	• Associated with beating of the heart
• It may be localised or diffuse	• It is localised to precardial region
• Occurs at slower frequency	• Higher rate of frequency, occurs with each beat
• Disappears with holding of breath	• Does not disappear

Other Miscellaneous Sounds

There are certain sounds heard following some manoeuvres:

1. **Succussion splash:** It is a splashing sound produced by movement of fluid in a cavity or hollow viscus containing both fluid and air so as to allow the movement of fluid. The sound sometimes may be loud enough to be appreciated by the patient.

   Method (Fig. 2.18): Define the upper border of dullness in lateral chest wall along the mid-axillary line in sitting position. Now place the diaphragm of stethoscope at this point and shake the patient vigorously from side to side (⇄). A splashing sound is audible with every jerk (Fig. 2.18). Sometimes, splashing sound can be heard without stethoscope. The **causes** are:
   i. Hydropneumothorax/pyopneumothorax
   ii. A large cavity containing thin fluid and air
   iii. Eventration of diaphragm with herniation of stomach into the thorax on left side

2. **Post-tussive suction.** When signs of a lung cavity are present, then patient is asked to cough violently. A sucking inspiratory sound heard over the chest following coughing is called *post-tussive suction.* It is heard over a cavity which is thin-walled and compressible. It carries no significance.

3. **Coin test** (Fig. 2.19): In hydropneumothorax, at the junction of air and fluid, the metallic quality of the sound produced by striking one coin over another placed on the chest can be heard appreciably at the diametrically opposite side of the chest wall.

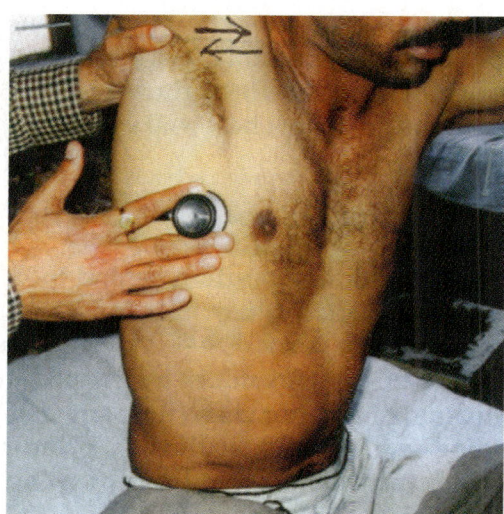

Fig. 2.18: Elicitation of succussion splash.

4. **Pneumothorax click/mediastinal crunch:** It is a clicking or crunching sound produced by pneumomediastinum (air in mediastinum) with each heartbeat, heard along the left sternal border. It is due to sudden movement of the air by systolic contractions of the heart.
5. **Forced expiratory time (FET):** It is a parameter of severity of airway obstruction. The patient is asked to expire forcibly with mouth open after a full inspiration. The examiner note the time of expiration by listening over the chest with stethoscope. Normal FET, is less than 4 seconds, more than 6 seconds indicates airway obstruction.

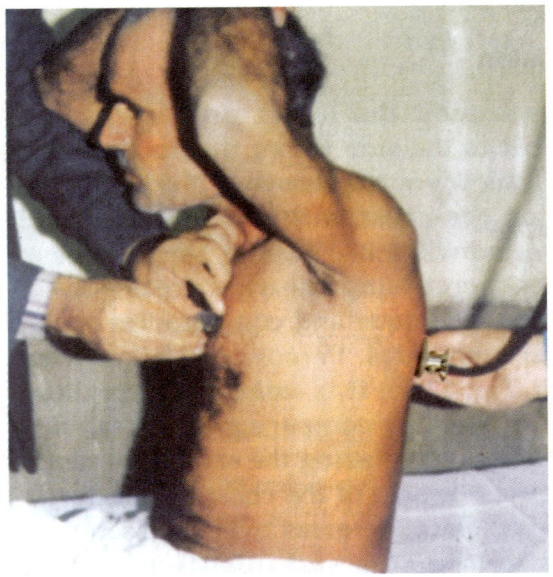

Fig. 2.19: Coin test. Place the coin on the anterior chest and strike the coin with another coin. Place the stethoscope on posterior chest diametrically opposite to the coin to hear the metallic sound.

6. **D'Espine sign:** Whispered sounds heard below the T3 vertebra in a patient with mediastinal mass is called *D'Espine sign*.

EXAMINATION OF THE POSTERIOR CHEST

It has to be carried out in similar fashion as examination of anterior chest. Therefore, the specific findings pertaining to the posterior chest wall will be highlighted here only.

☞ Inspection

Stand behind the patient and inspect from the midline position.

- *Observe the shape of the chest for asymmetry or deformities.*
  In addition to the deformities mentioned under the examination of anterior chest, note any deformity of the spine (e.g. *gibbus, scoliosis*), prominence of scapulae (*scoliosis, winging of scapulae in myopathy*).
- *Observe skin and subcutaneous tissue for swelling or nodules, purpuric spots and bruises.*
- *Observe the type of breathing.* Note abnormal retraction of the intercostal spaces during inspiration.
- *Observe the respiratory movements and expansion of the chest.* Note any abnormality on one side or both sides of the chest.

☞ Palpation

As you palpate the chest, focus on areas of tenderness and abnormalities in the overlying skin, respiratory movements and chest expansion. Compare the tactile vocal fremitus on both sides and note any abnormality either on one side or on both the sides.

Note any widening or narrowing of the intercostal spaces on either side of the chest.

☞ Percussion

For percussing the lower posterior chest, stand somewhat to the side rather than behind the patient. This will allow you to place your pleximeter finger more firmly on the chest and your plexor will be more effective and will make a better percussion note.

When percussing the two areas, use the same percussion technique and compare the corresponding areas on both sides. Percuss or strike twice in each location (Fig. 2.20) It is easier to detect differences in percussion note by comparing one area with another rather than by percussing the same area repeatedly.

Percuss one side of the chest and then the other at same level. Omit the areas over the scapulae. Identify and locate the area and quality of any abnormal percussion note.

The sites for percussion are represented in Fig. 2.20.

☞ Auscultation

The areas to be auscultated are same as used for percussion (Fig. 2.20B).

Points to be noted are same as discussed in auscultation of anterior chest, i.e. breath sounds, vocal resonance and added sounds.

Examination of Respiratory System

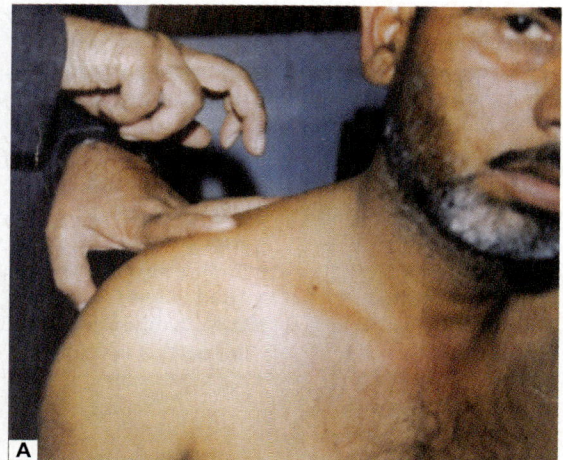

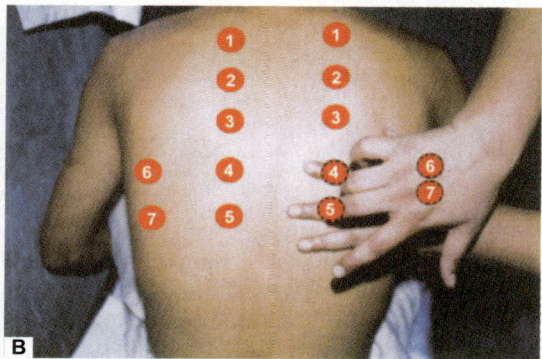

Figs 2.20A and B: Percussion. (A) Method and point of start of percussion and auscultation on the back; (B) Final stages of percussion and areas to be percussed and auscultated are labelled.

DIFFERENTIAL DIAGNOSIS

I. DIFFERENTIAL DIAGNOSIS OF VARIOUS LUNG LESIONS

The differential diagnosis among various pulmonary conditions based on physical signs is presented in Table 2.13.

II. DIFFERENTIAL DIAGNOSIS OF ACUTE DYSPNOEA

Acute onset dysponea may be pulmonary or cardiac origin.

i. First establish clinically whether it is of pulmonary or cardiac origin (Table 2.14).
ii. Then try to establish the cause of dyspnoea (Table 2.15).

BRIEF SYNOPSIS OF COMMON RESPIRATORY DISEASES

PNEUMONIC CONSOLIDATION

Definition: It is defined as solidification of the lung due to inflammation of the lung parenchyma distal to terminal bronchioles. It is produced by inhalation of microbes from the air (e.g. tubercular pneumonia), or aspiration of organisms from nasopharynx (pneumococcal pneumonia), or haematogenous spread from a distant site of inflection (e.g. *Staphylococcus pneumoniae*) and direct spread from contiguous site of infection or following penetrating injuries.

The *infective agents* are:
- Bacterial, e.g. streptococcal, *H. influenzae*, pneumococcal, staphylococcal, Mycoplasma gram-negative, Bacteroides, Legionella.
- Viral [respiratory viruses, influenza ($H_1 N_1$)]
- Fungal (Aspergillus)

Predisposing Factors

1. Old age: Alcoholism, smoking
2. COPD, bronchiectasis, chronic venous congestion of lungs (congestive heart failure)
3. Endotracheal intubation or tracheostomy
4. Immunosuppression (diabetes, cancer, steroid HIV infection), neutropaenia
5. I.V. drug abuse (*Staph. pneumoniae*)
6. Thoracic cage abnormalities (kyphoscoliosis)
7. Altered consciousness, e.g. epilepsy, head injury, anaesthesia
8. Surgery on upper respiratory tract.

Classification

i. *Primary*: The lung is healthy
ii. *Secondary*: The lung is diseased or immunocompromised.

Depending on the anatomical site, it may be
- Segmental, lobar and bronchopneumonia.

Clinical Features

1. Sudden onset of fever, cough, haemoptysis and pain chest (pleuritic)
2. Shaking chills and rigors
3. Tachypnoea, tachycardia, diaphoresis.

Signs (read Table 2.13)

Diagnosis is confirmed by X-ray chest.

BRONCHIECTASIS

It is defined as an abnormal and irreversible dilatation of bronchi, manifesting clinically as pulmonary

TABLE 2.13: Differential Physical Signs Clue to the Diagnosis of Respiratory Disorders

Sign	Lobar consolidation	Lobar collapse	Fibrosis/bronchiectasis	Cavity or lung abscess	Pleural effusion	Pneumothorax (closed)	Acute or chronic bronchitis	Bronchial asthma	Emphysema
1. Shape of the chest	N	Retraction on the side involved	Retraction on the side involved	N or slight retraction to the side involved	N	N	N	N	Hyper-inflated shaped
2. Chest wall movement	Reduced on the side involved	Reduced on the side involved	Reduced on the side involved	Slightly reduced on the side involved	Reduced or absent on the side involved	Reduced or absent on the side involved	N	Bilateral diminished	Bilateral diminished
3. Expansion of chest	Reduced on the side involved	Reduced on the side involved	Reduced on the side involved	Reduced or absent on the side involved	Reduced or absent on the side involved	Reduced or absent on the side involved	N	B/L reduced	B/L reduced
4. Activity of extra respiratory	A	A	A	A	A	A	P	P	P
5. Position of trachea and mediastinum	N	Shifted to the side involved	Shifted to the side involved	Shifted to the side involved	Shifted to opposite side	Shifted to opposite side	N	N	N
6. AP and transverse diameter	N	N	N	N	N	N	N or abnormal	N	Abnormal AP > T
7. Vocal fremitus	Increased on the side involved	Reduced or absent on the side involved	Increased over the area involved	Increased over the area involved	Reduced or absent on the side involved	Reduced or absent on the side involved	N	N	N or reduced on both side
8. Percussion note	Dull on the side involved	Dull on the side involved	Impaired over the area involved	Impaired over the area involved	Stony dull on the side involved, rising dullness, may be present	N or hyper-resonant	N	N or hyper-resonant	Hyper-resonant
9. Breath sounds	High-pitched bronchial over the area involved	Diminished or absent over the area involved	Low-pitched bronchial over the area involved	Amphoric bronchial over the area involved	Absent or diminished over the area involved	Absent or diminished on the side involved	B/L vesicular with prolonged expiration	B/L vesicular with prolonged expiration	B/L vesicular with prolonged expiration
10. Intensity of breath sounds (vocal resonance)	Increased over the area involved and *bronchophony* and *whispering pectoriloquy* present	Decreased over the area involved	Increased over the area involved	Increased over the area involved, *whispering pectoriloquy* present	Decreased over the area involved	Decreased on the side involved	N	N	N or diminished
11. Added sounds	Fine crackles early, coarse crackles appear later on the area involved	None	Coarse crackles on the area involved	Coarse crackles on the area involved	Pleural rub in some cases over the area involved	None	Rhonchi with some coarse crackles on both the sides	Rhonchi/wheezes mainly expiratory and high-pitched	Expiratory rhonchi/wheezes

Abbreviations: N = normal; B/L = bilateral; P = present; A = absent; AP = antero-posterior; T = Transverse.

suppuration (cough with massive sputum). It may be *congenital* (cystic) or *acquired* (tubular, cylindrical). The common **causes** are:
 i. *Infections*: Bacterial, viral and fungal infections.
 ii. *Obstructive bronchiectasis*. It is localised bronchiectasi distal to obstruction by a tumour, foreign body, COPD and bronchostenosis.
 iii. *Non-infective causes*
   - Allergic bronchopulmonary aspergillosis
   - α_1-antitrypsin deficiency
   - Cystic fibrosis
   - Kartagener syndrome
   - Young syndrome (azoospermia, sinusitis)

Symptoms
- Chronic cough with massive sputum, haemoptysis
- Postural and diurnal variation of cough and sputum.
- Dyspnoea
- *Systemic features*, i.e. fever, weight, loss, anaemia, weakness
- Recurrent pulmonary infections with recurrent pleuritic pain
- Oedema feet due to hypoproteinaemia, amyloidosis of kidney or cor pulmonale.
- *Complications* include meningtis, brain abscess, septicaemia.

Signs (read Table 2.13)

Diagnosis is confirmed by radiology and bronchoscopy.

LUNG ABSCESS

It is defined as collection of purulent material (pus) in a necrotic localised area of lung parenchyma, commonly in right lower lung.

Causes
Necrotising infections, i.e. bacterial, anaerobic, tubercular, fungal, etc., *embolic infarction* with cavity formation, *malignancy lung*, Wegener's granulomatosis, coal miner's pneumoconiosis are its common causes.

TABLE 2.14: Differentiation Between Cardiac and Pulmonary Dyspnoea

	Cardiac dyspnoea	*Pulmonary dyspnoea*
History	1. Clinical evidence of heart disease	1. Clinical evidence of respiratory disease
Symptoms	1. Acute onset	1. Gradual onset except when there is an acute exacerbation of COPD or acute asthma
	2. Associated symptoms such as chest pain, orthopnoea, palpitation, diaphoresis (sweating) etc.	2. Associated symptoms of cough, wheeze, haemoptysis, stridor
	3. A previous history of left ventricular failure	3. Previous history of repeated attacks of asthma or chronic bronchitis
	4. Paroxysmal attacks of dyspnoea (PND) are common, relieved by sitting or recumbent position	4. PND is less common, is relieved by cough and expectoration
	5. Wheezing less frequent	5. Wheezing is marked and even audible
	6. Dyspnoea is marked with less unproductive cough	6. Dyspnoea is less marked with troublesome productive cough
Signs	1. Tachycardia, tachypnoea, cyanosis (both central and peripheral)	1. Tachypnoea, tachycardia and central cyanosis are less marked
	2. Percussion note may be dull at bases	2. Hyper-resonant or dull or impaired note may be present
	3. Trachea central and normal in length	3. Trachea central or shifted
	4. Normal chest	4. Abnormal chest
	5. Crepitations at the bases with a few rhonchi	5. Diffuse rhonchi and crepitations
	6. Apex beat is normal or displaced	6. Apex beat may not be visible or normal or displaced
	7. Breath sounds normal (vesicular)	7. Vesicular breath sounds with prolonged expiration
	8. 3rd heart sound may be present (gallop rhythm)	8. No 3rd heart sound
	9. Murmurs may be present	9. No murmur, rub may be present

TABLE 2.15: Differential Diagnosis of Acute Severe Dyspnoea

Condition	History	Signs
1. Left ventricular failure (pulmonary oedema)	Previous cardiac disease or chest pain, orthopnoea, PND and palpitation. There is pink frothy sputum	• Central cyanosis, cardiomegaly, 3rd heart sound • JVP—normal or raised • Sweating, tachycardia, gallop rhythm • Cold extremities • End-inspiratory crackles at bases
2. Massive pulmonary embolism	• Recent surgery or other risk factors • Chest pain • Haemoptysis • Deep vein thrombosis	• Central cyanosis • ↑ JVP, loud P_2 • Signs of shock • Unilateral oedema • Calf tenderness • Pleural rub may be heard
3. Acute bronchial asthma	• History of previous episode • History of asthma medication • Wheeze • Allergy/hypersensitivity to dust/pollens/smoke	• Tachycardia • Pulsus paradoxus • Cyanosis (late) • JVP normal • Diffuse rhonchi (rales), sonorous • Forced expiratory time (> 6 sec)
4. Acute exacerbation of COPD	• Long duration of history of cough (> 2 years) • Repeated hospital admissions • History of smoking • Mucoid or mucopurulent sputum	• Cyanosis • Signs of COPD (barrel-shaped chest, intercostal indrawing, pursed lips breathing) • Signs of CO_2 retention (warm extremities, bounding pulse, flapping tremors) • Bilateral crackles and rales
Pneumonia	• Fever, cough, chest pain and haemoptysis	• Raised temperature • Signs of consolidation • Pleural rub may be present • Cyanosis, if widespread disease
Psychogenic (anxiety)	• Previous episodes • Acute anxious events precipitate it	• No cyanosis • No signs of heart or lung disease • Hyperventilation • Anxious looks • Carpopedal spasms

Symptoms
- Fever, cough with massive purulent or mucopurulent sputum.
- Postural and diurnal variation of cough and sputum.
- Haemoptysis and halitosis (foetid breath)
- Pain chest (pleuritic)

Signs (read Table 2.13)

Complications: They are empyema, meningitis, brain abscess, secondary amyloidosis, malnutrition/hypoproteinaemia, involvement of other parts of lung/other lung and recurrent haemoptysis.

Diagnosis is confirmed by X-ray and sputum for culture and sensitivity.

BRONCHIAL ASTHMA

It is defined as allergo-inflammatory disorder of lung parenchyma produced by hypersensitive response to various allergens resulting in reversible narrowing of air passages.

Acute severe asthma: It is a continuous state of asthma where patient is not symptom-free in between attacks of asthma.

It is caused by allergens (atopic) and nonallergens (nonatopic). The common precipitating allergens are:
- Air-borne pollutants (smoke, NO_2, SO_2, ozone)
- Grass or flower pollen
- Animal danders and feathers
- House dust
- Mite present in carpets, sofa furnishings
- Insect webs, cockroach, antigens
- Fungal spores

Nonatopic asthma occurs in adults and differs from atopic (childhood) asthma (Table 2.16).

Symptoms
- Attacks of cough and wheezing, dyspnoea and tightness of chest.

TABLE 2.16: Important Points of Differentiation between Two Clinical Types of Asthma

Atopic (extrinsic or childhood)	Nonatopic (intrinsic adulthood)
• Episodic, sudden onset	• Nonepisodic, chronic or continuous asthma
• Early onset or childhood asthma	• Late onset or adult asthma
• More wheeze, less cough	• More productive cough, less wheeze
• Mostly seasonal	• Mostly non-seasonal
• Attacks may be precipitated at any time of the day or night or exercise	• Mostly attacks occur at night (nocturnal asthma). It is not exercise induced
• Positive family history for an allergic disorder	• No family history
• Skin tests for hypersensitivity are positive	• Skin tests are negative
• Sodium cromoglycate is most effective	• Not effective

- The duration of attack varies from hours to days and even to weeks.
- Morning dipping of symptoms is common.
- May be seasonal or nonseasonal.
- Attacks are precipitated by allergen or triggered by nonallergens, e.g. smoke, tobacco, cold, viral infections, drugs, anxiety and exercise (exercise induced asthma).
- Acute exacerbations of symptoms by infection and allergen are common.

Tetrad of symptoms, i.e. chest tightness, wheeze, cough and exertional dyspnoea are diagnostic clues.

Physical signs (read Tables 2.13 and 2.15)

CHRONIC OBSTRUCTIVE PULMONARY DISEASE (COPD)

Chronic obstructive pulmonary disease (COPD) is characterised by irreversible obstruction to the airflow throughout the lungs. It includes chronic bronchitis and emphysema.

Chronic bronchitis is defined as cough with expectoration on most days at least three consecutive months in a year for more than two consecutive years. Therefore, it is duration of cough which makes the diagnosis likely.

Emphysema is defined as irreversible dilatation of alveoli or bullae formation due to rupture of alveoli, leading of hyperinflated lungs.

Smoke, atmospheric and industrial pollutants, infections (e.g. upper respiratory infections), physical factors (e.g. dampness, exposure to fog) and genetic and familial (i.e. α_1-antitrypsin deficiency lead to emphysema) factors are its aetiological factors.

Symptoms

- A long history of more than 2 years justifies the definition of chronic bronchitis
- Cough and expectoration
- Dyspnoea on exertion
- Wheezing
- Haemoptysis
- Chest tightness, chest discomfort

Physical Signs

Signs of chronic bronchitis	Signs of emphysema
1. Cyanosis	1. Excavation of suprasternal notch
2. Presence of wheezes/rhonchi	2. Barrel-shaped chest
3. Crackles (coarse)	3. Purse-lip breathing
4. Vesicular breathing with prolonged expiration	4. Decreased chest movements and expansion
	5. Hyper-resonant note
	6. Cardiac dullness obliterated
	7. Liver dullness is pushed down
	8. Decreased breath sounds

Gold Criteria for COPD Severity (Box 2.7)

Box 2.7 Gold Criteria for COPD Severity

Gold stage	Symptoms	Severity	Spirometry
0	+	At risk	Normal
I	+	Mild	• $FEV_1/FVC < 0.7$ • $FEV_1 \geq 80\%$ predicted
II	+	Moderate	• $FEV_1/FVC < 0.7$ • FEV_1 50 to 79% predicted
III	+	Severe	• $FEV_1/FVC < 0.7$ • FEV_1 30 to 49% predicted
IV	+	Very severe	• $FEV_1/FVC < 0.7$ • $FEV_1 < 30\%$ predicted or $FEV < 50\%$ predicted with respiratory failure or Signs of right heart failure

How to decide the dominance between chronic bronchitis and emphysema (Table 2.17)?

TABLE 2.17: Salient Clinical Features of Two Components of Chronic Obstructive Pulmonary Disease (COPD)

Feature	Predominant emphysema (pink puffers)	Predominant bronchitis (blue bloaters)
1. Age (in years) at diagnosis	Late elderly (60+)	Early elderly (50+)
2. Dyspnoea	Severe	Mild
3. Cough	Follows dyspnoea	Precedes dyspnoea
4. Sputum	Minimal, mucoid	Copious, purulent
5. Infection	Less frequent	More frequent
6. Cyanosis	Absent or present terminally	Present and common
7. Cor pulmonale	Rare, hence called pink puffers	Common, hence called blue bloaters
8. Secondary polycythaemia	Uncommon	Common

Diagnosis is confirmed by radiology and arterial blood gas analysis.

TUBERCULAR CAVITY

Tuberculosis is a chronic infective disorder caused by *Mycobacterium tuberculosis*. The primary lesion is *Ghon's focus* along with hilar lymphadenopathy. If the primary lesion does not heal completely, it can lead to post-primary tuberculosis manifesting as a *tubercular cavitary* lesion in the lung.

Symptoms
- Cough with expectoration, haemoptysis
- Dyspnoea
- Tightness/pain chest or chest discomfort
- Weakness/weight loss and fatigue.
- Constitutional symptoms, i.e. fever, lassitude, night sweats.

Signs (read Table 2.13)
- Retraction of the chest with crowding of the ribs on the side or site involved.
- Shift of trachea to same side
- Dull percussion note
- Coarse crackles/crepitations
- Post-tussive suction in a thin-walled compressible cavity
- Cavernous or amphoric bronchial breathing.

Diagnosis is made on clinical symptoms and signs confirmed by sputum examination, sputum culture and radiology.

PULMONARY EMBOLISM

It is defined as an acute hemodynamic disturbance due to occlusion of pulmonary vasculature by an embolus or emboli. The embolus may be a detached thrombus from veins (DVT, CHF) and heart (right-sided endocarditis, AF) or it may be nonthrombotic such as fat embolism (bone trauma/fracture), amniotic fluid embolism (caesarean section), tumour (choriocarcinoma) or air embolus (pulmonary barotrauma).

Predisposing factors include postpartum period, congestive heart failure, 'In-plaster' injuries or fracture of lower limb bones, prolonged immobilisation, oral contraceptives, thrombophlebitis (rare), varicose veins of legs, obesity, hypercoagulable state.

Symptoms
1. *Triad of pulmonary embolism*, i.e. pleuritic chest pain, pleural rub and haemoptysis.
2. Associated wheezing, dyspnoea and cyanosis can occur but is uncommon.
3. Massive pulmonary embolism produces *'acute cor pulmonale'* while repeated multiple embolisation over a long period results in *chronic cor pulmonale*.

Signs
1. *Signs of a pulmonary infarct*
   - Tachycardia, tachypnoea
   - Pleural rub, wheezes (rhonchi)
   - Signs of segmental collapse or atelectasis or pleural effusion
   - Crackles
2. *Signs of acute cor pulmonale*
   - Hypotension or shock
   - Raised JVP
   - Cyanosis
   - Loud P_2 with wide splitting
   - An ejection systolic murmur at P_2 area
   - Signs of RV hypertrophy
3. *Signs of chronic cor pulmonale*
   (It is discussed separately)

Diagnosis suspected clinically is confirmed by pulmonary angiography, diffusion and perfusion scan and D-dimers levels in blood.

CRYPTOGENIC FIBROSING ALVEOLITIS (IDIOPATHIC PULMONARY FIBROSIS)

This is common interstitial lung disease of unknown aetiology with characteristic clinical, radiological and pathological features. An acute progressive form of this disease is known as *Hamman-Rich syndrome*. The disease runs a progressive downhill course with development of respiratory failure, pulmonary hypertension and cor pulmonale.

Symptoms
- Dry cough, progressive dyspnoea and cyanosis.
- Clubbing of the fingers and toes.

Signs
- Cyanosis and clubbing
- Bilateral chest retraction
- Chest expansion is poor
- Numerous bilateral end-inspiratory crackles
- Ultimately pulmonary hypertension develops leading to *chronic cor pulmonale*.

Diagnosis is confirmed by radiology and lung function tests.

PULMONARY COLLAPSE

Atelectasis or collapse is defined as 'airless with shrinkage' of a part or the whole lung. It may be *central collapse* due to obstruction of a major bronchus by bronchial adenoma/carcinoma/lymph node/foreign body/mucus plug, etc. or it may be *peripheral collapse* due to small bronchial obstruction by mucus plugging/emboli/asthma/eosionophils, etc.

Symptoms
- Dry cough, fever, breathlessness
- Dyspnoea, tachypnoea
- Malaise, night sweats, weight loss and evening rise of temperature if tuberculosis is the cause.

Physical Signs
- Orthopnoea, tachypnoea, tachycardia.
- Central cyanosis.
- Shift of trachea to the side involved.
- Flattening/depression of the part of chest involved with crowding of ribs and narrowing of intercostal spaces.
- Diminished movement/expansion of the part of chest involved.
- Vocal fremitus is decreased over the part/side of the chest involved.
- Dull/impaired percussion note.
- Absent breath sounds with no added sounds if major central bronchus is obstructed.

or

Bronchial breathing, increased vocal resonance with bronchophony/whispering pectoriloquy, if peripheral bronchus is obstructed.

BRONCHOGENIC CARCINOMA

It is common malignant tumour of the bronchus. The *causative factors* include:

1. Cigarette smoking (active or passive)
2. Occupational exposure (i.e. asbestos, industrial products, ionising radiation)
3. Genetics (point mutation of *K-ras* gene)

Types
Pathologically, it may be
1. Squamous cell carcinoma
2. Small cell anaplastic (oat cell) carcinoma
3. Adenocarcinoma
4. Large cell carcinoma
5. Mixed/combined type

Symptoms
1. *Symptoms of primary tumour,* i.e. cough, haemoptysis, dyspnoea, wheeze, stridor.
2. *Symptoms of intrathoracic extrapulmonary extension*
   - Pleural pain (pleurisy), pleural effusion
   - Rib pain/erosion
   - Tracheal obstruction (*stridor*) oesophageal compression (*dysphagia*) recurrent laryngeal nerve compression (*hoarseness*), Horner's syndrome (compression of cervical sympathetic), *superior vena caval obstruction* (chemosis, suffusion and puffiness of face), *monoplegia* (Pancoast's tumour—aptical tumour involving brachial plexus), *pericardial effusion* or *cardiac temponade*.
3. *Paraneoplastic syndromes,* i.e.
   - Cushing's syndrome (ACTH production by the tumour)
   - Hyperparathyroidism (PTH secretion)
   - Hypoglycaemia (secretion of insulin-like peptide)
   - Myasthenic-myopathic syndrome (Eaton-Lambert syndrome)
   - Hypertrophic pulmonary osteoarthropathy
   - Polycythaemia (erythropoietin production by the tumour)
   - Acanthosis nigricans

Physical Signs
- General weakness, malignant cachexia
- Supraclavicular lymphadenopathy
- Hypertrophic osteoarthropathy of wrists and ankles (grading IV clubbing).
- Signs are variable depending on the structures involved, i.e.
  ◆ Signs of collapse if major bronchus involved.
  ◆ Signs of pleural effusion if pleura involved
  ◆ Signs of superior vena cava obstruction (chemosis, periorbital oedema, suffusion, raised JVP).

Physical Signs, Symptoms, Diagnosis and Differential Diagnosis

- ◆ Mediastinal compression, Horner's syndrome, recurrent laryngeal nerve palsy, diaphragmatic paralysis.
- ◆ *Pancoast tumour* causing wasting of small muscles of hand, rib erosions (rib tenderness), Horner's syndrome and signs of mass lesion in upper lobe.

Diagnosis and Differential Diagnosis

Diagnosis is confirmed by radiology (chest X-ray, CT scan/MRI), pleural fluid cytology and biopsy (lymph node/lung).

Differential diagnosis. It comes into differential diagnosis of most of the pulmonary conditions due to varied manifestations.

PLEURISY

Inflammation of the pleura is called *pleuritis* or *pleurisy*. It may be dry or with effusion.

Causes of Dry Fibrinous Pleurisy
- Peumonias
- Pulmonary infarct
- Pulmonary tuberculosis
- Bronchiectasis/lung abscess
- SLE and rheumatoid arthritis
- Bronchial carcinoma
- Uraemia
- Viral pleurisy (epidermic myalgia, Bornholm disease)
- Idiopathic

Symptoms
- Cough, fever and chest pain (pleuritic pain). It is common in children and young adults.

Signs
- The affected chest wall muscles are tender.
- Restriction of the movements on the side of the chest involved.
- Pleural rub on auscultation.

PLEURAL EFFUSION

Collection of fluid more than normal (50–150 ml) in the pleural cavity is called *pleural effusion*. Fluid more than 300 ml is detected on USG and more than 500 ml is detected clinically.

Causes

Transudative pleural effusion	Exudative pleural effusion
• Congestive heart failure	• Tuberculosis and empyema thoracis
• Constrictive pericarditis	• Malignancy lung
• Nephrotic syndrome	• Mesothelioma
• Cirrhosis of liver	• Pulmonary infarct
• Hypoproteinemia	• Postmyocardial infarction (Dressler's syndrome)
• Hypothyroidism	• SLE, RA
	• Lymphoma, chylothorax
	• Rupture of amoebic liver abscess into pleura

Clinical Features

Symptoms
- Cough, fever, sputum
- Dyspnoea
- Symptoms of dry pleurisy (fever, pleuritis pain and haemoptysis) may precede pelural effusion.

Signs
Read Table 2.13

Diagnosis and Differential Diagnosis

Diagnosis is confirmed by chest X-ray and pleural fluid aspiration.

Differential diagnosis rests between various conditions leading to pleural effusion, characteristic of pleural fluid (exudate/transudate) and fluid cytology (Tables 2.18 and 2.19).

TABLE 2.18: Characteristics of Pleural Fluid

Constituent	Transudate (> 1.1 g/dl)	Exudate (< 1.1 g/dl)
Proteins	<3.0 g% or < 50% of serum proteins	>3.0 g% or >50% of serum protein
Pleural fluid LDH/ serum LDH ratio	Low	High (more than two-thirds)
pH	> 7.3	< 7.3 (inflammatory)
Glucose	Normal	Low
Cells (WBC)	<1000/mm^3	Usually > 1000/mm^3
Gross appearance	Thin, clear	Thick, contain sediments, straw-coloured and forms cobweb on standing in tuberculosis

EMPYEMA THORACIS

Definition: Collection of pus or pus-like material in the pleural cavity is called *empyema thoracis* (*pyogenic pleural effusion*).

Causes

Traumatic	Nontraumatic
A. Penetrating chest injury	A. Chest diseases
	• Pneumonia
B. Iatrogenic	• Tuberculosis
• Thoracic surgery	• Lung abcess
• Following pleural aspiration	• Bronchiectasis
	• Mediastinitis
• Intercostal tube drainage	B. Osteomyelitis of ribs or vertebrae
	C. Extrathoracic sepsis
	• Rupture of subphrenic or liver abscess

Symptoms

- Fever with chills and rigors
- Symptoms of toxaemia (tachypnoea, tachycardia sweating)
- Pleuritic chest pain, cough and sputum (purulent)
- Dyspnoea

Physical Signs

A. *Signs of empyema thoracis with obstructed bronchus*
- All signs of pleural effusion (read pleural effusion) with signs of toxaemia (fever, tachypnoea, tachycardia, diaphoresis)

B. *Signs of empyema thoracis with patent bronchus (bronchopleural fistula)*
- Signs of hydro/pyopneumothorax (read hydropneumothorax) i.e. shifting dullness with succession splash absent breath sound on the side/site involved.
- Signs of toxaemia as described above.

TABLE 2.19: Differential Diagnosis of Pleural Effusion

Cause	Appearance of fluid	Nature of fluid	Predominant cell type in fluid	Other features
Tuberculous	Serous or straw-coloured. Forms a *cobweb* on standing	Exudate	Lymphocytes	• Positive tuberculin test • Pleural biopsy shows granulomatous lesion • Culture for AFB may be positive
Malignant	Serous or haemorrhagic	Exudate	Serosal cells, lymphocytes and malignant cells	• Positive pleural biopsy (< 50% cases) • Evidence of malignant disease elsewhere
Congestive heart failure	Serous, straw-coloured	Transudate	Few serosal cells	• Evidence of heart failure or cor pulmonale • Response to diuretics
Pulmonary infarction	Serious or blood stained	Exudate	RBCs and eosinophils	• Presence of DVT • Factors predisposing to venous thrombosis • Haemoptysis
Nephrotic syndrome	Serous, straw-coloured, occasionally chylous	Transudate	Mesothelial cells	• Massive oedema, puffiness of face • Massive proteinuria • Ascites common
Cirrhosis of liver	Serous or straw-coloured	Transudate	Endothelial cells	• Past history of hepatitis • Signs of portal hypertension (ascites, splenomegaly oedema, caput medusae, oesophageal varices on radiology and haematemesis)
Hypoproteinaemia	Serous	Transudate	–	• Signs of protein and vitamins deficiency • Evident cause of protein loss, i.e. diarrhoea, malabsorption malnutrition • Pitting pedal oedema • Thin wasted muscles
Empyema thoracis	Purulent (pus-like)	Exudate	Neutrophils, pus cells	• History of fever, toxaemia • History of chest injury/pleural aspiration • History of lung suppuration (lung abscess, bronchiectasis)

Differential Diagnosis of Empyema Thoracis

When empyema thoracis resolves, its healing leads to thickened pleura, hence it has to be differentiated from thickened pleura.

The differentiating features are tabulated in Table 2.20.

TABLE 2.20: Differentiating Features between Thickened Pleura and Empyema Thoracis

Thickened pleura	Empyema thoracis
• No signs of toxaemia	• Signs of toxaemia present
• Chest is retracted on the side involved	• Normal chest
• Trachea is shifted to same side	• No shift, if shifted, it will be to opposite side
• Intercostal spaces narrow	• Normal intercostal spaces
• Impaired percussion note	• Stony dull note
• Breath sounds are diminished	• Breath sounds absent

PNEUMOTHORAX

It is defined as presence of air in the pleural space. It may be *closed*, *open* and *tension* (valvular) pneumothorax.

Symptoms

Closed type	Open type	Tension type
Asymptomatic, mild dyspnoea, chest discomfort on the affected side	• Dyspnoea which increases on deep breathing • Symptoms of infection, i.e. fever, tachycardia, tachypnoea and sweating present	• Marked breathlessness • Orthopnoea • Tachypnoea • Tachycardia • Chest tightness • Shock or collapse

Signs (read Table 2.13)
- In **small pneumothorax**, there may be no physical sign.
- On the side of **moderate or large pneumothorax**, there will be fullness of chest with wide intercostal spaces, shift of trachea and mediastinum to opposite side, diminished movement and expansion and hyper-resonant note. In **closed pneumothorax**, the breath sounds are markedly diminished; in **open pneumothorax** (*bronchopleural fistula*), on the other hand, there is amphoric bronchial breathing with increased vocal fremitus and vocal resonance and presence of whispering pectoriloquy.
- In tension pneumothorax, there will be cyanosis, raised JVP, tachypnoea, tachycardia, prominent hyper-resonant chest with decreased expansion and movement. There is shift of trachea and mediastinum to the opposite side. Breath sounds are absent.

Diagnosis is confirmed on radiology.

BRONCHOPLEURAL FISTULA (OPEN PNEUMOTHORAX/HYDROPNEUMOTHORAX)

A communication between a bronchus with pleural cavity is called *bronchopleural fistula*. Since this communication is open with the atmosphere, it is called *open pneumothorax*, hence is likely to produce either *hydropneumothorax* (collection of air and fluid) or *pyopneumothorax* (collection of purulent fluid with air). **Open pneumothorax is caused** by:
1. Tubercular cavity rupturing into pleural space/cavity.
2. Trauma to chest or barotrauma.
3. Following lung resection.
4. Rupture of bulla/bleb into pleural space.

Causes of Hydropneumothorax
1. Rupture of subpleural tubercular cavity discharging its contents into pleural space.
2. Penetrating chest injuries.
3. Following cardiac surgery.
4. Iatrogenic, i.e. introduction of air during aspiration of fluid.

Causes of Pyopneumothorax
- Necrotising pneumonia leading to empyema thoracis with patent bronchus.
- Lung abscess rupturing into the pleural space.
- Secondary infection of hydropneumothorax.

Symptoms and Signs

The open pneumothorax presents either hydropneumothorax or pyopneumothorax; the difference in clinical features between hydropneumothorax and pyopneumothorax is presence of infection in the later, hence, symptoms of toxaemia will be present. The similarities and dissimilarities between the two are:

Hydropneumothorax	Pyopneumothorax
Symptoms	
History of dyspnoea at rest, cough, chest pain/heaviness of chest, splashing sound during walking and jumping	History of fever, cough, sputum, haemoptysis, dyspnoea, chest pain/heaviness of chest. Sound of fluid movement in the chest during walking

Contd.

Hydropneumothorax Signs	Pyopneumothorax
Fever absent	Fever present
Normal look	Toxic look
Breathless at rest	Breathlessness at rest with marked tachypnoea
No tachycardia	Tachycardia present
Cyanosis may or may not be present	Cyanosis is usually present
No clubbing	Clubbing of fingers present
Trachea shifted to opposite side	Trachea shifted to opposite side
Accessory muscles of respiration not working	Accessory muscles of respiration working
A definite horizontal level between dull note below and hyper-resonant note above	No such clear cut level. Level is ill-defined
Succussion splash present	It may be present, but absent in case the pus is thick
Coin test positive	It may be positive
Tingling (crack pot) sounds on auscultation	No such sound
Amphoric bronchial breathing	Amphoric bronchial breathing may or may not be present if pus is thick

MEDIASTINAL COMPRESSION/MEDIASTINAL MASS/SUPERIOR VENA CAVA SYNDROME

Compression of structures (trachea, oesophagus, bronchus, nerves and blood vessels) in the superior mediastinum is called *superior mediastinal compression syndrome*. It is mostly associated with superior vena cava obstruction, hence, also called superior vena cava syndrome.

Causes
1. Bronchogenic carcinoma.
2. Mediastinal lymphadenopathy (tubercular, lymphoma, malignancy)
3. Retrosternal goitre, thymoma
4. Aortic aneurysm
5. Oesophageal carcinoma

Symptoms
- Cough, dyspnoea, dysphagia, hoarseness of voice
- Swelling of face (chemosis), redness of eye (conjunctival suffusion), visual disturbance
- Swelling of upper extremities

Physical Signs
1. Face oedematous, eyes chemosed, conjunctival redness.
2. Neck veins engorged, JVP raised, neck veins nonpulsatile. Lymph nodes may be enlarged depending on the cause.
3. Hoarseness of voice
4. Prominent central part of the chest with prominent veins over the upper part. Blood flow in the veins is from above downwards.
5. Dullness beyond one or both sides of sternum (widening of mediastinal dullness).
6. There may be signs of collapse of the lung if bronchogenic carcinoma is the cause.
7. Mediastinal crunch in case of mediastinal emphysema.

Unit III

Cardiovascular System

- Symptoms and their Analysis
- History
- Physical Signs on General and Systemic Examination
- Diagnosis and Differential Diagnosis
- Brief Synopsis of Cardiovascular Disorders

SYMPTOMS AND THEIR ANALYSIS

The symptoms are given in Box 3.1.

Box 3.1 Symptoms Of Cardiac Disorders

- Chest (cardiac) pain
- Dyspnoea, orthopnoea and paroxysmal nocturnal dyspnoea (PND)
- Palpitations
- Swelling (oedema) of feet and the body
- Syncope, tiredness and fatigue
- Nocturia
- Anorexia, nausea and vomiting
- Cough, sputum and haemoptysis
- Cyanosis

CHEST (CARDIAC) PAIN

Cardiac chest pain is an unpleasant sensation or discomfort perceived by the patient due to stimulation of sensory nerve endings and pain receptors in the heart. Pain over the anterior chest wall is a common symptom of cardiovascular and non-cardiac diseases.

Non-cardiac chest pain occurs due to involvement of lung and pleura (respiratory diseases) muscles (myalgia), nerves (neuralgia), oesophagus (GI tract disorders) and skin (eruptions).

Sites of Pain

- Central pain over the chest localised to retrosternal or substernal region pointed out by the patient by putting a fist/fingers over the sternum is frequently associated with organic heart disease but can be extracardiac in origin due to involvement of GI tract and superficial structures, e.g. skin, muscles, nerves and bones.
- Precordial pain (pain localized to precordium) occuring during exertion and relieved by rest is due to angina unless proved otherwise.
- Left inframammary pain (peripheral chest pain) occurring at rest is mostly functional in origin called *cardiac neurosis*. Patient can localize the exact site of pain by putting a finger at the site.

Causes of Chest Pain

I. Cardiac causes
- Angina pectoris (stable/unstable)
- Myocardial infarction
- Aortic dissection
- Pericarditis
- Mitral valve prolapse
- Valvular heart disease
- Aortic aneurysm/dissection
- Shoulder–hand syndrome

II. Respiratory causes
- Pleurisy
- Pneumonia
- Massive lung collapse
- Pneumothorax
- Pulmonary embolism
- Lung carcinoma
- Mediastinitis, pneumomediastinum, mediastinal growth and mediastinal emphysema.

III. Gastrointestinal causes
- Oesophagitis
- Gastro-oesophageal reflux disease (GERD)

- Hiatus hernia
- Cardia achalasia
- Diffuse oesophageal spasms, oesophageal obstruction.

IV. Neuromuscular and rheumatological causes
- Intercostal neuralgia (zoster infection)
- Myositis, fibromyalgia, epidemic myalgia
- Costochondritis (Teitz's syndrome), caries/metastases, rib fracture
- Cellulitis, mastitis (breast pain)

V. Referred pain
- Intra-abdominal disease, e.g. peptic ulcer, cholecystitis, liver abscess, pancreatitis
- Premenstrual tension, menopause
- Pain of cervical and upper thoracic disc disease

VI. Psychogenic pain (cardiac neurosis)
- Functional/non-organic pain

Symptom Analysis

Ask about the following

Q. Onset (acute or chronic)
- It is *acute* in angina, myocardial infarction aortic dissection and pericarditis. *Chronic* chest pain is mostly non-cardiac in origin.

Q. What is its exact site?
- Central (retrosternal) or peripheral mammary or inframammary pain on left side occurs in myocardial and pericardial disease.
- Central chest pain (isolated) is common in GI disorders, costochondritis.
- Peripheral chest pain is mainly due to lung and pleural diseases, neuromuscular causes. It can be referred pain or functional pain.

Q. What is its character, e.g. dull, severe, stabbing, tearing, etc.?
- Pressing or constricting pain occurs in angina. Patient puts the fist across the chest to describe it.
- Stabbing pain across the chest between the two shoulder blades occurs in dissecting aneurysm of the aorta.
- Sharp pain, worst on breathing and bending is pleuritic pain.
- Poorly localised dull central pain indicates expanding mediastinal tumour.

Q. Is it radiating to some other sites?
- Pain of angina or of myocardial infarction may radiate to shoulders or arms or into the neck or jaws. Pain radiating to interscapular region indicates aortic dissection.
- Pain referred to left shoulder indicates diaphragmatic pleurisy/liver or subphrenic abscess.

Q. Is there any precipitating or relieving factor(s)?
- Effort or exertion or excitement precipitates anginal pain which is relieved on rest or by use of sublingual nitrate.
- Pain associated with overeating, recumbency relieved by sitting or use of antacid indicates pain of oesophageal spasm/GERD/hiatus hernia.
- Pain occurring on lying to one side which gets relieved on turning to other side is pleural pain (dry pleurisy).
- Pain aggravated by movements and relieved by rest is muscular pain.
- Pain aggravated by coughing, sneezing or deep breathing, straining is due to thoracic cage disease (costochondritis, neuritis).
- Pain occurring on lying down and relieved on bending forward in sitting position is pericardial pain (pericarditis).

Differential Diagnosis of Chest Pain
Read Table 3.1

DYSPNOEA, ORTHOPNOEA AND PAROXYSMAL NOCTURNAL DYSPNOEA

Dyspnoea
It is defined as an uncomfortable subjective awareness of one's own breathing. Dyspnoea is a common symptom of both cardiovascular and respiratory diseases.

Orthopnoea
It is defined as dyspnoea on lying down which gets relieved on sitting or propped up position. It is due to the effect of recumbency which increases venous return and lungs congestion in the presence of LVF. It is a symptoms of LVF. Dyspnoea occurring in upright position relieved by recumbency is called *platypnoea*. It is just reverse of orthopnoea, occurs in right to left intracardiac shunts.

Paroxysmal Nocturnal Dyspnoea (PND)
As the name suggests, it is episodic dyspnoea which occurs at night during sleep and awakens the patient from sleep. To get relief from it, patient has to sit up and recline on a chair or sit up on the bed reclining forward with legs dangling by the side of bed or have to walk to an open window to get fresh air. The attacks of PND indicate left ventricular failure or pulmonary oedema.

TABLE 3.1: Differential Diagnosis of Chest Pain/Discomfort

Disorder	Mechanism	Site	Quality, severity and timing	Aggravating factors	Relieving factors	Associated features
Cardiovascular						
Angina pectoris	Reversible myocardial ischaemia due to atherosclerosis of coronary artery or coronary vasospasm	Retrostrenal or across the anterior chest, radiating to the arms (left), neck, shoulders, lower jaw, or upper abdomen	Pressing, squeezing, tightness or heaviness in chest usually of mild to moderate intensity, perceived as discomfort rather than pain. Duration is short, i.e. 1–3 min (may be up to 10 minutes)	Exertions, cold, heavy meals, psychological stress act as precipitating factors	Rest and nitroglycerine	Nausea, vomiting, sometimes dyspnoea
Myocardial infarction	Irreversible prolonged myocardial ischaemia resulting in muscle damage/necrosis	Same as above	Same as above Except pain is more severe and prolonged (20 minutes to several hours)	No aggravating factor. Risk factors include obesity, smoking, diabetes, hypertension, stress, high lipid levels	No relieving factor except nitrates	Nausea, vomiting, perspiration, exhaustion, weakness, hypotension
Pericarditis	Irritation of pericardium and of adjacent pleura	Precordial, may radiate to the tip of shoulder and to the back	Sharp, cutting (knife-like), often severe and persistent	Breathing, change in posture, coughing, lying down	Forward bending or sitting forward may give some relief	Fever and symptoms of underlying illness, pericardial rub is present
Aortic dissection	Formation of a dissecting channel within layers of aortic wall allowing the passage of blood	Anterior chest radiating to the neck, back or abdomen	Tearing pain which is severe and persistent. Abrupt onset	Hypertension	No relieving factor	Symptoms of the underlying cause. Syncope, haemiplegia, paraplegia Aortic diastolic murmur of aortic regurgitation may appear
Pulmonary						
Acute bronchitis	Inflammation of large bronchi and trachea	Upper sternum or on either side of the sternum	Burning, mild to moderate intensity	Coughing	Sputum expulsion	Symptoms of the underlying cause
Pleuritis	Inflammation of parietal pleura	Anterior chest wall overlying the area of pleurisy	Sharp, cutting (knife-like), often severe and persistent	Breathing, coughing, movement of the trunk	Lying on the involved side may relieve it	Symptoms of the underlying cause
Gastrointestinal						
Reflux oesophagitis	Inflammation of the oesophageal mucosa	Retrosternal, may radiate to the back	Burning or squeezing pain, mild to moderate	Large meal; bending,	Antacids and nitrates, lying down	Heartburn, sour eructation, acid taste in mouth

Contd.

Disorder	Mechanism	Site	Quality, severity and timing	Aggravating factors	Relieving factors	Associated features
Contd.						
Diffuse oeso-phageal spasm	A motility disorder of oesophagus	Retrosternal, may radiate to the back, arms, and jaw	Burning or squeezing of mild to moderate intensity	swallowing of food, cold liquid, emotional stress	Antacids and nitrates	-do-
Myalgia/Teitz's syndrome	Variable, unclear	Often below the left breast or along the costal cartilage or elsewhere	Stabbing, sticking or dull aching or fleeting nature. Severity variable	Movements of chest, trunk, arms aggravate it. There may be local tenderness	-	
Psychogenic						
Anxiety neurosis (cardiac neurosis)	Unclear	Precordial, below the left breast or across the anterior chest	Stabbing, sticking or dull-aching. Variable intensity, fleeting nature	May follow stress or effort	Mental rest and anxiolytics, psychotherapy	Hyperventilation, palpitations, weakness, anxious look

Recumbency, stimulation of ADH during sleep and diminished sympathetic nervous system activity during sleep lead to overloading of the failing myocardium resulting in pulmonary congestion and PND.

Grading of Dyspnoea

New York Heart Association (NYHA) Classification/ Grading

NYHA functional classification is as follows:

Class I (grade I) : Dyspnoea occurring at severe and unaccustomed exercise/activity
Class II : Dyspnoea on moderate exertion
Class III : Dyspnoea during mild exertion/activity
Class IV (grade IV) : Dyspnoea at rest

Causes

I. Causes of dyspnoea at rest
- *Respiratory causes*, e.g. bronchial asthma, pneumothorax, ARDS, acute exacerbation of COPD, pulmonary embolism, pneumonia laryngeal obstruction.
- *Cardiac causes*, e.g. left heart failure (pulmonary oedema).
- *Metabolic causes*, e.g. metabolic acidosis of diabetes, salicylate poisoning and uraemia.
- *Cheyne-Stokes breathing* due to cerebrovascular disease.
- *Hyperventilation syndrome* (psychogenic)
- *Thyrotoxic crisis*

II. Dyspnoea on exertion
- *Cardiovascular diseases*, e.g. valvular, hypertensive, ischaemic heart diseases and cardiomyopathies.
- *Pulmonary diseases*, e.g. chronic bronchitis, bronchial asthma, chronic obstructive pulmonary disease (COPD), lung collapse, pulmonary fibrosis (restrictive lung disease), pickwickian syndrome (obesity).
- Anxiety, neurocirculatory asthenia, anaemia
- Increased intra-abdominal pressure due to ascites, pregnancy

III. Causes of orthopnoea
- Cardiac failure due to any cause
- Respiratory diseases with markedly decreased vital capacity, e.g. severe COPD, asthma, etc.

IV. Causes of PND
- Acute left ventricular failure
- Bronchial asthma
- Obstructive sleep apnoea

Symptom Analysis

Ask about the following

Q. **Is breathlessness acute in onset? Is it exertional or occurs at rest?**
- The causes of acute onset breathlessness on exertion have already been listed.
- Breathlessness of chronic onset and of long duration occurs in pleural effusion, anaemia, COPD, interstitial lung diseases, pulmonary fibrosis and kyphoscoliosis.

Cardiovascular System

Q. **Is dyspnoea episodic or recurrent?**
- Recurrent attacks of dyspnoea with morning dipping in a specific season indicate bronchial asthma

Q. **What is the grade of dyspnoea?**
- NHYA grading of dyspnoea has already been described.

Q. **Does dyspnoea has any relation to posture?**
- Dyspnoea on lying down getting relieved on sitting indicates orthopnoea (acute left heart failure, acute exacerbation of asthma, COPD, etc.).

Q. **Ask about history of snoring.**
- Dyspnoea with snoring indicates obstructive sleep apnoea.

Q. **Ask about associated features.**
- Wheezing with dyspnoea indicates asthma or COPD.
- Dyspnoea without wheeze indicates interstitial lung disease, pulmonary fibrosis.
- Coughing, wheezing and dyspnoea indicate acute bronchitis, respiratory infection.
- Palpitation with dyspnoea indicates cardiovascular diseases, e.g. hypertension, valvular and ischaemic heart disease or cardiomyopathy.
- Obesity with dyspnoea indicates hypoventilation syndrome (pickwickian syndrome).

Q. **Is breathing abnormal?**
- Cheyne-Stokes breathing with dyspnoea occurs in cardiovascular and respiratory diseases, CNS disorder, etc.

Q. **Ask about fever.**
- Fever with dyspnoea indicates infective cardiovascular or respiratory disorder.

Q. **Does the patient sleep with many pillows behind the head?**
- It indicates orthopnoea.

PALPITATION

Definition: It is defined as undue awareness of heartbeat. Patient describes it as thumping, pounding, fluttering, jumping and racing or bumping of the heartbeat.

Causes

I. Physiological
- During exertion, excitement, fever, excessive intake of tea and coffee, pregnancy, exhaustion and asthenia.

II. Pathological
- *Cardiovascular causes*, e.g. valvular heart disease, hypertension, congenital heart diseases, arrhythmias (premature beats, paroxysmal atrial tachycardia, supraventricular tachycardia (SVT), atrial fibrillation or flutter) and aortic aneurysm.
- *Endocrinal diseases*, e.g. thyrotoxicosis, phaeochromocytoma.
- *Blood disorders*, e.g. anaemia.
- *Pulmonary causes*, e.g. pneumothorax, pneumonia, lung collapse/fibrosis, mediastinal tumour.
- *Abdominal causes*, e.g. ascites, pregnancy, GI infection.
- *Drugs and poisons*, e.g. alcohol, digitalis, thyroid hormones, atropine, ephedrine, adrenaline, etc.

Symptom Analysis

Ask about the following

Q. **Onset.**
- It is insidious in onset in valvular heart disease and sudden in onset in paroxysmal tachycardia.

Q. **Ask about history of joint pain and fever.**
- Joint pain and fever (John's criteria) suggest acute rheumatic fever.

Q. **Ask about history of taking excessive tea, coffee or drugs.**
- Excessive tea, coffee and drugs are known to produce ventricular or atrial ectopics.

Q. **Is palpitation episodic?**
- Episodic or intermittent palpitation indicates paroxysmal tachycardia. Regular fast heart rate (palpitation) indicates anxiety, thyrotoxicosis, hypertension.

Q. **What is the duration of palpitation?**
- Paroxysmal tachycardia or ectopic beats may last for seconds, or may continue for hours or days.

Q. **What are its relieving factors?**
- Holding of breath, gagging or putting the fingers into the mouth or lowering of the head may stop attacks of paroxysmal atrial tachycardia.

Q. **Ask about associated features.**
- Tremors, sweating, heat intolerance, loss of weight and emotional instability indicate thyrotoxicosis or anxiety neurosis.
- Accompanying dyspnoea indicates heart disease; while cough, and sputum along with palpitation indicate respiratory disease.
- Flushing, headaches, sweating and palpitation suggest phaeochromocytoma.

SYNCOPE

Definition: It is defined as transient loss of consciousness due to fall in blood pressure leading to decreased cerebral perfusion. This symptom usually occurs when person is upright/standing, gets aborted by lying down. The patient describes the syncope as light-headedness.

Causes and Mechanisms

I. Syncope due to decreased cerebral perfusion
- *Hypersensitive carotid sinus* (carotid sinus syncope) due to cervical disease or tight cervical collar.
- *Vasovagal attack* (common faint) due to unusual seen, i.e. accident, sudden death of near or dear or emotional or painful stimuli.
- *Postural hypotension* due to diabetes, parkinsonism, old age, drugs.
- *Hypovolaemia* due to blood loss (haemorrhage) or fluid loss (dehydration or diuretic therapy.
- *Valsalva manoeuvre* (deliberate), i.e. during bending, weight lifting, trumpet playing.
- *Cerebral syncope* due to cerebrovascular disease, TIA, cerebral trauma.
- *Cough* and *micturition* syncope.

II. Syncope due to reduced/inadequate cardiac output (cardiac syncope)
- *Obstructive cardiac lesions*, i.e. aortic or pulmonary stenosis, pulmonary hypertension, hypertrophic cardiomyopathies, mitral or tricuspidal stenosis, atrial myxoma, ball valve thrombus.
- *Arrhythmias*
  i. *Tachyarrhythmias*, e.g. PSVT, AF, VT and VF
  ii. *Bradyarrhythmias*, e.g. sick sinus syndrome, complete heart block (Stokes-Adams attacks).

III. Syncope due to metabolic causes
- *Hypoxia* (pulmonary diseases, Fallot's tetralogy)
- *Hypoglycaemia*.
- *Hyperventilation syndrome*.

IV. Psychogenic (hysterical)

Symptom Analysis

Ask about the following

Q. Age and sex.
- A simple faint can occur at any age. Carotid sinus syncope is more common in middle and old age. Hysterical fainting and hyperventilation occur in young girls and young women.

Q. Ask about any precipitating cause.
- Acute pain, unpleasant scene, excess heat, prolonged standing (policemen) can precipitate *vasovagal syncope*.
- *Cough syncope* occurs in heavy smokers, and obstructive airway diseases.
- *Micturition syncope* occurs due to straining at micturition in patients with benign enlargement of prostate, cancer prostate.
- *Hypersensitivity carotid sinus* occurs due to stimulation of carotid sinus in the neck by tight cervical collar, stooping, bending or on turning the head.
- *Exertional syncope* occurs in obstructive cardiac lesions.

Q. Do symptoms of syncope occur during standing or sitting?
- Syncope usually occurs during standing, bending, straining but Stoke-Adams attack occurs during lying down or sitting or in any position.

Q. Ask about the time of its occurrence.
- Morning syncope on sitting up in the morning indicates postural syncope.

Q. Are their any premonitoring symptoms?
- Weakness, nausea, pallor, sweating indicate vasovagal syncope (simple faints).
- There is no premonitory symptoms in cardiac syncope.
- Uneasiness, dizziness, numbness and tingling of hand and feet are common in psychogenic syncope.

Q. Ask about history of head injury.
- Head trauma (brain concussion) can lead to syncope.

Q. Ask about blood loss (history of piles, malena, menorrhagia, etc.).
- Acute blood loss and anaemia can lead to syncope.

Q. Ask about history of drug being taken or taken just before it.
- Nitrates, hypotensive drugs and insulin are notorious to cause syncope.

Q. Ask about any other accompanying features.
- *Dyspnoea and palpitation*. They are common accompaniment of cardiac syncope.
- *Mental confusion, perspiration, apprehension* are common in hypoglycaemia.
- *Tetany* is common in hyperventilation syndrome
- *Vertigo, giddiness, memory defects, transient neurologic deficits* are common in TIA and vertebrobasilar insufficiency.

Cardiovascular System

- *Nausea, yawning, epigastric discomfort* are common in vasovagal attacks.

Q. Does syncope occur in the presence of someone?
- *Syncope occurring only in the presence of someone* indicates hysterical syncope.

NOCTURIA
Definition: It is defined as nocturnal frequency of micturition and patient is waken up from sleep to pass urine.

Causes
In several conditions in which there is increased frequency of micturition or diuresis, there may be change in the pattern of micturition. Normally in health 2/3 of urine volume is formed during the day and one-third during night (sleep). In certain diseases, this pattern of formation of urine is changed, i.e. night urine formation equals or exceeds day urine formation, hence, leads to nocturia. The *causes* are:

1. Diabetes mellitus, diabetes insipidus
2. Chronic renal failure
3. Congestive heart failure
4. Enlarged prostate
5. Use of long-acting diuretic

Symptom Analysis
Ask about history of passing urine at night, its frequency and volume of urine.

FATIGUE
(It has been discussed already).

ANOREXIA, NAUSEA AND VOMITING
(**Read it as a symptom in gastroenterology**). However, in cardiac failure it is due to hepatic and GI tract congestion or due to drugs (digoxin, etc.).

COUGH, SPUTUM AND HAEMOPTYSIS
(**Read them under respiratory symptoms**). However, in cardiology, these symptoms occur due to congestion of the lung due to left heart failure of any cause.

OEDEMA (SWELLING)
It is defined as collection of fluid in the interstitium either due to increased hydrostatic pressure (cardiovascular causes) or decreased oncotic pressure (hypoproteinemic causes, e.g. nephrotic syndrome, cirrhosis and malnutrition/malabsorption) or due to increased capillary permeability, venous or lymphatic obstruction.

Causes
(Read General Physical Examination in the Unit I). However, congestive heart failure due to any cardiovascular disease leads to pitting oedema at various sites discussed below.

Sites of oedema in heart disease
- Ankle oedema, oedema feet and legs (common site).
- Sacral oedema, e.g. oedema over the back, buttocks and sacrum and parietal oedema (oedema of the abdominal wall) occur when generalised anasarca develops.

Symptom Analysis
Ask about the following

Q. Onset of oedema.

Q. When does it appear?
- Morning facial oedema indicates renal oedema (renal disorder) while in CHF oedema occurs on feet during the day. If patient is in CHF and bed riddened, then it appears on the sacrum and the back.

Q. Postural relation.
- Oedema disappears on lying down. Raising the legs on pillows relieve oedema of CHF.

Q. History of tightening of socks/shoes, etc.
- Oedema leaving marks of socks or tightening of shoes indicate pitting oedema which can be demonstrated by putting pressure over the ankle.

Q. What is ditstribution of oedema?
- Generalised oedema involves the whole body while local oedema (venous or lymphatic obstruction) involves the part involved.

Q. Is it associated with swelling of abdomen (ascites)?
- Ascites with oedema indicate CHF, nephrotic syndrome, cirrhosis of liver, hypoproteinaemia, etc.

Q. Is it associated with cough, sputum and dyspnoea?
- Cough, sputum and dyspnoea with oedema suggest CHF or cor pulmonale.

Differential Diagnosis (Read Unit I)

HISTORY

Present History
- Ask the present complaints and write them in chronological order.
- Analyse the symptoms with *mode of onset, progression, aggravating or relieving factors, associated*

fever and *other symptoms*. (Read symptom analysis in the beginning.)

Past History

Ask about
- History of rheumatic fever (fever, polyarthritis, tachycardia, subcutaneous swellings, rash, involuntary movements).
- History of sore throat or skin or urinary infection.
- Recurrent respiratory infection since childhood (cogenital heart disease).
- History of cyanotic spalls (cyanotic congenital heart disease).
- Recent dental extraction, throat surgery, genitourinary instrumentation (bacterial endocarditis).
- History of hypertension, diabetes mellitus, ischaemic heart disease or any other intercurrent illnesses.

Family History

Ask about
- Hypertension, ischaemic heart disease, congenital heart disease, rheumatic fever, syphilis, sudden death (hypertrophic cardiomyopathy).
- Consangunity between parents

Personal History

Ask about
- Habits, e.g. smoking, alcoholism, sexual habits.
- Bowel or bladder disturbance
- Menstrual history and history of previous pregnancies in females, maternal rubella (fever, rash) infection.

Treatment History

Ask about
- Drug taken in the past, being taken at present.
- Penicillin prophylaxis
- Diuretics

GENERAL PHYSICAL EXAMINATION

It includes:
1. Build, stature, nourishment, BMI
2. Cyanosis
3. Anaemia/polycythaemia
4. Malar flush over cheeks
5. Eyes for ophthalmos, blue sclera, fundus, jaundice
6. Neck for lymphadenopathy, thyroid enlargement, JVP and carotid pulsations.
7. Painful finger tips, gangrene of toes and fingers
8. Palmar erythema, Janeway lesion.
9. Splinter haemorrhages
10. Temperature of extremeties (warm/cold)
11. Clubbing of fingers and toes
12. Vital signs, e.g. pulse, BP and body temperature
13. Oedema feet

BUILD, STATURE, NOURISHMENT AND BMI

☞ *Look at build, stature, nourishment, BMI, etc.*

- *Short stature* and *growth retardation* in children suggest congenital heart disease.
- *Brachydactyly and polydactyly* are seen in chromosomal syndrome with congenital heart diseases such as Turner and Down syndromes.
- *Fingerised thumb (thumb resembles a finger)*: It is seen in *Holt-Oram syndrome*.
- *Fingers clenched with index finger crossing over the third finger*: It is seen in *Edward syndrome* (trisomy 16–18) with congenital heart disease.
- *Tall stature, arachnodactyly, brachydactyly and polydactyly*: Arachnodactyly (long slender finger), suggest Marfan's syndrome, homocysteinuria.
- *Excessive degree of emaciation* can occur in severe chronic congestive heart failure.
- Increased BMI (>30 kg/m^2) indicates obesity, can be associated with ischaemic heart disease.

CYANOSIS

It refers to bluish discolouration of skin and mucous membrane due to presence of reduced haemoglobin of 5 g or more. It can be central or peripheral or mixed.

☞ *Look for central as well as peripheral cyanosis*

Central cyanosis (to be seen on under surface of tongue, palate and oral mucosa)

It is due to mixing of deoxygenated blood from the right side with oxygenated blood from the left side in right to left intracardiac shunts. It is seen in cyanotic congenital heart disease and Eisenmenger's syndrome.

Peripheral cyanosis (to be seen on peripheral parts, lips, nails, tip of nose, ear lobule)

It is due to supply of deoxygenated blood to the peripheral parts due to extraction of O_2 from the blood during slow circulation in congestive heart failure and shock syndrome. It can occur locally due to vasospastic disorders (acrocyanosis, Raynaud's phenomenon, cold hypersensitivity).

Mixed cyanosis: It is a combination of the two, seen in congestive cardiac failure.

Red cyanosis: It is seen in erythrocytosis or polycythemia.

Differential cyanosis: Cyanosis when present appears both in upper and lower extremites. It is called *differential* when it is either present in upper extremities not in the lower extremities (aortoarteritis) or present in the lower extremities not in upper extremities (reversed coarctation of aorta).

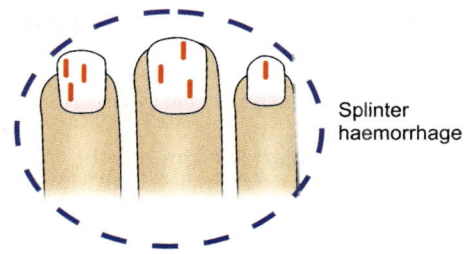

Fig. 3.1: Splinter haemorrhage.

ANAEMIA

☞ *Look for anaemia (tongue, mucous membrane, nails, lips, palmar creases and conjunctivae), polycythaemia (suffused face and conjunctivae)*
- Anaemia in cardiovascular diseases is due to bacterial endocarditis, haemoptysis due to left heart failure.
- Anaemia itself can precipitate or aggravate heart failure.
- Polycythaemia can occur in cyanotic congenital heart disease.

FACE, HANDS AND FINGERS

☞ *Look at the face for malar flush*
- It is a bluish hue (colour) seen over the malar prominences of the cheeks in fair-flexioned persons having mitral stenosis. It indicates low cardiac output due to severe mitral stenosis.

☞ *Look for painful finger tips (Osler's nodes) and gangrenous fingers/toes*
- Tender nodular spots over tips of the fingers (*Osler's nodes*) and gangrenous fingers indicate embolisation of peripheral vessels in patients with infective endocarditis or vasculitis.

☞ *Look for palmar erythema and Janeway lesion*
- Redness of hypothenar and thenar eminences is called *palmar erythema* or *Janeway lesion*, occurs due to vasculitis in patients with infective endocarditis.

☞ *Look for splinter haemorrhage (Fig. 3.1) under nail's bed*
  These are flame-shaped or linear haemorrhages under the nailbed, seen in infective endocarditis.

☞ *Look for temperature of extremities (hands)*
- With the help of back of the hand cold extremities in warm environment indicates CHF.
- Warm and moist extremities indicate thyrotoxic heart disease, phaeochromocytoma.

☞ *Look for clubbing of the fingers/toes*
- It is seen congenital heart disease, Eisenmenger's syndrome and subacute bacterial endocarditis.
- Grades of clubbing (read respiratory system).

SKIN

☞ *Look at the skin for pigmentation, xanthomas/xanthelasmas*
- **Bronze pigmentation** suggest haemochromatosis as a cause of cardiomyopathy if suspected.
- **Xanthelasmas/Xanthomas** are due to dyslipidaemia associated with ischaemic heart disease.

EYES

☞ *Look for the jaundice, exophthalmos, blue sclera, fundus*
- *Jaundice* in cardiac disease can be due to hepatitis, hepatic congestion (CHF), cardiac cirrhosis, etc.
- *Exophthalmos* suggest thyrotoxic heart disease.
- *Blue sclera* suggests osteogenesis imperfecta with aortic regurgitation.
- *Exudate, hemorrhoge on fundus* indicate hypertensive heart disease, Roth's spots indicate infective endocarditis, retinal pulsations occur in AR and corkscrew retinal arteries are present in coarctation of aorta.

NECK

☞ *Examine the neck for jugular venous pulse as well as pressure, lymphadenopathy and thyroid enlargement*

☞ *Examine carotid pulsations.*

Jugular Venous Pulse and Pressure (JVP)

The neck veins (internal and/or external jugular veins) are used to analyse the venous waveforms and to estimate the jugular venous pressure (JVP). Usually, the right internal jugular vein is the best for both the purposes:

- Since there are no venous valve between right atrium and the internal jugular vein, hence, degree of distension of the veins directly represents the pressure in the right atrium called JVP.
- The internal jugular vein can only be examined when the neck muscles are relaxed. The external jugular vein is visible but it is not reliable because it is prone to kinking and obstruction.
- The venous pulsations in the neck when the veins are invisible create confusion with carotid pulsations. The differentiation between the two is tabulated in Table 3.2.

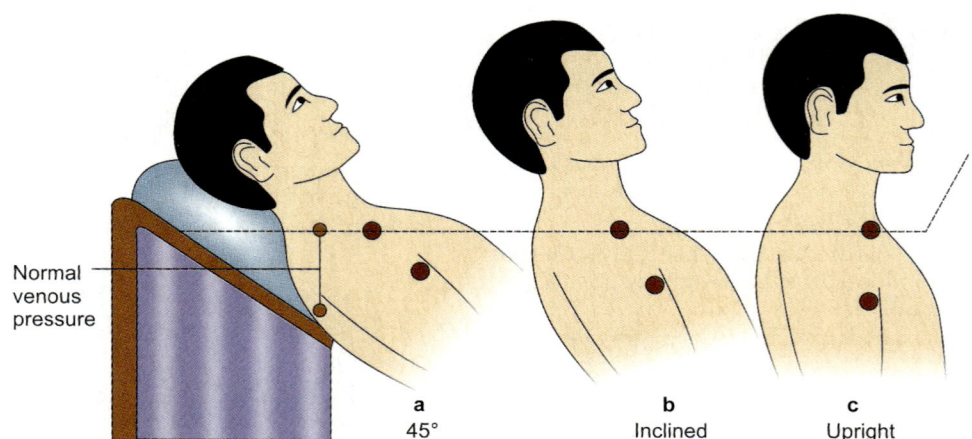

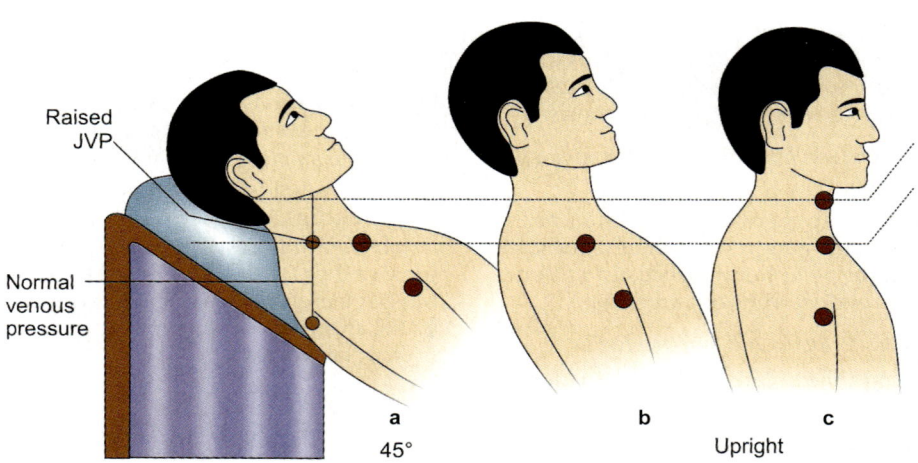

Fig. 3.2: Jugular venous pulsations and jugular venous pressure.

Upper: Normal jugular venous pressure. In normal subjects, when body is inclined to 45° to the horizontal, (a) the venous pulsations are just visible in the internal jugular vein just above the clavicles. (b) As patient tries to adopt upright position, the distance between the right atrium and sternal angle remains constant, regardless of the position of the thorax. However, in sitting (upright) position, (c) the venous pulsations, become hidden behind the clavicle which is just situated equivalent to the sternal angle. Therefore, for JVP, the inclination of 45° is must to see the venous pulsations.
Lower: Raised jugular venous pressure (↑JVP). When JVP gets elevated, the internal jugular vein becomes full and venous pulsations appear in the neck which can be appreciated. To differentiate them from carotid pulsations, perform hepatojugular reflux which not only makes the veins prominent but gives an idea of upper column of pulsations. The JVP is measured as vertical distance between top of the pulsations and sternal angle. When JVP is markedly elevated the venous pulsations get hidden behind the angle of jaw, hence, it is beyond measurement.

Cardiovascular System

TABLE 3.2: Differentiation between Jugular Venous and Carotid Artery Pulsations

Internal jugular pulsations	Carotid pulsations
• Better visible than palpable	• Better palpable than visible
• Not palpable	• Palpable
• They exhibit rapid inward movement	• They exhibit rapid outward movement
• Two peaks are seen per heartbeat in sinus rhythm	• A vigorous thrust with a single peak is seen per heartbeat
• Pulsations can be obliterated by pressure at root of the neck	• Pulsations remain unaffected by such pressure
• Level of pulsations changes with position, i.e. falls as the patient becomes upright	• Position does not have any such effect
• Level of pulsations usually descends with inspiration	• Pulsations not affected by inspiration
• Veins can be made prominent with abdominal pressure (abdominojugular reflux)	• Abdominal pressure has no effect

Normal Jugular Venous Pressure (JVP)

The normal mean right atrial pressure is < 9 cm of H_2O or < 8 mmHg. Since the sternal angle (angle of Louis) is approximately 5 cm above the right atrium, therefore, the normal jugular venous pulse should not extend beyond 4 cm above the sternal angle (Fig. 3.2) When a normal person sits upright the pulse is hidden behind the clavicle and sternum. When the patient is propped up to 45°, the top of the pulsations is normally just at the level of the clavicle. If pulsations are not seen at this position, then a normal right atrial pressure is confirmed by applying pressure over the centre of the abdomen for 5–10 seconds (abdominojugular reflux). This manoeuvre increases the venous return to right side of the heart and leads to transient rise in right atrial pressure of 1–3 cm which is reflected in the height of jugular venous pulse.

In contrast, when jugular venous pressure is raised, reclination up to 60° or even 90° may be required to see the pulsations which may be hidden behind the angle of the jaw. In all these positions, the sternal angle usually remains about 5 cm above the right atrium, hence is a reference point as illustrated in Fig. 3.2.

Waveforms

The jugular venous pulse waveform requires experience. It has two positive waves; a wave and v wave, and two descents x and y. There is a third positive wave called 'c' wave which is not visible (Fig. 3.3).

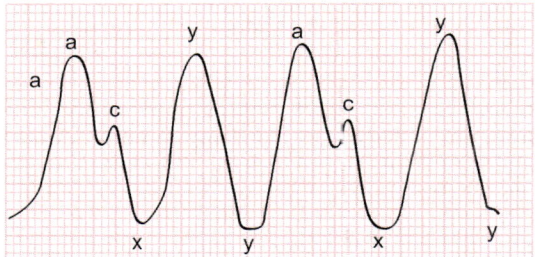

Fig. 3.3: The waveforms of jugular venous pulse.

The **'a' wave** or first positive wave occurs due to right atrial contractions just before the first heart sound.

- The 'a' wave becomes prominent in pulmonary hypertension, pulmonary stenosis, and tricuspid stenosis. **Giant 'a' wave (cannon wave)** occurs due to forceful atrial contractions against closed tricuspid valve, is seen in complete heart block, supraventricular nodal tachycardia and ventricular tachycardia.
- The 'a' wave is absent in atrial fibrillation.

The **'c' wave**, is a wave produced by bulging of the tricuspid valve into right atrium as right ventricular pressure rises. It is not visible on JVP.

The **'v' wave** is the third positive wave produced by the increasing volume of blood into the right atrium during ventricular systole when the tricuspid valve is closed.

Tricuspid regurgitation causes the v wave to be more prominent while tricuspid stenosis diminishes it.

The **x descent** is the first negative wave that follows a wave (c is not visible). This is produced by atrial relaxation.

It is accentuated in constrictive pericarditis but is diminished in right ventricular dilatation.

The combination of a prominent 'v' wave and obliteration of 'x' descent produces a single large positive wave with y descent called 'vy' collapse, characteristically seen in tricuspid regurgitation.

The **'y' descent** is the second negative wave produced by the opening of the tricuspid valve and the subsequent rapid inflow of the blood into the right ventricle.

- A sharp *y* descent is seen in patients with constrictive pericarditis, or with right-sided heart failure.
- A slow *y* descent indicates obstruction to the right ventricular filling, is seen in patients with tricuspid stenosis or right atrial myxoma.

Remember. The absent venous pulsations with prominent dilated neck veins are characteristically seen in *superior mediastinal compression* or *superior vena cava obstruction.*

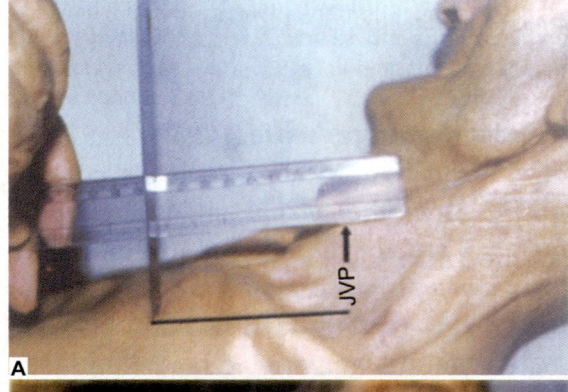

Method of Examination of Jugular Venous Pulse and Measurement of JVP

The steps are as follows:
1. Make the patient supine comfortably with the head resting on a pillow.
2. Raise the head of the patient to 45° in supine position by putting the pillows behind the head or by raising the head end of the bed or examining table.
3. Turn the patient's head slightly away from the side you are inspecting. Use good source of light for examination.
4. Inspect the neck veins from the side of the patient.
5. Identify the internal jugular pulsations especially on the right side. Focus on the pulsations and note the highest point of pulsations, if necessary, by means of abdominojugular reflux.
6. Measure the JVP (Fig. 3.4A) by vertical distance in centimeter between the top of venous pulsations and the sternal angle. This distance measured in centimeters above the sternal angle is the JVP. If JVP is markedly raised, make the patient to sit and measure the JVP and describe it in sitting position. If still raised, say JVP is raised beyond the angle of jaw, hence not measured (Fig. 3.4B).

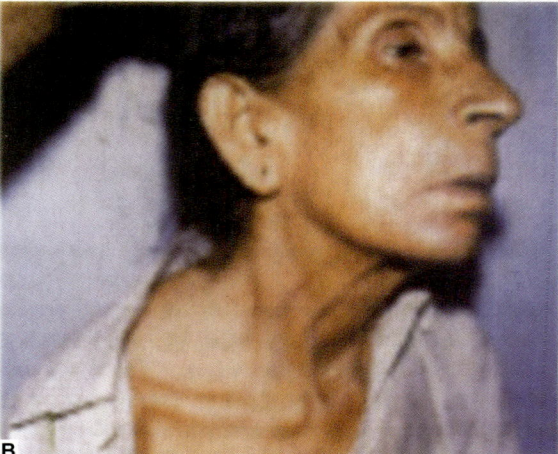

Figs 3.4A and B: Measurement of JVP. (A) Actual measurement at 45°, it is raised; (B) Markedly raised JVP beyond measurement say, JVP is raised up to the angle of jaw and above.

Causes of raised JVP
1. Right-sided heart failure (cor pulmonale) or congestive cardiac failure (Fig. 3.4A).
2. Constrictive pericarditis, pericardial effusion.
3. Tricuspid stenosis.
4. Superior vena cava obstruction (JVP is raised but pulsations may be absent).

Causes of low JVP
- Shock
- Hypovolaemia
- Dehydration

Remember. Sometimes JVP is markedly raised beyond the angle of the jaw even on sitting position, so upper level cannot be defined, then say it is beyond measurement even after sitting position. (Fig. 3.4B).

7. Now read just the position of the patient, if necessary, to make the waveforms clearly visible.
8. Now identify the pattern of waveforms (*a*, *v* and *y*) of venous pulsation and note any abnormality.

Effect of Respiration on JVP

Normally, the JVP decreases during inspiration, the paradoxical rise of JVP during inspiration (opposite to normal decrease) is called *Kussmaul's sign.* It is most often seen in constrictive pericarditis, severe right-sided failure or right ventricular infarction.

In patients with *chronic obstructive pulmonary disease* (COPD), venous pressure may be elevated on expiration only. The veins collapse on inspiration. This finding indicates congestive heart failure.

Unilateral distension of the external jugular vein is usually due to local kinking or obstruction.

Abdominojugular reflux test/ manoeuvre

In patients suspected of having right ventricular failure with normal JVP at rest, the abdominojugular reflux test may be helpful to detect latent or incipient right heart failure. It is performed by applying firm pressure with the palm of the hand over the abdomen for 10 seconds or more. In normal persons, this manoeuvre does not alter JVP significantly but when incipient or compensated right heart failure is present, the upper level of the pulsations usually increases, hence, test is said to be *positive*.

The Carotid Pulsations

After measuring the JVP, move onto assessment of carotid pulsations in the neck. The carotid pulse is useful for detecting stenosis or regurgitation of the aortic valve and in evaluation of a case with stroke.

☞ Look at the carotids for quality of upstroke, its amplitude and feel for contour, and presence or absence of any thrill and hear for bruit.

Method. To assess the amplitude and contour, the patient should be lying comfortably on the bed with the head of bed elevated to 30°. Inspect the neck for carotid pulsations. These may be visible just medial to sternomastoid muscles. Then place your right index and middle fingers (or left thumb) on the right carotid artery in the lower third of the neck, press posteriorly and feel for pulsations (Figs 3.5A and B).

Caution: Avoid pressing the carotid sinus which lies at the level of the top of the thyroid cartilage. Pressure on the carotid sinus may cause reflex bradycardia or hypotension.

Never press both carotids simultaneously as this may reduce blood supply to the brain and induce syncope.

Abnormalities

- Delayed carotid pulsations on one side felt in a patient with stroke indicate an atherosclerotic narrowing leading to cerebral embolism.
- Delayed carotid upstroke occurs in aortic stenosis.
- A carotid bruit with or without thrill in a middle aged or older person suggests artherosclerotic aortic stenosis.

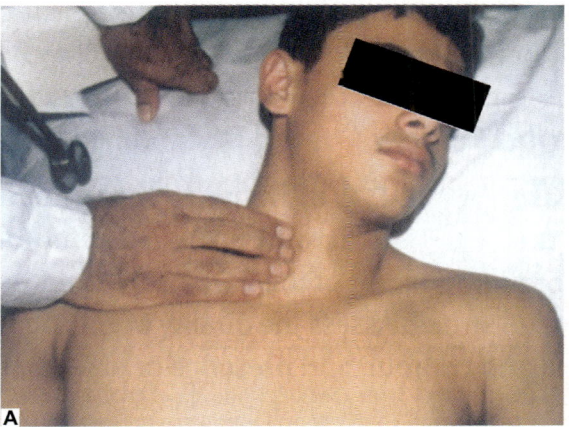

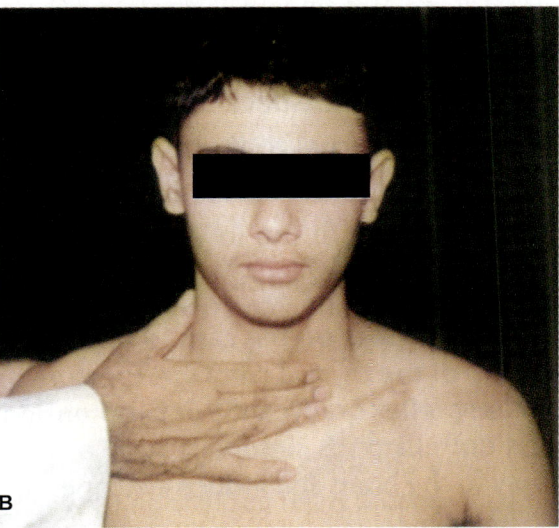

Figs 3.5A and B: Method of palpation of carotid pulse. (A) Palpation by index and middle fingers; (B) Palpation of the opposite carotid.

- An aortic ejection systolic murmur may radiate to the carotid artery and sound like a thrill.

Neck for Lymphadenopathy

The examination of neck lymph nodes has been described with three significance in Unit I.

Examination of Trachea (read Unit II on respiratory system).

VITAL SIGNS

The Arterial Pulse

Definition: It is a wave produced by cardiac systole which traverses through the arterial tree and felt easily at peripheral vessels. It is felt best at the radial artery (*radial pulse*) because of its superficial position. Radial pulse on both the sides should be palpated simultaneously. Various pulses and their site of palpation are depicted in Table 3.3. The method of palpation is depicted in Box 3.2.

TABLE 3.3: Various Pulses and their Site of Palpation

1.	Radial pulse	It is felt at the front of wrist just medial to styloid process of the radius. It is best felt with the person's forearm slight pronated and wrist somewhat flexed
2.	Brachial pulse	In the cubital fossa
3.	Carotid pulse (Figs 3.5A and B)	In the neck at the upper end of thyroid cartilage along sternomastoid
4.	Femoral pulse	In the femoral triangle of thigh with the leg slightly abducted and foot externally rotated
5.	Popliteal pulse	In the popliteal fossa in supine position both hands encircling the knee and supporting it on each side
6.	Posterior tibial	In the groove between the medial malleolus and tendoachilles by curving the fingers around the ankle
7.	Dorsalis pedis	Front of foot just below the ankle

☞ *Examine the pulse for*
- Rate
- Rhythm
- Equality
- Condition of the vessel wall
- Radiofemoral dalay
- Any abnormal character (Table 3.4 and Fig. 3.7)

  I. *Rate:* Count the beat for at least half a minute, preferably for full one minute if pulse is regular. Its pulse is irregular, always count the pulse for full one minute.

Pulse rate >100/min is called *tachycardia* and <60/min is called *bradycardia*. Normal pulse rate varies between 60 and 90/min (average 72/min) in normal healthy adults.

  II. *Rhythm*: Normal rhythm of pulse is regular called *sinus rhythm*.
  Pulse deficit: Calculate the pulse deficit, if pulse is irregular.
  It is the difference between the heart rate and pulse rate (heart rate always being higher than pulse rate). Pulse deficit occurs when heart rate is irregular and some feeble beats are not transmitted to the pulse, therefore, always count the heart rate with the stethoscope when

Box 3.2 Palpation of Various Pulses

Pulses *Method (Fig. 3.6)*

1. **The brachial artery** is palpated in the antecubital fossa by compressing it against the humerus. The examiner should use the index, middle fingers or thumb of opposite hand. With your free hand, flex the elbow to varying degree to get optimal pulsations (Fig. 3.6A).

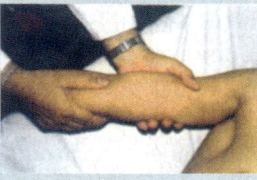
Fig. 3.6A: Examination of brachial pulse with thumb.

2. **The carotid artery** is palpated in the neck by gently compressing it against the transverse process of cervical vertebrae when the patient is resting on the bed or couch. Use the left thumb for right carotid and *vice versa*. *See Fig. 3.5*

3. **The femoral pulse** is palpated in the thigh between the iliac crest and the pubic ramus by compressing the artery against the underlying femur (Fig. 3.6B).

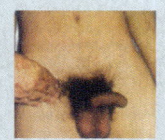
Fig. 3.6B: Palpation of femoral artery pulsations

4. **The popliteal artery** is palpated in the popliteal fossa while the patient lies supine. With the knee flexed at an angle of 120°, the finger tips are used to palpate the artery while the thumb rests on the patient's patella (Fig. 3.6C).

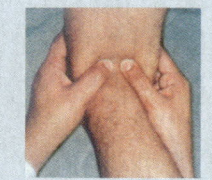
Fig. 3.6C: Palpation of popliteal artery pulsations

5. **The posterior tibial** is palpated behind the medial malleolus of the tibia with the foot relaxed between plantar and dorsiflexion (Fig. 3.6D).

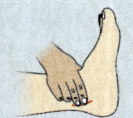
Fig. 3.6D: Palpation of posterior tibial artery

6. **The dorsalis pedis.** It is palpated on the dorsum of foot by compressing it against tarsal bone. The left dorsalis pedis is palpated with fingers of right hand and *vice versa* (Fig. 3.6E).

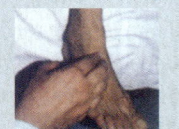
Fig. 3.6E: Palpation of dorsalis pedis artery pulsations

heart rate is irregular, i.e. in atrial fibrillation, ventricular ecotpics and sinus arrhythmia.

- Normally there is no *pulse deficit*
- Irregularity of the pulse related to respiration, i.e. pulse increases during inspiration, decreases on expiration is called *sinus arrhythmia*.
- Irregularity may be regular due to regular dropping of beats, for example in pulsus bigeminus, every second beat is dropped, pulsus trigeminus in which every third beat is missing. Similarly in fixed second degree heart block, the beats are missed regularly producing regularly irregular pulse.
- Irregularly irregular pulse indicates *atrial fibrillation, ventricular ectopics, sinus arrhythmia, supraventricular ectopics* and *variable second degree heart block.*

III. *The volume:* It is the amplitude of the pulse felt by the palpating finger. It depends on the force of contraction of heart (*systolic pressure*) and relaxation of the blood vessel (*diastolic pressure*), therefore, *pulse pressure* (difference between systolic and diastolic BP) decides the volume. **Good volume pulse** occurs when pulse pressure exceeds 40 mmHg and **low volume** when it decreases to <20 mmHg.

Causes of good volume or collapsing pulse are
- Aortic regurgitation (AR), sometimes in mitral regurgitation and PDA
- High output states, e.g. anxiety, thyrotoxicosis, anaemia, fever, pregnancy, complete heart block, beriberi, Paget's disease, AV fistula, cirrhosis of liver and cor pulmonale.

Causes of absent radial pulse
- Aberrant (abnormally placed) radial pulse—a congenital anomaly.
- Previous surgical cut down and artery tied off incidentally at surgery.
- Brachial artery or radial artery catheterisation or embolisation.
- Subclavian artery stenosis
- Cervical rib
- Blalock-Taussig shunt surgery
- Takayasu arteritis

Causes of low volume pulse are
- Shock, dehydration
- Cardiac tamponade, chronic constrictive
- pericarditis
- Myocarditis, dilated cardiomyopathy, CHF, acute MI.

- Aortic stenosis, mitral stenosis, coarctation of aorta
- Tachyarrhythmias

Remember: A varying volume pulse is either pulsus alternans or pulsus paradoxus (Read table 3.4 on characteristic pulses.)

IV. *Character:* The normal character of a pulse is rapid rise, rounded peak and a rapid fall. It has a percussion (P) and a tidal wave (T), a dicrotic wave and a notch 'D' (Fig. 3.7A). Some abnormal pulses with their characteristics pulses and associated conditions are described in Table 3.4.

V. *Condition of arterial wall:* Normally the vessel wall is not palpable. With advanced age, the arteries become thick and hard as rigid tubes and become palpable, e.g. in atherosclerosis. The condition of the vessel wall is estimated by flattening the artery by digital pressure, then the empty vessel is rolled up, down and sideways with palpating fingers.
- Normally all the peripheral pulses are equally felt simultaneously on both the sides. Abnormally pulse may be delayed due to pulse inequality.

VI. *Pulse equality*
- *Radioradial delay* means one of the radial pulses is delayed when both the radial pulses are palpated simultaneously. The causes are:
  1. Anomalous abnormal course of radial artery
  2. Preductal coarctation of aorta
  3. Aortitis
  4. Dissecting aneurysm of aorta
  5. Peripheral embolisation.
- *Radiofemoral delay* means femoral pulse is delayed as compared to radial pulse when both are palpated simultaneously on one side. Both the femoral pulses are classically delayed in:
  i. Postductal coarctation.
  ii. Aortitis
  iii. Takayasu syndrome (block at bifurcation of aorta (saddle-shaped embolus)
- *Femoral radial delay:* The radial pulses come after the femoral, i.e. just reverse to radiofemoral delay, indicates reverse coarctation of aorta (atherosclerosis or aortitis).

VII. *Capillary pulsations* **(Quinke's sign)**
Arterial pulsations can be transmitted to the dilated capillaries to the subcapillary venous

TABLE 3.4: Differential Diagnosis of Pulse

Pulse (Figs 3.7A to I)

Normal: It has a fairly rapid rise, rounded top and fairly steep fall. It has a rapid rising percussion (P) wave, a rounded tip, a tidal (T) wave, a notch (N) and a dicrotic (D) wave

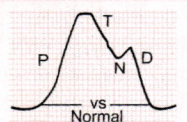
Normally seen (Fig. 3.7A)

Anacrotic. It is a slow rising, small volume, well-sustained pulse. It is now-a-days called **pulsus tardus**. An 'anacrotic notch (AN) between percussion (P) and tidal wave (T) is present. It is seen in aortic stenosis

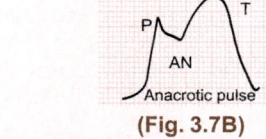
Anacrotic pulse
(Fig. 3.7B)

Collapsing or water hammer or corrigan pulse. It is characterized by a rapid upstroke (forceful, high percussion wave) which gives a tap to the palpating finger similar to feeling of a water-hammer, followed by rapid downstroke producing collapsing character. The method of palpation of water hammer pulse is described in Fig. 3.7C
• The causes of good volume/collapsing pulse have been described already
It is demonstrated by holding, say the right hand with your left hand and palpate the right radial pulse with right index middle and with finger after raising the hand above the heart level

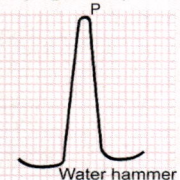
Fig. 3.7C: Collapsing pulse

Pulsus parvus. It is low volume ill-sustained pulse, differs from pulsus tardus where pulse is low-volume but well sustained. It is seen in mitral stenosis

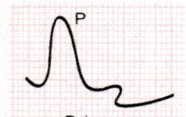
Pulsus parvus
(Fig. 3.7D)

Pulsus bisferiens. It is a double peak pulse. The first peak is due to quick rising percussion wave (P) and second one is due to delayed tidal wave (T), with a notch (N) in between, thus both the peaks have same amplitude. It is felt in AR alone, AS and AR and hypertrophic cardiomyopathy (HCM)

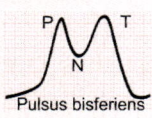
Pulsus bisferiens
(Fig. 3.7E)

Dicrotic pulse. It is characterized by two palpable waves, one in systole and one in diastole, separated by an accentuated normal dicrotic notch. It is felt in high grade fever and dilated cardiomyopathy

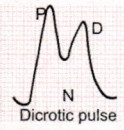
Dicrotic pulse
(Fig. 3.7F)

Pulsus alternans: Large and small volume pulses alternate. It is felt in dilated cardiomyopathy and CHF

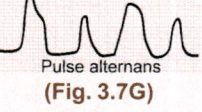
Pulse alternans
(Fig. 3.7G)

Pulsus bigeminus or trigeminus or quadrigeminus: The pulse is regularly irregular due to fixed unifocal extrasytoles coming after every normal beat or after every two or three normal beats with the usual pause after the extrasystole. It occurs when multiple ectopics have fixed pattern

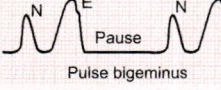
Pulse bigeminus
(Fig. 3.7H)

Pulsus paradoxus: Volume of pulse decreases during inspiration and increases during expiration. It is felt in pericardial effusion, shock, acute asthma, etc.

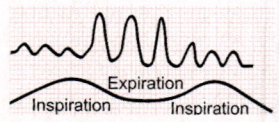
(Fig. 3.7I)

plexus in patients with wide pulse pressure (i.e. >60 mm).

Capillary pulsations can be demonstrated in the following ways:
1. By applying gentle pressure at the tip of the nail and observing the nailbed for rhythmic pulsations/flush.
2. It can also be demonstrated by transilluminating the ear tip or finger or thumb tip by a torch light shading the part observed with flexed fingers.
3. By gently pressing the mucous membrane of the lips by a glass slide.

Causes
1. *Capillary dilatation* due to hot weather, hot bath, fever, anaemia, pregnancy, thyrotoxicosis, etc.
2. *Cardiac conditions with wide pulse pressure,* i.e. AR, systolic hypertension, complete heart block.

VIII. *Digital throbbing.* It is detected by approximating the fingers of your right hand to those of patient's right hand. It has same significance as capillary pulsations.

IX. *Capillary refill:* it is done in the same way as for capillary pulsations. In this you have to measure the time in seconds required for the pink colour to appear. Balanch the nail and observe the refill after releasing it and note the time in seconds.

Normal time is < 1 sec. Time taken > 3 sec indicates peripheral vascular disease.

X. Other peripheral pulses

☞ *Look for the various peripheral arterial pulses as discussed under examination of peripheral vascular system.*

- Pain or diminished pulses suggest arterial insufficiency, hence, look for postural colour changes. (Read examination of peripheral vascular system.)

The Temperature

☞ *Record the temperature if person is febrile*

Fever or rise in temperature in a patient with cardiovascular disease indicates rheumatic fever, infective endocarditis, pericarditis, myocarditis and atrial myxoma. Certain systemic infections, e.g. typhoid fever, influenza may be associated with fever and cardiac complication, e.g. myocarditis. Certain systemic disorders may be associated with fever and cardiovascular manifestation such as SLE, rheumatoid arthritis, etc. Even when heart is not affected, fever can lead to tachycardia and collapsing pulse with wide pulse pressure.

Respiration

☞ *Record the respiratory rate and type of breathing if the patient is breathless*

Tachypnoea and dyspnoea are common accompaniments of left heart failure. *Cheyne-Stokes breathing* can occur in CHF.

Blood Pressure (BP)

It is the pressure exerted by the column of blood on lateral walls of the vessels during cardiac systole and diastole. Systolic BP indicates force of cardiac contraction and diastolic BP indicates vessel wall resistance.

Clinically the BP is measured by a mercury/aneroid sphygmomanometer. To measure the BP accurately, one must choose a cuff of appropriate size, i.e. 12–14 cm for an average adult and the length of the cuff should be about 80% of upper arm circumference (almost long enough to encircle the arm).

If aneroid instrument is used, recalibrate periodically before use because it becomes inaccurate with repeated use.

Technique (Fig. 3.8). The examination sequence is as follows:
- Ideally ask the patient to avoid smoking or drinking caffeinated beverages for 30 minutes before BP is measured, and person should rest for at least 5–10 minutes.
- Support the arm comfortably at about heart level
- Remove all the clothing from the arm.
- Apply the cuff to the arm and identify the brachial pulse.
- Inflate the cuff until the pulse is impalpable. Note the pressure on the manometer which is rough estimate of systolic pressure.
- Now inflate the cuff another 20–30 mmHg above and listen through the stethoscope over the brachial artery.
- Deflate the cuff slowly until the regular heart sounds (*Korotkoff sounds*) can be heard. This is systolic pressure.
- Continue to deflate the cuff slowly.
- Record the point at which the sounds just disappear or get muffled. It is diastolic BP. Occasionally the muffled sounds persist, in which case, the point at which they first become muffled gives the diastolic BP.

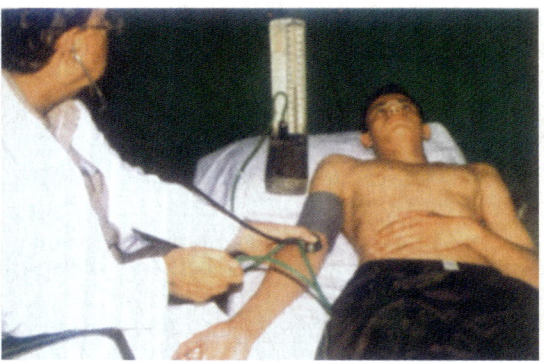

Fig. 3.8: Measurement of blood pressure.

In some people, muffling point and the disappearance point are further apart. Occasionally as in aortic regurgitation, the sounds never disappear. If there is more than 10 mmHg difference in muffling and disappearance point, record both figures as 150/80/68 mmHg.

Blood pressure should be taken in both arms at least once. Normally there may be a difference of 5 mmHg and sometimes up to 10 mmHg, beyond this, it is abnormal, hence, repeated measurements are to be taken in case of abnormality.

In case of wide pulse pressure (suspected AR), BP should also be measured in the lower limbs. It is higher (> 40 mmHg) than upper limb called *Hill's sign*.

Definitions of Normal and Abnormal Level

Blood pressure varies with excitement, stress and environment. Repeated measurements are required before a patient should be identified as hypertensive. In some patients, the measurement of just BP by the doctor as soon as the patient approaches the doctor cause BP to rise—called *white coat hypertension*. This may come to normal after sometime when the patient is relaxed and as soon as he/she comes out of doctor's chamber. Ambulatory BP monitoring helps to distinguish these patients from those with sustained hypertension.

Recently, the VIIIth Joint National Committee (JNC VIII) has retained the recommendations of JNC VII. On prevention, detection, evaluation and treatment of hypertension, has defined normal and abnormal values of BP (Box 3.3). According to it, 120/80 mmHg is taken as upper limit of normal. BP <140/90 mmHg should not be treated except lifestyle modification. Normal pulse pressure (difference between systolic and diastolic) is around 20–30 mmHg.

In patients taking antihypertensive treatment or elderly patients or patients with symptoms of faintings or syncope, or patients with depletion of blood volume, take the BP in *supine, sitting* and *standing* positions (unless contraindicated). Normally, as the patient rises from the lying down to a standing position, systolic pressure falls slightly or remains unchanged, while diastolic pressure rises slightly. Another reading after 1 to 5 minutes of standing may identify *orthostatic hypotension*, if missed by earlier readings. The repetition is especially useful in elderly. A fall in systolic BP > 20 mmHg especially when accompanied by symptoms (syncope) indicates *orthostatic (postural) hypotension*.

In suspected coarctation of aorta, it is useful to compare the systolic BP in the arm with that in the leg on same side when the patient lies prone and an 18 cm cuff is used above the knee to measure the systolic BP over the popliteal artery. The difference is noted.

- BP is higher in the arms than the legs in coarctation of aorta.

Box 3.3: JNC VII Classification of Hypertension

Category	Systolic (mmHg)	Diastolic (mmHg)
Normal	<120	<80
Prehypertension	120–139	80–89
Hypertension		
First stage	140–159	90–99
Second stage	≥ 160	≥ 100

Precautions

- In anxious and apprehensive patients, BP should be taken after relaxation.
- In obese patients, a wider cuff (15 cm instead of 12.5 cm) may be used. For thin patients, a pediatric cuff may be used.
- In patients with an arrhythmia, i.e. ectopics or atrial fibrillation, determine several observations and take a mean of those readings.

OEDEMA

☞ *Look for oedema*

Compare one foot and leg with the other, noting their relative size and the prominence of veins, tendons and bones.

Oedema causes swelling that may obscure the veins, tendon and bony prominences.

Cardiovascular System

☞ *Check for pitting oedema (Figs 3.9A and B)*

If you suspect oedema, measurement of the legs may help you to identify it.

A difference of more than 1 cm just above the ankle or 2 cm at the calf is unusual in normal persons and suggests oedema.

To demonstrate the pitting oedema, press over the medial malleolus by a thumb for 15 seconds and look for a pit on removal of the thumb (Fig. 3.9).

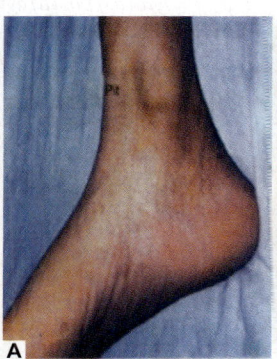 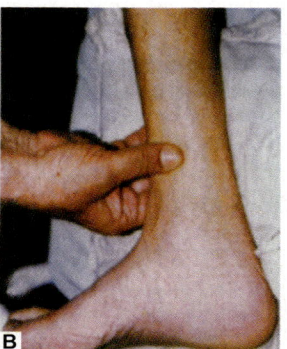

Figs 3.9A and B: Demonstration of pitting ankle oedema. (A) Swollen right leg and ankle; (B) Pressure over the medial malleolus by a thumb till nail blanches for 15 seconds produces a pit on removal of the thumb.

SYSTEMIC EXAMINATION OF CARDIOVASCULAR SYSTEM

It is done under: (i) *Inspection*; (ii) *Palpation*; (iii) *Percussion*, and (iv) *Auscultation*.

☞ INSPECTION (TO LOOK AT)

Position

The patient is made to lie comfortably at 45° on the bed couch with shoulders horizontal and chest fully exposed. The examiner should stand or sit on the right side facing the patient.

A tangential inspection of the chest with the patient recumbent either from one side of both the sides or from the foot gives valuable information regarding precordial pulsations and swellings. Note the following features of chest.

1. Size, shape and type of chest

This part is dealt during the inspection of respiratory system. *Scoliosis, straight back syndrome (normal concavity of upper dorsal column is lost), kyphoscoliosiss, pectum excavatum* may have important bearing on the heart, hence must be noted.

2. Shape of precordium:
Normaly chest is bilaterally symmetrical. Buldging or retraction of the chest can occur due to:

a. *Skeletal deformities*, i.e. scoliosis, kyphoscoliosis lead to asymmetry of chest, shoulders and nipples.
  - Backward sternal bulge, i.e. *pectum excavatum* pushes the heart to the left simulating heart disease.
  - Flat chest/shield chest in a female suggests *Turner's syndrome* with or without conigenital heart disease (coarctation of aorta).

b. *Disease of lungs and pleura (pneumothorax, pleural effusion midiastinal growth)* can lead to chest deformity.

c. *Diseases of heart and pericardium* such as *ventricular hypertrophy, pericardial effusion, congenital heart disease* may produce bulging of precordium.
  - Localised bulge of a part of precordium may be due to *ventricular aneurysm*. Upper body parts including chest are well developed than the lower part of the body (legs and trunk are thin) in *coarctation of the aorta*.
  - Pericardial flattening or retraction may be seen in pericardial adhesions (constrictive pericarditis) or lung collapse or fibrosis.

3. *Scar:* Look for the scars and note its site.
  - *Midline sternotomy scar* indicates coronary artery bypass surgery or valvotomy.
  - *A mark of needle prick with or without cotton swab* over the precordium indicates tapping of the pericardial effusion.

4. *Apex beat:*
Cardiac impulse is a circumscribed systolic outward and forward thrust of the heart imparted to the precordium. *Apex beat* is, thus, the lowermost and outermost point of the cardiac pulsation seen or felt.

Normal apex beat being less the 2.5 cm in diameter lies in the 5th intercostal space within midclavicular line in an adult in the sitting position.

  - The apex beat is observed for (i) *presence or absence*, (ii) *location* (normally placed or displaced), (iii) *whether localized or diffuse*, (iv) whether *single or double*, and (v) for other characteristics.

Normal variation of apex beat
- In thin and narrow chested elderly persons, it may sometimes be seen in 6th intercostal space.
- It may be displaced up and outwards by eventration of the diaphragm or raised diaphragm.

Abnormalities of apex beat
- They are confirmed on palpation but can be noted on inspection. They are:

i. Nonvisible apex beat
- Apex beat is not visible in obese persons and women with heavy breasts, patients with pleural/pericardial effusion, emphysema and dextrocardia. It may be hidden under a rib.

ii. Displacement of apex beat
a. Apex beat may be displaced further to left by extraneous forces which may pull the heart to same side, i.e. *pneumectomy, collapse of the lung/lung fibrosis*.
b. It may be pushed to opposite side (*pneumothorax, pleural effusion*).
c. It may be displaced upwards by *ascites*, an *abdominal tumour, eventration of diaphragm*.
d. Left ventricular hypertrophy (AR, MR) displace the apex beat down and out where as right ventricular hypertrophy shift it outwards only.
e. *Congenitally displaced apex beat*. Apex beat is formed by the left ventricle, hence lies on the left side. In dextrocardia it lies on the right side than the left.

iii. Extent of apex beat
- The normal apex beat is less than 2.5 cm in diameter and occupies single intercostal space. When apex beat occupies a larger area (more than one space) it is called *diffuse apex beat*. Diffuse apex beat occupying two or three spaces make the precordium shaky. Diffuseness of apex beat is due to:
  a. Normal in thin chest person.
  b. Hyperkinetic states (anaemia, thyrotoxicosis, AR, AV fistula, etc.)
  c. Severe valvular regurgitation (AR or MR)
  d. Left to right shunts
  e. Hypertrophic or dilated cardiomyopathy
  f. Collapse of the lung

iv. Force of apex beat
Apex beat with good force visible over 2–3 spaces is called *hyperkinetic* and with less force (*imperceptible*) is called *hypokinetic*. The **causes** of hyperkinetic apex beat are same as diffuseness of apex beat as listed above.
The **causes** of *hypokinetic impulse* are:
- Shock (hypovolaemia)
- Myocarditis
- Myocardial infarction.

v. Double apex beat
It is characteristic of hypertrophic obstructive cardiomyopathy (HOCM) in which LV forming the apex is divided into two chambers by hypertrophied interventricular septum resulting in double apex beat.

5. Other pericardial movements
i. *Left parasternal pulsation* may be seen in massive right ventricular hypertrophy due to any cause. This may be associated with a heave on palpation.
ii. *See-saw (rock and roll) movements of precordium* are observed in massive hypertrophy of one of the ventricles either right or left.
iii. *Systolic retraction of precordium* (sucking of precordium) is seen in adhesive pericarditis, tricuspid regurgitation, etc.

6. Other pulsations of the chest wall
- *Upper sternal pulsations* are seen in aneurysm of ascending aorta or aortic arch, aortic root dilatation (Marfan's syndrome) and marked AR.
- *Pulsations in second and third left intercostal spaces* are due to dilatation of pulmonary artery/conus in PDA and left to right shunts and aneurysm of descending aorta.
- *Prominent and pulsating vessels* in the *upper part of chest both front (infraclavicular region) and back (interscapular region)* are best seen in coarctation of aorta when patient bends forward.
- *Suprasternal pulsations*. Pulsations in the suprasternal notch are fairly common in apparent thin normal individual. Pulsations are also seen in hyperkinetic conditions already described. In addition, pulsations occur in aortic arch aneurysm, aortic regurgitation, unfolded aorta and anomalous right subclavian artery.
- *Epigastric pulsations*. They are also seen in thin persons normally but occur abnormally in abdominal aortic aneurysm, right ventricular hypertrophy and hemangioma of the liver.

☞ PALPATION (TO FEEL)
Palpation is done to confirm the findings of inspection.
Palpate the apex beat over the precordium.

Method: The apex beat is preferably palpated in the sitting position. The palpation is done by flat hand (*palmar palpation*) which must be warmed (by rubbing against each other) and put on different areas of precordium. The localization of the apex beat is done with the tip of the index finger or tips of the second and third fingers of the right hand. It is often necessary to manually displace the breast upwards in females for palpation of apex beat.

What is apex beat?
The pulsations palpable over the precordium only indicate ventricular trust (right/left), does not mean

the apex beat. Hence, the apex beat mean most lateral or outer most point of the cardiac impulse felt by the palpating finger.

The **characteristics** of normal apex beat are:
1. It lies within 10 cm from the midsternal line inner to midclavicular line.
2. It occupies only one intercostal space.
3. It just comes as an upward thrust, touches the finger and goes back (*up-touch-go apex beat*).

I. Abnormal Palpable Apex Beats

1. *Heaving or sustained apex beat:* It means the apex beat lifts the palpating finger slowly and sustains it for a moment. It indicates left ventricular hypertrophy due to any cause (e.g. AS, hypertension).
2. *Hyperdynamic/hyperkinetic apex beat:* It is a diffuse forceful apex beat palpable over a wider area (2–3 spaces) of precordium. It represents hyperdynamic left ventricle due to volume overload. This is seen in MR, AR, left to right shunts and cardiomyopathy.
3. *Tapping apex beat:* Apex beat is felt as a sharp, systolic tap. Actually it is nothing but a palpable first heart sound. This is felt characteristically in mitral stenosis.
4. *Double apex beat:* It is bifid apex beat where two systolic thrusts are felt. This is characteristic of hypertrophic obstructive cardiomyopathy (HOCM).
5. *Ill sustained but forceful apex beat (slapping apex beat).* The apex beat just slaps the palm and go back. It indicates hyperkinetic circulation, seen in fevers, thyrotoxicosis and after exercise or excitement.
6. *Nonpalpable apex beat:* Apex beat may not be visible or palpable in certain conditions already mentioned during inspection. Sometimes, hypokinetic apex beat may also not be palpable.
7. *Paradoxical apex beat:* The outward movement of some part of precordium over and above the apex beat—*a paradox*, hence, called paradoxical apex beat. This paradoxical apex beat occurs when LV fills and expands during systolic contraction of the ventricle in ventricular aneurysm.

II. Parasternal Heave

The pulsations or lift felt in the parasternal area is called *parasternal heave*. It may be left or right parasternal heave.

a. *Left parasternal heave*: It occurs both during volume and pressure overloading of left ventricle.
b. *Right parasternal heave*. The heaving of right parasternal area occurs in left ventricular hypertrophy, chronic cor pulmonale, left to right shunts. Thus, heave is nothing but represents either the hyperdynamicity or hypertrophy of the ventricle lying behind the sternum.

III. Other Pulsations Felt

- *Pulsations of aortic aneurysm or unforded aorta* may be felt right of the sternum.
- *Intercostal pulsations due to coarctation of aorta.* They are best felt than seen in the interscapular regions when patient bends forwards with arms by the side thus stretching the skin of the back.
- *Epigastric pulsations.* They are felt by keeping one finger below the xiphisternum and pressing it a little backwards and upwards. Alternative method is to palpate the epigastrium by putting 2–3 finger in epigastrium. They are produced by (i) right ventricular hypertrophy, (ii) aortic aneurysm and (iii) *pulsatile liver*. They can occur normal in thin persons.

The differences between right ventricular and aortic pulsations in epigastrium are
1. The right ventricular pulsations are felt as downward movements while aortic pulsations are up and down movements.
2. Parasternal heave is invariably associated with RVH not with aortic pulsations.
3. Put the two fingers in epigastrium to feel the pulsations and note whether the fingers are separated or just lifted. These are separated in aortic pulsation. No such separation occurs with RV pulsations rather fingers are lifted and pushed downwards.

Pulsatile liver. An expansile pulsations of the liver occurs in TR or TS, which can be palpated by bimanual method (read clinical methods by DR SN Chugh) in which one hand is placed over the lower anterior chest and other is placed over posterolateral part of chest. The separation of the hands by impulses felt by both hands indicate pulsatile liver.

The differences between pulsatile liver and aortic pulsations transmitted to liver are
a. The pulsations transmitted from the aorta (aortic aneurysm) will disappear when patient assumes knee-elbow position while that of pulsatile liver persist.
b. Pulsatile liver is associated with raised JVP, '*vy*', collapse and parasternal lift.
c. Signs of pulmonary hypertension may be present/associated with pulsatile liver.

IV. Thrills

Palpate for the thrill over the precordium
- A thrill is defined as a vibratory sensation felt over the area of the heart or aorta.

They resemble sensations from the throat of a purring cat. In fact, they indicate loud palpable murmurs, help in the localization of the maximum intensity of a murmur when normal column of blood flows through a normal defect.

Method: They are best palpated by just placing lightly the palm of the hand over the area of the thrill. They get obliterated by pressure. The following features should be noted about the thrill.
   a. *Site of maximum palpability.*
   b. *Its extent*
   c. *Whether systolic/diastolic/continuous*
   d. *Radiation to other sites*

The various thrills, site of production and their radiation are represented in Table 3.5.

V. Palpable Pericardial Rub

Palpate the pericardial rub at precordial area

- A friction or scratching sound produced by the friction between two layers of pericardium is called *friction rub*. It may be palpable as well as audible. It is best heart in mid-precordial region with held respiration. If it changes its character with respiration, it is called *pleuropericardial rub*.

Causes of Pericardial Rub
- *Infective pericarditis* (bacterial, viral, fungal and parasitic)
- *Autoimmune pericarditis,* e.g. SLE, RA, acute rheumatic pancarditis.
- *Drug-induced pericarditis,* e.g. hydralazine, procainamide, isoniazid, anticoagulant, Dressler's syndrome.
- *Postmyocardial infarction.*
- *Traumatic, bleeding disorders.*
- *Metabolic,* e.g. uraemia, hypothyroidism
- *Miscellaneous,* e.g. radiation, sarcoidosis, amyloidosis, etc.

N.B. Pericardial rub may mimic a continuous murmur; hence has to be differentiated (Box 3.4).

Box 3.4: Differences between Pericardial Rub and a Continuous Murmur

Pericardial rub	Continuous murmur
• Rubbing or scratching sound	• Soft, musical, machinery sound
• Heard either in systole or diastole	• Heard both in systole and diastole
• Best heard in sitting position with held respiration when patient leans forward	• Heard in all positions
• Associated with pain	• No pain
• Inconsistent and intermittent in character, i.e. appear and disappear	• Consistent character

VI. Palpable Heart Sounds

Palpate the precordium for heart sounds

Heart sounds are produced by vibrations of opening and closing of the heart valves, and if these vibrations get accentuated, the sound becomes loud and becomes palpable, for example; in severe mitral stenosis, the first heart sound is accentuated and becomes palpable. Aortic component of second heart sound in aortic area gets accentuated and becomes palpable in systemic hypertension. In syphilitic aortitis, aortic component is accentuated and becomes *tambour-like sound.*

TABLE 3.5: Thrills, their Nature, Site of Production and Radiation

Thrill and its nature	Lesion	Site of production	Radiation
I. Systolic thrill	• MR	Apex	Left axilla
	• VSD	Lower part of sternum	Rt side of sternum
	• Pulmonary stenosis	Pulmonary area (second left intercostal space)	—
	• Aortic stenosis	Aortic area (second right space)	Neck vessel
II. Diastolic thrill	Mitral stenosis	Apex (in left lateral position)	—
	Aortic regurgitation	Aortic area (2nd right and 3rd left)	—
III. Continuous thrill	Patent ductus arteriosus (PDA)	Left first intercostal space below the clavicle	—
IV. Noncardiac thrill	Coarctation of aorta	Interscapular area over the collateral vessels	—

Tracheal Tug

Feel for the tracheal tug in suprasternal notch
- A downward pull or tug felt with each heartbeat by the fingers placed on both the sides of carotid and applying firm upward pressure is called *tracheal tug*. This is felt in aortic aneurysm. With each heartbeat, aneurysm depresses the left bronchus downwards which in turns pulls down the trachea.

☞ PERCUSSION (TO ELICIT THE NOTE OF RESONANCE)

Percussion is method of examination which interprets the amount of resistance encountered on subjecting the chest to a series of strokes or taps with the fingers placed in the intercostal spaces or with a special instrument.

In this method, resonance of the chest is analysed for *pitch*, *intensity* and *character* of the sound. A special attention is paid to the resistance encountered during percussion. The chest becomes *dull* (sound is imperceptible with maximum resistance encountered during percussion when fluid or solid growth or a consolidated part of lung is present). It becomes *hyper-resonant* (chest vibrates easily with audible sound and no resistance is encountered during percussion) when either the lungs are hyper-voluminous (*emphysema*) or air is present in the pleural cavity (*pneumothorax*).

Methods of Percussion

1. *Direct* where strokes are discharged directly at the chest wall. This method is used for percussion over the clavicles in special circumstances.
2. *Indirect* where strokes are discharged on the fingers placed on the chest wall. This method of percussion is employed routinely.

Rules of percussion (read clinical methods in medicine by DR SN Chugh).

Aims and Objectives of Percussion

i. To define the percussion note, i.e. *normal*, *abnormal* (hyper-resonant, dull, stony dull, impaired).
ii. To define the cardiac borders. The dullness beyond the normal cardiac dullness indicates pericardial effusion.
iii. To define the upper borders of the liver and liver span.
iv. Area of supracardiac dullness, i.e. 2nd left space in pulmonary hypertension and area of slight dullness over the upper part of sternum and 2nd right intercostal space in aortic aneurysm, mediastinal tumour and substernal goitre.

Note. Now-a-days, the value of percussion in clinical medicine is limited just to define the upper border of liver and demonstrating the hyper-resonant lungs in emphysema. In cardiology, it is considered as useless exercise because the area of cardiac dullness on percussion, is doubtful.

Defining the Cardiac Dullness/Borders

A. Left Cardiac Border

The left cardiac border is defined first of all by percussing the fifth left interspace from the axilla inwards/towards the sternum. A definite impairment or change of note from normal resonant note appears as the apex of the heart is reached. This is noted. Normally, it corresponds to the apex beat. Similarly, the left border is percussed in the third and fourth space.

The normal left border in adult lies about 7–9 cm from the midsternal line in the 5th interspace and 3½ to 4 cm in the third space.

B. Right Cardiac Border

The reliability of defining the right border of the heart is doubtful because of vibrating qualities of the sternum. However, in gross enlargement of the heart, the right border dullness can be appreciated. It is defined by percussing 3rd and 4th right intercostal spaces from midclavicular line towards sternum noting the change in note, i.e. resonant to dull.

Normally right border of heart lies just lateral to the right border of sternum, however, dullness beyond 0.5 cm from the right sternal border indicates gross heart enlargement or pericardial effusion. Besides this percussion is carried out in the second interspace both to the right and left of sternum to determine dullness due to pulmonary hypertension (left second space) and aortic aneurysm (right second space).

Abnormalities of Cardiac Dullness

Left border of cardiac dullness may be displaced further to left beyond normal in left ventricular hypertrophy, pericardial effusion and due to mediastinal shift in left lung collapse/fibrosis/pneumonectomy or pushed by right-sided pleural effusion and pneumothorax.

Defining Upper Border of the Liver

(*Read Respiratory System*)
It is defined by percussing the right side of the chest in midclavicular line from the second

intercostal space downward till a change of note is felt. This space indicates the upper border of the liver dullness.

Normal liver dullness lies in 5th intercostal space. It may be pushed down by right pleural effusion or pneumothorax.

Liver Span

(*Read Examination of Abdomen*)

Liver span is enlarged due to hepatomegaly in CHF/pericardial effusion.

☞ AUSCULTATION (TO HEAR)

Auscultation is method of hearing sounds over the precordium, across the great vessel and over the vascular areas (tumour, thyroid). The heart sounds are produced by closure and opening of the heart valves, movement of the myocardium during rapid filling phase and by the flow of blood into the ventricles and across the normal and abnormal valves and vascular sounds over the communication or a defect or rumor, thyroid (Graves' disease) and aneurysm of great vessels.

Aims of Auscultation

- To hear heart sounds, their character, intensity and splitting.
- To hear adventitious sounds/murmurs, if present then to note their intensity, character, grade and radiation.

- *Any change with alteration in position or with exercises.*

Surface Marking of Heart Valves and Areas of Auscultation

The heart valves are diagrammatically represented in Fig. 3.10 with surface marking. The auscultation is done in Z-shaped manner starting from mitral to tricuspid, pulmonary and aortic areas.

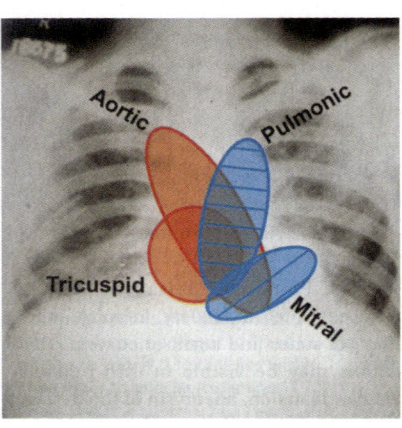

Fig. 3.10: Surface marking of the heart valves for auscultation in Z-shaped manner, i.e. mitral area at apex, tricuspid area at 4th intercostal space, left sternal border, pulmonary area (2nd left interspace) and last of all aortic area (A1 at right second intercostal space).

TABLE 3.6: Normal Heart Sounds

Heart sounds	Area to be auscultated	Abnormality
• **First heart sound.** It is produced by closure of mitral and tricuspid valves	• At the apex (5th intercostal space inner to midclavicular line)	• *Loud Ist sound* is heart in MS, left to right shunt, and hyperdynamic circulation • *Intermittent loud 1st sound (cannon sound)* is heard in complete heart block • *Variable intensity of Ist sound* is heard in AF • *Muffled sound* occurs in MR, TR and calcified valves
• **Second heart sound.** The sound is produced by closure of aortic valve (aortic component) and pulmonary valve (pulmonary component)	• Aortic components heard over aortic area (second right and third left interspace) and pulmonary component (P_2) is heard over left second intercostal space	• *Loud second sound* occurs in systemic hypertension (A_2 is loud), and pulmonary hypertension (P_2 is loud) • *Decrease in intensity of second sound* occurs in aortic stenosis, aortic regurgitation and pulmonary regurgitation and pulmonary stenosis
• **Third heart sound.** It is produced by tensing of the myocardium during rapid filling phase	• Heard with the bell of stethoscope (low-pitched sound) at the apex	• Normally heard in children, young adults and pregnant women • It is heard in mitral, aortic and tricuspid incompetence and in dilated cardiomyopathy
• **Fourth heart sound.** It is produced by atrial contractions during late diastole	• Heard over the right/left sternal border with bell of stethoscope (low-pitched sound)	• It is present in systemic hypertension, AS, hypertrophic cardiomyopathy, IHD and acute MR

Heart Sounds

- Listen to the heart sounds over the designated area (Table 3.6) and note their *intensity* or *pitch* and *splitting*.

High-pitched sounds (S_1, S_2, opening snap and systolic murmurs and aortic diastolic murmur) are low intensity sounds, best heard with diaphragm of stethoscope.

Low-pitched sounds (S_3, S_4 and mitral diastolic murmur)

- These are high intensity sounds heard on the chest wall by the bell of stethoscope loosely applied.
- Note the regularity of the heart for rhythm. If the pulse rate is irregular, then count the heart rate over the apex. Note the difference between the heart rate and pulse rate called *pulse deficit*.

Normally there is no pulse deficit. Pulse deficit indicates either extrasystoles or atrial fibrillation (AF).

Triple rhythm and gallop rhythm: When the third or fourth heart sound becomes prominent and loud, the cadence produced by the three heart sounds is called *triple rhythm*. As already mentioned, triple rhythm (presence of 3rd heart sound) is normal in children, young adults and pregnant women. Abnormally it is present in congestive heart failure and in other conditions mentioned in Table 3.6. When triple rhythm is associated with tachycardia, it is called *gallop rhythm*. When 3rd and 4th heart sounds appear together in gallop rhythm, it is called *summation gallop rhythm* (summation effect of 3rd and 4th sounds).

- *Effect of exercise.* When rhythm is irregular, then to differentiate between multiple ectopics and atrial fibrillation, the patient is made to exercise the legs, if condition allows, on the bed. He/she lies and sits ups, repeats this leg exercise for 4–5 times.

Atrial fibrillation becomes more irregular while multiple ectopics either disappear or decrease in number. Heart block is generally not altered.

Splitting of the Heart Sounds

Split first heart sound. The mitral valve closes earlier than tricuspid, hence, split is natural but not appreciated clinically due to a very short interval of separation. However, if split is present and appreciated, it is not indicative of heart disease, but a sign of right bundle branch block which is mostly congenital.

Split second heart sound: The splitting of the second sound is appreciable because aortic (A_2) and pulmonary (P_2) components are widely separated and both the components are audible in the pulmonary area (P_2), hence, splitting is best heard at or close to pulmonary area, i.e. 2nd left interspace close to the sternum. The normal and abnormal splitting of 2nd heart sound and their causes are presented in Fig. 3.11.

Atrial fibrillation has to be differentiated from multiple ectopics (Box 3.5).

Box 3.5 Multiple Ectopic vs Atrial Fibrillation

Ectopics	Atrial fibrillation
• Occasionally irregular	Irregularly irregular
• Pulse deficit is <10/bpm	Pulse deficit >10/bpm
• Exercise abolishes them	No effect of exercise
• 'a' wave is present in JVP	No effect of exercise 'a' wave is absent on JVP

Adventitious (Added) Sounds

Auscultate for any adventitious sound

- *The audible ejection clicks.* These are high-pitched sounds produced by opening and closing of the semilunar valves in patients with valvular stenosis (aortic, pulmonary) and over the great vessel dilatation (aortic root and pulmonary artery dilatation). These clicks indicate pliable valves, hence, become absent when the valve gets calcified.
- *Non-ejection midsystolic clicks.* These are the sounds produced by column of blood passing through incompetent mitral/tricuspid valve or its apparatus (redundant chordae tendineae) resulting in its prolapse. These are heard in mitral and tricuspid valve prolapse either at the apex or along the left sternal border and they are influenced by the manoeuvres which have been discussed with murmurs.
- *Metallic (prosthetic) sounds.* These are high-pitched sounds produced by mechanical heart valves during opening and closing. These are heard in the area of replaced valve, i.e. at apex in mitral valve and second right space in aortic valve replacement.
- *Opening snap (OS).* As the name suggests, it is high-pitched snappy diastolic sound produced by restricted opening of the stenosed valve. It occurs when the valve is thickened and stenosed but pliable. It occurs about 0.09 to 0.12 second after the second heart sound (between S_2 and S_1). This is produced due to sudden doming of mitral valve apparatus during diastole when the LV attempts to suck left atrial blood into the LV cavity. During this doming, the anterior leaflet bulges downward with a snap.

Diagram

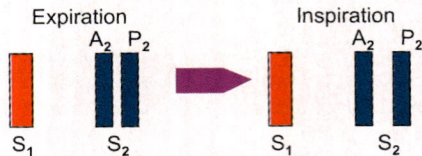

Normal or physiological split widens in inspiration and narrows in expiration.

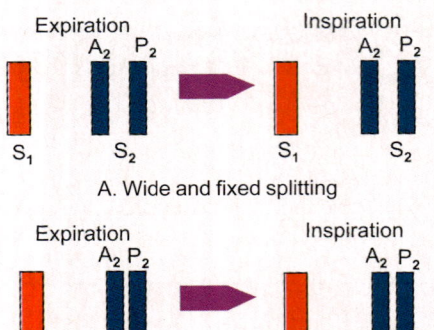
A. Wide and fixed splitting

B. Narrow and fixed splitting

Fixed splitting of second heart sound. The splitting does not change during inspiration and expiration. It may be wide and fixed or narrow and fixed.

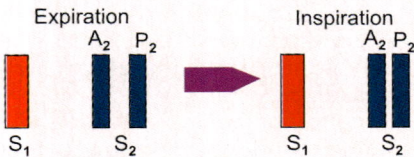

Reversed or paradoxical splitting (e.g.) splitting occurs maximally in expiration and decreases during inspiration. Even in inspiration, splitting is so narrow that it may appear as single S_2 as shown in diagram.

Cause(s)

Seen in normal individuals. A single sound (S_2) in inspiration is normal in adults

Wide and fixed splitting is characteristic of atrial septal defect (ASD).

Wide but not fixed splitting occurs in right ventricular hypertrophy due to pulmonary stenosis and right bundle branch block.

In pulmonary hypertension, splitting may be normal, narrow or wide, depending on its cause and pulmonary vascular resistance.

Reversed splitting occurs in left ventricular outflow obstruction, a large aorto-pulmonary shunt, systolic hypertension, left bundle branch block.

Fig. 3.11: Splitting of second heart sound.

Significance

1. It signifies that valve leaflets are mobile even though valve is stenosed.
2. The *"second sound–OS interval"* (interval between second heart sound and the opening snap) is a guide to the severity of MS. The nearer the OS to second heart sound, more severe is the stenosis. This interval also decreases after exercise, in tachycardias and AF besides MS.
3. The OS becomes absent when the valve is calcified or chordae tendineae and papillary muscles are dysfunctional due to matting or fusion.
4. OS becomes absent when moderate mitral regurgitation is associated with mitral stenosis. With mild mitral regurgitation the OS may persist in patients with MS.

Characteristics of OS

1. It is sharp, snappy clicking sound audible after second heart sound.
2. It is best heard over the fourth intercostal space along the left sternal border.
3. It is best heard with diaphragm of stethoscope.
4. It is accentrated by exercise.
5. No effect of deep inspiration. It does not change during AF, i.e. persists despite AF.
6. It is usually accompanied by loud S1.
7. It persists after mitral valvotomy due to sub-valvular fusion.

Differential diagnosis of OS

Following conditions have to be differentiated from OS.

1. *Loud split second sound.* OS is best heard at the *apex along left sternal* border and standing

increases the distance between OS and S_2, (S_2–OS interval increases). On the other hand, loud split S_2 is heard best at 2nd left space and split increases during inspiration.

2. *Pericardial knock* (read it below)
3. *Tumour flop* of left atrial myxoma. The flop changes with change in the position of the patient from sitting to supine.
4. *Ball valve thrombus* that moves freely from LA into LV, hence, murmur changes with position.

Other causes of OS

1. *Mitral regurgitation*. Though mitral regurgitation is known to produce absence of OS but when anterior leaflet is thickened and rigid and posterior leaflet remains mobile, OS can occur. This is an exceptional situation in MR.
2. *Subendocardial fibroelastosis* which is also associated with stiff and fibrosed mitral valve.
3. *Left atrial myoxma* (10% cases). Myxoma occludes mitral valve intermittently and produces OS.
4. *Large left to right shunts*, e.g. large VSD, PDA, etc. and after Blalock-Taussig operation for tetralogy of Fallot.
5. *Hyperdynamic circulation*, e.g. thyrotoxicosis.

OS of tricuspid valve (tricuspid snap)

It is rare and seldom heard because of invariable presence of MS (mitral snap). It is heard along the right sternal border in the 4th intercostal space with bell. It indicates tricuspid stenosis (congenital or acquired associated with MS), left to right shunt in ASD and sometimes in chronic constrictive pericarditis involving the tricuspid valve in constriction (a constriction band around tricuspid valve).

- *Pericardial knock (rub):* It is a superficial high-pitched scratching sound heard best with patient leaning forward during expiration. It is heard both during systole and diastole at left sternal border with the bell of the stethoscope. It is a characteristic sign of acute pericarditis. Its intensity varies from time to time with resolution or progression of pericarditis.

Vascular Sounds and Extraneous Sounds

Sometimes, vascular sounds may be audible normally over the right carotids.

Pistol shot sounds. These systolic sounds are heard over the great vessels in patients with gross AR. These are produced due to sudden rush of blood through a large peripheral vessel due to gross reduction in peripheral resistance.

Extraneous sounds (muscular sounds, crepitations): These are sounds produced by extraneous structures which mimic heart sounds and murmurs, e.g., muscular sounds (rumbling or roaring) or hairy crepitations (due to rubbing of the chestpiece with hairs on the chest). These hairy crepitations can be minimised either by moistening or shaving of hair.

Arterial bruit. Bruit can be heard over a narrow blood vessel (renal artery stenosis) and a dilated blood vessel (aortic aneurysm). For renal bruit auscultate the abdomen with stethoscope placed just above and lateral to umbilicus on each side or over the costophrenic angles on each side on the back.

For bruit over the aortic aneurysm, place stethoscope just lateral to umbilicus on either side.

MURMURS

Definition: A murmur is defined as an auditory sound or vibrations produced as a result of turbulence set up by the rapid flow of blood through the valves (normal or narrowed), or a defect or chordae tendineae and dilated great vessels.

Significance

1. The presence of murmur does not imply a heart disease as innocent murmurs are commonly associated with normal heart.
2. Serious heart disease can occur in the absence of murmurs, i.e. MI, congenital heart disease, etc.
3. The intensity of the murmur does not correlate with the severity of heart lesion. However, the length or duration of a murmur is better indicator of severity and prognosis than the intensity.
4. A murmur heard over the heart (precordium) need not necessarily be of cardiac origin. It could be of extracardiac origin.
5. A very loud murmur or cooing murmur usually indicates organic heart disease.
6. Diastolic murmur is always organic in origin while systolic murmur may be organic as well as innocent.
7. A stenotic or regurgitant murmur need not be valvular in origin, they can be produced due to relative or functional stenosis or regurgitation due to rapid large blood flow through a normal valve. These are called *functional murmur*.
8. Left-sided murmurs usually occur due to acquired heart disease while the right-sided murmurs are usually due to congenital heart disease (pulmonary and tricuspid).

Pathogenesis and Pathophysiology

They occur mainly due to three mechanisms, i.e.
1. High velocity flow causing turbulence through a valve (narrow/normal), a cardiac defect, or

a vessel or an abnormal communication, for example, patent ductus which acts as a tube of uniform calibre.
2. Setting up of vibrations by a turbulent flow under hemodynamic conditions (*benign murmurs*).
3. Backflow of blood through a regurgitant (incompetent) valve produce diastolic murmurs.
4. Continuous flow through extracardiac or intracardiac shunts producing continuous systolic as well as diastolic gradient results in continuous murmurs.
5. The vibration of loose, soft structures such as torn cusps, chordae tendineae or loose chordae tendineae or papillary muscles result in production of murmurs.

☞ *Listen to the murmur over different areas (mitral, aortic, pulmonary and tricuspid)*

One has to describe the murmur under the following heads:
1. *Timing of the murmur* (whether systolic or diastolic)
2. *Intensity/loudness/pitch*
3. *Site where it is best heard*
4. *Quality/character* (soft, harse, rough and rumble, cooing, etc.)
5. *Radiation* to any site
6. *Grade of the murmur* (whether associated with thrill)

Classification and Causes of Murmurs (Table 3.8)

I. Timing of Murmur

Depending on the timing, they can be *systolic, diastolic and continuous murmur*.

The main differences between systolic and diastolic murmurs are given in Table 3.7.

TABLE 3.7: Distinguishing Features of Two Commonly Encountered Murmurs

Systolic murmur	Diastolic murmur
• Soft and blowing	• Rough and rumble (mitral) or blowing (aortic and pulmonary)
• Crescendo-decrescendo	• Decrescendo in character
• Shows radiation. Mitral murmurs radiate to left axilla and aortic to neck vessels	• Nonradiating
• They are ejection systolic, midsystolic, pansystolic and late systolic	• Early and mid-diastolic
• Appears between 1st and 2nd heart sounds	• Appears between 2nd and 1st heart sounds

Whether a murmur is systolic or diastolic, is decided by its timing with apex beat or carotid pulse. Therefore, while hearing the murmur, fingers must be put on carotid pulse to time it. Carotid pulse normally coincides with first heart sound. A systolic murmur is heard between 1st and 2nd heart sounds. A diastolic murmur is heard between 2nd and 1st heart sounds, i.e. during diastole. A continuous murmur is heard both in systole and diastole.

II. The Loudness or Intensity of Murmurs

It is graded on a scale of 1–6. The murmur associated with a thrill is graded IV loud murmur. **Grade I** is difficult to hear and **Grade VI** is heard with stethoscope without touching the chest, i.e. by lifting the stethoscope for a smallest distance from the chest. The grading of murmur is as follows:

Grade I : Murmur is faint and audible with difficulty.
Grade II : Soft, faint but heard easily with the stethoscope.
Grade III : Moderate intensity.
Grade IV : Loud murmur associated with thrill.
Grade V : Very loud with thrill, may be heard when the stethoscope is partly off the chest.
Grade VI : Heard with stethoscope without touching the chest.

Systolic murmurs: The ejection or midsystolic murmurs are associated with ventricular outflow obstruction, occur in early or midsystole and exhibit crescendo-decrescendo character. *Pansystolic* murmurs extend from 1st heart sound throughout systole with constant intensity, hence, also called *holosystolic*. Late systolic murmurs occur during the end of systole.

Diastolic murmurs: Mid-diastolic murmurs occur due to turbulent flow across mitral and tricuspid valves during diastole. Early diastolic murmur occurs due to regurgitation of blood flow from aortic and pulmonary valves into the heart. They are decrescendo and blowing in character.

Benign systolic (physiologic) murmurs: The characteristics of benign systolic murmurs are:
- They do not occur beyond early or midsystole.
- They are soft and musical
- Mostly midsystolic or ejection systolic
- Heard at the left sternal edge
- They do not radiate
- Not associated with thrill
- No other cardiac abnormality

Continuous murmurs: These usually result from combination of systolic and diastolic flow across a communicating channel between heart and a vessel or between two vessels having different pressures. These murmurs start with the onset of systole, pass through the systole with increasing intensity and, then pass through 2nd heart sound to enter into diastole (*waxing and waning character*). These murmurs represent constant gradient during systole and diastole. They are heard in patients *with patent ductus arteriosus, aortopulmonary window, an arteriovenous fistula, coronary arteriovenous fistula and communication between sinus of Valsalva and right side of the heart.*

The types of murmurs, their location and conditions in which they are produced are given in Table 3.8.

TABLE 3.8: Classification and Causes of Murmurs

I. **Systolic murmurs**
   A. **Ejection systolic (Fig. 3.12A)**
      i. *Normal or reduced flow through stenotic valve*
         - Aortic valvular stenosis
         - Pulmonary valvular stenosis
      ii. *Abnormal rapid flow through normal valves (innocent flow murmurs)*
         - Fever
         - Athletes
         - Pregnancy
         - High cardiac output states, e.g. beriberi, thyrotoxicosis, Paget's disease, AV fistula, etc.
         - Atrial septal defect (pulmonary flow murmur)
      iii. *Other causes*
         - Hypertrophic cardiomyopathy (obstruction of left ventricular outflow—subvalvular stenosis)
         - Acute aortic regurgitation (aortic flow murmur)
   B. **Midsystolic murmur (Fig. 3.12B)**
      - Mitral valve prolapse. There is an associated midsystolic click.
   C. **Pansystolic (Fig. 3.12C)**
      - Mitral regurgitation
      - Tricuspid regurgitation
      - Ventricular septal defect
      - Leaking mitral or tricuspid prosthesis
      - Mitral valve prolapse
      - Rupture of chordae tendineae in acute MI
   D. **Late systolic murmur (Fig. 3.12D)**
      - Papillary muscle dysfunction

II. **Diastolic murmurs**
   A. **Early diastolic (Fig. 3.12E)**
      - Aortic regurgitation
      - Pulmonary regurgitation (Graham-Steell's murmur)
   B. **Mid-diastolic (Fig. 3.12F)**
      - Mitral stenosis
      - Tricuspid stenosis
      - Austin-Flint murmur of functional mitral stenosis
      - Carrey-Coombs' murmur of mitral valvulitis
   C. **Late diastolic or presystolic (Fig. 3.12G)**
      - Pre-systolic murmur is heard in mild MS, while pre-systolic accentuation of MDM indicates moderate to severe MS

III. **Continuous murmur (Fig. 3.12H)**
   - PDA
   - Aortopulmonary window
   - Rupture of sinus of Valsalva into right atrium
   - Coronary arteriovenous fistula

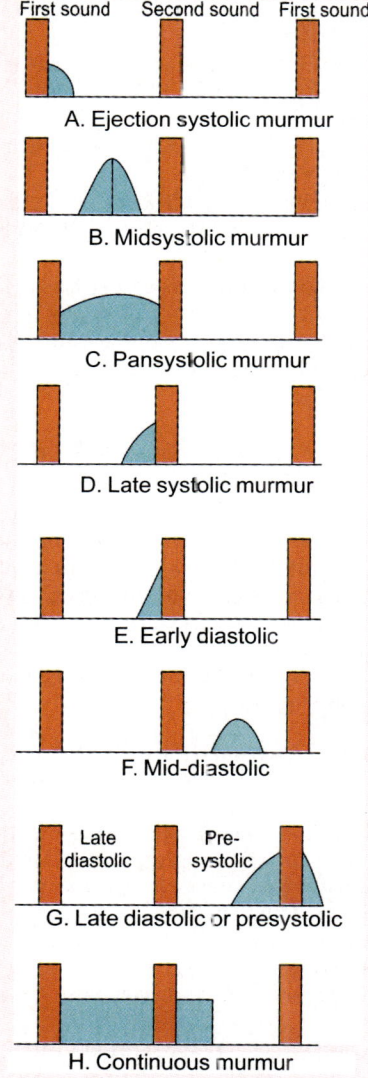

Figs 3.12A to H: Classification of murmurs.

III. Site of Production (Site of Maximum Intensity)

It is determined by auscultation as it may suggest the site of production, e.g., mitral diastolic murmur has maximum intensity at the apex. The pansystolic murmur heard at 3rd and 4th interspace across the sternum indicates left to right shunt of VSD.

IV. Character or Quality of Murmur

The quality of murmur may be characteristic enough to permit an immediate recognition of its nature, e.g.
- Rumbling diastolic murmur of MS is like a sound produced by a wooden cart going over cobblestones.
- Continuous machinery murmur of PDA is like a train-in-tunnel (*Gibson's murmur*).
- Soft blowing early diastolic murmur of AR resembles to *"sucking of breath"* or *"sound of a whispered R"*.
- *Musical or sea-gull murmur* of papillary muscle or chordae tendineae rupture resemble a *vibrating band*.
- Loud, rough, harsh, rasping or grating murmur occur in AS.

Rule: As a rule, regurgitant murmurs are soft and blowing while stenotic murmurs are harse, rough, rasping or rumbling.

Effects of certain physiological and pharmacological interventions on heart murmurs

Certain manoeuvres that increase or decrease the blood flow across the valves alter the intensity of the murmur (Table 3.9). Right-sided murmur increases due to increase in venous return to the heart during inspiration. The systolic murmurs of hypertrophic cardiomyopathy (HCM) and mitral valve prolapse (MVP) become louder with Valsalva manoeuvre and during standing.

Extent of murmur (area of distribution): The murmur may be *localized* to a small area (as in MS) or *diffuse* (as in MR) or *widely heard* (as in coarctation of aorta). When a murmur over the precordium is widely heard involving the two or more valves area, then one has to decide whether it is a single murmur or two distinct murmurs. The dispute is easily settled by tracing the murmur with auscultation inch by inch from one valve area to other, noting the intensity and character of the murmur.

- If there is an alteration in intensity (increase or decrease) but no change in quality or character of the murmur, then probably same murmur is being heard at both the places.
- If on the other hand, the character and pitch of the murmur at two different areas is different, then there is possibility of two distinct murmurs.

TABLE 3.9: Effects of Certain Manoeuvres on Heart Murmurs

Manoeuvre	Effect
Respiration	• *Right-sided murmurs* of TR, PS, TS and PR increase during inspiration. • *Left-sided murmurs* become louder during expiration
Valsalva manoeuvre This procedure helps to differentiate murmur of hypertrophic obstructive cardiomyopathy (HOCM) from aortic stenosis (AS). It helps to identify a prolapsed mitral valve	Most murmurs decrease in length and intensity. Two murmurs that become louder include systolic murmurs of HOCM and mitral valve prolapse (MVP). The systolic murmur of aortic stenosis decreases which differentiates it from HOCM
Positional change	With standing (decreased venous return, i.e. preload and decreased vascular resistance) most murmurs diminish but systolic murmur of HOCM becomes louder while that of MVP increases in length and intensity (click moves earlier systole and murmur lengthens). With squatting (increased venous return as well as peripheral vascular resistance) there is decrease in the intensity of murmur of HOCM and MVP but increase in the intensity of murmur of aortic stenosis (AS). In left atrial myxoma, the mid-diastolic murmur varies from supine to lateral position. Some murmurs (e.g. diastolic murmur of AR) are better heard in stooped forward position
Exercise	Murmurs due to rapid blood flow across normal valve (innocent murmur) or obstructed valves (e.g. MS, PS) become louder with both isotonic and isometric (hand-grip) exercise
Pharmacological interventions	During amylnitrate inhalation (hypotensive response), the murmurs of MR, VSD and AR decrease while murmur of aortic stenosis increases. The response in MVP is biphasic (first softer and then louder than normal). The phenylepinephrine (vasoconstrictor) tends to produce opposite effects

V. Radiation or Direction of Selective Propagation

The following factors are determinants, i.e.:
1. The louder the murmur, further it is transmitted, e.g. loud murmur of AS may not only be heard over the neck but head also.
2. The murmur if loud can be conducted through muscles and bone. The conduction of the murmur through bone is transmission of murmur of VSD across the sternum and murmur of PS heard over the clavicle.
3. *Direction of flow transmits the murmur:* This factor plays a role in transmission/radiation/conduction of the murmur of aortic stenosis (AS) to the neck vessels and downward conduction of the aortic regurgitant murmur along the left sternal border. The best example of radiation of the murmur along the flow of blood is mitral regurgitant murmur which radiates to the left axilla.

VI. Pitch

Pitch depends on the velocity of blood flow as well as pressure head at the site of production of murmur. High velocity and a large pressure difference across the aortic valve in AR produces high-pitched but low intensity murmur, while low velocity with a small pressure gradient at mitral valve in MS produces a low-pitched high intensity diastolic murmur. Pitch is just inverse to intensity. High pitch means intensity is low.

VII. Presence of Thrill

Thrills are palpable murmurs, hence, are associated with low frequency or harsh murmurs, denote stenotic or obstructive lesion (e.g. MS, AS, PS). On the other hand, thrill is absent with high-pitched or high frequency, blowing murmurs. Presence of thrill indicates loud murmur (grade IV on scale of VI).

OTHER BENIGN MURMURS

Flow murmurs: Not all murmurs are produced by a structural heart disease, some of them may arise due to abnormal rapid flow across a normal valve. These are called *flow murmurs*. These are common across the aortic and pulmonary valves (read innocent murmurs). These murmurs do not radiate and are localized.

Pulmonary flow murmurs (*ejection murmurs*) are most commonly heard in children, young adults, athletes and aortic murmurs (atherosclerosis) in the elderly. They also occur in high output states.

Mammary souffle: Many women have a sound over the engorged breasts like murmur heard both in systole and diastole during late pregnancy and during lactation. It indicates increased blood low in their breasts. It is not only heard over the breasts but also heard in the 2nd and 3rd interspace on either side of the sternum. The souffle is *soft systolic to and fro or continuous sound like murmur* heard during supine position. The sound or murmur gets obliterated when pressure is applied to the stethoscope.

Venous hum: These are continuous murmur heard both in systole and diastole, soft in character, heard above the medial third of clavicle. They arise from the jugular veins commonly in children and young adults hence murmur is increased in intensity in the erect position, deep inspiration and diastole. The murmur decreases with recumbency and can be obliterated by pressure on the jugular veins. A cervical venous hum is common in patients on chronic hemodialysis. Venous hum around the umbilicus is heard in cirrohsis of liver (*Cruveilhier-Baumgarten syndrome*).

Arterial bruits: Murmurs occurring at the site of arterial occlusion are called *bruits*. The supraclavicular arterial bruits produced by carotid artery occlusion are best heard over supraclavicular fossa and carotid vessels in patients with embolic stroke. Since this bruit may be transmitted down to aortic or pulmonary area, hence, is to be differentiated from murmur of AS, PS and ASD. Remember that the bruit unlike the above mentioned murmur of AS, PS, ASD has maximal intensity over supraclavicular fossa and carotid vessels not in aortic or pulmonary area.

Murmurs due to chest deformities: Benign midsystolic murmurs are likely to be produced when antero-posterior diameter of the chest is reduced (*pectum excavatum and straight back syndrome*). The murmur is heard at left sternal border. Severe kyphoscoliosis can produce an ejection systolic murmur at the pulmonary area. The murmur in severe deformity of chest may produce even late systolic, soft and loud murmur resembling MVP. The murmur decreases in intensity on inspiration and in sitting position.

DIFFERENTIAL DIAGNOSIS OF MURMURS

I. EJECTION SYSTOLIC (ES) OR MIDSYSTOLIC MURMURS

A. Aortic Systolic Murmur

The murmur is produced due to a pressure gradient across the valve. It starts with opening of the aortic valve, may or may not be associated with an ejection click or thrill.

Causes

The main cause of aortic ejection systolic murmur is obstruction to the left ventricular outflow tract which may occur either at *subvalvular, valvular* or *supravalvular level*:

I. *Causes of subvalvular stenosis*
   - A discrete congenital fibrous band or a diaphragm with a central hole
   - Hypertrophic obstructive cardiomyopathy (HOCM)

II. *Causes of valvular stenosis*
   - Congenital AS
   - Acquired AS (rheumatic)
   - Degenerative AS (old age)
   - Hypertensive aortic sclerosis

III. *Supravalvular aortic stenosis*
   - William's syndrome (congenital)
   - Coarctation of aorta (congenital or acquired)

IV. *Functional aortic stenosis (flow murmur)*
   - Medial cystic necrosis (Marfan's syndrome)
   - Syphilitic aortitis
   - Aortic aneurysm

The differentiation and characteristic of murmur in different aortic stenotic lesions is presented in Table 3.10. In addition to the features mentioned in Table 3.10, age of patient is also a differentiating

TABLE 3.10: Differential Conditions Associated with Aortic Systolic Murmur

Clinical feature	Congenital AS			Acquired AS	HOCM	Functional AS
	Valvular	*Subvalvular*	*Supravalvular*			
1. Facial appearance	Normal	Normal	Elfin facies with pegged molar teeth	Normal	Normal	Normal
2. Pulse	Slow rising with sustained peaking	Slow rising and carotid stronger than left	slow rising sustained peak	Slow rise and double pulse peak	Bisferiens	Good volume
3. BP (pulse pressure)	Low systolic (narrow pulse pressure)	Low to normal (normal pulse pressure)	Hypertension (normal pulse pressure)	Low systolic (narrow pulse pressure)	Wide pulse pressure	High systolic and wide pulse pressure
4. Apex beat	Sustained	Sustained and single	Normal	Sustained may be down and out	Sustained or illustained, may be double	Hyperkinetic
5. Thrill (systolic in aortic area)	May be present	Absent	Absent	Present	Absent	May or may not be present
6. Ejection click	Characteristic	Rare	Rare	Uncommon	Rare	Uncommon
7. Maximum intensity of ESM	Second right intercostal space (A_1 area)	Second right intercostal space (A_1 area)	First right intercostal space (above A_1 area)	Second right (A_1) or 3rd left (A_2 area) interspace	Left sternal edge or apex	Second right space
8. Radiation	Localized or radiate to carotids	Localized	Localized	Radiate to carotids	No radiation	May radiate to neck
9. Splitting of second (S_2) heart sound	Normal	Normal	Narrow, there may be single sound	Single sound or paradoxical splitting	Paradoxical splitting or single sound	Wide splitting
10. Intensity of S_2 (aortic component)	Decreased or normal	Decreased or normal	Loud	Absent A_2	Normal or decreased	Normal
11. Murmur of AR	Common	Common	Uncommon	Common	Rare	Common
12. Calcification	Uncommon	Uncommon	Rare	Common	Rare	Rare

A_1 : Aortic area one, A_2 : Aortic area two, AS : Aortic stenosis, AR : Aortic regurgitation, S_2 : Second heart sound, ESM : Ejection systolic murmur.

feature as congenital lesions are more common in younger age while degenerative and hypertensive conditions occur in old age. Hypertension is a feature of hypertensive aortic stenosis (hemodynamic stress) as well as coarctation of aorta. Radiofemoral delay is another characteristic feature of coarctation of aorta with formation of collaterals over the interscapular region.

B. Pulmonary Systolic Murmur

Causes

1. Murmur due to right ventricular outflow tract obstruction (pulmonary stenosis) usually congenital, may be valvular or infundibular (subvalvular) or of pulmonary branches.

Isolated infundibular stenosis is usually associated with large VSD. Isolated infundibular stenosis with intact septum is rare entity.

Differentiation between valvular and infundibular pulmonary stenosis

- In valvular pulmonary stenosis, there is an ejection click and an ejection systolic murmur while in infundibular stenosis with intact septum, there is no ejection click and murmur is faint. Thrill is present in valvular stenosis, absent in infundibular stenosis.
- P_2 (pulmonary component of S_2) is absent in valvular stenosis but not in infundibular stenosis.
- Splitting of the S_2 is wide in PS due to delayed closure of pulmonary valve. It is more wider in valvular than infundibular stenosis.
- Signs of Fallot's tetralogy, i.e. (i) VSD (pansystolic murmur across the sternum. (ii) overriding of the aorta producing cyanosis (due to mixing up to oxygenated and unoxygenated blood), (iii) infundibular stenosis, and (iv) right ventricular hypertrophy will be present.

Remember. Pulmonary valvular stenosis produces RV heave while it is absent in Fallot's tetralogy inspite of RVH. This is due to the fact that shunt in Fallot's tetralogy is bidirectional and balanced.

2. **Murmur due to branch stenosis of pulmonary artery:** There is an ejection systolic murmur with a thrill (grade IV) at the upper left sternal border which is widely transmitted to chest, back and axillae. With more peripheral artery stenosis, systolic ejection murmur is replaced by even continuous murmur due to continuous gradient.

3. *Ejection systolic murmur of ASD or VSD (left to right shunt):* In ASD and VSD, the pulmonary ejection murmur is a flow murmur due to over-filling of right ventricle which empties into pulmonary artery. The murmur is loud with early peaking. There is no ejection click or thrill. In addition, there can be another mid-diastolic flow murmur (rumble) across the tricuspid valve in ASD, while in VSD, there will be an additional pansystolic murmur with or without thrill (*maladie*).

Remember. The murmur in left to right shunt depends on the pulmonary vascular resistance, i.e. the lower the resistance, the louder and longer will be the murmur while if resistance is high, the murmur shortens and may even become absent if shunt is reversed (right to left shunt do not produce murmur).

Note: The splitting of second heart sound is wide and fixed in ASD while it is wide and not fixed (variable) in VSD.

4. **Murmur due to pulmonary arterial hypertension:** Reactive pulmonary hypertension in MS produces a loud P_2, narrow splitting of S_2 and an ejection systolic murmur. There may be a *Graham-Steell murmur* (diastolic murmur) also due to functional AR. In hyperkinetic pulmonary hypertension due to VSD and ASD, the murmur is functional flow murmur without thrill and associated with wide splitting of S_2 (read above).

C. Functional Systolic Murmurs

i. *Murmur due to hyperkinetic circulation.* It occurs in severe anaemia, fever, thyrotoxicosis, cirrhosis of liver and high output states where there is increased flow of blood through both the ventricles and their outflow tracts, therefore, the murmur may be present either in aortic area (A_1 and A_2) or in the pulmonary area (more common here). These murmurs are associated with other signs of high cardiac output, i.e. good volume pulse (may be collapsing), wide pulse pressure, hyperkinetic apex beat and widely split P_2. They are not associated with thrill. They are of no consequence, hence, also called *benign murmurs*.

ii. *A benign systolic murmur of straight back syndrome* is associated with a click and wide splitting of second heart sound, hence, can be confused with ASD and PS.

D. Peripheral Systolic Murmurs

These are the murmurs heard over the big vessels, i.e. aorta (aortic aneurysm) carotid artery (stenosis or severe AR) or over the collaterals in coarctation of aorta (murmur becomes softer and disappears when collateral are compressed) and aortic-coronary artery bypass.

E. Vascular Murmur
A systolic murmur (bruit) may be heard over thyroid due to increased vascularity.

II. PANSYSTOLIC MURMURS

Causes
1. Mitral regurgitation
2. Mitral valve prolapse (MVP)
3. Tricuspid regurgitation
4. Ventricular septal defect (congenital or acquired following MI)
5. Leaking mitral or tricuspid prosthesis
6. Rupture of chordae tendineae in acute MI.

Differential Diagnosis

1. **Mitral regurgitation:** The pansystolic murmur of MR is maximally heard over the apex. It is soft and blowing in character, gets transmitted to the axilla or inferior angle of the left scapula. It is commonly associated with thrill in organic MR.

   In severe MR, there can be an additional diastolic flow murmur due to rapid flow of large volume of blood from the left atrium to left ventricle in rapid filling phase. This may be associated with a third heart sound (S_3).

   Note: If MR murmur is suspected, look for the other signs of MR (read MR).

2. **Mitral valve prolapse:** The murmur often is midsystolic or late systolic but can be holosystolic. It is best heard at the apex, has a tendency to have late systolic crescendo. It is often accompanied by an ejection click due to which MVP is known as *click-murmur syndrome* (*Barlow's syndrome*).

   The murmur is produced by billowing of a mitral valve cusp (posterior or anterior or both). The murmur radiates either anteriorly over the precordium or to the left axilla depending on the valve cusp prolapsed.

   Inspiration, standing phase of Valsalva, standing and *amylnitrate* result in early onset of click and a longer murmur.

   The *squatting* and *release phase of valsalva manoeuvre* move the click away from the S1 and murmur becomes short.

   The click has been shown to occur at the time of maximal prolapse of the valve on echocardiography, therefore, in MR due to slackening of more than one chordae tendineae there may be more than one click (multiple clicks).

3. **Tricuspid regurgitation:** Tricuspid regurgitation TR is mainly secondary to pulmonary hypertension due to any cause (mitral valve disease, primary pulmonary hypertension, cor pulmonale, etc.).

   The characteristics of murmur of TR are
   i. It is best heard at lower right sternal edge.
   ii. It increases with inspiration (right-sided murmur increase during inspiration due to increased venous return). This point differentials it from murmur of MR which becomes fainter during inspiration.
   iii. Murmur in severe TR may be associated with signs of RVH and raised JVP with *vy* collapse and pulsatile liver.
   iv. The murmur may radiate to apex and mimic MR.

4. **Ventricular septal defect (VSD):** The murmur in VSD is loud, harsh, pansystolic, often associated with thrill, heard with maximum intensity in 3rd and 4th left intercostal space across the sternum.

   The intensity and duration of the murmur depends on the pulmonary vascular resistance. As the pulmonary vascular resistance increases, the murmurs goes on becoming shorter and shorter in systole and may not be heard when patient develops *Eisenmenger's complex* (VSD with reversed shunt. Similarly advanced age decreases the gradient across the defect also, may not produce murmur or may produce short systolic murmur.

5. **Murmur of dysfunction** of papillary muscles or chordae tendineae producing an acute MR in patients with acute MI or infective endocarditis.
   The characteristics of the murmur are
   - The murmur may be pansystolic with midsysolic crescendo or may be short systolic. It resembles murmur of MVP.
   - There will be history or other evidence of acute MI or endocarditis.
   - The murmur radiates to axilla or back in case of prolapse of anterior cusp.
   - The murmur will be directed anteriorly over the precordium or toward base of aorta if posterior cusp prolapses.
   - There will be other signs of MR, i.e. good volume pulse, widely split second heart sound and hyperkinetic apex beat.

6. **Infective endocarditis** involving right side, e.g. drug (heroin addicts) users or congenital heart disease.
   - The murmur is decrescendo pansystolic cooing murmur heard over left sternal border.

- It retains all the characterstics murmur of TR, i.e. it increases in inspiration and associated with other signs of TR.

7. **Dilated cardiomyopathy:** It is characterized by dilated chambers of the heart with mitral and tricuspid regurgitation due to dilated mitral and tricuspid rings. There will be two murmurs:
   1. Pansystolic murmur of MR with all its characteristics.
   2. Pansystolic murmur of TR may or may not be conspicuous. If present, it also shows all the characteristic or TR.
   3. The patient has dilated heart (apex beat down and out).
   4. Though MR and TR both may be present, but there are no signs of pulmonary hypertension (loud P_2, narrowly split S_2, ejection systolic or Graham Steell murmur). This differentiates it from rheumatic MR leading to TR through pulmonary hypertension (signs of pulmonary hypertension present).

DIASTOLIC MURMURS

A. Mid-diastolic murmur
B. Early diastolic murmur

A. MID-DIASTOLIC MURMUR (MITRAL AND TRICUSPID MURMURS)

Mid-diastolic murmurs are organic as well as functional in origin. Organic murmurs are usually associated with thrill, while functional may or may not be.

Causes

I. **Obstruction to AV valves (organic murmur)**
   - Mitral stenosis and tricuspid stenosis
   - Atrial myxoma
   - Atrial ball valve thrombus
   - Mitral valvulitis (Carey Coombs' murmur)

II. **Increased flow across normal AV valves (functional murmur)**
   a. Increased flow through mitral valve in left to right shunt, e.g. VSD, PDA
   b. Increased flow across the tricuspid valve, e.g. ASD, tricuspid regurgitation, Ebstein anomaly, pulmonary hypertension with cor pulmonale
   c. Increased flow through both valves
      - Dilated cardiomyopathy producing MR and TR (flow mid-diastolic murmur)
      - Severe anaemia
      - Pregnancy
      - Hyperthyroidism

d. Back regurgitation of aortic flow in AR produces *Austin-Flint murmur*.

Differential Diagnosis

1. **Mitral stenosis (MS):** The characteristics of mid-diastolic murmur in MS are:
   - The murmur is low-pitched mid-diastolic rough and rumble.
   - Best heard at apex with bell of the stethoscope in left lateral position in held expiration. There is presystolic accentuation.
   - The murmur may or may not be associated with the thrill.
   - *Other signs of MS*, e.g. loud first sound, opening snap usually accompany the murmur.
   - In the presence of atrial fibrillation, the presystolic accentuation of mid-diastolic murmur disappears.
   - When pulmonary hypertension develops, opening snap and murmur become less loud.
   - Silent MS is possible which means patient has MS but murmur is not audible. The murmur becomes less audible or unaudible in MS in following conditions, i.e.
      - Calcified mitral valves (calcific MS)
      - Severe pulmonary hypertension with RV hypertrophy and low cardiac output
      - Severe degree of emphysema.

2. **Tricuspid stenosis (TS):** Isolated TS is rare in rheumatic heart disease. TS is usually associated with TR in RHD. The murmur of TS has same characteristics as that of MS. The important feature of this murmur is that it increases with inspiration.
   - The murmur is usually associated with thrill if rheumatic heart disease is the cause.
   - JVP is usually raised and 'a' wave on JVP is prominent (*cannon wave*).

3. **Carey Coombs' murmur (rheumatic fever):** It is soft low-pitched mid-diastolic murmur heard at the apex. The other characteristics are:
   - It is transient.
   - It is neither associated with thrill or OS nor loud first heart sound.
   - It is associated with acute rheumatic carditis leading to mitral valvulitis (oedema and thickening of mitral valve cusps).
   - Other Jones criteria of *acute rheumatic fever*, i.e. fever, leukocytosis, raise ESR and polyarthritis are present.

4. **Left atrial myxoma:** It is benign tumour of the atrium, may be pedunculated or sessile. It is

mainly associated with constitutional symptoms, i.e. fever, arthralgia, syncope, etc. The main presenting symptoms include *dyspnoea*, *palpitation* and *embolisation*.

The mid-diastolic murmur in atrial myxoma is due to obstruction of mitral valve by the mobile pedunculated tumour, therefore, the characteristics of the murmur are:

1. The intensity of the mid-diastolic murmur varies, often strikingly with the change in position, i.e. best heard during sitting position and less audible in supine (lying down) position.
2. It is not associated with other features of MS.
3. A systolic murmur of MR may be audible as tumour interferes with mitral valve closure.
4. A *tumour plop* (a late diastolic sound) may also be audible after S_2.
5. First heart sound (S_1) may be split due to delayed mitral valve closure.

5. **Austin-Flint murmur:** In severe AR, regurgitant jet of aortic back flow strikes the anterior leaflet of mitral valve resulting in its partial closure leading to a mid-diastolic murmur called "*Austin-Flint murmur*".
   - The murmur is mid-diastolic, arises at mitral valve and heard at apex.
   - It is not associated with other signs of MS, i.e. OS, loud first heart sound or a thrill. Instead it is associated with other signs of severe AR, i.e. a collapsing pulse, wide pulse pressure, dancing carotid, pistol shot sounds, Quinck's sign, Durozieus murmur, Hill's sign, etc.

6. **Ball valve thrombus:** In mitral valve disease, a ball valve thrombus may develop in left atrium which at times if near to the mitral valve may produce a mid-diastolic murmur similar to atrial myxoma. The murmur has all characterstics of murmur of left atrial myxoma.

7. **Mid-diastolic flow murmurs**
   a. *Mitral mid-diastolic flow murmur.* In left to right shunts, i.e. VSD and PDA, the increased volume and flow of blood from left atrium (overloaded left atrium) through normal mitral valve to left ventricle produces a mid-diastolic murmur at the apex in PDA and at the left sternal edge in VSD. These murmurs become shorter when pulmonary hypertension develops (loul P_2, narrow split S_2 and Graham Steell murmur).

   Similary, in severe MR, the left atrium receives blood from the lungs as well as from the left ventricle during systole, gets overburdened, therefore, when it empties its large volume of blood into left ventricle, produces *functional (flow) mid-diastolic murmur* which accompanies the pansystolic murmur and other signs of MR.

   b. *Tricuspid diastolic murmur. In left to right shunts,* e.g. ASD; a mid-diastolic murmur is heard when shunt in ASD is large (2 : 1). It is usually associated with an other ejection systolic murmur across the pulmonary valve due to large flow across it.

   In TR due to pulmonary hypertension or in TR of Ebstein anomaly, a mid-diastolic murmur (flow murmur) is heard along with pansystolic murmur of TR and both the murmurs increase during inspiration.

N.B. The mid-diastolic murmur besides the soft and blowing pansystolic murmur in MR does not indicate organic mitral stenosis unless or until other sings of MS are present. It can be due to functional MS due to severe MR alone.

B. EARLY DIASTOLIC MURMUR

These are the murmurs produced by regurgitation of blood through the semilunar valves during diastolic. These are:
1. Aortic diastolic murmur of AR
2. Pulmonary diastolic murmur (Graham Steell murmur of PR).

I. Aortic Diastolic Murmur of AR

It is an early diastolic murmur, starts with the second heart sound, increases in intensity (crescendo) to attain the peak, then decreases in intensity (decrescendo) hence called "**crescendo-decrescendo murmur**".

- The murmur is soft and faint in rheumatic AR but is high-pitched and blowing in non-rheumatic AR sounding like pouring of water or a *whispered* "*R*".
- Murmur of severe acute AR may be transmitted to the apex, it is loud, high-pitched and musical murmur (*see-gull or cooing murmur*) suggestive of torn or retroverted cusps.
- *Site of maximal intensity* is A_2 area (left third space) in AR due to syphilis, aortic aneurysm, aortic dissection while in congenital AR due to bicuspid aortic valve, it is heard in right second space and associated with thrill and an ejection click.
- *Transmission of murmur*: It may be localized to aortic area (A_1 and A_2) or may be heard at the apex and the whole precordium if loud.
- Being high pitched murmur, it is best heard with chestpiece of stethoscope pressed firmly against the chest wall when the patient bends

forward and holds the breath during expiration (*respiratory effect*).
- *Effect of manoeuvre*: Murmur increases in intensity with squatting, isometric exercise (*handgrip*) or after administering a vasopressor.
- Other murmurs heard in severe AR are
  i. A moderately loud ejection systolic flow murmur resembling see-saw due to augmented stroke output across the deformed valve into the aorta.
  ii. *Austin-Flint murmur* (mid-diastolic mitral murmur): It has already been discussed.
  iii. *Durozieus murmur* (systolic murmur over the femorals when compressed proximally and a diastolic murmur when compressed distally)
- Other signs of AR may be present
  - *Water-hammer pulse*: Dancing carotids (*Corrigan's sign*) or *pulsus bisferiens* (severe AR)
  - *De Musset's sign* (nodding of head with each beat)
  - *Quincke's sign* (capillary pulsations in nailbed on light compression or mucous membrane by glass side compression)
  - *Pistal shot sounds* over the femorals
  - *Hill's sign* (systolic BP of lower limbs, i.e. over popliteal is more than 20 mm than systolic BP in upper limbs, i.e. over brachial)

II. Pulmonary Regurgitation (Graham Steell Murmur)

- The murmur is an early diastolic murmur, heard in pulmonary area, i.e. left second and third space, conducted downwards along the left sternal border.
- It is due to regurgitation of blood through the pulmonary valves secondary to pulmonary hypertension (primary or secondary), hence, is associated with other signs of pulmonary hypertension (loud P2, narrowly split S_2, right ventricular heave).
- It resembles an early diastolic murmur of AR in all its characteristics hence, has to differentiated from it (Table 3.11).

CONTINUOUS MURMURS

Definition: As the name suggests, the murmur is present throughout the cardiac cycle both during systole and diastole because of continuous flow of blood across the defect.

Causes

I. Shunt fistula between a high pressure and a low pressure chamber, i.e.

TABLE 3.11: Differences Between AR and PR

Physical sign	AR	PR
Murmur	An early diastolic, heard in right second or left third space, increases on expiration (left sided murmur)	An early diastolic murmur heard in left 2nd space, increases on inspiration (right-sided murmur)
	The murmur is high pitched, heard while bending forward	The murmur can be heard in supine as well as in sitting position
Associated features	All peripheral signs of AR are usually present	Sings of pulmonary hypertension may be present
Parasternal heave	Left ventricular heave	Right ventricular heave
Additional heart sounds	S_3 may be present	S_4 may be present
'a' wave on JVP	Not prominent	Prominent 'a' wave

- Peristent ductus arteriosus (PDA)
- Rupture of sinus of Valsalva into RA or RV
- Coronary artery fistula to a cardiac chamber or pulmonary vessel.
- Dissecting aneurysm with fistulous communication with RA.
- Postoperative (Blalock-Taussig operation)
- Pulmonary arteriovenous fistula
- Aortopulmonary window

II. Continuous flow of blood through a narrowed vessel
- Coarctation of aorta
- Aortic arch syndrome
- Peripheral pulmonary artery stenosis (congenital or acquired)
- Bronchial artery dilatation associated with pulmonary atresia or collateral formation in coarctation of aorta.

Differential Diagnosis of a Continuous Murmur

1. **Murmur of PDA:** It is a continuous machinery murmur heard just below the clavicle on left side in first or second intercostal space just lateral to sternum.
   - It is *waxing* (increases in intensity at the end of systole and early diastole) and *waning* (whole diastole) in character.
   - It starts with the first heart sound, passes through the second heart sound (S_2).
   - The murmur is accentuated during expiration and after exercise.
   - It is commonly accompanied by thrill.

- If pulmonary hypertension develops (*Eisenmenger's complex*), then diastolic gradient disappears, hence, murmur remains only systolic.
- Other signs of PDA, i.e. a paradoxically split S_2, a mitral mid-diastolic flow murmur and a third heart sound (rapid ventricular filling) may be present.

2. **Aortopulmonary window murmur:** The murmur has all the characteristics of murmur heard in PDA. The only difference is that the site of the murmur is second left interspace or just lower to it (3rd left space).
3. **Rupture of sinus of Valsalva aneurysm into RA or RV:** The aneurysm of sinus of Valsalva is congenital in origin due to weakness of supporting tissue. Rupture occurs from the right and noncoronary sinus into the right atrium (common) or right ventricle (uncommon) in all cases after the age of 20 years either spontaneously or following trauma or severe exertion commonly in females. The characteristics of the murmur are:
   - The murmur is heard maximally at the lower left sternal border.
   - The murmur *waxes* during diastole and *wanes* during systole. This point differentiates it from the murmur of PDA or AV fistula.
4. **Coronary artery aneurysm and fistula:** There is a communication between a coronary artery with either the right atrium or ventricle leading to a superficial continuous murmur associated with thrill. The characteristics that differentiate it from murmur of extracardiac shunts are:
   - It is superficial and heard along the left sternal border.
   - Murmur is associated with thrill.
   - Since the coronary artery filling occurs during diastole, hence, pressue gradient is more during diastole, therefore, the murmur gets accentuated during diastole instead of during systole as occurs in extracardiac shunts.
   - The murmur decreases with Valsalva manoeuvre.
5. **Continuous murmur due to severe arterial stenosis.**
   i. *Coarctation of aorta*: It produces a constant gradient across the narrowed segment both during systole and diastole, resulting in a continuous murmur over upper part of sternum which peaks in late systole (crescendo) and then goes into diastole.

> *Remember.* In coarctation, a continuous murmur can be heard over the collaterals formed in the interscapular region.

ii. *Pulmonary artery stenosis or pulmonary artery branch stenosis with dilatation of collateral bronchial vessels:* In this condition, the murmur is heard over the posterior as well as anterior chest wall. The murmur can be heard all over the chest (front and back) in severe pulmonary artery stenosis due to enlargement and dilatation of bronchial vessels.

iii. *Thoracic aortic aneurysm*: It can cause a continuous murmur due to narrowing of the pulmonary artery by compression caused by aortic aneurysm.

iv. *Aortic arch syndrome* (*Takayasu's syndrome*): In this syndrome, collaterals form between the intercostals branches of descending aorta and branches of subclavian artery, therefore, a continuous murmur is heard anteriorly above the right or left clavicle.

In addition to the murmur, the intercostal vessels are pulsatile.

Conditions Simulating a Continuous Murmur

- Venous hum
- Mammary souffle

These have already been discussed during auscultation.

PHYSICAL SIGNS OF DIFFERENT CARDIOVASCULAR CONDITIONS

I. **Differential signs of valvular heart diseases** (Table 3.12)

II. **Differential signs of cardiomyopathies** (Table 3.13)

JONES CRITERIA (RHEUMATIC FEVER)

Rheumatic fever is a multisystem disorder that typically follows an episode of sore throat (streptococcal) and usually presents with fever, anorexia, joint pains and lethargy. Fleeting polyarthritis is common presentation, occurs in 75% of patients; other features include *skin rashes, carditis, subcutaneous nodules* and *chorea*. The Jones criteria for diagnosis are given in Box 3.6.

Clinical Significance

In a patient suspected of rheumatic heart disease, past history of sore throat, joint pains (fleeting character), fever and skin rash must be asked. For evidence of rheumatic fever one should look for:
- *Sore throat, lymphadenopathy, fever*
- *Swelling of large joint(s)*, if any
- *Erythema marginatum*, i.e. red macules with pale centre (appear as red rings). They are seen on the trunk and extremities (Fig. 3.13). They may not be visible in dark-complexioned persons.

Cardiovascular System

TABLE 3.12: Physical Signs in Various Common Valvular Heart Diseases

Physical signs	Mitral stenosis	Mitral regurgitation	Tricuspid regurgitation	Aortic stenosis	Aortic regurgitation	Pulmonary stenosis	Pulmonary hypertension and pulmonary regurgitation
Pulse	Low volume	Good volume	Normal volume	Anacrotic	Good volume collapsing pulse	Poor volume	Poor volume
Blood pressure and pulse pressure	Low systolic Low pulse pressure	High systolic, wide pulse pressure	Normal	Low systolic, low pulse pressure	High systolic, low diastolic, wide pulse pressure	Low systolic, low pulse pressure	Low systolic, low pulse pressure
Jugular venous pulse (JVP)	'a' wave absent, if atrial fibrillation present	'a' wave absent, if atrial fibrillation present	Y collapse with 'v' wave prominent (VY collapse)	Normal wave pattern	Normal wave pattern	Giant 'a' wave seen	Prominent 'a' wave
Other pulsations	Epigastric pulsations due to RVH may be present Pulsations of pulmonary artery in left second space present	Pulmonary artery pulsations in 2nd left space present	Epigastric RV pulsations present Liver is pulsatile	No other pulsations	Diffuse pulsations over precordium Epigastric aortic pulsations may be present	Epigastric RV pulsations may be present	Epigastric RV pulsations present Pulmonary artery pulsations in left 2nd space present
Parasternal heave	Left parasternal heave	Left parasternal heave	Right parasternal heave	No heave	Left parasternal thrust may be present	Right parasternal heave	Right parasternal heave
Palpable thrill	Diastolic thrill at apex in left lateral position	Systolic thrill at apex in supine or sitting position	Systolic thrill may or may not be present	Systolic thrill at 2nd right interspace	Diastolic thrill at 2nd right and 3rd left interspace	Systolic thrill at 2nd left interspace	No thrill
Heart sounds	Loud Ist sound Second sound normal, accentuated if pulmonary hypertension present	Ist sound muffled 2nd sound normal, accentuated, if pulmonary hypertension present	Ist sound muffled Second sound accentuated or normal	Ist sound normal Aortic component of S_2 weak or absent	Ist sound normal Second sound feeble due to weak A_2	Ist sound normal P_2 (pulmonary component of S_2) is absent	Ist sound normal Second sound loud
Click	Absent	Mid systolic click in MVP (mitral valve prolapse called *click murmur syndrome*)	Absent	An ejection click	No click	An ejection click	No click

Contd.

Contd.

Physical signs	Mitral stenosis	Mitral regurgitation	Tricuspid regurgitation	Aortic stenosis	Aortic regurgitation	Pulmonary stenosis	Pulmonary hypertension and pulmonary regurgitation
Murmurs	A mid-diastolic rough and rumble murmur heard at apex with diaphragm of stethoscope in left sternal position	A pansystolic murmur at apex radiating to axilla in supine position A mid-diastolic murmur may also be audible in severe MR (flow murmur)	A pansystolic murmur over right parasternal edge or epigastrium A mid-diastolic flow murmur like that of MR may be audible	A diamond-shaped crescendo decrescendo murmur at second right space (A_1) or 3rd left space (A_2) audible when patient bends forward and in held expiration. Murmur radiates to neck vessel	An early diastolic murmur heard in second right interspace or 3rd left interspace (A_2 area) in sitting position with patient bending forward and during held expiration	An ejection systolic murmur (ESM) in pulmonary area (second left interspace) Murmur increases during inspiration	An early diastolic murmur (Graham Steell murmur) at 2nd left interspace
Opening snap	Usually present	May sometimes be present	Absent	Absent	Absent	Absent	Absent
Split second sound	Narrow split	Narrow split	Normal or narrow split	Single second sound	Normal split	Wide split due to delayed P_2 component	Narrow split
S_3 *(third heart sound) or* S_4 *(fourth heart sound)*	—	S_3 may be present and audible	S_4 may be present or audible	—	S_3 may be audible	—	S_4 may sometimes be audible

Cardiovascular System

TABLE 3.13: Differential Clinical Signs of Cardiomyopathies

Physical signs	Dilated cardiomyopathy	Hypertrophic cardiomyopathy	Restrictive cardiomyopathy
Pulse	Normal to low volume	Pulsus bisferiens or jerky pulse	Low volume pulse
BP	Normal or low systolic	Normal	Low systolic
Jugular venous pulse	'VY' collapse due to TR	Prominent 'a' wave	Normal wave pattern
Apex beat	Down and outside the midclavicular line, single apex beat	Double apex beat, or well sustained apex beat.	Normally located single apex beat
Parasternal heave	Present	Present	Absent
Epigastric pulsations	Present due to RVH	Absent	Absent
Heart sounds	Normal/feeble	Normal	Normal
Third heart sound	Present	Absent	Absent
Fourth heart sound	Absent	May be present	Present
Murmurs	• Pansystolic murmur in mitral area radiating to axilla (left) • Pansystolic murmurs in tricuspid area increases with inspiration	A mid-systolic or an ejection systolic murmur at 3rd or 4th space along left sternal border accentuated by standing and on Valsalva, becomes softer on squatting	There may be no murmur

Box 3.6: Jones Diagnostic Revised Criteria for Rheumatic Fever

Major
- Carditis
- Polyarthritis
- Chorea
- Erythema marginatum
- Subcutaneous nodules

Minor
- Fever
- Arthralgia
- Previous history of rheumatic fever or rheumatic heart disease
- Raised ESR, or positive C-reactive protein
- Leucocytosis
- First degree or second degree AV block on ECG

Interpretation. The diagnosis is suggested by
- Two or more major criteria *plus*
- One major and two or more minor criteria *plus*
- Evidence of preceding streptococcal infection is also required such as increased ASO titre, positive throat culture for group A streptococci or other antistreptococcal antibodies or echocardiographic evidence of endocarditis.

- *Subcutaneous nodules.* Palpate for small painless nodules over the bony prominences and tendons on the extensor surface of forearms and legs. These nodules are smaller than those of rheumatoid arthritis.
- *Involuntary movements (chorea).* Look for wide flunging dancing irregular movements of extremities. These usually recover and may be accompanied or followed by rheumatic carditis.

- *Arthralgia.* A migratory polyarthritis involving one or two large joints is common at presentation. A corollary about *"it licks the joint and bites the heart"*, is true and widely accepted for acute rheumatic fever.

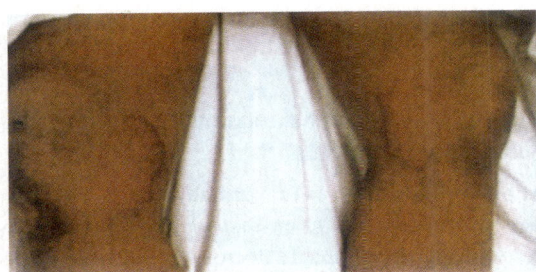

Fig. 3.13: Erythema marginatum in a patient suspected to be a case of acute rheumatic fever. Note the red macules with serpiginous borders over the swollen knee joints.

Acute Rheumatic Activity

A patient of chronic rheumatic heart disease is prone to another attack of rheumatic fever if not treated with penicillin as prophylaxis. Rheumatic activity in such cases of chronic valvular heart disease should be suspected when fever is present along with one or two manifestations of John's criteria.

CONGENITAL HEART DISEASE

Congenital heart disease (prevalence rate about 1%) present at birth (pulmonary atresia, PDA) or in

TABLE 3.14: Differential Signs of Congenital Heart Diseases

Physical signs	Patent ductus arteriosus (PDA)	Atrial septal defect (ASD)	Ventricular septal defect
Pulse	Good volume, may be collapsing	Normal pulse	Normal pulse
Normal BP and pulse pressure	Normal BP, wide pulse pressure	Blood pressure as well as pulse pressure normal	High systolic, pulse pressure may be wide
Jugular venous pulse	Normal	Normal	Normal
Apex beat	Normally placed, heaving in character	Normal	Dynamic or hyperkinetic and diffuse
Parasternal heave	Absent	Left parasternal	Left parasternal
Pulmonary artery pulsation	Present, visible	May not be visible	Present, visible
Thrill	Continuous or systolic thrill at left second intercostal space	No thrill	A systolic thrill across the sternum
Murmur	A continuous machinery murmur starting from the first heart sound and extending through the second heart sound, waxing and waning in character.	• An ejection systolic flow murmur in second left intercostal space • A mid-diastolic flow murmur, at left sternal (tricuspid area)	A pansystolic murmur at 3rd and 4th intercostal spaces across the sternum
Heart sounds	Both the heart sounds normal, merged with the murmur	Heart sounds normal	Normal heart sounds
Splitting of second sound (S_2)	There may be reversed splitting of S_2	Wide and fixed splitting	Wide but not fixed splitting
Crackles and rales	May be present due to lung congestion	May or may not be present	Usually present due to lung congestion

later life, either detected incidentally during stress or pregnancy. Aetiology is unknown but maternal infections (*rubella*), chromosomal defect (*trisomies, monosomy*), connective tissue disorders (*Marfan's syndrome*) and *maternal alcohol abuse* are considered some of incriminating factors. Certain teratogenic drugs also predispose to them.

Symptoms and Signs

Most of the congenital health diseases are asymptomatic or remain asymptomatic for longer time. They may be *cyanotic* (cyanosis present at birth or appear in later life such as Fallot's tetralogy) or *acyanotic* (ASD, VSD, PDA). Most of the children or adults with congenital health disease are either tall (*Marfan syndrome*) or short stature. There may be growth retardation and intellectual impairment in children. The **physical signs** in three common acynotic congenital heart diseases are presented in Table 3.14.

INFECTIVE ENDOCARDITIS

Infective endocarditis is a microbial infection of mural endocardium, heart valve(s), i.e. native or prosthetic or lining of a blood vessel or a congenital defect by bacteria (*streptococci, Staph. aureus, HACEK organisms, anaerobes*), rickettsia and fungi. It may be *acute* or *subacute*. It occurs spontaneous following septicaemia or may be provoked by dental extraction, instrumentation and procedures. Vegetations are formed by fibrinous clot and the organism, which are fragile and prone to embolisation. An immune complex mechanism involves the kidneys (*glomerulonephritis*), joints (*arthritis*), blood vessels (*vasculitis*). Anaemia is also a characteristic feature. The physical signs of infective endocarditis are presented in Table 3.15.

Diagnosis of infective endocarditis is suspected when fever and signs of toxaemia appear in a patient with congenital heart disease or rheumatic heart disease. The diagnosis is confirmed by Duke Criteria. Virtually out of three blood culture taken one hour apart from a patient who is not on antibiotic therapy, if two are positive, it is diagnostic of infective endocarditis in 98% cases.

Cardiovascular System

TABLE 3.15: Physical Signs of Infective Endocarditis

I. General physical signs

- Toxic look, patient is febrile and weak, there may be tachypnoea, tachycardia
- Skin may show purpuric spots, ecchymosis, Janeway lesions, palmar erythema
- JVP may be raised
- Clubbing of the fingers, digital gangrene, coldness of extremities
- Splinter haemorrhages
- Roth's spots in the eyes and subconjunctival haemorrhages
- Loss of peripheral pulses

II. Systemic signs

- Anaemia, oedema may be present
- Haematuria (embolic or immune complex glomerulonephritis)
- Splenomegaly
- Haemoptysis, chest pain, pleural rub (pulmonary infarct)
- Toxic encephalopathy and meningitis (septicaemia)

CONGESTIVE HEART FAILURE (CHF)

It refers to congestion of all viscera due to heart failure. **Heart failure** refers to inability of the heart to cater the demands of oxygen to all the tissues. Congestive heart failure includes both left and right heart failure.

Diastolic heart failure refers to decreased filling of ventricles due to left ventricle thickening and LVH as a result of hypertension, AS or AR or left ventricular stiffening due to ischaemia.

Systolic heart failure refers to decreased muscle contraction due to myocarditis, myocardial infarction, drugs, dilated cardiomyopathy, alcohol abuse. Ultimately diastolic heart failure also results in systolic heart failure.

Causes

1. Diseases of myocardium, i.e. myocarditis, cardiomyopathies, MI
2. Valvular heart diseases (mitral and aortic valve diseases)
3. Congenital heart disease
4. Hypertensive heart disease
5. Thyrotoxic heart disease

The congestive heart failure in a patient with heart disease is precipitated by *infections, arrhythmias, drugs, hypertension, salt intake*, etc., hence, it is mandatory to look for symptoms and signs of CHF in each and every patient of heart disease (Fig. 3.14).

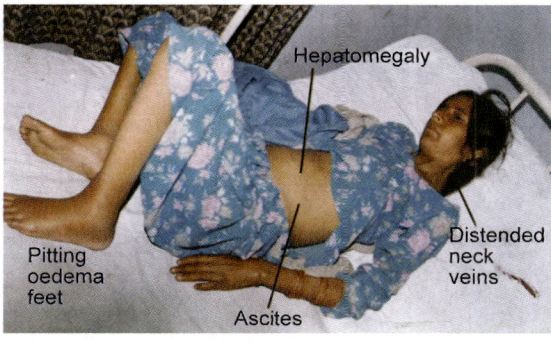

Fig. 3.14: Congestive heart failure (CHF).

Diagnosis. It is mainly clinical supported by investigations, i.e. radiology and echocardiography.

Framingham criteria for diagnosis of CHF (Table 3.16).

Left heart failure is a separate entity, includes failure of left ventricle to pump sufficient blood leading to congestion of lungs. The *causes* include valvular heart disease (mitral and aortic), ischaemic heart disease, hypertension, HOCM, endomyocardial fibrosis, left ventricular endocarditis. The symptoms and signs are given in Table 3.17.

TABLE 3.16: Physical Signs of CHF

Major criteria	Minor criteria
• Paroxysmal nocturnal dyspnoea (PND)	• Peripheral pitting oedema
• Distended neck veins	• Nocturnal cough
• Raised JVP	• Dyspnoea on exertion
• Cardiomegaly	• Hepatomegaly
• Rales	• Pleural effusion (hydrothorax)
• Acute pulmonary oedema	• Reduced vital capacity (one-third of normal)
• S_3 gallop	
• Positive hepatojugular reflux	

TABLE 3.17: Physical Signs of Left and Right Heart Failure

Physical signs of left heart (ventricular) failure	Physical signs of right heart failure
• Dyspnoea, orthopnoea, paroxysmal nocturnal dyspnoea	• Raised JVP
	• Puffiness of face
	• Cardiomegaly
• Cardiomegaly	• Hepatomegaly (tender)
• S_3 gallop	• Ascites
	• Pitting oedema over the feet and legs

Contd.

Contd.

- Crackles and rales at both bases of lungs
- Pleural effusion, hydrothorax
- There may be tachypnoea, tachycardia
- Vital capacity is reduced to one-third of normal
- There may be an evident cause, i.e. valvular, congenital, hypertensive, cardiomyopathy, ischaemic thyrotoxic heart disease, etc.
- Right-sided S_3 gallop
- Parasternal heave

CHRONIC COR PULMONALE

Chronic cor pulmonale is defined as right ventricular enlargement/hypertrophy due to diseases of the lungs, pulmonary vessels and thoracic cage. Right heart failure (congestive heart failure) is a complication rather than manifestation.

Causes include; chronic obstructive pulmonary disease (COPD), interstitial lung diseases, pulmonary embolism, kyphoscoliosis, primary pulmonary hypertension (PPH), etc.

Symptoms and signs include that of basic respiratory disease, i.e. cough, sputum, dypnoea, cyanosis, haemoptysis and that of right heart failure (Table 3.18).

TABLE 3.18: Physical Signs of Chronic Cor Pulmonale (Right Heart Failure)

- Signs of the disease causing cor pulmonale, i.e. COPD, PPH, etc.
- Orthopnoea, i.e. patient sits with hands on the cardiac table and legs dangling/hanging from the bed to relieve breathlessness
- Cyanosis
- Distended neck veins and raised JVP
- There may be '*vy*' collapse on jugular venous pulse
- Positive hepatojugular reflux, peripheral pitting oedema and ascites (may be present)

Diagnosis is confirmed by radiology, blood gas analysis and echocardiography.

Differential Diagnosis

Differential diagnosis of both CHF and cor pulmonale lies within its causes because they are complications of all heart diseases (CHF) and respiratory diseases (cor pulmonale).

ISCHAEMIC HEART DISEASE (IHD)

The ischaemia of the heart due to coronary artery disease is called *ischaemic heart disease* or *coronary artery disease*. Ischaemia of heart may be due to occlusion of coronary arteries (atherosclerosis, thrombus, embolism) vasospasm, or endarteritis or relative ischaemia due to increased demands (thyrotoxicosis, ventricular hypertrophies) or small vessel disease (syndrome X).

Risk factors include old age, smoking, alcohol, hypertension, obesity, hypercholesterolaemia, hyperhomocysteinemia, sedentary habits and low levels of antioxidants. Clinically IHD manifests as *angina pectoris* (stable or unstable), *acute coronary syndrome* and *myocardial infarction*. The **characteristic symptom** is anginal pain (i.e. exertional pain relieved by rest or by nitrates). There is usually no physical sign in uncomplicated disease except a soft systolic cooing murmur of papillary muscle dysfunction in some cases. Signs appear when a complication develops.

Diagnosis is pure clinical, confirmed on ECG, exercise testing, echocardiogram and coronary angiography.

Differential Diagnosis

It comes into the differential diagnosis of chest pain which has already been discussed under symptoms related to cardiovascular system.

PERICARDITIS

Inflammation/infection of pericardium by a large variety of agents including infective agents is called *pericarditis*. Pericarditis is caused by *bacteria* (tuberculosis, pyogenic), *virus* (coxsackie, echo, etc.), *fungi* (histoplasmosis), *parasite* (Echinococcus), sarcoidosis, uraemia, SLE, RA, trauma, radiation, myxoedema, and drugs. It also occurs following rheumatic fever and myocardial infarction or postcardiotomy syndrome (*Dressler's syndrome*).

It is characterised by a *triad* comprising of (i) retrosternal/precordial pain radiating to left shoulder increased by coughing/sneezing and supine position, (ii) a pericardial rub (palpable or audible), and (iii) fever associated with myalgia or arthralgia.

The **diagnosis** is purely clinical and differential diagnosis is chest pain due to any cause (read differential diagnosis of chest pain).

PERICARDIAL EFFUSION AND CARDIAC TEMPONADE

Collection of fluid more than normal (50–150 ml) in the pericardial cavity is called *pericardial effusion*. When pericardial fluid is enough to cause reduction

Cardiovascular System

in the diastolic filling of the heart, the condition is called *cardiac temponade*.

Pericardial effusion may be transudate, exudate, pus, blood or chyle. Pericardial effusion can develop following pericarditis due to any cause, hence, causes of both pericarditis and pericardial effusion are same, i.e. infections, neoplastic pericardial disease, uraemia, tuberculosis and following cardiac surgery.

It is characterised by dyspnoea on lying down relieved by sitting up, cough, chest discomfort, difficulty in swallowing, etc.

Physical signs include:
1. Pulsus paradoxus
2. Distended neck veins, raised JVP and positive Kussmaul's sign
3. Signs of CHF, i.e cyanosis, oedema feet, ascites, hepatomegaly.
4. Nonpalpable and nonvisible apex beat, a palpable pericardial rub (may or may not be present) widening of the cardiac dullness, soft or muffled heart sounds, audible pericardial rub and a patch of bronchial breathing beneath the angle of left scapula (*Rotch's sign*).
5. Signs of cardiac temponade may be present if pericardial effusion is large, i.e. pulsus paradoxus, rising JVP, falling BP, tachypnoea, tachycardia, pale and anxious looking face, cyanosis and patient sitting on the edge of bed, bending forwards and legs dangling along the bedside.

Diagnosis is made on clinical grounds and confirmed on radiology and echocardiography.

THE PERIPHERAL VASCULAR SYSTEM

Causes of Peripheral Vascular Disease

I. **Acute arterial ischaemia**
   A. *Thrombosis*, e.g. atherosclerotic obliteration, thromboangiitis (Buerger's disease), arteritis (connective tissue disease, giant cell and Takayasu's arteritis), myeloproliferative disease (polycythaemia) and hypercoagulable states.
   B. *Embolic*, e.g. cardiac origin (valvular disease, prosthetic valve, AMI, AF with atrial thrombus, infective endocarditis, cardiomyopathy, left atrial myxoma); atherosclerotic plaques (in aorta or big vessels), trauma and arterial spasm.

II. **Chronic arterial disease**
   - Atherosclerotic obliterans
   - Thromboangiitis obliterans
   - Arteritis, e.g. connective tissues, disorders, temporal arteritis (giant cell) and Takayasu's disease.
   - Miscellaneous, e.g. trauma, entrapment, congenital arterial narrowing.

Symptoms of Occlusive Arterial Disease

A. **Lower limb symptoms**
   i. Acute lower limb ischaemia presents with *pain, paraesthesias, paralysis, pallor, pulselessness* and *perishingly cold limb* (denoted by 6 Ps). Any one or all of them may be present. Any "cold limb" could be ischaemic, hence, must be evaluated. Differentiation of acute embolic from thrombotic occlusion is important (Table 3.19) because treatment and prognosis are different.

B. **Chronic ischaemia of limb**
   There are four well-defined stages of lower limb ischaemia, i.e.
   i. Asymptomatic
   ii. Intermittent claudication

TABLE 3.19: Acute Limb ischaemia (Thrombosis vs Embolism)

Clinical feature	Embolism (Fig. 3.15)	Thrombosis
1. Onset	Sudden (seconds or minutes)	Hours
2. Severity	Complete occlusion (no collaterals)	Incomplete occlusion (collaterals)
3. Embolic source present	Yes (atrial fibrillation common)	No
4. Previous claudication	Absent	Present
5. Central pulses present	Yes	No
6. Upper limb affected	Commonly (25%) leg:arm (3:1)	Rare leg:arm (10:1)
7. Palpation of artery	Soft, tender	Hard, calcified
8. Bruits	Absent	Present
9. Contralateral leg pulses	Present	Absent
10. Multiple sites	Up to 15% (sometimes)	Rare
11. Diagnosis	Clinical	Angiography
12. Treatment	Embolectomy, warfarin	Thrombolysis
13. Prognosis	Loss of life > loss of limb	Loss of limb > loss of life

iii. Rest pain
iv. Tissue loss (ulceration/gangrene)
  i. *Asymptomatic lower limb ischaemia* is identified by a reduced ankle brachial pressure index (ABPI). It is common in middle aged and elderly. Such patients are also at high risk of developing complications.
  ii. *Intermittent claudication* refers to cramp-like muscle pain in calf, buttock or thigh on walking which is rapidly relieved by taking rest.

Male patients with gluteal claudication, due to internal iliac disease, are almost invariably impotent. Enquiry into sexual activity should be made if not told by the patient.

The term claudication just denotes pain in the leg on walking, could also be due to neurological and musculoskeletal disorder of the lumbar spine (neurogenic claudication) and due to venous outflow obstruction from the leg (venous claudication). However, all these claudications are much less common than arterial claudication and can easily be distinguished on history and examination (Table 3.20).

Symptom Analysis
Ask about the following
- Have you ever had any pain or cramping in your legs on walking or exercise?
- How far can you walk without pain?
- Does the pain get better with rest?
- Ask also about coldness, numbness, or pallor in the legs or feet or loss of hair over the anterior tibial surfaces.

iii. *Night/rest pain:* It may be initial presentation PAD. The patient goes to bed and is woken up after 1–2 hours by pain in the foot, usually in the in-step. This is due to loss of beneficial effects of gravity on limb perfusion on recumbency. Sleep also precipitate ischaemia by decreasing heart rate, BP and cardiac output. Patients usually get relief by hanging their leg out of bed by getting up and walking around. When the patient returns to bed symptom recurs.

iv. *Tissue loss* (ulceration and/or gangrene). It is due to critical limb ischaemia. In such cases, minor injury will fail to heal and provide a portal of entry for bacteria leading to gangrene and/or ulceration. Without revascularisation, the ischaemia will rapidly progress.

The Physical Examination
☞ Look for the following signs
- Anaemia and cyanosis
- Signs of cardiac failure
- Direct or indirect evidence of vascular disease (Box 3.7 for signs and their related vascular disease).

A thorough search sould be made for these signs in addition to the detailed examination of arterial pulses.

EXAMINATION OF VASCULAR SYSTEM
Assessment of the peripheral vascular system relies primarily on **inspection** of the arms and legs, **palpation** of pulses, and a search for oedema or an arterial bruit.

TABLE 3.20: The Clinical Characteristics of Arterial, Neurogenic and Venous Claudication

Feature	Arterial	Neurogenic	Venous
Cause	Stenosis or occlusion of major limb arteries	Lumbar nerve root or cauda equina compression (spinal canal stenosis)	Obstruction to the venous outflow of the leg due to iliofemoral venous occlusion
Site of pain	Calf, but may involve high and buttock	Ill-defined. Whole leg pain, may be associated with numbness and tingling	Whole leg pain, bursting in nature
Lateralisation	Unilateral, can be bilateral	Often bilateral	Nearly always unilateral
Onset	Gradual, occurs after walking some distance	Often immediate after walking or even standing up	Gradual, occurs from the moment walking starts
Relieving factors	Cessation of walking abolishes pain immediately	Relief is achieved on bending forwards and stop walking. May have to sit to obtain full relief.	Elevation of leg relieves discomfort
Colour	Normal or pale	Normal	Normal or increased

Cardiovascular System

Box 3.7	Common Signs Suggested Vascular Diseases
Sign	*Suggested vascular disease*
1. Hands and arms	
• Nicotine stains	• Smoking
• Purple discoloration	• Atheroembolism from a subclavian aneurysm
• Pits and healed scars on finger pulps	• Secondary Raynaud's phenomenon
• Cyanosis and visible nail-fold capillary loops	• Scleroderma and the CREST syndrome
• Wasting of small muscles of the hands	• Thoracic outlet syndrome
2. Face and neck	
• Corneal arcus and xanthelasma	• Hypercholesterolaemia
• Horner's syndrome	• Carotid artery dissection or aneurysm
• Hoarsenss of voice and bovine cough	• Recurrent laryngeal nerve palsy from a thoracic aortic arch aneurysm
• Prominent veins in the neck and over shoulder and anterior chest	• Axillary/subclavian vein occlusion
3. Abdomen	
• Epigastric umbilical pulsations	• Aortoiliac aneurysm
• Mottling of abdomen	• Ruptured abdominal aortic aneurysm or saddle embolism occluding aortic bifurcation
• Evidence of weight loss	• Visceral ischaemia

Examination Sequence

Inspection

☞ *Inspect both the arms (hands, fingertips, nailbeds, skin) and legs (feet, toes) for size, symmetry, change in temperature, colour of the skin and nailbeds. Note any area of pigmentation, rashes, scales, ulcer (Fig. 3.15) or gangrene:*

- Purple fingertips suggest atheroembolism
- Cyanosis of fingertips indicate scleroderma and CREST syndrome
- Pigmentation over the finger may be due to nicotine smoking in smokers
- Coldness of limbs indicate limb ischaemia
- Ulcer (gangrene of the fingertip) indicates embolism or Buerger's disease.

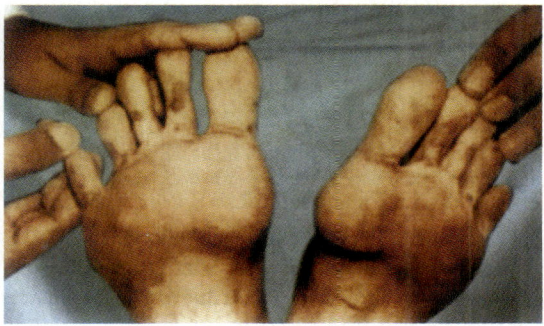

Fig. 3.15: Feet in a patient with bacterial endocarditis. Note digital embolisation (gangrene).

Palpation

i. Palpate upper limb vessels
ii. Palpate lower limb vessels

Measure the blood flow or grade the volume of the pulse as follows:

Normal	+
Reduced	±
Absent	–
Aneurysmal	++

Note: If the examiner is in any doubt about which pulse is being felt (i.e. his or her own or patient's pulse), it is useful for the clinician to palpate his or her own pulse at the same time. Lack of synchronization implies that it is the patient's pulse.

☞ *Now palpate for the lymph nodes (axillary, epitrochlear, cervical and inguinal) for any enlargement.*

- Lymph node enlargement in lymphoma. Leukaemia may occlude limb vessels.

☞ *Perform tests for vascular insufficiency of upper limbs, if suspected.*

1. **The Allen's test for patency of ulnar and radial arteries.** Ask the patient to make a tight fist of one hand. Compress both the radial and ulnar arteries between your thumb and fingers at the wrist (Fig. 3.16A). Now ask the patient to open the hand into a relaxed and slightly flexed position. The palm becomes pale in this position (Fig. 3.16B).

   Patency of the radial artery may be tested by releasing the radial artery while still compressing the ulnar (Fig. 3.16 C). Palm flushes within a few seconds. Paleness of palm indicates occlusion of radial artery or its branches.

   Release your pressure over the ulnar artery. If artery is patent the palm flushes within

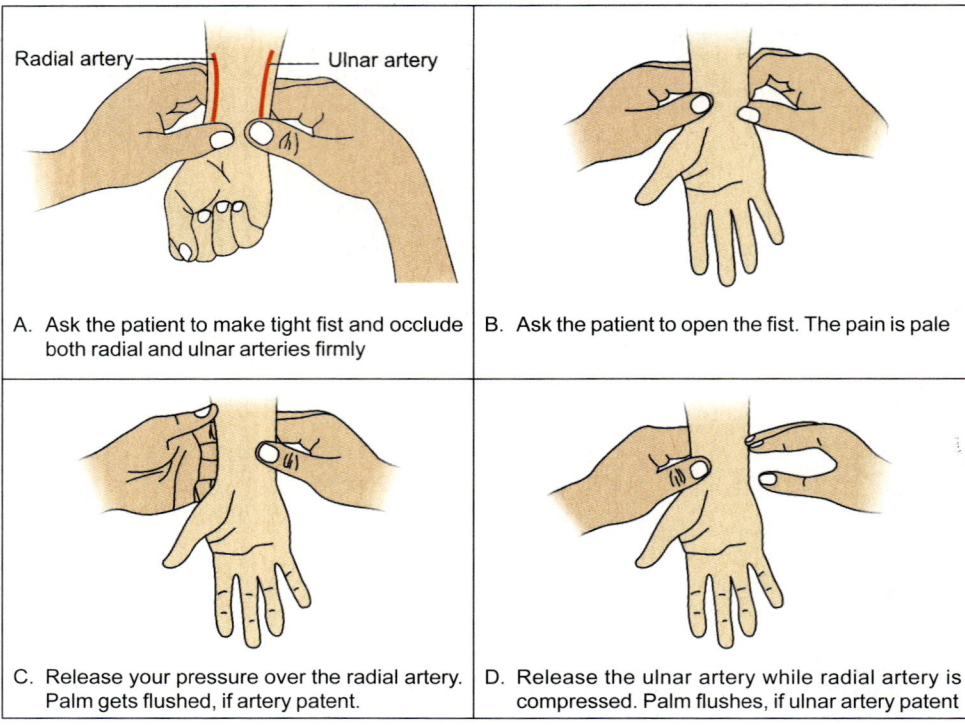

Figs 3.16A to D: The *Allen* test for patency of the vessel.

3–5 seconds (Fig. 3.16D). Persisting pallor indicates occlusion of ulnar artery or its distal branches.

2. **Adson's test:** This is performed for presence of subclavian artery compression by a cervical rib or scalenus anticus muscle (*thoracic outlet syndrome*). While the patient is sitting, palpate the radial pulse on the affected side (i.e. there is pain or diminished pulse on that side). Then patient is asked to inhale and hold the breath and turn his chin upwards and towards the affected side. A decrease in or absence of radial pulse indicates positive test for subclavian artery compression.

3. **Postural colour changes for chronic arterial insufficiency (Buerger's test):** If pain or diminished pulses suggest arterial insufficiency, look for postural colour changes. Raise both the legs while the patient is lying supine to about 60° until maximal pallor of the feet develops usually within 60 seconds. In this position, a slight pallor is normal response, but marked pallor suggests arterial insufficiency.

Now ask the patient to sit up with legs dangling down. Compare both feet, noting the time required for return of normal pink colour (usually returns within 10 seconds) and filling of veins of the feet (normally fill within 15 seconds).

The abnormal response indicates arterial insufficiency.

> Persistence of rubor (dusky redness) on dependency indicates positive test for arterial insufficiency.

Normal responses accompanied by diminished arterial pulsations indicate that a good collateral circulation has developed around the arterial occlusion.

Colour changes may be difficult to see in darker-skinned persons.

Palpations of Various Peripheral Pulses

☞ Palpate the various pulses of upper and lower limbs for pulsations (*normal, increased, diminished or absent*)

The arterial pulses are detected by gently compressing the vessel against some firm underlying structure such as bones. The method of palpation of various pulses is illustrated in Box 3.2 and Fig. 3.6.

RELATED SYSTEMIC EXAMINATION

The Heart
- Examine the heart for any evidence of vascular heart disease or ischaemic heart disease that predisposes to atrial or mural thrombosis which may lead to systemic embolisation (Fig. 3.17).
- Record the systolic blood pressure in the upper and lower limbs to calculate the ankle/brachial pressure index or ratio (ABPI).
- Auscultate the abdominal aorta or any other major vessel, i.e. carotid artery for any bruit (Fig. 3.18).

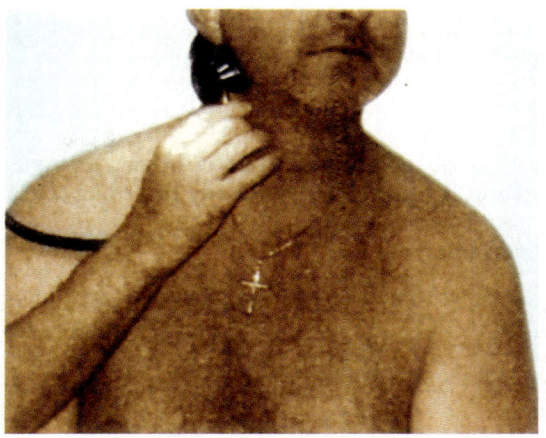

Fig. 3.18: Carotid artery auscultation for bruit. Note that the bell of the stethoscope is placed gently on the skin overlying the angle formed by the sternocleidomastoid muscle and the lower jaw.

Measurement of Ankle/Brachial Pressure Index (ABPI)

Measurement of ABPI is useful in assessing the severity of chronic lower limb ischaemia. This index has predictive value in the healing of the ischaemic ulcers.

It is performed using a hand-held Doppler and a sphygmomanometer. The probe is held over the three pedal arteries (posterior tibial, dorsalis predis, perforating peroneal) in turn while a BP cuff wrapped round the ankle is inflated. The pressure at which Doppler signal disappears gives the systolic BP in that artery. The ratio of the highest pedal artery pressure to highest brachial artery pressure (BP recording) is ABPI.

> Normally the ABPI index is ≥1.0 in supine position (ankle systolic BP is equal to or higher to brachial systolic BP) while in patients with various types of occlusive PAD, the index in below 0.9 and in some cases below 0.5.

In diabetics, crural arteries are hard and incompressible, hence, may falsely raise the pedal pressures, and thus the ABPI. In such circumstances, an alternative is to "*isolate*" the artery while elevating the foot. The height above the bed in centimetres at which the Doppler signal disappears is approximately equal to the perfusion pressure in mmHg.

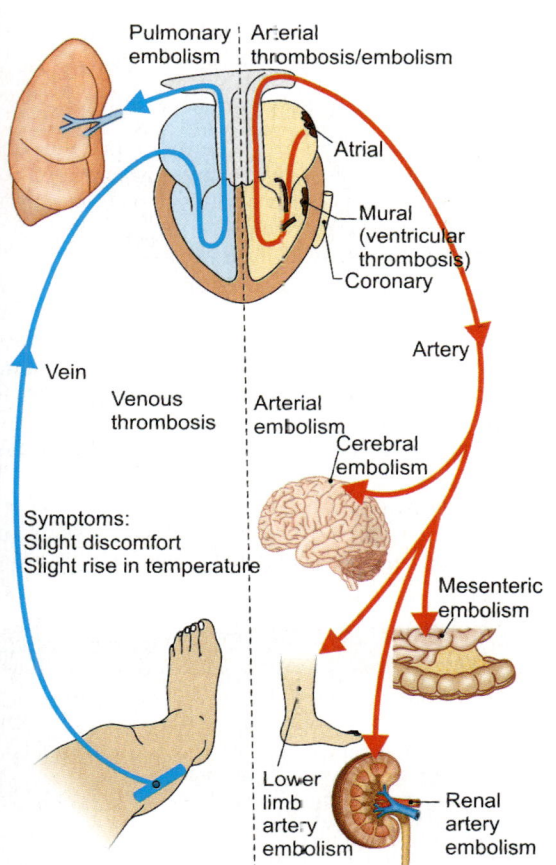

Fig. 3.17: Thrombosis and embolism.
1. Right side of figure shows venous thrombosis of leg and its embolism.
2. Left side of figure shows arterial thrombosis (mural left ventricular or atrial) and its subsequent embolism to organs and limb vessels.

THE ABDOMEN

☞ Look at the abdomen for aortic pulsations and auscultate for any bruit.

Note: Auscultate all the major vessels for bruit if there is an evidence of diminished pulsations.

THE NERVOUS SYSTEM

Examine the nervous system for any neurological deficit. Vascular disease may present with *transient ischaemic attacks (TIA), stroke* or *multi-infarct dementia.*

A significant proportion of strokes and TIAs are due to atheroemboli originating from a tight atherosclerotic stenosis or the origin of internal carotid artery. The signs of internal carotid artery occlusion include ocular (loss of vision in the ipsilateral eye—called *amaurosis fugax*) often described by the patient as a curtain coming across the field of view lasting for a few minutes. Less commonly there may be permanent monocular blindness and cerebral/hemispheric signs such as hemiplegia, hemianaesthesia and dysphasia (if dominant hemisphere is affected).

Vertebrobasilar arterial insufficiency presents with *giddiness, collapse, with or without loss of consciousness, transient occipital blindness* or *complete loss of vison* in both the eyes.

Patients with subclavian artery stenosis or occlusion proximal to the origin of the vertebral artery may experience vertebrobasilar symptoms, as part of the *subclavian steal syndrome.* This happens when the arm is exercised. The increased blood supply to the arm is met by stealing the blood from posterior cerebral circulation producing symptoms and signs of vertebrobasilar insufficiency. Signs of this include asymmetry of pulses and BP in the arms and sometimes a bruit over the subclavian artery in the supraclavicular fossa may be heard.

BRIEF SYNOPSIS OF PERIPHERAL VASCULAR DISEASES

Buerger's Disease

This is an inflammatory obliterative arterial disease different from atherosclerosis. It presents in young (<30 yr) male smokers and characteristically affects the peripheral arteries giving rise to intermittent claudication in the feet or rest pain in the fingers and toes. This disease has a strong genetic basis.

The condition also affects the veins, and superficial thrombophlebitis is common. Wrist and ankle pulses are usually absent but brachial and popliteal pulses are characteristically palpable. Arteriography shows narrowing or occlusion of arteries below the knee with relatively healthy vessels above that level. The condition usually remits if patient stops smoking. In severe disease, there may be ulceration and gangrene of the toes (Fig. 3.19).

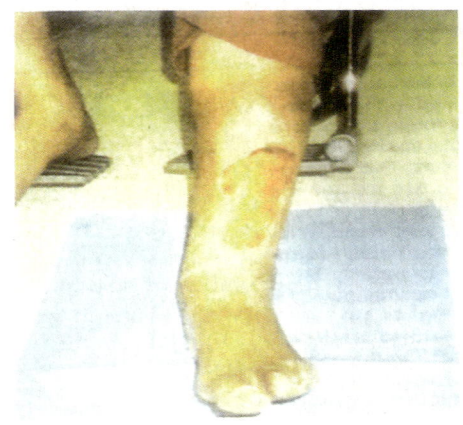

Fig. 3.19: Buerger's disease.

Vascular occlusion by embolism or vasculitis: There may be involvement of big vessels due to embolism and small vessels in vasculitis.

VASOSPASTIC DISORDERS

Vasospastic disorders involve the small vessels (arteries and arterioles), hence, are characterized by changes in the skin colour and temperature rather than intermittent claudication and gangrene. The various vasospastic conditions are given in Box 3.8.

1. **Raynaud's phenomenon (Fig. 3.20).** It is the commonest vasospastic disorder characterised by brief, intermittent triphasic colour response, i.e. *pallor, cyanosis* and *redness of the digits* due to constriction followed by dilatation of small vessels (arteries, arterioles) precipitated by exposure to cold or emotional stress. This could be:
   - *Primary* (*idiopathic* called *Raynaud's disease*) owing to vasospasm of digital vessels of unknown cause.

Box 3.8 Common Vasospastic Conditions

1. **Raynaud's phenomenon**
   - Primary (Raynaud's disease)
   - Secondary due to connective tissue disease, occlusive arterial disease, hypothyroidism, phaeochromocytoma.
2. **Livedo reticularis**
   - Primary
   - Secondary to connective tissue disease, vasculitis, myeloproliferative disorders.
3. **Acrocyanosis**
4. **Chronic pernio syndrome (chilblains)**
5. **Reflex sympathetic dystrophy**

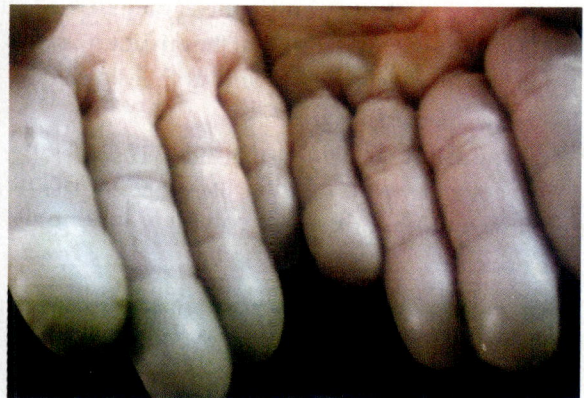

Fig. 3.20: Raynaud's phenomenon after immersion of the hand in cold water.

- *Secondary (Raynaud's syndrome)* is due to digital artery obstruction caused by:
  - Connective tissue disease (most commonly systemic sclerosis)
  - Vibration injury (secondary to use of power tools)
  - Atheroembolism from a proximal source such as subclavian artery aneurysm.

Initial evaluation includes:
- History of tricolour response precipitated by cold and emotion
- Drug history includes intake of beta blockers and ergot preparation
- Allen's test
- Look for thoracic outlet compression.

2. **Livedo reticularis:** It is purplish mottling of skin due to spasm of the dermal arterioles, seen commonly in lower extremities and is more prominent in cold weather. Recurrent ulceration around the ankle may occur in primary livedo reticularis.

3. **Acrocyanosis:** It is characterized by coldness and cyanosis (bluish discolouration) of the acral parts (hands, fingers, feet and toes). It is always a primary and commonly occurs in women. Cyanotic heart disease and methaemoglobinaemia must be excluded before making the diagnosis.

4. **Chronic pernio syndrome:** It results from cold injury and is characterized by abnormal reaction of the blood vessels to changes in environmental temperature. There are often erthematous, cyanotic, haemorrhagic or ulcerative lesions of the toes during the colder months, and they disappear in warm whether.

5. **Reflex sympathetic dystrophy:** It is probably a neurological disorder that occurs following trauma, characterized by pain, oedema, warmth, hyperhidrosis, coldness and colour changes.

ANEURYSMAL DISEASE (ABDOMINAL AORTIC ANEURYSM—AAA)

Aortic aneurysm is commoner in men than in women, occurs after the age of 65 years. The presenting complaints include *abdominal and/or back pain or pulsations*. Many patients may remain asymptomatic until aneurysm ruptures. Usually a mural thrombus in the aneurysm often leads to complete obstruction and distal embolisation.

In the extremities, the most common aneurysms encountered are in the femoral, popliteal and subclavian artery.

Clinically abdominal aortic aneurysm presents with a pulsatile mass in the epigastrium. A pulsatile mass below the umbilicus suggests an iliac artery aneurysm.

The **diagnosis** of ruptured aortic aneurysm is made by the classical features of *abdominal and/or back pain, pulsatile abdominal mass* and *hypotension*.

Atheroembolism may arise from abdominal arch aneurysm and lead to *"blue leg toe syndrome"* characterized by purple discolouration of the toes/forefoot.

THE VENOUS SYSTEM

Clinical Symptoms

Venous disease is much more common in the legs than in the arms. It usually presents in one of the four following ways:
1. Deep vein thrombosis (DVT) with pain and swelling.
2. Superficial thrombophlebitis with rednessness, pain and swelling.
3. Varicosity of veins (dilated tortuosity of the veins over the part/limb) resulting in venous ulceration and pigmentation.
4. Chronic venous insufficiency.

Symptom Analysis

1. **Pain** of deep vein thrombosis is deep seated and associated with pitting oedema below the level of obstruction. The superficial venous thrombophlebitis produces a red, painful area overlying the vein involved.

   Patient with uncomplicated varicose vein may complain of an aching pain/discomfort in the leg, itching and a feeling of swelling due to prominence of venous system. **Symptoms** are aggravated by prolonged standing and are worst towards the end of the day. Varicose ulceration is painless, but if pain occurs, it is relieved by elevation of the limb.

2. **Swelling.** It is associated invariably with deep vein thrombosis and deep venous reflux. It may be present with varicose veins.
3. **Discolouration:** Deep blue/black to purple or even red discolouration may be complained on the medial aspect of the lower part of the leg by the patients suffering from chronic venous insufficiency. The discolouration is due to deposition of haemosiderin in the skin leading to lipodermatosclerosis.
4. **Ulceration:** A venous ulcer occurs on the lowest dependent part especially the ankle in patients with varicose vein. This is associated with pigmentation around it. Patients with venous ulceration may not seek medical attention for many years. Bleeding from the ulcer and secondary infection at the site of ulcer are common.

Q. Ask about nature of pain or discomfort.
Q. Ask about itching or swelling of leg(s).
Q. Ask about aggravated and relieving factors.
Q. Ask about any pigmentation or discolouration.
Q. Is there any ulceration or exudation from the leg ulcer?

THE HISTORY

Ask about the following in a patient with venous system disease.
- Onset of the symptoms and profession (farmers, policemen).
- Recent bed rest or operation on the leg or pelvis
- Recent travel (e.g. long air flight)
- Prolong forced immobilization, especially following bone fracture, trauma, plaster of Paris splintage.
- Pregnancy or history of delivery or history of taking oral contraceptive.
- Previous deep vein thrombosis
- Family history of thrombosis
- Recent central vein catheterisation, injection of drugs or prolonged IV drip through a cannula in the upper limb (for superficial thrombophlebitis).
- History of weight loss (if patient has recurrent thrombophlebitis due to suspected malignancy).

EXAMINATION OF VENOUS SYSTEM

It is done under two heads:
1. Inspection
2. Palpation

☞ Inspection

- Examine the legs with the patient standing and then lying supine.
- Expose the limbs adequately and inspect it for swelling, any superficial venous dilatation and tortuosity. Look the skin for any colour change or ulcer.

☞ Palpation

- Palpate the limbs for any differences in the temperature.
- Elevate the limb to about 15° above the horizontal and note the rate of venous emptying.
- If appropriate, perform the Trendelenburg test.

BRIEF SYNOPSIS OF VENOUS DISORDERS

I. DEEP VEIN THROMBOSIS (DVT)

Deep vein thrombosis commonly involves the legs (Fig. 3.21) than the arm (axillary vein thrombosis). The precipitating and predisposing facotrs for deep vein thrombosis are given in Table 3.21. The incidence of deep vein thrombosis is increasing because of greater use of indwelling central venous catheters.

TABLE 3.21: Deep Vein Thrombosis; Predisposing and Precipitating Factors

Predisposing factors	Precipitating factors
• Venous statis	• Congestive heart failure
• Oral contraceptives	• Orthopedic procedure (total hip replacement.
• Prolonged bed rest or immobilization	• Malignancy (e.g. pancreas, lung, ovary, testes)
• Hypercoaguable state	• Nephrotic syndrome
• Old age	• SLE and antiphospholipid syndrome
• Smoking	• Inflammatory bowel disease
• Pregnancy	• Polycythaemia
• Dehydration	• Protein C and S deficiency
	• Homocystinuria

Clinical Features

The clinical features of DVT of lower limb (leg) and upper limb (arm) are given in Table 3.22.

Homan's sign (Fig. 3.22): It is unreliable diagnostic sign of DVT of leg where increased resistance or pain occurs during dorsiflexion of foot. It is now-a-days not performed due to risk of dislodgement of thrombus.

Differential Diagnosis

DVT must be differentiated from a variety of disorders that cause unilateral leg pain or oedema such as:

Cardiovascular System

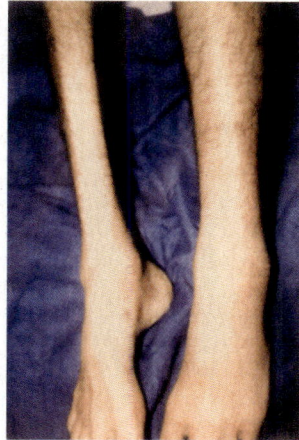

Fig. 3.21: Deep vein thrombosis of left leg. Note the swelling over the foot.

- Muscle rupture
- Muscle haematoma due to trauma or haemorrhage
- A ruptured popliteal cyst
- Lymphoedema. The skin over the oedema is thickened, indurated and pigmented (brawny). The oedema is non-pitting.
- Postphlebitic syndrome. It results from acute recurrent deep vein thrombosis.

Complications

- Chronic venous insufficiency and ulceration
- Pulmonary embolism. It can occur even without symptoms of venous thrombosis.

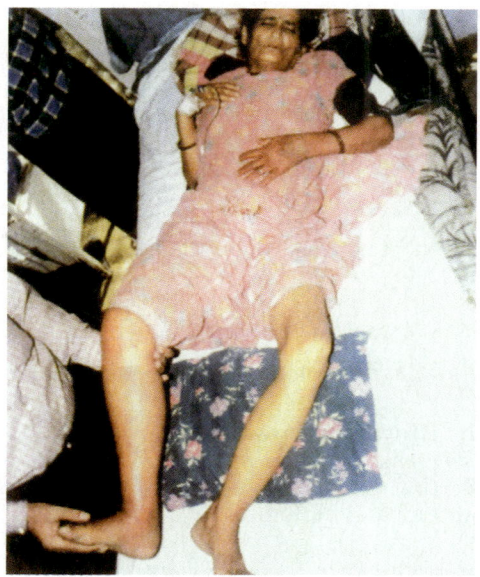

Fig. 3.22: Homan's sign.

II. SUPERFICIAL VENOUS THROMBOPHLEBITIS (Fig. 3.23)

This is usually sterile inflammation of superficial veins, may be associated with intraluminal thrombosis. The most common cause is central indwelling catheters or needles used for intravenous fluids. Sometiems, it is secondary to trauma or carcinoma of pancreas (recurrent superficial thrombophlebitis). Primary superficial venous thrombosis is often seen in pregnancy, postpartum state and in thromboangiitis obliterans.

TABLE 3.22: Clinical Manifestations of DVT of Leg and Arm

Feature	DVT of leg	DVT of arm
Veins involved	Illiac, femoral or popliteal	Subclavian or axillary vein
Pain	Calf pain, increases during walking	Arm pain exacerbated by activity especially occurs on holding the arms above the head
Tenderness	Calf tenderness on squeezing the calf	Arm tenderness on squeezing
Swelling	Unilateral leg oedema	Unilateral arm oedema
Warmth	Present	Present
Increased tissue turgor	Present	Present
Skin colour	In some patients, a cyanotic hue presents due to deoxygenated haemoglobin in stagnant vein—a condition called *phlegmasia cerulea dolens*. In others, there may be pallor due to increased interstitial tissue pressure—a condition called *phlegmasia alba dolens*.	The skin is often cyanosed and mottled especially on dependency
Visible distended veins	Distension of superficial veins over the calf and around the ankle or over foot	Superficial distended veins acting as collaterals are seen in the upper arm, over the shoulder and anterior chest wall
Palpable vein	A cord may be felt in the calf region	A cord may be felt in the arm region

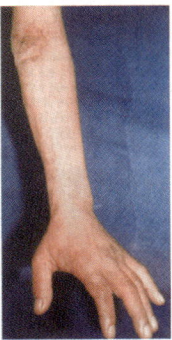

Fig. 3.23: Superficial venous thrombophlebitis.

The **clincial features** include *dull aching pain, swelling, erythema* and *induration* along the vein involved. There may be associated *fever* and *chills* as constitutional symptoms.

III. VARICOSE VEINS AND CHRONIC VENOUS INSUFFICIENCY

Varicose veins are defined as abnormally dilated, tortuous superficial veins of the lower extremities involving commonly the saphenous vein and its branches (Fig. 3.24A).

Trendelenburg test (Fig. 3.24B)

It is done to assess the valvular competence in both the communicating veins and saphenous venous system.

Method
- Start with the patient lying supine
- Elevate the limb to empty the superficial veins by "milking" the leg.
- With the leg still elevated, the upper end of the vein is then occluded by finger pressure on the saphenous opening. The saphenous opening lies 2–3 cm below and 2–3 cm lateral to pubic tubercle.
- While the examiner maintains this pressure, the patient stands.
- If the valves (saphenofemoral junction) are incompetent the veins will fill rapidly from above (retrograde filling) when the pressure is released.

Results
1. Rapid filling of the superficial veins while the saphenous vein is occluded indicates incompetent valves in the communicating system.
2. Positive Trendelenburg test indicates saphenofemoral junction incompetence.

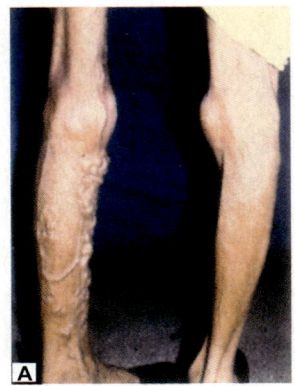

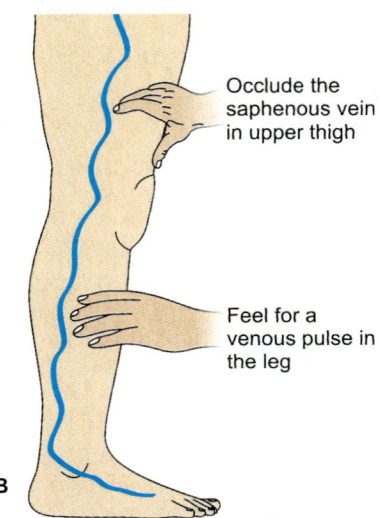

Fig. 3.24: Varicose veins. (A) The dilated and tortuous veins of the left leg indicate varicose vein; (B) Trendelenburg's test for valve incompetence.

Types
1. **Primary:** The primary incompetency of venous valves is of unknown cause. This may be inherited. Incompetent valves of the perforating veins in the thigh and lower limbs, communicate the pressure from the deep veins to superficial veins and make them to swell elongated and tortuous. Pregnancy and prolonged standing (e.g. in policemen, farmers) are common precipitating factors.
2. **Secondary:** This is due to damage to the venous valves due to neoplasms or thrombophlebitis.

Symptoms and Signs
The varicosity of veins may be asymptomatic, but if symptoms occur, then patients usually complain of a dull ache or pruritus. The involved veins are dilated

and tortuous (Fig. 3.24A). In long standing cases, chronic venous insufficiency develops producing skin changes in the lower leg, e.g. varicose eczema, lipodermatosclerosis (brownish discolouration and in duration), venous ulcerations due to sustained venous stasis and increased pressure.

IV. CHRONIC LEG ULCERATION

Deep vein thrombosis is a common cause of chronic venous insufficiency, which, in turn, is the commenest cause of leg ulceration (Fig. 3.25). Vast majority of the leg ulcers can be ascertained by clinical examination (Table 3.23).

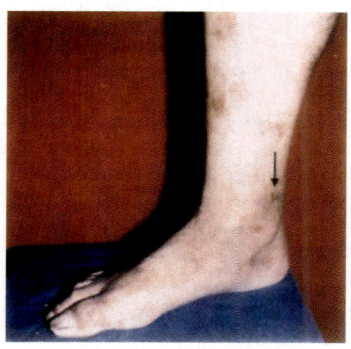

Fig. 3.25: Chronic venous ulceration and pigmentation. Note the oedema of leg, venous ulceration (↓) and pigmentation of right foot and leg.

TABLE 3.23: Differentiation Between Various Trophic Ulcers

Feature	Arterial insufficiency	Chronic venous insufficiency	Neuropathic ulcer
Site	Toes, feet or in areas of trauma	Around the ankle	Pressure points in areas with diminished sensation, as in diabetic neuropathy
Skin around the ulcer	No callous, excess of pigment, may be atrophic	Pigmented	Calloused
Pain	Severe unless neuropathy present	Not severe	Absent, hence, ulcer often goes unnoticed
Associated gangrene	May be present	Absent	Absent in uncomplicated ulcer
Other signs	Decreased pulses, pallor of the foot on elevation, dusky rubor on dependency	Oedema, pigmentation, stasis, dermatitis	Decreased sensation and absent ankle jerk

Unit IV

The Urogenital System and Sexually Transmitted Diseases

- Symptoms and their Analysis
- History
- Physical signs on General and Systemic Examination
- Diagnosis and Differential Diagnosis
- Brief Synopsis of Urogenital Disorders

I. COMMON URINARY SYMPTOMS

Renal disease especially chronic renal failure may be totally asymptomatic, detected incidentally by the presence of an *anaemia, hypertension, proteinuria* or *raised blood urea*. The symptoms of renal disease which bring the patient to a doctor are given in Box 4.1.

Box 4.1	Common Symptoms Pertaining to Urinary System
• Loin pain (renal pain)	• Increased frequency
• Dysuria	• Burning micturition
• Oliguria/anuria, polyuria/nocturia	• Puffiness of face and oedema
• Haematuria	• Symptoms of uraemia, e.g. pallor, nausea, vomiting
• Hesitancy, retention of urine, retention with overflow	• Fatigue/tiredness
• Urinary incontinence	

LOIN PAIN/RENAL PAIN/URETERIC PAIN

The pain in loin or renal area arises either due to large kidneys or due to obstruction to the flow of the urine or due to inflammation/infection around the renal area. The pain due to renal disorder is constant and localized, may radiate down toward groin or up to the chest.

Causes

1. Large kidneys due to hydronephrosis, pyonephrosis, polycystic kidney disease, etc. The pain due to these diseases is dull dragging flank pain.
2. Acute glomerulonephritis
3. Perinephric abscess
4. Obstruction to flow of urine by a stone, clot or a tumour.

Pelviureteric/ureteric pain is felt in the lumbar region radiates down to the groin, testes or labia, is due to ureteric spasm, stone, tumour, retroperitoneal fibrosis.

Symptom Analysis

Q. Is pain severe or dull aching?
- Acute severe renal/ureteric pain is colicky in nature.

Q. Ask about history of loin pain (back pain) and its radiation.
- Loin pain indicates renal disease, i.e. large kidneys, glomerulonephritis, kidney stone or tumour.
- Lumbar pain radiating down to groin testes or labia indicates ureteric pain.

Q. Does pain occur during initiation or at the end or during whole act of micturition?
- Pain in the beginning of micturition indicates urethral disease and during the end of micturition indicates prostatic or urinary bladder disease.
- Renal/ureteric pain occurs throughout the act of micturition.

Q. Ask about associated haematuria.
- Read the causes of haematuria.

Q. History of strangury or dysuria.
- Dysuria indicates bladder, urethral or prostatic disease.

- Q. **History of symptoms of uraemia, e.g. pallor, nausea, vomiting, pruritus, lassitude, fatigue.**
  - Uraemia occurs ultimately in most of renal disorder.
- Q. **Ask about the aggravating and relieving factors.**
  - Hot water bottle may relieve ureteric or renal pelvis spasm.
  - Exercise, dehydration, exertion may precipitate renal/ureteric colic.

OLIGURIA/ANURIA

Definition: *Oliguria* is defined as urine output less than 400 ml/day in an average adult. It signifies urine formation not the urine volume collected. The collection of urine without spilling or catheterised urine is necessary to define oliguria.

Anuria means urine output less than 50 ml/day or patient may not pass urine at all. Bladder either does not contain urine or the amount of urine is <50 ml on catheterisation.

The **causes** of oliguria and anuria are same (Box 4.2).

Box 4.2 Causes of Oliguria and Anuria

Oliguria
1. **Pre-renal causes,** e.g. hypovolaemia, heart failure, renal artery stenosis/occlusion
2. **Renal causes** include acute glomerulonephritis, drug/nephrotoxins
3. **Post-renal,** e.g. stone, tumour, retroperitoneal fibrosis

Anuria
1. Complete bilateral urinary tract obstruction
2. Total renal artery or venous occlusion
3. Bilateral renal cortical necrosis
4. Acute glomerulonephritis
5. Severe shock

Symptom Analysis

Ask about

- Q. **Onset, i.e. acute or slowly developing.**
  - Acute onset of oliguria occurs due to fluid/blood loss and acute nephritic syndrome. Slowly developing oliguria is a complication of congestive heart failure and due to post-renal causes.
- Q. **Is there a history of haematuria?**
  - Haematuria with oliguria indicates acute GN, renal/ureteric stone, renal artery stenosis, renal tumour.
- Q. **History of fluid loss (diarrhoea/vomiting/diuresis/sweating), blood loss (trauma, menorrhagia, hematemesis/haematuria/epistaxis/hemoptysis).**
  - Fluid loss/blood loss can cause hypovolaemia and hypotension that lead to oliguria.
- Q. **Ask about nephrotoxic durgs/poison.**
  - Nephrotoxic drugs/poison, i.e. recent radio contrast use, nephrotoxic antibiotic, i.e. (aminoglycosides, beta-lactam) or anticancer (cisplatin, cyclosporin), NSAIDs, sulpha drugs, rifampicin, captopril, etc. can produce ARF hence oliguria.
- Q. **History of fever, sore throat, rash, etc.**
  - Streptococcal sore throat with fever and rash (skin involvement) can cause oliguria due to post-streptococcal GN.
- Q. **Ask about history of renal colic.**
  - Bilateral renal/ureteric stone can cause oliguria by blocking urinary tract (obstructive uropathy).

POLYURIA

Normal urine output is 800–2500 ml/day. Urine output varies with diet, temperature and fluid intake.

Polyuria refers to urine output >3 L/day provided patient is not on high fluid intake or diuretics.

Nocturia means excessive amount of urine passed at night.

Causes

1. *Physiological*, e.g. high, fluid intake, excessive intake of tea and coffee.
2. *Diabetes insipidus*
   - Pituitary adenoma
   - Nephrogenic diabetes insipidus due to polycystic disease and interstitial disease of kidneys, drugs, toxins, multiple myeloma and renal amyloidosis.
3. Systemic disease (osmotic diuresis)
   - Chronic renal failure
   - Diabetes mellitus
   - Hyperparathyroidism
4. *Osmotic diuresis* due to mannitol
5. *Salt and water diuresis* due to salt losing nephropathy and diuretics
6. *Psychogenic*, e.g. primary polyuria, polydipsia syndrome.

Symptom Analysis

- Q. **Ask about amount of urine passed. What is the nature, i.e. clear, turbid?**

- A patient of diabetes insipidus and psychogenic polyuria passes a large amount of crystal clear urine (urine of low specific gravity).
- Urine of diabetes mellitus contain sediments, hence, is not clear.

Q. Is patient on a diuretic?
- Diuretic therapy is a common cause of polyuria.

Q. History of high fluid intake, tea, coffee, etc.
- They cause physiological polyuria.

Q. History of renal disease.
- Chronic renal failure and interstinal renal disease produce polyuria due to loss of concentrating and diluting capacity of the kidneys.

Q. Ask about nephrotoxic drugs.
- Drug and toxin may cause tubular damage, hence, cause polyuria.

Q. History of diabetes, multiple myeloma, hyperparathyroidism.
- All these diseases cause polyuria.

Q. Does that patient complain of swollen face and leg with polyuria?
- Puffy face and oedematous legs with polyuria indicate nephrotic syndrome.

HAEMATURIA

Definition: *Haematuria* means passage of blood (RBCs) in the urine. It may produce red discolouration called *macroscopic haematuria* or may not produce discolouration called *microscopic haematuria*.

Causes
1. *Renal disease*, e.g. glomerulonephritis (GN), interstitial nephritis, polycystic kidney disease and renal stone/tumour or trauma, Alport syndrome.
2. *Ureteric stone/neoplasm.*
3. *Cystitis, bladder stone/trauma/tumour, schistosomiasis.*
4. *Urethritis, urethral injury* (catheter induced).
5. *Prostatitis, benign enlargement of prostate, prostatic cancer.*
6. *Bleeding* (purpura) or *coagulation disorder* (hemophilia)/anticoagulant therapy, leukaemia.
7. *Systemic disorders*, e.g. polyarteritis nodosa, SLE, infective endocarditis, hypertension.

Symptom Analalysis

Q. Ask about the age.
- Bladder stone is common in children. Renal calculous, malignant tumours and hypertension are common causes of hematuria in adults while prostatic cancer and hypertrophy are common in the elderly.

Q. Ask about history of anticoagulant use.
- Positive history establishes the cause.

Q. Ask about history of hypertension or cardiovascular disease.
- Hypertension and SABE (embolic nephritis) can lead to haematuria.

Q. Ask about the quantity of blood lost.
- Blood loss is profuse in bladder and kidney tumours while small in prostatic tumour and following trauma.

Q. Ask about the relation of haematuria to act of micturition.
- The relation of haematuria with act or phase of micturition establish the source of bleeding.
- Haematuria occurring at the beginning of micturition indicates urethra or prostate as the source of bleeding.
- Haematuria throughout the act of micturition resulting in the entire specimen of urine containing blood indicates either the renal or ureter as the cause of bleeding.
- Haematuria at the end of micturition (i.e. first sample of urine passed is clear) indicates cystitis or bladder as the source of bleeding.

Q. Ask about the frequency of micturition.
- Increased frequency of micturition indicates disease of bladder, ureter or renal pelvis (pyelitis).
- Decreased frequency and oliguria with haematuria suggest acute glomerulonephritis.

Q. Ask about pain during micturition.
- *Painful micturition* indicates urinary tract colic (stone in kidney, ureter and bladder), cancer bladder and crystalluria.
- *Painless haematuria* indicates renal neoplasm, glomerulonephritis, hydronephrosis, renal tuberculosis, enlarged prostate and prostatic cancer. It is seen in certain systemic diseases, i.e. SLE, purpura.

Q. Ask about associated symptoms.
- Fever, hypertension, sore throat, haematuria indicate acute GN.
- Purpuric spots, joint pain and haematuria indicate Henoch-Schölein purpura.
- Rash, anaemia, HT, lymphadenopathy with haematuria suggest SLE.
- Renal/ureteric colic with haematuria suggests stone in the urinary tract.

INCREASED FREQUENCY OF MICTURITION

Increased frequency of micturition means patient goes for micturition many times but the total output of urine remains normal, hence, 24-hour urine output differentiates it from polyuria.

The increased frequency of micturition occurs due to irritative lesion in the urinary tract, i.e. from kidney to urinary bladder.

Causes
1. *Renal causes*, e.g. pyelitis, pyelonephritis, urinary tract infection.
2. *Ureteric causes*, e.g. ureteric stone
3. *Bladder causes*, e.g. cystitis, bladder stone and tumour.
4. *Prostatic causes*, e.g. prostatitis, benign hypertrophy of prostate, prostatic cancer.

Symptom Analysis

Ask the following

Q. Is it associated with pain?

Q. Is increased frequency of urine nocturnal?

Q. Is there any history of associated haematuria, dysuria?

Q. Is there any associated symptom?

URINARY INCONTINENCE

Definition: Involuntary passage of urine is called *urinary incontinence*.

Dribbling of urine means leakage of a small amount of urine either due to raised intra-abdominal pressure during straining, coughing or sneezing or due to local causes such as cystocoele, rectocoele, weak pelvic floor, neurogenic bladder and prostate enlargement.

Causes
Incontinence of urine occurs either due to neurological causes or non-neurological causes.

I. Neurological causes
- *CNS disorder*, e.g. stroke, trauma, brain tumour, parkinsonism, dementia.
- *Cord lesion*, e.g. spinal cord compression, multiple sclerosis.
- *Peripheral nerve lesion*, e.g. diabetes mellitus, pelvic fracture.

II. Non-neurological causes
  i. *Weakness of sphincter* mechanism leading to *stress incontinence*.
   - Incontinence due to this mechanism occurs in postmenopausal women during exertion, straining or stress, laughing, coughing, sneezing, etc.

  ii. *Detrusor instability* leads to *urge incontinence*. The *causes* include; urinary tract infection, bladder stones, cystitis.

  iii. *Post-micturition dribbling/incontinence* (occurs following transurethral resection).

  iv. *Overflow incontinence* is insensible incontinence, occurs with distended bladder, bladder neck obstruction, urethral stricture, enlarged prostate.

  v. *Total incontinence*, e.g. ureterovaginal fistula, vesicovaginal fistula, neurogenic bladder, post-prostectomy incontinence.

  vi. *Antisocial or functional incontinence* occurs in those individuals who have lost ability to appreciate the need to pass urine. They can pass urine at any place at anytime.

Symptom Analalysis

Q. **Ask about the age of the patient.**
- Stress incontinence is common in old post-menopausal women.

Q. **Does it occur due to stress (laughing, coughing, straining at stool, etc.)?**
- Incontinence in old post-menopausal women, commonly occurs due to stress.

Q. **Is it overflow incontinence?**
- Overflow incontinence occurs with distended bladder, bladder neck obstruction, urethral stricture, enlarged prostate, spinal cord compression.

Q. **Is it total incontinence?**
- Read the causes of total incontinence.

Q. **Does the patient suffer from stroke, brain tumour, dementia, parkinsonism?**
- All the conditions can lead to urinary incontinence.

Q. **Since when the patient has not passed urine?**
- Holding of urine for longer period is called *retention*. Retention can lead to overflow incontinence.

Q. **Does the patient has suprapubic distress?**
- Retention urine produces suprapubic distress.

Q. **History of diabetes.**
- Diabetes can lead to incontingence due to neurogenic bladder (autonomic dysfunction).

Q. **Ask about the neurological and non-neurological cause of retention.**
- Read the causes of incontinence.
- History of prostectomy or transurethral resection.
- Prostatectomy and TUR.

Q. Is there a history of dribbling of urine?
- Dribbling incontinence occurs following transurethral resection for enlarged prostate.

DYSURIA

It means pain urethra during and after micturition and sometimes in suprapubic region.

Causes

It may occur acutely producing distress.
1. *Urethral causes*, e.g. urethritis (gonococcal), balanitis, trauma, stricture.
2. *Prostatic causes*, e.g. prostatitis, prostate cancer, BEP (benign enlargement of prostate).
3. *Bladder causes*, e.g. cystitis, bladder stone.
4. *Uterine*, e.g. fibroid, cancer.

Symptom Analysis

Ask about the following

Q. Ask about the pain during or after the act of micturition.
- Pain during micturition is called *dysuria*. Read the causes of dysuria

Q. Ask about the history of urethritis and sexually transmitted diseases.

Q. Ask about frequency of micturition or urinary retention (for prostatic disease).

Q. Ask about suprapubic pain and painful micturition (bladder diseases)

Q. Ask about menstrual irregularity menorrhagia (uterine disease).

URINARY RETENTION

Holding of urine in the urinary bladder is called *retention*. It may occur acutely producing distress. Chronic retention of urine may be followed by overflow incontinence.

Full bladder on percussion confirms urinary retention.

Causes

I. **Neurological,** e.g. diabetic autonomic neuropathy, parasagittal neoplasm of the brain, stroke, spinal cord compression due to any cause.
II. **Non-neurological** (obstructive uropathy)
- Obstruction to urinary flow will lead to retention. Obstruction can occur at any of the following levels.
    1. *Urethral obstruction* due to stone, stricture, urethral valve, trauma, etc.

2. *Bladder outflow obstruction*, e.g. bladder neck obstruction due to stone, enlarged prostate, bladder tumour, ureterorectocoele.

Symptom Analysis

Ask about the following

Q. Has the patient any suprapubic distress?

Q. History of diabetes, spinal cord disease or trauma.

Q. History of bladder stone, stricture (instrumentation, trauma).

Q. History of rectocoele, ureterorectocoele.

OTHER URINARY SYMPTOMS/TERMS

HESITANCY

Patient hesitate to pass urine immediately. He/she wait for sometime before passing urine. It is due to urinary tract obstruction.

Symptom Analysis

Q. Ask about spinal cord disease.
- **Thin stream/diminished stream.** The urine is passed with a thin stream. This indicates partial obstruction to flow of urine (prostate hypertrophy).

Q. Ask about history of bladder stone, stricture and BEP.

URGENCY

- The patient feels and/or has urge to pass urine without any delay.

PRECIPITANCY

- If the patient does not find a suitable place to pass urine, then she/he wets herself or himself.

Q. Ask about history of incontinence, prostate surgery, menopause, pelvic surgery, repeated pregnancies.

FACIAL PUFFINESS

Puffiness of face or periorbital oedema are interchangeably used to describe the oedema of upper and lower eyelids bilaterally with facial oedema.

Causes

1. *Renal*, e.g. acute nephritic syndrome, nephrotic syndrome.
2. *Liver disease*, e.g. cirrhosis of liver.

3. *Hypoalbuminaemia* due to malabsorption, malnutrition.
4. *Cardiac disease*, e.g. CHF, pericardial effusion.
5. *Mediastinal causes*, e.g. mediastinal compression, superior vena cava obstruction.
6. *Endocrinal causes*, e.g. Cushing's syndrome, hypothyroidism.
7. *Miscellaneous*, e.g. angioneurotic oedema.

Symptom Analysis

Q. Ask about the morning puffiness of face.
- Morning puffiness of face and pitting pedal oedema indicate renal disorder.

Q. History of discolouration of urine, oliguria.
- Dark-coloured urine and oliguria indicate acute nephritic syndrome.

Q. History of cardiac disease and congestive heart failure.
- All cardiac diseases leading to CHF result in puffiness of face.

Q. History of oedema feet/leg and distension of abdomen.
- Puffiness of face associated with oedema feet and legs, and ascites indicate generalised anasarca.

Q. Is there history of chronic liver disease or cirrhosis?
- Chronic liver disease and cirrhosis result in periorbital oedema.

Q. History of chronic diarrhoea/malabsorption.
- Chronic diarrhoea and malabsorption can result in periorbital oedema due to hypoproteinaemia.

Q. History of cough, stridor/hoarseness.
- Puffiness of face, conjunctival congestion, stridor or hoarseness of voice indicate superior mediastinal compression.

Q. History of anaemia, hypertension.
- Anaemia, hypertension along with puffiness of face suggest chronic renal failure.

Q. History of wasp/bee sting
- Wasp and bee sting produce angioneurotic oedema.

SYMPTOMS OF URAEMIA

Advanced chronic renal disease may progress to renal failure leading to symptoms of uraemia. The symptoms in uraemia result due to retention of nitrogenous and other toxic waste products. The symptoms are nonspecific and variable. They are:

1. *General symptoms*, e.g. lethargy, mental confusion.
2. *Neurological*, e.g. muscle cramps, peripheral neuropathy, epileptic seizures, myoclonus, coma.
3. *Cardiovascular*, e.g. hypertension, pericarditis, Arrhythmias, CHF.
4. *Respiratory*, e.g. Kussmaul's breathing (acidotic breathing), pleurisy, pneumonia, non-cardiogenic pulmonary oedema.
5. *Dermatological*, e.g. pallor, dry scaly (uraemic) skin or uraemic frost over the face, shallow pigmentation, pruritus, half and half nails.
6. *Gastrointestinal*, e.g. nausea, vomiting, anorexia, haematemesis, uremic smell.
7. *Haematological*, e.g. anaemia, haemorrhagic tendencies.
8. *Metabolic and endocrinal*, e.g. osteomalacia, renal osteodystrophy, impotence, amenorrhoea.
9. *Urinay*; puffiness of face, polyuria/oliguria, generalised anasarca, acid-base and electrolyte disturbance.

Causes

The **common causes** are:
1. Diabetic kidney disease, hypertensive kidney disease, SLE.
2. *Kidney diseases*
   - Acute nephrotic and nephritic syndrome
   - Glomerular diseases.
   - Cystic kidney diseases
   - Tubulointerstitial diseases.
   - Urinary tract infection and urinary tract obstruction (obstructive uropathy).

Symptom Analysis

Q. Ask about the history of chronic renal disease.
- History of renal disease >6 months indicates chronic disease, while acute renal failure develops within days to weeks.

Q. Ask about the systemic symptoms of uraemia.
- Nausea, vomiting, anorexia, headache, fits, diminished vision, dyspnoea, etc.

Q. Ask about the change in urine volume.
- Change in volume of urine, i.e. oliguria suggests ARF; while polyuria suggests CRF.

Q. Ask about swelling of face (periorbital oedema) in the morning. Ask about swelling of feet.
- Anaemia, oedema and hypertension indicate chronic renal failure (uraemia).

The Urogenital System and Sexually Transmitted Diseases

General Commentary about Urinary Symptoms

- *Dysuria, frequency* and *urgency* suggest the disorders of the lower urinary tract (bladder, prostate, and urethra). Commonly, it is due to urinary tract infection, tumour, calculi and urinary tract obstruction.
- *Dysuria* with *urethral discharge* indicates *gonorrhoea*.
- *Dysuria with stranguary* indicates acute bladder neck obstruction due to a stone or blood clot.
- *Painless haematuria* in an adult is usually due to benign bladder papilloma or a renal, bladder or prostatic carcinoma.
- *Change in colour of the urine after standing* (fresh voided urine is of normal colour) indicates acute intermittent porphyria.
- *Polyuria* alone is due to renal disease, *polyuria*, *polydipsia* and *polyphagia* indicate diabetes, *polyuria* and *polydipsia* suggest diabetes insipidus and psychogenic polydipsia. *Polyuria* and *nocturia* suggest cardiac failure.
- *Reduced force of urinary stream and thinning of urinary stream* in males suggest bladder outlet obstruction (prostate enlargement, urethral stricture).
- *Hesitancy, double voiding* (need to pass urine again within a few minutes of micturition), dribbling after micturition, increased frequency and nocturia due to incomplete bladder emptying or complete urinary retention are symptoms of prostatic outflow obstruction.
- *Stress incontinence* (leakage of urine in response to coughing, sneezing, or laughing) occurs in multiparous women due to weakness of pelvic floor muscles.

II. SYMPTOMS OF SEXUALLY TRANSMITTED DISEASES (STDs)

- Males complain of *urethritis* with pain during micturition and *discharge per urethra* or *genital ulcer lesion*. They may complain of masses in groin (*lymphadenopathy*)
- Females complain of *excessive vaginal discharge*, (*purulent in gonorrhea*), *white and curdy* (*candidiasis*), frothy and yellow during intercourse.

Symptom Analysis

Q. Ask about pain during micturition, i.e. in the beginning, during whole micturition or at the end (Read Loin Pain in the beginning of the Unit).

Q. Ask about discharge per urethera in male (white curdy, purulent) and vaginal discharge (germs, foul smelling purulent) in females.

Q. Ask about masses in the groin (Read inguinal lymphadenopathy)

Q. Ask about extra-marital contact.

Q. History of use of condoms or tampons.

Q. History of genital hygiene after sexual act.

Q. History of homosexuality.

HISTORY

Present History

Ask about the following

- Complaints or the symptoms, their onset, duration, progression and write them in chronological order.
- Analyse the symptoms in details.
- Find out the aggravating and relieving factors.
- Ask about the associated symptoms.
- Ask about symptoms of complications of renal disease, i.e. uraemia or renal failure.

Past History

Ask for

- Renal colic or loin pain (intermittent colic due to stone or clot due to haematuria).
- Polyarthritis (gout, rheumatoid arthritis, SLE)
- Hypertension and diabetes (diabetic nephropathy).
- Long history of chronic suppurative lung disease or tuberculosis (tuberculosis of kidney, amyloidosis).
- Malaria or filarial infection (nephrotic syndrome, chyluria).
- Poisoning, snakebite or insect stings and bites.
- Surgery, instrumentaion/catheterisation
- Sexually transmitted diseases.
- Sore throat or skin disease with secondary bacterial infection.
- Complications during pregnancy.

Family History

In certain heritable and developmental renal disorders which get transmitted from parent to offsprings, the family history provides an important clue to presence of some or many of the manifestations in the index patient and in other members of the family. These disorders are:

1. *Cystic renal diseases*, e.g. polycystic kidney disease (autosomal dominant or autosomal recessive), tuberous sclerosis, von Hippel-Lindau disease and medullary sponge kidney or medullary cystic disease.
2. *Hereditary nephritis* (Alport's syndrome)
3. *Hereditary metabolic disorders* (e.g. Bartter's syndrome, Alport's syndrome, familial urate nephropathy).

4. *Hereditary renal tubular defects.*
5. *Hereditary systemic disorders* with involvement of kidneys, e.g. diabetes, hypertension, Wilson's disease, familial Mediterranean fever, sickle cell disease.
6. *Vesicoureteric reflux disease.*

Personal History

Marital status and occupation should be asked for:
- Sewerage workers are predisposed to leptospirosis.
- Aniline dye exposure—uroepithelial tumour.
- Hot atmosphere calculous disease.

Drug History

The kidneys play a major role in the excretion of many drugs, and has rich vascular supply, hence, is susceptible to the effects of various drugs/toxins. Exposure to these toxins may be accidental or deliberate. The drugs causing nephrotoxicity are given in Box 4.3, their history of intake must be asked in each and every case of renal disease.

Box 4.3 Nephrotoxic Drugs/Toxins

Drugs
1. Antibiotics, e.g. aminoglycosides, penicillins, cephalosporins, vancomycins, tetracyclines
2. Sulphonamides
3. Antifungal, e.g. amphotericin
4. Antiviral, e.g. acyclovir
5. Antimitotics, e.g. cyclosporin, cisplatin, cyclophosphamide, methotrexate, cytosine arabinoside, thioguanine, 5-fluorouracil
6. NSAIDs, or aspirin or phenacetin (analgesic nephropathy)
7. Diuretics
8. Rifampicin T
9. Pentamidine
10. Lithium
11. Heroin-induced nephropathy
12. Occupational exposure to chemicals

Toxins
- Heavy metals, e.g. lead, mercury, cadmium, gold, pencillamine
- Chemical and plant toxins, e.g. $CuSO_4$, mushroom poisoning
- Metabolic toxins, e.g. hyperuricaemia, hypercalcaemia, hyperoxaluria, cystinosis, Fabry's disease

Sexual History

The sexual history is important for sexual dysfunction as well as for sexually transmitted diseases (Box 4.4) in young adults. Although such topics are often avoided by patients because of embarrassment, it is particularly important to interview and examine the patient in privacy and with confidentiality.

The history should explore the two important aspects:

Box 4.4 Sexually Transmitted Diseases (Causative Agents)

1. **Bacterial**
   - Syphilis (*T. pallidum*)
   - Gonorrhoea (*N. gonorrhoeae*)
   - Lymphogranuloma venereum (*Chlamydia trachomatis*, LGV 1–3 serovars)
   - Chancroid (*H. ducreyi*)
   - Granuloma inguinale (*Calymmatobacterium granulomatis*)
   - Bacterial vaginosis
   - Non-specific genital infection (ureaplasma, Mycoplasma)
2. **Viral**
   - Genital herpes (herpes simplex virus 1 and 2)
   - Genital warts (human papillomavirus)
   - Molluscum contagiosum (molluscum contagiosum virus)
   - AIDS and related disease (human immunodeficiency virus)
   - Hepatitis (virus A, B, C and delta viruses)
3. **Fungal**
   - Thrush/moniliasis/candidiasis
4. **Protozoal**
   - Trichomoniasis (*T. vaginalis*)

1. *Sexual function and activity*: Ask about sexual activity and whether they have any of the disorders known to predispose to sexual dysfunction, i.e. diabetes, alcoholism, chronic renal failure, marital difficulty or psychological disorder.
2. *To explore the possibility of sexually transmitted diseases* as listed in Box 4.4. The points to be asked are:
   a. History of premarital, extramarital or marital exposure and date of last exposure.
   b. How many sexual partners have you had in the last 12 months?
   c. How many of your partners have been males and how many females?
   d. How many of your partners have casual relationship?
   e. Do you use condom most of the time, all of the time, or not at all?
   f. Have you ever suffered from a sexually transmitted disease?

Males: Ask for any problem with sexual drive, erection, penetration, ejaculation or orgasm.

Females: Ask for any problem with sexual drive, pain during intercourse (dyspareunia) or orgasm.

A history of intercourse with homosexual or bisexual men, I.V. drug users or with persons living in or from an area of high HIV endemicity may suggest AIDS as the cause.

The type of sexual practice must be asked such as:
- Straight sex (peno-vaginal intercourse)
- Oral sex (oro-penile intercourse)
- Gay sex (oro-anal sex) or (peno-anal intercourse)

Nature of sexual partner, i.e. prostitute, call girl, foreigner must be asked.

Hepatitis B and HIV infection are common in practising peno-anal or peno-vaginal intercourse.

MENSTRUAL AND OBSTETRICS HISTORY

Ask about the following
- Age of menarche
- Age of menopause, if appropriate
- Use of contraceptive drugs or device, or hormone replacement therapy
- Date of the first day of last menstrual period
- Frequency, duration and regularity of menses
- Blood loss during menses, i.e. scanty or heavy.

The normal age of menarche varies from the ages between 10 and 15 years. Failure to menstruate at all by this age indicates *primary amenorrhoea*.

The normal age of the menopause varies between 45 and 55 years. *Secondary amenorrhoea* may be due to pregnancy, systemic illness, hyperprolactinaemia, androgens excess or hypopituitarism. It could be psychological also.

The obstetric history includes details of all pregnancies, successful or otherwise, and any problem experienced during pregnancy such as hypertension or urinary infection. If a woman has never conceived, it is appropriate to ask whether this was by choice or whether difficulties in conceiving have been experienced.

If a female complains of vaginal discharge, then ask about its *colour, consistency* and *odour* (foul smell indicates anaerobic infection).

Points to be asked in obstetric history are
- Number of pregnancies and live births, miscarriages and termination.
- Any health problem during pregnancies or after delivery.
- Were the previous deliveries vaginal or caesarean?
- Were forceps or episiotomy used?
- Ask about medical disorders complicating pregnancy such as anaemia, hypertension, diabetes mellitus, thyroid disease or urinary infection.

Vaginal bleeding following intercourse could be due to cervical erosions, polyp or carcinoma.

The presence of vaginal discharge, or intermenstrual, postcoital or postmenopausal bleeding is an indication for gynaecological assessment and examination.

EXAMINATION

It includes:
1. General physical examination
2. Examination of the abdomen and other systems
3. Examination of genitalia.

GENERAL PHYSICAL EXAMINATION

☞ *Look for consciousness. Is there any disturbance in consciousness?*

Consciousness in renal disease may be disturbed due to uraemic encephalopathy as a result of retention of waste substances or uraemic toxins.

☞ *Look for pallor or anaemia at different sites.*

Anaemia in renal disorders occurs due to (i) depressed erythropoiesis, haematuria, bleeding or coagulation defect, and/or (ii) reduced production of erythropoietin in CRF, and/or (iii) hypoplasia of marrow due to uraemic toxins, and/or (iv) shortened span of RBCs (haemolysis).

☞ *Look at the mouth and tongue: Note any abnormality.*

- Buccal mucosa is pale in anaemia.
- Tongue and mucous membrane are dry in dehydration, renal failure
- White deposits (oral candidiasis) and ulceration of the mouth are seen in severely ill patients or patients receiving steroids or immunosuppressive drugs, fungal infections.

☞ *The skin: Look for any abnormality.*

- Steroid facies seen due to steroid therapy in nephrotic syndrome.
- *Facial puffiness* may denote nephritic or nephrotic syndrome.
- Dry, pale and flaky skin are seen in uraemia.

- Uraemic frost (dirty brown appearance of skin) looks like dandruff on the forehead and is due to crystallisation of urea from the sweat. It is seen in terminal uraemia.
- Bruises or purpura suggest a bleeding or coagulation defect.
- A *butterfly rash* over face indicates SLE with renal involvement (Fig. 4.1).
- Scratch marks or excoriation of skin indicates pruritus.
- The lustre and laxity of the skin can be demonstrated by pinching the skin between finger and the thumb. Skin turgor or lustre is lost in dehydration.
- Subcutaneous calcium deposits in skin may occur due to hyperparathyroidism which may ulcerate.
- Scars of vascular access surgery may be seen in forearms or ankles and the veins over dorsum of the hands may be dilated as a result of arteriovenous anastomosis constructed in the forearm in patients undergoing dialytic therapy (haemodialysis).
- Scars of lithotripsy for crushing of stone may be noticed (Fig. 4.2).
- Pitting oedema of the ankles, scrotum and oedema of the genitalia may be present. This is due to hypoproteinaemia in renal disorders (e.g. nephrotic syndrome).
- Wart and skin cancers are common in immunosuppressed patients with renal transplant.

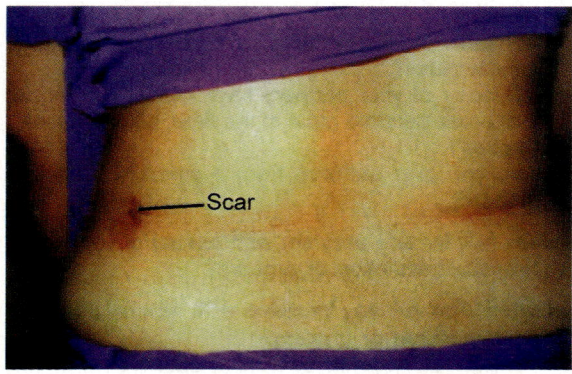

Fig. 4.2: A lithotripsy scar in left renal area.

☞ *Examine the growth and development especially in children.*

The growth is retarded and puberty delayed in children suffering from chronic renal failure.

☞ *Deformity. Look for it, if present.*

- The *renal rickets* may cause valgus or varus deformity of the knees ('*knock knees*' or '*bow legs*', Fig. 4.3), ankles swelling or beading of costochondral junctions (*rickety rosary*) and proximal muscle weakness so that patient is not able to get up from squatting position without levering up with the arms.
- Renal osteodystrophy in CRF results in deformities.
- *Shortening of distal phalanges*. Shortening of fingers due to shortening of terminal phalanges may occur as a result of resorption of bone secondary to hyperparathyroidism in chronic renal failure. There may be softening of the vertebrae with consequent curvature of the spine (*Rugger-Jersey spine*) and loss of height may cause a rounded shoulder appearance.

☞ *Examine the extremities and note any abnormality.*

- *Flapping tremors* of outstretched hands may be seen in uraemia (uraemic flaps). There may be sporadic twitchings of the limbs and muscle cramps.
- *Restless leg*—an uncontrolled desire to move their legs continuously may be seen in patients with CRF undergoing dialysis.

☞ *Examine the nails. Note any abnormality*

- White and opaque nails (*leuconychia*) are sometimes seen in nephrotic syndrome or CRF.

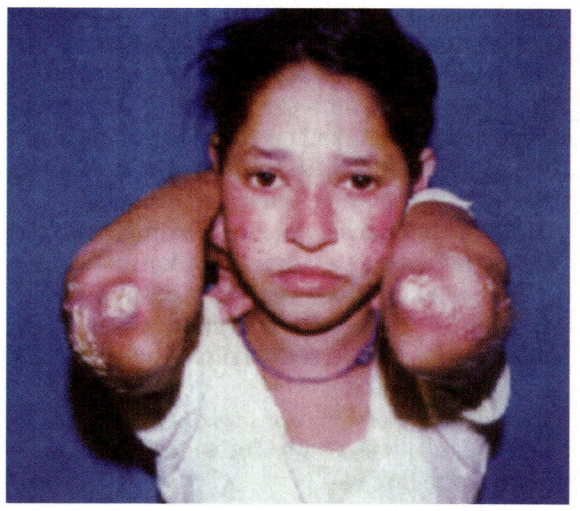

Fig. 4.1: Puffiness of face (periorbital oedema) due to SLE induced nephrotic syndrome.

The Urogenital System and Sexually Transmitted Diseases

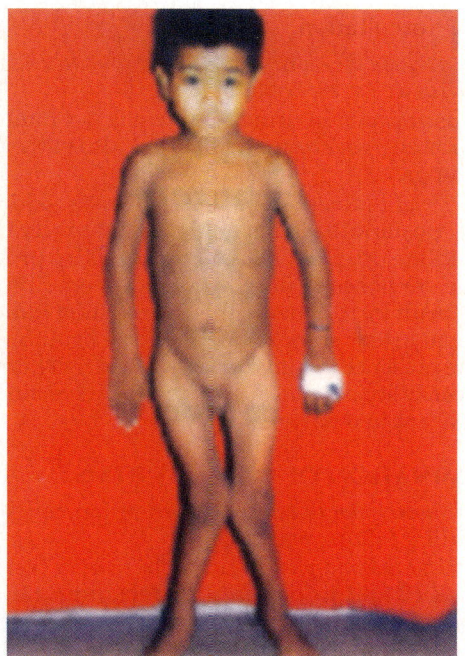

Fig. 4.3: Knocked knees in a child with renal rickets. Note the bowing of the legs also.

- *Nail dysplasia* with multiple osseous abnormalities (elbow and patella) are seen in Nail-Patella syndrome—an autosomal dominant disorder of kidney (hereditary nephropathy).
- *Half and half nails.* Lower half white and upper half brown of a nail called *half and half syndrome* is seen in chronic renal failure (Fig. 4.4).

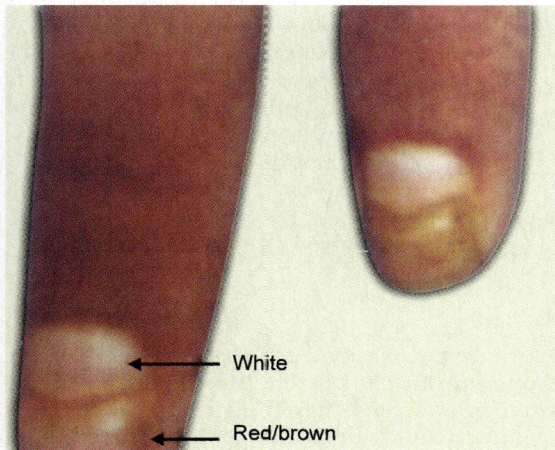

Fig. 4.4: 'Half and half nails' in a patient with chronic renal failure.

☞ *The eyes:* Note any abnormalities in the eyes.

- Pain and redness of eyes may be caused by local deposits of calcium due to hyperparathyroidism.
- Thin curved white lines in corneoscleral junction (*band keratopathy*) may occur due to hyperparathyroidism.
- Haemangioblastomas of retina occur in *von Hippel-Lindau disease.*
- Blurring of vision or visual loss may occur due to *hypertensive retinopathy* or retinal vascular thrombosis.
- Macular flecks and recurrent corneal erosions are seen in Alport's syndrome.
- Retinal changes (exudates, haemorrhage retinopathy) may occur due to hypertension, diabetes and vascular disorders.

☞ *The Ear:* Examine the ears for deafness.

Sensorineural deafness may be present in patients with *Alport's syndrome* (consisting of proteinuria, haematuria, renal failure and ocular abnormalities) and other forms of hereditary renal disease. It can be due to aminoglycoside toxicity in renal diseases.

☞ *Vital signs:* Record pulse, BP, temperature and respiration.

- *Hypertension* is common in acute glomerulonephritis, chronic parenchymal kidney disease, renal vascular disease and polycystic kidney disease.
- *Hyperventilation (increased respiratory rate)* is seen in acute and chronic renal failure due to metabolic acidosis (*Kussmaul breathing*).
- Fever indicates UTI or infection of kidneys.

EXAMINATION OF ABDOMEN (UROGENITAL SYSTEM)

☞ **1. Inspection**

Look for any mass or generalised distension.

☞ *Look at renal angle on the back of abdomen for fullness.*

- A bulge in lumbar region on one side or both sides may be seen in polycystic kidney diseases hydronephrosis, etc. The renal angle is full due to renal mass.
- A bulge in one or both lumbar regions on the front of abdomen may also be seen due to renal mass.

- Generalised anasarca produces distended abdomen.

☞ **2. Palpation**

Palpate the kidneys by bimanual palpation.
- Normal kidneys, especially right one which is lower than the left due to presence of liver, may sometimes be felt in thin persons with relaxed abdomen.
- The palpable, enlarged kidneys are always abnormal, except compensatory hypertrophied kidney in response to removal of the other kidney.
- The **causes** of enlargement of kidneys as well as palpation of a renal lump and its differential diagnosis has been discussed in the examination of abdomen (Unit VI).
- *The characteristics of distended bladder* due to delayed micturition, outlet obstruction or neuropathy (neurogenic bladder) have also been discussed in Unit VI.
- *Fullness of renal angle and tenderness of kidneys* (renal area) or *bladder* (suprapubic area) may occur due to enlargement of kidney and overdistended bladder.

- Renal angle becomes full on palpation due to enlargement of kidney(s) due to any cause.
- Tenderness of renal angle is due to perinephric abscess, following renal biopsy, renal infarction (sickle cell crisis).
- Bladder is full and tender due to cystitis or urinary tract obstruction.

Remember. It should be remembered that a transplanted kidney lies in the iliac fossa, where it can be felt as a firm swelling underneath the skin and anterior abdominal musculature.

- *Diffuse oedema of the abdominal wall* which indents or pits on pinching the abdominal wall or by pressure of the stethoscope. Sacral and pedal oedema may be caused by salt and water retention, hypoproteinaemia due to nephrotic syndrome and chronic renal failure.

☞ **3. Percussion**

Percussion in urinary system disorders is done
 i. To diagnose pulmonary complications such as pneumonia and pleural effusion.
 ii. To diagnose ascites (perform fluid thrill and shifting dullness) in nephrotic syndrome or CRF.

☞ **4. Auscultation**
- *Auscultate the kidneys around the umbilicus on each side as well as the renal angle*

Auscultation in urinary system is not limited to the kidneys (renal vasculature) but also of the heart and lungs.
- *Arterial bruits* may be heard over the kidneys, i.e. posteriorly (renal angle) or anteriorly in the midline on either side of umbilicus by pressing the stethoscope in relaxed abdomen. Presence of bruit in patients with hypertension indicates renal artery stenosis. Ileofemoral bruit implies the presence of atherosclerosis and increases the possibility of renal artery stenosis when no bruit is heard in renal area.

EXAMINATION OF OTHER SYSTEMS

1. *Cardiovascular system* for hypertension, congestive cardiac failure, pericarditis.
2. *Pericardial and pleural rubs.* These may be heard in CRF and in patients undergoing dialysis, and sometimes in conditions, such as systemic lupus erythematosus and vasculitis where kidney, heart and lungs are involved as a part of multisystemic involvement.
3. *Respiratory system* for Kussmaul's breathing, crackles at the bases (uraemic lungs), pleural effusion (pleural rub).
4. *Gastrointestinal system* for bloody diarrhoea, adynamic ileus, uraemic breath.

EXAMINATION OF GROIN AND GENITALIA

☞ **Inspection and Palpation of the Groin**

Inspection of the groin for the hernial sites has been described during examination of abdomen. Look for swelling and for cough impulse.
- Normally, when patient coughs and raises the intra-abdominal pressure, a non-expansible impulse is transmitted to the palpating hand which may be confused with small reducible inguinal hernia in unexperienced hand.

A bulge that appears on straining (coughing) suggests a hernia **(Fig. 4.5)**.

Method

Ask the patient to stand up in front of you, turn him to one side and inspect the site of swelling. Note whether it descends into the scrotum or not. Now ask him to cough loudly and look for *cough impulse* (*expansile impulse*) and try to decide whether it is above or below the inguinal ligament. If a cough impulse produces a bulge on inspection, it suggests

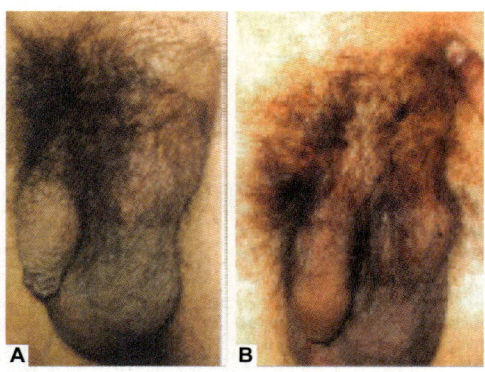

Figs 4.5A and B: Inguinal hernia. (A) Cough reflex. The hernia reappears on standing and coughing. It increases in size and becomes prominent during coughing; (B) The inguinal hernia is direct on palpation.

hernia, so move to that side where the lump is present in the groin and stand by the side and a little behind the patient. If right groin is being examined, support the patient by putting left hand on the right buttock, and fingers of the right hand being placed over the inguinal canal. Ask the patient to strain (cough) and feel for an expansile impulse, if present, indicates hernia.

Now decide whether it is inguinal or femoral hernia.

Palpate for an inguinal hernia by placing your fingers or thumb on the anterior thigh in the region of the femoral canal (Fig. 4.5). Ask the patient to cough or strain down again. Note whether thrust is imparted to the fingers/thumb above or below the inguinal ligament. A swelling and thrust below the inguinal ligament in the region of femoral and indicate femoral hernia.

If hernia is confirmed to be inguinal, then proceed to decide.

1. *Whether it is direct* (Fig. 4.5) *or indirect* (this has also been discussed in inspection of abdomen: Hernias, Unit VI).
2. *Is the hernia fully reducible or not?* It is clinically important because non-reducible hernias are prone to strangulation. The best way to demonstrate it is to ask the patient to lie down; if protuberance disappears, hernia is reducible. You can also ask the patient about its reducibility, and if need to be confirmed, then ask the patient to reduce it himself.
3. *What are the contents of hernial sac?* The gut produces gurgle, is soft and compressible on palpation; while omentum in the sac feels firmer and doughy.

Differential Diagnosis of Inguinal Hernia

The conditions that mimic inguinal hernia include:
- A large hydrocoele of tunica vaginalis
- A large cyst of the epididymis
- An undescended testis (scrotum will be empty in this condition)
- A lipoma or a hydrocoele of the spermatic cord.

Read all these conditions under the examination of scrotum.

Differential Diagnosis of Femoral Hernia

In addition to inguinal hernia, the other conditions to be kept in its differential diagnosis include:
- A lipoma in femoral triangle
- A pulsatile aneurysm of the femoral artery
- A sphenovarix is a swelling containing varicose veins, hence, a bluish tinge is imparted to the swelling. The swelling disappears on lying down and a venous hum may be heard over it.
- A psoas abscess (mass is fluctuant and compressible)
- An enlarged lymph node. Look for any evidence of infection in the areas it drains (i.e. feet, legs, thigh, scrotum, pudendal or perineal areas). If inflammatory in origin, it will be tender and skin temperature be raised (acute lymphadenitis).

EXAMINATION OF THE MALE GENITALIA

THE PENIS

Inspection

☞ *Note the size of the penis, the presence or absence of the prepuce and the position of the external urethral meatus. Examine the penile shaft for warts, ulcers, burrows and excoriated papules of scabies and rashes.*
- The abnormalities of penis are given in Table 4.1.

TABLE 4.1: Abnormalities of the Penis

Venereal warts (*condyloma acuminatum*, Fig. 4.6). Venereal warts are rapidly growing excrescences that are moist and often malodorous. They result from infection by papillomavirus.

Genital herpes: A cluster of small vesicles followed by painful non-indurated ulcers on red bases, suggests a herpes simplex infection. The lesion may occur anywhere on the penis.

Syphilitic chancre: A syphilitic chancre (Fig. 4.7) is an oval or round, dark red painless erosion or an ulcer with an indurated base usually associated with non-tender enlarged inguinal lymph nodes. Chancres may be multiple and may become painful due to secondary infection. Chancres are infectious.

Chancroid (Fig. 4.8): It is sexually transmitted disease caused by *H. ducreyi*, produces multiple tender ragged ulcers which bleed on manipulation.

Contd.

Contd.

Donovanosis (Fig. 4.9): It is called *granuloma venereum inguinale*; a sexually transmitted disease produces a single or multiple ulcers with granulation tissue. There is an associated inguinal lymphadenopathy.

Hypospadias: It is a congenital displacement of the urethral meatus to the inferior surface of the penis. A groove extends from the actual urethral meatus to its normal location on the tip of the glans.

Peyronie's disease: In this disease, there are palpable non tender hard plaques just beneath the skin, usually along the dorsum of the penis. The patient complains of crooked, painful erections.

Carcinoma of the penis: Carcinoma may appear as an indurated nodule or ulcer that is usually non-tender, common to men who are not circumcised in childhood and it may be masked by the prepuce. Any persistent penile ulcer must be suspected as malignant.

☞ *The prepuce (foreskin), if present, retract it or ask the patient to retract it. This step is essential for detection of any chancre and carcinoma. Smegma, a cheesy whitish material may accumulate normally under the prepuce.*

Phimosis (Fig. 4.10): It refers to tight prepuce that cannot be retracted over the glans.

Paraphimosis (Fig. 4.11): It refers to tight prepuce that, once retracted, cannot be returned. Painful oedema of glans ensues.

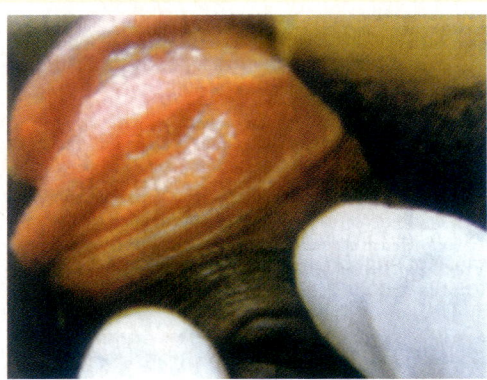

Fig. 4.8: Chancroid. Note multiple, tender, dirty looking (ragged) ulcers which bleed on manipulation.

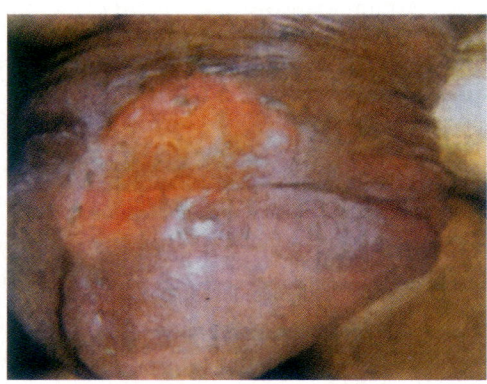

Fig. 4.9: Donovanosis. Note the red ulcer with lot of granulation tissue at the base.

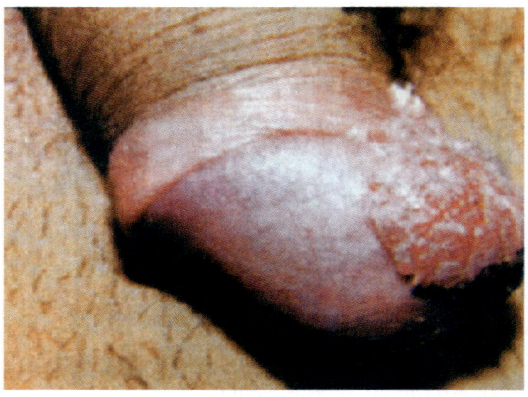

Fig. 4.6: Venereal wart (condyloma acuminatum).

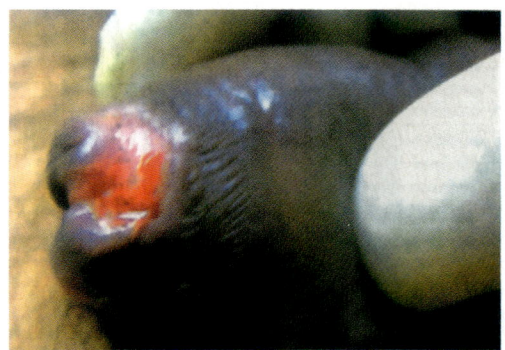

Fig. 4.7: Primary syphilis. A chancre on glans penis.

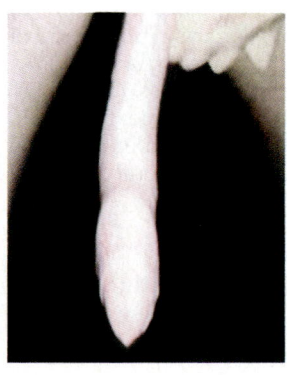

Fig. 4.10: Phimosis. Note the significant erythema and swelling.

The Urogenital System and Sexually Transmitted Diseases

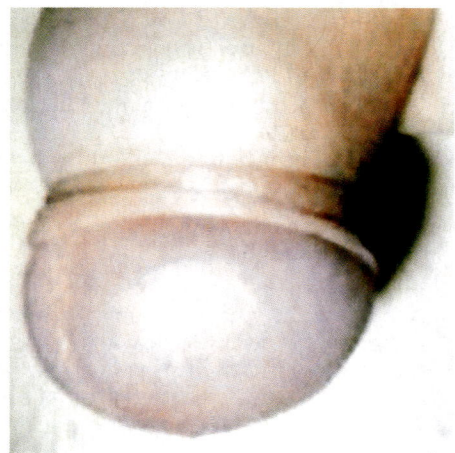

Fig. 4.11: Paraphimosis. Severe oedema of the glans is the result of paraphimosis and the glans becomes ischaemic.

☞ Look at the glans for any ulcer, scar, nodule or signs of inflammation.

Balanitis is inflammation of the glans leading to pain and redness.
Balanoposthitis means inflammation of both the glans and prepuce.

☞ Check the skin around the base of the penis for excoriation or inflammation. Look for nits or lice at the base of the pubic hair.

Pubic or genital excoriations suggest the possibility of lice or scabies.

☞ Note the site of urethral meatus—normal or displaced.

Hypospadia (Table 4.1) is a congenital, ventral displacement of the meatus on the penis.

☞ Compress the glans gently between your index finger and the thumb. This manoeuvre will open the urethral meatus. Look at the meatus for inflammation, urethral discharge, narrowing (stricture) and warts.

Normally there is no discharge per urethra. Profuse yellow discharge occurs in gonococcal urethritis (Fig. 4.12); white or clear discharge occurs in non-gonococcal urethritis.

- If the patient reports a discharge but you do not see any, in such a situation, ask him to strip and milch the shaft of the penis from its base to the glans. Alternatively, you can do it yourself. This manoeuvre may bring the discharge out of the meatus for examination. Have this discharge on glass slide for examination as well as for culture.

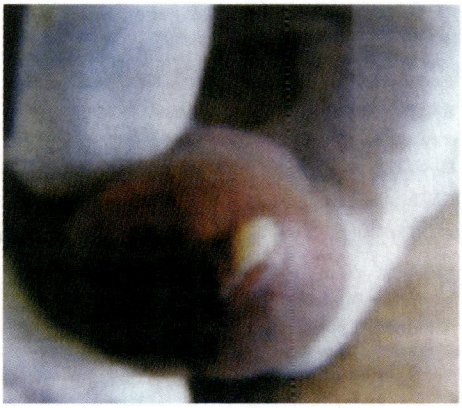

Fig. 4.12: Gonococcal urethritis. Note the thick white or creamy discharge coming out of the urethral meatus.

Palpation

☞ Now palpate the penis between your thumb and first two fingers for any tenderness or induration.

Palpation of the shaft may be omitted in a young asymptomatic male patient.

Induration along the ventral surface of the penis suggests a urethral stricture or possibly a carcinoma. Tenderness of penis suggests periurethral inflammation secondary to urethral stricture.

If you retract the foreskin, replace it before proceeding onto the examination of scrotum.

THE SCROTUM AND ITS CONTENTS

Inspection

☞ Look at the scrotal skin for any redness, swelling or ulcer. Lift up the scrotum so that you can see its under (posterior) surface.

- Scabies causes erythematous nodular lesions on the scrotum and glans penis.
- Ulceration can result from a gumma or from fungating tumour of the testes.
- White scaly lesion over scrotum indicates seborrhoeic dermatitis (Fig. 4.13).

Palpation

☞ Palpate the testis in the scrotum as follows
- Place the right hand below the scrotum and palpate both the testes separately.
- Now fix each testis between the hands and the fingers (Fig. 4.14); support the posterior aspect of the testis with middle, ring and index fingers of both the hands, the right hand being inferior.

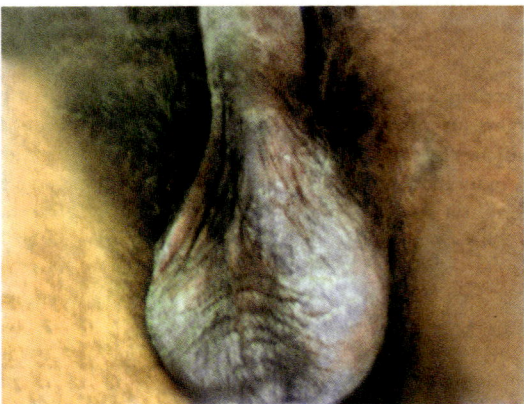

Fig. 4.13: Seborrhoeic dermatitis of the scrotum.

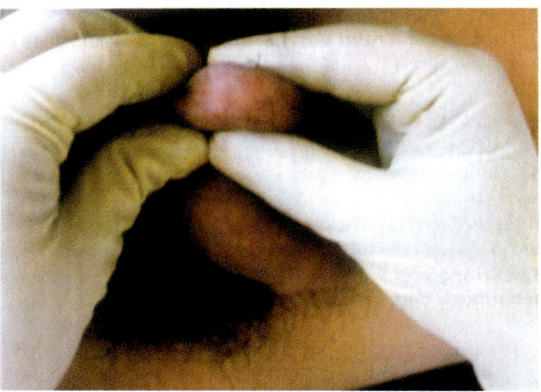

Fig. 4.14: Palpation of testis.

Palpate the anterior surface of the testis with the index finger and thumb of each hand, lateral border with index finger and medial border with the thumb.
Note the *size, shape, consistency, tenderness*. Feel for any nodules or irregularities. Pressure on the testis normally produces a deep visceral pain.
- Now gently palpate the upper pole of the testis by approximating the index finger and the thumb of the left hand, pushing the testis inferiorly.
- Next move the testis upwards by reversing the movements of the hands and gently approximating the index finger and the thumb of the right hand. This will allow you to palpate the lower pole of testis.

Normal testes are equal in size, varying between 3.5 and 4 cm in length, soft in consistency.

☞ *Palpate the epididymis and spermatic cord as follows*
- Palpate the epididymis at the upper pole of the testis posteriorly. The head is felt between the left thumb anteriorly and the index and middle fingers posteriorly. It is soft and nodular structure of about 1 cm in length.
- Palpate the tail of epididymis at the inferior pole of the testis. It is felt between the thumb and fingers of the right hand. The tail is also soft, coiled tubular structure.

Note: Occasionally epididymis may be situated anteriorly.

- Finally palpate the spermatic cord with the left hand. Then exert gentle downward traction on the testis by placing the fingers of right hand behind the scrotum and the thumb placed anteriorly. Palpate the spermatic cord including the vas deferens inside it between your thumb and fingers of the left hand from the epididymis to the superficial inguinal ring (Fig. 4.15). Note any nodules or swelling.

The vas deferens feels like a thick piece of string inside the spermatic cord.

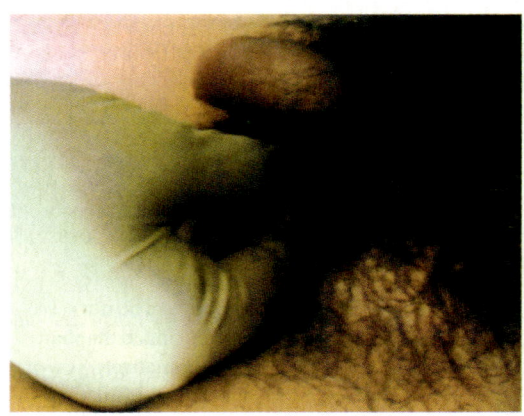

Fig. 4.15: Palpation of spermatic cord.

- Repeat the process on the other side to palpate epididymis and spermatic cord of other side.

Transillumination test. Any swelling in the scrotum other than the testicles can be evaluated by transillumination. After darkening the room, shine the beam of a strong flashlight from a torch from behind the scrotum though the mass. Look for transillumination of light across the mass as a red glow through a piece of folded paper (Fig. 4.16).

In cystic swellings or swellings containing fluid as in hydrocoele, the transillumination test is positive; while in swellings containing blood or tissue, such as normal testis, a tumour or most hernias, the test is negative.

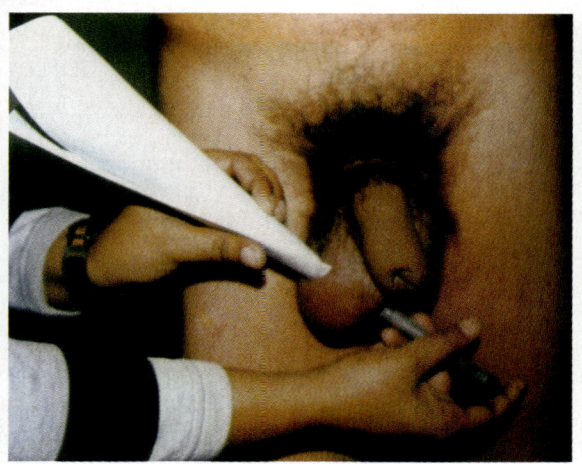

Fig. 4.16: Transillumination test in a patient with hydrocoele. The test is positive.

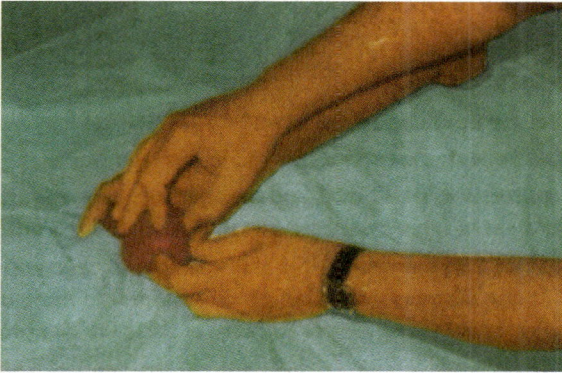

Fig. 4.17: Fluctuation test in a cystic scrotal swelling. Hold the swelling with fingers and thumb of both hands at two opposite ends. Now compress (or tap) the swelling on one side by one index finger (displacing finger) and feel the impulse on the other end by another index finger (watching finger).

DIFFERENTIAL DIAGNOSIS OF A SCROTAL SWELLING

The three ways used for accurate diagnosis and differential diagnosis of a scrotal swelling are inspection, palpation and transillumination.

Inspection

☞ *Look at the scrotal swelling*

- Expose the groin and scrotum fully. Look for any abnormality or swelling.
- If a swelling is present, proceed to determine the following characteristics on palpation.
  1. *Can one get above the swelling?*

     To decide it, **palpate** the neck of the scrotum between fingers and thumb and determine.
     - Whether finger and thumb can be approximated or not. If they can be approximated (nothing is felt in between them) then the swelling is limited to spermatic cord (i.e. one can get above the swelling). If cannot be approximated then swelling is arising from the above, i.e. groin, and may be inguinoscrotal hernia (one cannot get above the swelling).
  2. *Is the swelling cystic or solid?* This is decided by palpation (fluctuation test, Fig. 4.17) as well as by transillumination (Fig. 4.16).
  3. Whether *transillumination* is positive or negative? Transillumination of light across the swelling indicates it to be cystic in nature (i.e. an epididymal cyst or a hydrocoele of tunica vaginalis). If the swelling is non-transilluminant, then it is solid, hence, palpate it again to decide whether it is *epididymis* (epididymitis produces a painful swelling) or *testis* (orchitis produces a painful swelling while malignancy is usually painless).
  4. *A postural relation*. A swelling that is inapparent on lying down but becomes apparent on standing could be a varicocoele. If swelling is cystic and feel like palpating a bag of worms, it is a varicocoele.

EXAMINATION OF FEMALE GENITALIA

Vaginal examination is not a routine. An informed consent and presence of a female attendant is mandatory during the examination. The vaginal examination should be avoided if the hymen is intact (unmarried girls) particularly as the information required can be gathered by digital examination of the rectum. Vaginal examination of a minor requires a written consent of a parent or guardian.

Indications for Vaginal Examination

  i. For cervical carcinoma surveillance
 ii. Vaginal discharge
iii. A pelvic mass
 iv. Symptoms of uterine prolapse
  v. Unexplained urinary tract obstruction
 vi. Suspected tubal pregnancy
vii. Postmenopausal bleeding
viii. Evaluation of rape victim irrespective of age.

Method: The important areas of examination are given in **Box 4.5**.

Physical Signs, Symptoms, Diagnosis and Differential Diagnosis

Box 4.5 Areas of Examination

External examination (Fig. 4.18A)
- Mons pubis
- Labia majora and minora
- Urethral meatus, clitoris
- Vaginal introitus
- Perineum

Internal examination (Fig. 4.18B)
- Vagina and its wall
- Cervix (cervical os)
- Uterus and ovaries
- Pelvic muscles
- Rectovaginal wall

Steps (Fig. 4.18)

1. Ask the patient to empty the bladder.
2. Position the patient comfortably on her back, with head and shoulders slightly elevated, arms at the sides or folded across the chest to the abdominal muscles with hips and knees flexed and thighs abducted.
3. Use a good source of light for illumination of the genitalia.
4. Use suitable gloves and lubricate the examining fingers.

☞ Examine the perineum, vulva, labia majora and minora for discharge, redness, swelling, excoriation, ulcers, (syphilitic chancre), warts (venereal warts) and other lesions (genital herpes). In rape and sexual abuse cases, look for signs of trauma.

- Group vesicles (white plaques) multiple painful present in the labia majora suggest genital herpes (Fig. 4.19).
- Excoriation or itchy, small red maculopapules suggest pediculosis pubis.

☞ Look for nits or lice at the bases of pubic hair.

- Redness and swelling of the vulva with excoriation is seen in vaginal thrush and trichomoniasis *Condyloma lata*, e.g. papular lesions in intertriginous areas may erode to form lesions in secondary syphilis (Fig. 4.20).
- Pearly white umbilicate papules around the anogenital region are seen in molluscum contagiosum (Fig. 4.21).

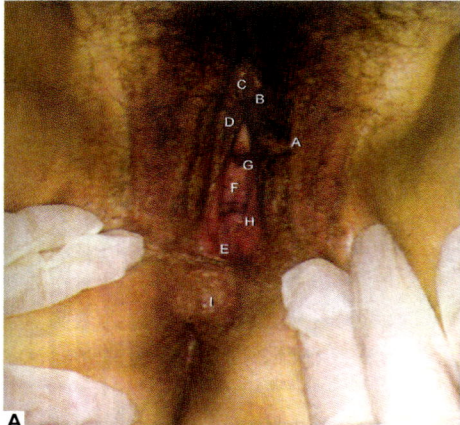
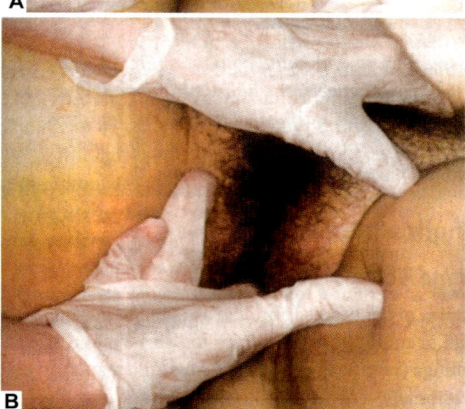

Figs 4.18A and B: Examination of female: **(A)** External examination; **(B)** Internal (vaginal examination). External genitalia. (A) Labia majora; (B) Labia minora; (C) Clitoris; (D) Urethra; (E) Fourchette; (F) Vagina; (G) Skene's adenitis; (H) Bartholin's glands; (I) Anus. **Bimanual examination (Lower Fig B):** The lubricant is applied to fingers which are inserted to palpate the cervix/proximal vagina, other hand used to palpate using a "hooking" manoeuvre to feel the uterus, then left and right lower quadrant to feel the adnexa.

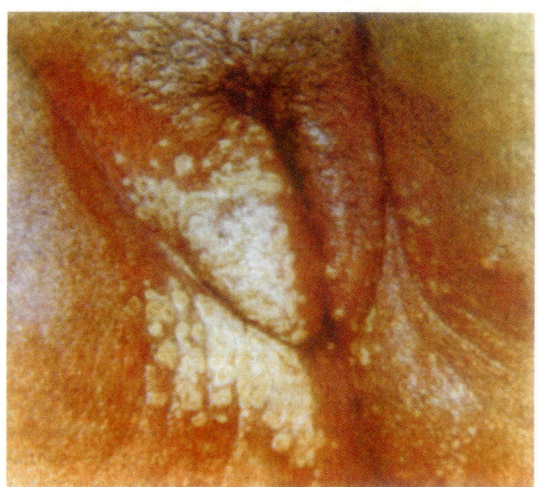

Fig. 4.19: Primary herpes genitalis. It is a sexually transmitted disease caused by *herpes simplex type 2 virus* (less commonly by type I). Multiple painful small grouped vesicles are present in the labia majora in females giving appearance of a white plaque.

- **Urethral caruncle** is a small, red benign tumour visible at the urethral meatus.
- **Prolapsed urethral mucosa** forms a red swollen ring around the urethral meatus.
- **Bartholin's gland abscess** (Fig. 4.22) is acutely formed hot, tender swelling caused by its infection with gonococci, *Chlamydia trachomatis*, etc. Look for the evidence of pus coming out of the duct or erythema around the duct opening.

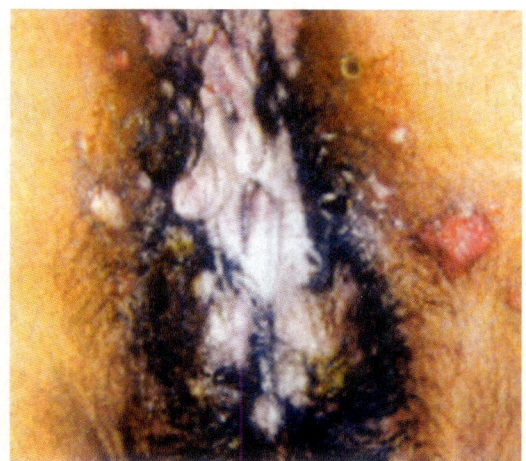

Fig. 4.20: Secondary syphilis. Note the condyloma lata in the intertriginous areas as papules eroding the skin. Mucocutaneous lesions are characteristic of secondary syphilis.

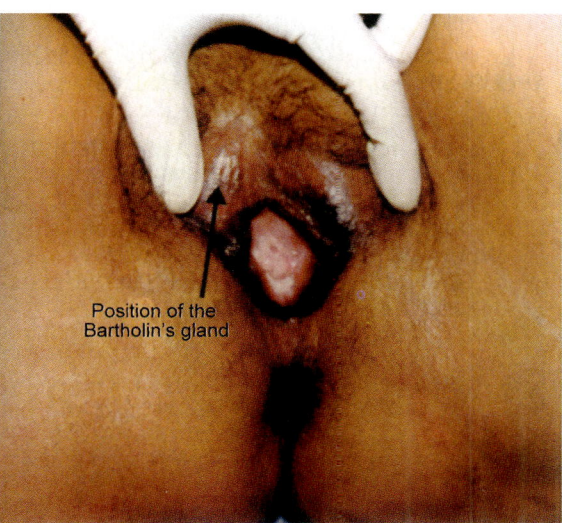

Fig. 4.22: Bartholin's gland abscess.

☞ Inspect the vaginal walls for any bulge or swelling or prolapse by asking the patient to strain down and then to cough.

Note the position and degree of any vaginal prolapse and the occurrence of any involuntary urinary incontinence on coughing.

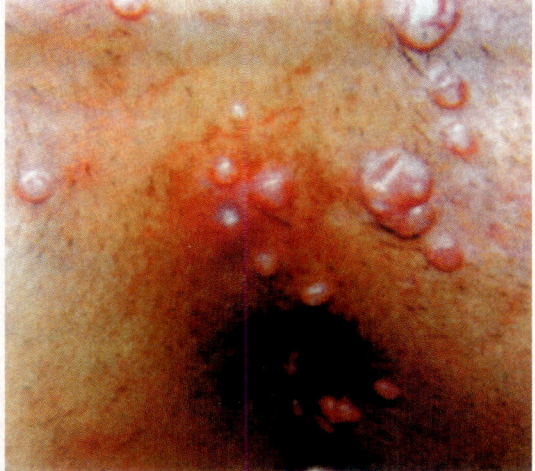

Fig. 4.21: Molluscum contagiosum is caused by *molluscum contagiosum virus*, may spread by endogenously from the GI tract in immunocompromised patients or sexually transmitted from one partner to other. It produces pearly white umbilicated papules.

☞ Separate the labia minora with the forefinger and thumb of the left hand, bringing into view the clitoris anteriorly, then the urethra, the vagina and the anus posteriorly.

Inspect for any evidence of discharge, ulceration, tumour or abnormalities of Bartholin's glands (normally they are not felt).

- **Clitoromegaly** occurs in musculinizing conditions.

- A **cystocoele** is a bulge of the anterior vaginal wall together with bladder above it and results from weakened supporting tissues. The upper two-thirds of the vaginal wall is involved.
- A **cystourethrocoele** is a bulge that involves the entire anterior vaginal wall together with the bladder and the urethra.
- A groove sometimes defines the border between urethrocoele and cystocoele, but not always present. A **rectocoele** is a herniation of the rectum into the posterior wall of the vagina resulting from a weakness or defect in the endopelvic fascia.

☞ Insert the index and middle finger of the right hand into the vagina and rotate the palm—upwards. Use only one finger if vaginismus (spasm of the vaginal muscles) or atrophic vaginitis makes the examination painful.

Palpate the cervix and note any tenderness on movements of the cervix.

Normal cervix points downwards and slightly backwards and feels like the tip of the nose.

Bimanual Palpation

☞ Now perform bimanual palpation (Fig. 14.18B) to identify the uterus between the hands and note its characteristics (*size, position, surface*). For this put two fingers in the anterior fornix, place the left hand flat on the abdomen above the pubis.
- If the uterus is not palpable; palpate with the fingers in the posterior fornix as uterus may be retroverted (read retroversion of the uterus).
- Palpate each lateral fornix in turn bimanually. Note any tenderness or swelling of the fallopian tubes or ovaries and the bladder anteriorly and the pouch of Douglas posteriorly.

Infection of fallopian tubes and ovaries may follow delivery of a baby or gynaecological surgery.

☞ Supplement digital examination of the vagina and cervix by a vaginal speculum.

Internal Examination by a Vaginal Speculum and taking a Cervical Smear (Figs 4.23A and B)

1. Gently insert a lubricated and warmed speculum into the vagina. Do not use a lubricant other than water if a cervical smear is to be taken.
2. Rotate the blades of speculum through 90° pointing the handle anteriorly if the patient is supine and posteriorly if in left lateral position.
3. Open the blades of speculum and identify the cervix (Fig. 4.23B).
4. Use the notched end of the spatula and rotate through 360° to scrape off a cytological sample from the *cervical os* (Figs 4.23A and B).
5. Spread the smear on the glass slide and fix it immediately with 50/50 mixture of alcohol and ether.
6. Swab any discharge from the urethra, vagina and cervix. Wipe the cervix and examine it for discharge, erosion, cervicitis, warts and ulcers.
7. Send one specimen for culture. Take another smear for direct microscopy; unstained smears are helpful to confirm trichomonial infection and stained smears to confirm gonorrhoea or thrust.

Warts on the cervix appear either as flat or papilliferous lesions. Take the smear for cervical cytology to detect dysplasia and cancer of the cervix. This is because there is strong association of cervical cancer with genital warts.

8. Remove the speculum after completion of the examination.

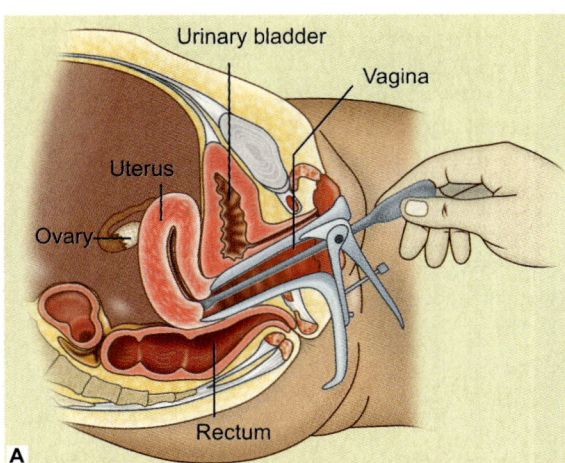

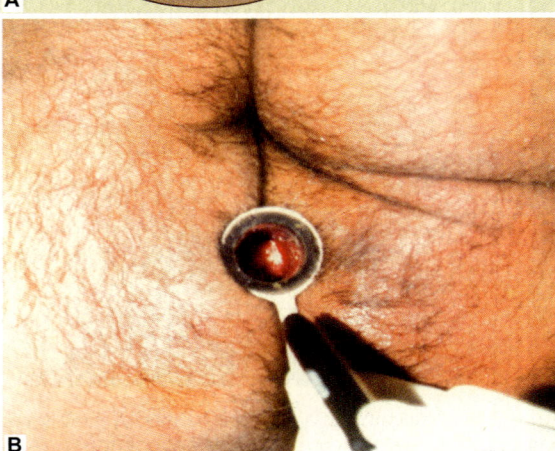

Figs 4.23A and B: (A) Method of taking the Papanicolaou (Pap) smears; (B) Cusco's speculum used to display the cervix for Pap smear as well as for examination.

BRIEF SYNOPSIS OF COMMON RENAL DISORDERS

1. **Acute renal failure:** The occurrence of recent decline of renal functions over days leading to oliguria or anuria constitute syndrome of *acute renal failure*. In contrast, when functional decline is noted over weeks instead of days, the renal failure is categorised as rapidly *progressive renal*

failure. In addition to *reduced GFR (oliguria), oedema, hypertension, abnormal electrolytes* and *urinary sediments* may be noted but are not specific to this syndrome. It is caused by *prerenal* (hypovolaemia), *renal* (renal diseases) and *postrenal* (obstructive uropathy) disorders.

2. **Acute nephritic syndrome:** It is characterised by acute onset of *oliguria, haematuria* (microscopic or macroscopic), *proteinuria* (<3 g/day), *hypertension, oedema* and *azotaemia* with *urine of high specific gravity, and smoky* in appearance. It invariably indicates acute glomerulonephritis due to any cause.

3. **Nephrotic syndrome:** It is defined as massive *proteinuria (>3.5 g/day), hypoalbuminaemia, periorbital or pitting pedal oedema, hyperlipidaemia* and *lipiduria* (passage of fat globules in urine) and *coagulopathy or hypercoagulable state* due to urinary losses of antithrombin C and S and hyperfibrinogenaemia.

Causes include *primary glomerular disease* (minimal, mesangioproliferative, membranous and membranoproliferative glomerulonephritis); *Secondary glomerular disease* (post-streptococcal, HIV, syphilis, malaria, leprosy), *neoplasms, systemic disorders* (SLE, vasculitis, amyloidosis, diabetes) and *toxaemia of pregnancy.*

4. **Chronic renal failure:** It is a clinical syndrome of uraemia occurring as a result of slow insidious irreversible deterioration of renal functions manifested by excretory, metabolic, neurological, haematological and endocrinal abnormalities. The **diagnosis** is made by clinical features (Fig. 4.24) and (i) *documentary evidence of uraemia* (raised blood urea and creatinine) for more than 3 months, (ii) *small contracted kidneys on radiology or USG*, (iii) *renal bone disease*, and (iv) *renal biopsy* for evidence of chronicity of the disease.

The occurrence of recent acute renal failure (e.g. oliguria, hypotension) on previously

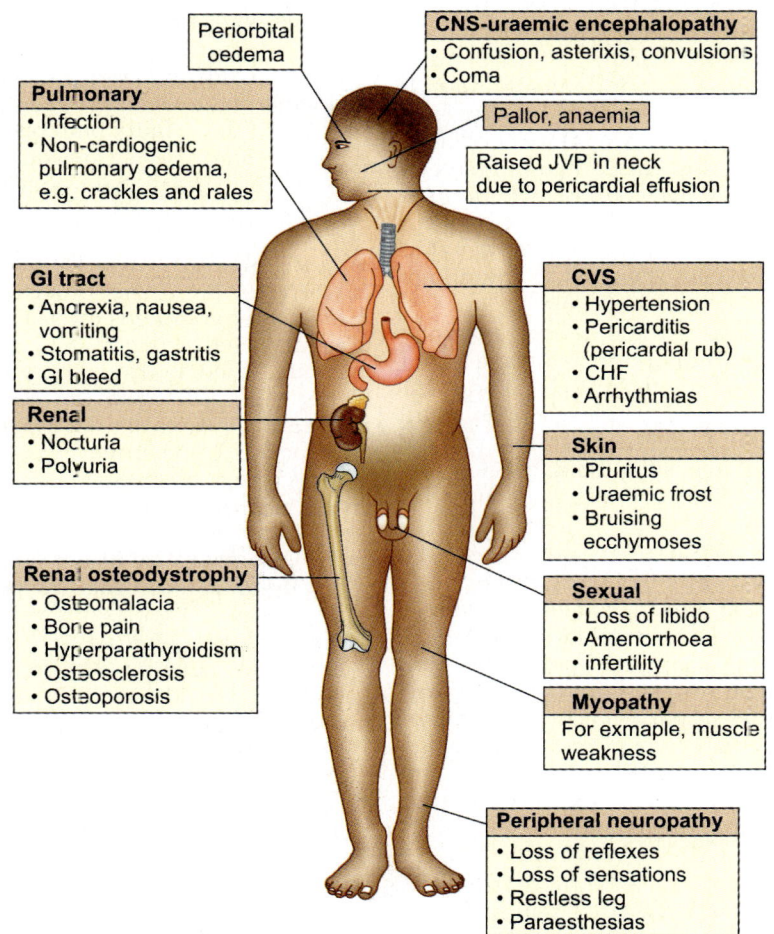

Fig. 4.24: Symptoms and signs of chronic renal failure (CRF).

compensated chronic renal failure has been termed as *acute on chronic renal failure*.

Anaemia, hypertension, hypocalcaemia, hyperphosphataemia; UTI, GI symptoms, electrolyte disturbance and renal osteodystrophy are some of the important clinical features of CRF in addition to low fixed specific gravity of urine and presence of broad hyaline casts (renal failure casts).

5. **Asymptomatic urinary abnormalities:** Detection of isolated haematuria, proteinuria or unexplained pyuria during screening procedures or routine medical check up for employment or life insurance purposes constitutes *asymptomatic urinary abnormalities*. Many cases of asymptomatic glomerular disease are diagnosed from these abnormalities. Most asymptomatic glomerular haematuria is due to IgA nephropathy (*Berger's disease*) or thin basement membrane (TBM) disease (*benign haematuria*). A rare but more ominous cause of isolated haematuria is hereditary nephritis (*Alport's syndrome*).

   Between 0.5 and 10% of the population have isolated proteinuria, a radiologically normal urinary tract and the absence of known renal disease. Majority of these patients excrete proteins of <2 g/day, and more than 80% have an excellent prognosis (*benign isolated proteinuria*). A minority (10–25%) are found to have persistent isolated proteinuria, some of whom develop progressive renal insufficiency over a period of one to two decades.

   Asymptomatic bacteriuria is defined as colony count >10^5/ml in midstream urine sample of healthy asymptomatic individual. About 1% children, 1% school girls, 0.03% school boys and men, about 1% non-pregnant women and 5% pregnant women have asymptomatic bacteriuria. Otherwise, such colony count in urine indicates urinary infection.

6. **Urinary tract infection:** It is characterised by *fever, dysuria, increased frequency* and *burning micturition*. It is common in females. It can occur in normal as well as abnormal kidneys. A midstream urine sample, appropriately collected under aseptic conditions, with colony counts >10^5/ml indicates urinary infection in symptomatic patients. Under certain conditions, colony counts between 10^2 and 10^4/ml in midstream sample or suprapubic aspiration of bladder may indicate urinary infection, needs further evaluation.

7. **Renal tubular defects:** Renal tubular defects (anatomical or functional) are either inherited or acquired. Anatomical defects such as *cystic diseases* (*polycystic and medullary cystic*) and *medullary sponge kidney*, are usually identified during investigations for haematuria, bacteriuria, flank pain or azotemia. USG and radiological techniques confirm the diagnosis.

   Functional renal tubular defects result in impaired secretion or resorption of electrolytes, H^+, HCO_3^- or organic solutes or decreased urinary concentrating and diluting activity. *Polyuria, nocturia, metabolic acidosis, disorders of fluid and electrolyte balance* are its clinical manifestations. Diagnosis is dependent on individual tubular functions. Tubular syndromes cause *pyuria, calculous disease, calcinosis, renal bone disease or renal failure*.

8. **Nephrolithiasis:** *Renal colic, painful haematuria, unexplained pyuria, dysuria* and *urinary frequency* raise the suspicion of a renal stone. Passage of stone, visualisation of a stone on X-ray or on removal at surgery or on cystoscopy confirms the diagnosis of stone disease. Stones detected on X-ray include calcium containing and cysteine stones, while uric acid stones are radiolucent.

9. **Urinary tract obstruction:** Oliguria, anuria, polyuria, nocturia, urinary retention, azotemia, slowing of the urinary stream, enlarged prostate, large kidneys, flank pain or tenderness, a full bladder after voiding are some of the diagnostic clues to urinary tract obstruction which is confirmed on investigations and radiology.

Anuria is almost always associated with complete bilateral urinary tract obstruction. *A palpable bladder* after voiding is caused by lower urinary tract obstruction (e.g. due to urethral stricture, tumour, stone, neurogenic cause and prostate hypertrophy). *Nocturia, increased frequency* and *outflow incontinence, hesitancy* also suggest **outflow obstruction**. Upper urinary tract obstruction may, at times, be asymptomatic especially when it is incomplete or unilateral.

10. **Adult polycystic kidney disease (APKD):** It is heredofamilial disorder characterised by cystic dilatations of tubules of the kidneys leading to their enlargement. APKD1 and APKD2 gene mutations are responsible for it. It is common in young and middle age, insidious onset with mass abdomen on one or both sides with flank pain. *Hypertension, haematuria, proteinuria, nocturia* are its cardinal features. *Urinary tract infection* is common. *Polycythaemia* can occur due to increased erythropoietin production.

Diagnosis is confirmed by positive family history, ultrasonography or CT scan.

Differential diagnosis: It rests on enlargement of kidney(s). The causes of a large kidney(s) are:

1. Unilateral/bilateral hydronephrosis or pyonephrosis
2. Adult polycystic kidney(s)
3. Solitary renal cyst (unilateral enlargement)
4. Renal tumour (unilateral)
5. Renal amyloidosis and diabetic nephropathy (bilateral).

BRIEF SYNOPSIS OF GENITAL DISEASES AND HERNIA

PROSTATITIS

It is caused by gram-negative bacilli or *Chlamydia trachomatis*. **Symptoms** are dysuria, increased urinary frequency and heistancy; **Signs** include tender, diffusely enlarged, boggy prostate, with epididymal tenderness.

BALANITIS

It is inflammation of the glans penis due to *Candida* or an autoimmune process. **Risk factors** include uncontrolled diabetes mellitus and chronic steroid use. **Symptoms and signs** include redness and swelling of the glans. It is commonly associated with paraphimosis.

BALANOPOSTHITIS

It refers to chronic oedema and inflammation of the glans and the foreskin, often due to moderate phimosis. **Symptoms and signs** include diffuse swelling of the glans penis and the foreskin with a phimosis. Purulent discharge from the prepuce may be present. It is commonly due to diabetes and paraphimosis.

PROSTATIC HYPERTROPHY

It is idiopathic increase in size of gland. It is a very prevalent condition with increasing age. **Symptoms** include *nocturia, urinary hesitancy, haematuria* and *increased frequency*. **On rectal examination**, the prostate gland is diffusely enlarged and without nodules. A distended bladder may be concurrent. **Complications** include recurrent urinary tract infections and obstructive nephropathy. **Diagnosis** is confirmed by ultrasonography.

CARDINOMA OF THE PENIS

Squamous cell carcinoma. Risk factors include *human papillomavirus infection*. **Symptoms and signs** include a painless, non-healing ulcer; in advanced cases, the ulcer is quite deep with enlargement of inguinal lymph nodes. Concurrent *condyloma acuminatum* is usually present. *Diagnosis* is confirmed by excisional biopsy.

PENILE ULCER (SYPHILITIC CHANCRE)

A single painless ulcer with raised edges and necrotic center located on the glans or shaft of the penis appearing 10 to 14 days after sexual exposure indicates syphilitic chancre. Multiple ulcers are found in 20 to 30% of patients. **Diagnosis** is established by *VDRL*, (Venereal Disease Research Laboratory) and MHA-TP (*microhemagglutinin Treponema pallidum*) tests. The *dark-field analysis* will also reveal spirochetes.

EPIDIDYMITIS/ORCHITIS

It is infection with *gram-negative bacilli* or *C. trachomatis*. **Symptoms and signs** include a tender swollen epididymis. In severe cases or with abscess there is a tender non-transilluminable nodule or a mass contiguous to the testis. Overlying scrotal oedema, erythema, warmth, and concurrently swollen boggy prostate may be present. **Diagnosis** is established by ultrasound with flow Doppler.

FEMORAL HERNIAS

It is defined as an anatomic defect in the fascia deep to the inguinal ligament, more common in females than males. The hernial sac passes out of the abdominal cavity into the anterior thigh, i.e. the femoral triangle via abnormal passage through the femoral canal, immediately posterior to the inguinal ligament. Because the defect size is usually small, it is easily incarcerated and strangulated. **Signs** include a soft mass in the anterior medial thigh deep into the inguinal ligament. The three discrete classes of hernias are *reducible, incarcerated,* and/or *strangulated*. Incarcerated hernias are non-tender and non-reducible. Strangulated hernias are tender, non-reducible and if there is bowel obstruction, then it is associated with concurrent abdominal distension with tympany.

FOURNIER'S GANGRENE

It is necrotising cellulitis and fascitis of scrotum and penis due to *mixed anaerobes* and *gram-negative rods*. **Risk factors** include uncontrolled diabetes mellitus and neutropenia. **Symptoms** include scrotal pain and swelling with signs of scrotal/penile oedema with crepitus, necrosis, and eschar formation.

HYDROCOELE

It is a fluid-filled mass within *tunica vaginalis*. **Symptoms and signs** include a chronic, smooth, firm, non-tender, and transilluminable mass in the scrotum, with a concurrent inguinal hernia. *Transillumination test* is positive. The fingers can get above the mass within scrotum. It can be unilateral or bilateral.

HYPOGONADISM

It is defined as decrease in testicular function resulting from either congenital (*Klinefelter*) or acquired causes (*cirrhosis* or *paramyxovirus infection*). **Symptoms** include facial immaturity, erectile dysfunction, and loss of libido. **Signs** include tall stature, facial alopecia, gynaecomastia, and a decrease in the size and firmness of the testes. Concurrent end-stage liver disease may be present. **Diagnosis** includes estimating serum testosterone and luteinizing hormone (LH)/follicle-stimulating hormone (FSH) levels; low testosterone levels and high FSH/LH levels indicate primary hypogonadism. For the congenital form, perform a karyotype for Klinefelter's syndrome.

INGUINAL HERNIA

It is due to defect in the connective tissue supporting the inguinal area, more common in men. **Indirect**: It is congenital form, with sac through internal and external rings into the scrotum or labium majus. **Direct:** It is an acquired form, with sac through Hesselbach's triangle in the abdominal wall. **Symptoms** are minimal unless there is incarceration or strangulation. **Signs** include a nontransilluminable soft mass in the scrotum adjacent to the spermatic cord that may be reduced. Incarcerated hernia is non-tender and non-reducible. Strangulated hernia is tender and non-reducible; a concurrent hydrocoele or distension with tympany of bowel obstruction may be present.

PARAPHIMOSIS

It is defined as retraction of the foreskin behind the glans with resultant oedema or ischaemia of the glans. **Risk factors** include phimosis, balanoposthitis, and forced retraction of the foreskin. **Symptoms and signs** include pain at the tip of the penis, swollen tender edematous glans; foreskin retracted and tightly bound around the circumference of the penis. Severe cases manifest with cyanosis or necrosis of the glans.

PHIMOSIS

It is defined as constricted prepuce (foreskin opening) due to old trauma or balanitis. **Symptoms and signs** include dysuria, urinary dribbling and inability to retract the foreskin with concurrent balanitis.

PROSTATIC NODULES/CARCINOMA

Nodular carcinoma of prostate is an adenocarcinoma. The patient will be asymptomatic. **Signs** include a non-tender, indurated nodule. **Diagnosis** includes a prostate-specific antigen (PSA) test and USG for residual urine and transrectal biopsy.

PURULENT URETHRITIS (GONORRHOEA)

It is a sexually transmitted infection by the organism called *Neisseria gonorrhoea* (Fig. 4.12) or *C. trachomatis*, or both. **Symptoms** include *dysuria*, *hesitancy* and *urgency*, and *pyuria*, a yellow crusty discharge on underpants/bed linens; the patient is usually sexually active. **Signs** include purulent discharge and swelling at the meatus. **Diagnosis** includes culture of discharge for *N. gonorrhoea* and *Chlamydia* species (spp.).

SPERMATOCOELE

It is a benign inclusion cyst adjacent to the testis in the spermatic cord. The patient is asymptomatic. **Signs** include a non-tender, transilluminable nodule in the superior epididymis.

TESTICULAR CARCINOMA

It is malignant neoplastic growth of germ cells. **Risk factors** include cryptorchidism, the abnormal retention of one or both of the testes within the abdomen. **Symptoms and signs** include a firm, non-tender, non-transilluminable nodule or mass adjacent to a testis; if ischaemia occurs, the mass may become acutely enlarged and tender. **Diagnosis** includes ultrasound, serum alpha fetoprotein (AFP) and beta human chorionic gonadotropin (β-hCG) tests.

VARICOCOELE

It is varicosity in the spermatic vein. The left side is more commonly affected because the left spermatic vein does not drain directly into the inferior vena cava. **Symptoms and signs** include a chronic, non-tender, nontransilluminable mass with a consistency of a *'bag of worms'* in the area around the vas deferens that decreases in size with scrotal elevation.

OVARIAN CYSTS AND TUMOURS

Ovarian cyst or a tumour presents as an adnexal mass arising from one side or both sides of pelvis, may extend out of pelvis. Cysts are smooth and compressible; while tumours are more solid and often nodular. Uncomplicated cysts and tumours are non-tender. Polycystic ovarian disease is an example of multiple cysts in ovaries.

Polycystic ovarian syndrome (PCOS) is a condition most often characterised by irregular menstrual periods, excess hair growth and obesity, but it can affect women in a variety of ways. Irregular or heavy periods may signal the condition in adolescence, or

PCOS may become apparent later when a woman has difficulty in becoming pregnant. *Diagnosis* is made by USG which shows large ovaries studded with numerous cysts (polycystic). These cysts are follicles, fluid-filled sacs that contain immature eggs.

RUPTURED TUBAL PREGNANCY

A ruptured tubal pregnancy spills blood into the peritoneal cavity, causing severe abdominal pain and tenderness. Guarding and rebound tenderness are sometimes associated. A unilateral adnexal mass may be palpable and tender. Fainting, syncope, nausea, vomiting, tachycardia and shock may be associated reflecting the haemorrhage. There will be prior history of amenorrhoea or other symptoms of pregnancy.

PELVIC INFLAMMATORY DISEASE (PID)

PID is most often a result of sexually transmitted infection of fallopian tubes (*salpingitis*) or of tubes and ovaries (*salpingo-oophritis*). It is caused by *N. gonorrhoeae*, *Chlamydia trachomatis* and other organisms. Acute disease is often associated with painful, tender adnexal masses with protective muscles spasm which usually makes it impossible to demarcate them. Movement of cervix produces pain. If not treated, a tubo-ovarian abscess may ensue.

UTERINE FIBROIDS

Myomas of the uterus (fibroids) are benign tumours, may be single or multiple, project from the surface as a swelling or swellings (nodules) which are firm and irregular in outline. Occasionally, a myoma projecting laterally may be confused with an ovarian tumour, a nodule projecting posteriorly can be mistaken for a retroflexed uterus. Submucus myoma project towards the endometrial cavity.

UTERINE PROLAPSE

Prolapse of the uterus occurs due to weakness of pelvic floor muscles, and is often associated with a cystocoele and rectocoele. In progressive stages, uterus becomes retroverted and descends down into the vaginal canal to the outside.

In first degree prolapse, the cervix is still well within vagina.
In second degree, cervix is at the introitus
In third degree prolapse (Fig. 4.25), the cervix and vagina are outside the introitus.

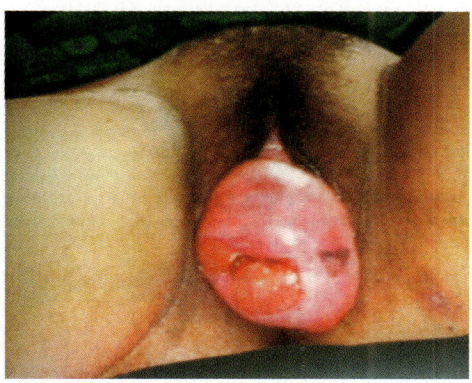

Fig. 4.25: Uterine prolapse.

RETROVERSION OF THE UTERUS

It refers to falling (tilting) backwards of the entire uterus, occurs normally in 1 out of 5 women. In mild cases, pelvic examination shows a cervix that faces forwards and uterus cannot be felt by bimanual examination. In marked retroversion, the body can be felt posteriorly either through the posterior fornix or through the rectum. A retroverted uterus is mobile and asymptomatic.

Unit V

Nervous System

- Symptoms Related to Neurological Disorders and their Analysis
- History
- General Physical Examination/Signs
- Systemic Examination
- Diagnosis and Differential Diagnosis
- Brief Synopsis of Neurological Disorders

COMMON SYMPTOMS

1. Headache
2. Involuntary movements
3. Seizure/convulsions
4. Vertigo/giddiness
5. Syncope
6. Facial pain/facial asymmetry
7. Symptoms related to cranial nerve paralysis
8. Speech disturbance
9. Disorders of consciousness (coma)
10. Motor symptoms, e.g. weakness or paralysis (hemiplegia, monoplegia, paraplegia, diplegia).
11. Sensory symptoms, e.g. paraesthesia, anaesthesia, allodynia, hyperpathia.
12. Gait abnormalities

HEADACHE

It means all aches and pains localised to the head. It occurs due to distortions, inflammation, distension, traction, displacement, involvement of pain sensitive structures, i.e.

- *Skin, subcutaneous tissue, muscles, arteries and periosteum* of the skull.
- *Intracranial dural venous sinuses* or veins.
- *Tissues of eyes, ears and nasal sinuses*.
- *Dura mater* at the base of brain and the arteries within dura- and pia-arachnoid mater.

Causes

The causes are classified in Table 5.1.

TABLE 5.1: A Practical Classification of Headache

1. **Acute primary headaches** (unknown cause)
   - Migraine
   - Tension-type
   - Benign exertional headache
   - Cluster headache
2. **Secondary headache** (secondary to some cause)

   A. Intracranial causes
   - Vascular disorders, e.g. embolic, thrombotic (arterial or venous), haemorrhagic, acute dissection
   - Infections, e.g. meningitis, encephalitis, brain abscess
   - Inflammation, e.g. vasculitis, arteritis
   - Tumours, e.g. benign and malignant (primary, metastatic)
   - Miscellaneous, e.g. benign intracranial hypertension, post-spinal and post-traumatic headaches

   B. Extracranial causes
   - Involvement of eye, ear, sinuses, teeth, neck and temporomandibular joint.

   C. Systemic illnesses and acute intoxications
3. **Neuralgias**
   - Trigeminal
   - Glossopharyngeal

Symptom Analysis

Ask about

Q. **Age, onset, frequency, duration and progress.**
- Acute onset of severe headache commonly suggests subarachnoid haemorrhage and meningitis.
- Progressively worsening headache suggests raised intracranial pressure or uncontrolled systemic disease.

- A chronic recurrent or episodic headache or chronic non-progressive daily headache indicates migraine, cluster headache or tension-type headache.
- The slowly evolving recurrent headache over weeks or months is either migraine or tension-type headache or it could even be due to unruptured aneurysm.
- Some headaches may be nocturnal or may occur at the same time of the day (*cluster headache*) or at specific occasion such as during menstruation or may increase towards the evening such as tension-type (*psychogenic*) headache.

The **age of the patient** is also a prime importance as migraine generally begins at a younger age, tension headache is more common in middle age and headache originating in older persons are usually due to organic causes.

The **frequency and duration of headache** also help to differentiate the episodic headaches from chronic progressive headaches. Many attacks of headache of short duration in a day would favour the diagnosis of *cluster headache* or *chronic paroxysmal hemicrania* (a variant of cluster headache).

Q. Site and quality of pain.
- Unilateral pulsating or throbbing headaches are usually vascular (*migraine* and *cluster headaches*).
- Bilateral diffuse dull headache is usually of tension-type (*psychogenic*).
- In secondary headaches of organic cause the nature, location and severity of headache depend on the structure involved.

Q. Are about any associated symptoms?
- Associated features such as nausea, vomiting flashes of light and noises along with headache suggest migraine.
- Fever, arthralgia and malaise suggest a systemic illness or meningitis.
- Transient visual symptoms (auras) are characteristic of migraine but can occur in transient ischaemic attacks, vascular anomalies or focal epilepsy secondary to space occupying lesions.
- Behaviour following an acute attack of headache distinguishes *migraine* (patient tries to sleep undisturbed in a dark room) from *cluster headache* in which a patient is up and moving about.
- Headache may be related to menstruation, more common in morning (hypertensive) and worst on bending (sinusitis related), may occur towards the evening (eye strain headache) or follow a period of inactivity (cervical pain).

Q. Are there any provoking and relieving factors?
- Primary headaches such as migraine can be triggered by various stimuli including food items and colours (chocolate).
- Headache due to intracranial pathology or raised intracranial tension worsens during coughing, straining or adopting the head in low posture.

INVOLUNTARY MOVEMENTS

These have been discussed under Motor System Examination.

SEIZURES/CONVULSIONS

Definition. The *epilepsies* are a group of disorders of cerebral functions characterised by chronic, recurrent, paroxysmal, non-synchronous discharges of cerebral neurons. *Seizure* is defined as an episode of neurological dysfunction. *Convulsions* are seizures accompanied by motor manifestations, i.e. limb jerking, incontinence, etc. Seizures need not be always convulsive.

Causes
I. **Primary** (idiopathic)
II. **Secondary** due to:
- *Head injury* (SAH, subdural haematoma)
- *Infections* e.g. encephalitis, meningitis, brain abscess, neurocysticercosis, syphilis.
- *Congenital abnormalities*, e.g. tuberous sclerosis, cerebral diplegia.
- *Degenerative brain disease*, e.g. cerebral atrophy.
- *Vascular disturbances*, e.g. CVA, hypertensive encephalopathy.
- *Drugs and toxins*, e.g. alcohol, barbiturates benzodiazepine, phenothiazines, etc.
- *Neoplasm*, e.g. brain tumour.
- *Metabolic disorders* e.g. hypoglycaemia, uraemia, hypocalcaemia, cerebral hypoxia, cerebral oedema.
- *Miscellaneous*, e.g. eclampsia, hysteria.

Symptom Analysis

Ask about the following

Q. The age.
- Age is important because hypoglycaemia, hypocalcaemia, acute infections are common causes of convulsions in children while space occupying lesions, neurocysticercosis and head injury are common in middle age and CVA, neoplasms are common in old age.

Q. History of head injury.
- Subdural haematoma and subarachnoid haemorrhage can lead to convulsions. The convulsions in head injury can occur at any time called *post-traumatic epilepsy*.

Q. What is the type of seizure? Is it generalised or focal? Take full description of the seizure either from the patient or from attendant who had witnessed the seizure.
- Generalised seizures suggest diffuse cerebral lesion while partial seizures indicate focal lesion, e.g. a cerebral tumour or a small infarct.

Q. Are attacks of convulsion recurrent?
- Recurrent attacks of convulsions occur in subdural haematoma, brain tumour, epilepsy, hypoglycaemic states and vascular events.

Q. Is aura or prodromata present?
- Aura is usually present in *grand mal seizure*. Unusual aura indicate focal lesion of the brain for example an olfactory aura indicate frontal lobe lesion, auditory aura suggests temporal lobe lesion and visual aura suggests occipital lobe lesion.

Q. Time of the day for seizure.
- Seizures just before or after waking indicate *grand mal epileptic seizure* because sleep deprivation precepitates attack.
- Seizures in front of someone at any time of the day is usually hysterical.

Q. Duration of convulsions.
- Short duration indicates infection, fever, hypoglycaemia, drugs or toxin, brain tumours, CVA as the cause.
- Long duration of convulsions (month to years) indicate idiopathic epilepsy, tuberous sclerosis, neurocysticercosis etc.

Q. History of transient paresis after an attack of convulsion.
- *Todd's paralysis* commonly follows focal seizures which subsequently recovers.

Q. Ask about the provoking factors.
- Omission of anticonvulsant treatment can precipitate an attack. Loud noise, listening to music, watching television, reading news paper etc can also provoke an attack.

Q. Past history.
- Ask about childhood infection, trauma, etc.

Q. Family history.
- Some patients may have positive family history of epilepsy.

Q. Drug treatment.
- Certain drugs can precipitate the attack (Read causes of convulsions).

Q. Dietary history
- Is patient vegetarian/non-vegetarian?
- *Neurocysticerosis* is common in non vegetarian than vegetarian.

FACIAL PAIN

Facial pain may be a neurologic symptom because of irritation of sensory trigeminal nerve supplying the face. It can be nonneurological (refered) due to involvement of other facial structures, i.e. teeth, skin or subcutanous tissue of face, temporomandibular joint, ear, skin, stylomastoid foramen, etc. Therefore, common **causes** of facial pain are:
1. Trigeminal neuralgia
2. Migrainous neuralgia
3. Post-zoster neuralgia.
4. Temporomandibular arthritis.
5. Otitis externa
6. Malocclusion of teeth.
7. Orbital pain
8. Atypical facial pain (psychogenic)
9. Parotitis/stone in parotid duct

Symptom Analysis

Q. Is facial pain paroxysmal and occurs in bouts?
- Bouts of facial pain are hallmark of trigeminal neuralgia.

Q. What is the nature of pain?
- Sharp lancinating unilateral pain distributed over the territory of one or more sensory divisions of a trigeminal nerve is characteristic of trigeminal neuralgia.
- Severe throbbing pain occuring around the eye in bouts associated with photophobia, lacrimation, conjunctival and nasal congestion suggests migrainous neuralgia (cluster headache).
- Dull, boring ache/pain over the face in anxious patients indicate psychogenic pain.

Q. Is pain related to chewing?
- Pain getting intensified on chewing or movements of jaw indicates either temporomandibular arthritis (*rheumatoid arthritis*) or malocclusion of the teeth or inflammation of stylomastoid foramen or parotitis (stone in parotid duct).

Q. Ask about the precipitants of pain.
- Pain triggered by touching, washing of face, shaving, brushing of teeth, cold breeze, eating, talking and use of cosmetics/lotions over the face indicate trigeminal neuralgia.

Q. History of vesicles around the ear, orbit and face.
- Vesicles/scar over the face indicate herpetic infection of trigeminal nerve.

FACIAL ASYMMETRY

It is a symptom of facial nerve palsy, hence, read the symptoms and signs of facial nerve palsy under cranial nerve examination.

VERTIGO OR DIZZINESS

Consciousness of disordered orientation of the body in space is called *vertigo* or *dizziness*. Patients usually describe it as *light-headedness, faintness, spinning, giddiness*, etc. Vertigo is an illusory or hallucinatory sense of self or environmental movement, most commonly due to disturbance of vestibular system.

Nystagmus is a common concomitant of vertigo. Vertigo may be *peripheral* (labyrinthine and vestibular causes) or *central* (brain stem and cerebellar lesions).

Causes
I. Peripheral Causes
1. *Involvement of middle ear*, i.e. labrinthitis, vestibular neuronitis, Ramsay Hunt syndrome, benign paroxysmal positional vertigo, Meniere's disease.
2. *Orthostatic hypotension* due to prolonged immobilisation, drugs, autonomic neuropathy, tabes dorsalis, multisystem atrophy, parkinsonian-like syndrome, hyponatremia, Addison's disease, etc.
3. *Cardiac syncope* due to low cardiac output as result of arrhythmias, Stokes-Adam attack and carotid sinus hypersensitivity.
4. *Hyperventilation syndrome.*

II. Central Causes
Neurological causes, e.g. Friedreich's ataxia, spinocerebellar atrophy, multiple sclerosis, cerebellopontine tumour, brain stem glioma, vertebrobasilar insufficiency, acute cerebellitis, basilar artery migraine, temporal lobe epilepsy.

Symptom Analysis
Ask the following
Q. Onset.
- Acute onset of vertigo suggests vestibular neuronitis, multiple sclerosis, drugs, brainstem infarction, cerebellar haemorrhage.

Q. Is it intermittent?
- Recurrent attacks of vertigo suggest benign positional vertigo, TIA, migraine, epilepsy and Meniere's disease.
- Persistent vertigo suggests drug effect, brainstem infarct, VIII nerve tumour, multiple sclerosis, posterior fossa tumour.

Q. Does it relate to change in head posture?
- Vertigo with change in posture indicates benign positional vertigo.

Q. Is there a history of deafness?
- Vertigo with deafness suggests Meniere's disease.

Q. Is there a history of trauma?
- Head injury (concussion) is a common cause of vertigo.

Q. What are percipitating factors?
- Vertigo precipitated by head movement indicates vertebrobasilar insufficiency, cervical spondylosis and carotid sinus syncope.

Q. Are there any associated symptoms?
- Associated nausea and vomiting suggest Meniere's disease, lateral medullary syndrome.
- Diplopia, facial, dysaesthesia, dysarthria indicate basilar artery insufficiency.
- Drop attacks without loss of consciousness indicate basilar artery insufficiency; while loss of consciousness indicates temporal lobe epilepsy.
- Vertigo with ataxia indicates labrinthine disease.

Evaluation
- The distinction between true vertigo and dizziness is made by *provocative test*, i.e. rapid rotation and abrupt cessation of movement in swival chair. This manoeuvre induces true vertigo (vestibular vertigo).
- Once, it has been established that it is true vertigo rather than dizziness, then find out whether it is central or peripheral.
- Patients with central vertigo can neither stand or walk and direction of fall is variable. Vertical nystagmus (up-beat or down-beat) is pathognomonic of central vertigo. It is not associated with nausea, vomiting, tinnitus and deafness. Most common cause of central vertigo is vascular insufficiency of brainstem (ischaemia/infarction) or basilar artery insufficiency supplying the cerebellum, hence, neurological involvement is common.
- A *peripheral cause* is suspected when there is history of ear discharge or pain, unilateral deafness or tinnitus. It is unidirectional nystagmus with slow component (phase) towards the affected ear and fast component away from (opposite to) the side of lesion. It is commonly

due to labyrinthine disorders. Postural instability is mild.
- *Positional vertigo* is precipitated by recumbent head position either to the right or to the left. It may be benign paroxysmal positional vertigo following head trauma or idiopathic, or may be central positional vertigo due to lesions in and around the fourth ventricle. The differences between the benign paroxysmal positional vertigo (BPPV) and central positional vertigo is that former is more common, severe and the symptoms are reproducible; while later is uncommon, is associated with nystagmus and other neurological symptoms, hence, is not reproducible.
    i. The time course and duration of vertigo also help in the diagnosis. Recurrent episodes of brief positional vertigo (lasting less than a minute) indicate benign positional or post-traumatic vertigo. It can be psychogenic.
    ii. On the other hand, recurrent spontaneous vertigo lasting for minutes/hours indicate Meniere's disease, vertebrobasilar insufficiency, migraine or autoimmune disease.
    iii. Spontaneous attacks of prolonged vertigo lasting for a day or longer suggest labyrinthitis, multiple sclerosis or an infarction in the vertebrobasilar artery territory.
- *Psychogenic vertigo*, usually a concomitant of agoraphobia (fear of large open spaces or crowd) should be suspected in patients distressed by their symptoms so much that they remain confined to the house (*house bound status*). It differs from the *organic vertigo* in which despite discomfort patients attempt to work. Organic vertigo is invariably accompanied by the nystagmus not the psychogenic.

NYSTAGMUS

It is defined *as to and fro rhythmic oscillatory movements of one or both eyes in any field or in all fields of gaze*. It is due to disturbance in ocular fixation. The degree and direction of nystagmus is defined by its fast phase movements.

Causes and Pathogenesis

Nystagmus occurs due to involvement of structures involved in maintaining the normal ocular posture. The causes are diseases of the eye (retina), ear (vestibular apparatus) cerebellum, ocular muscles and middle longitudinal fasciculus. The causes depending on its type are given in Table 5.2.

Symptom Analysis

It is analysed along with vertigo, hence, question to be asked is same both for vertigo and nystagmus. The nystagmus combined with vertigo indicates:
- It indicates organic vertigo.
- It also indicates central vertigo due to basilar artery insufficiency, brain stem infarct and cerebellar diseases.

TABLE 5.2: Causes and Types of Nystagmus

Type	Description	Causes
I. Jerky nystagmus		
• Horizontal	• Nystagmus in horizontal direction	• Labrinthine, cerebellar and brain stem dysfunction
• Vertical	• Nystagmus in up and down direction	• Brain stem infection, multiple sclerosis, encephalitis, syringobulbia, cerebellar tumour, phenytoin toxicity
• Rotatory	• Nystagmus around a temporary fixed anteroposterior axis in a circular manner	• Vestibular disease • Benign paroxysmal positional vertigo
II. Pendular nystagmus	• To and fro equal movements like a pendulum	• Poor vision in early age • Hereditary
III. Ataxic nystagmus	• Rhythm of nystagmus is dissociated (ataxic), i.e. inward movement in the adducting eye and irregular coarse nystagmus in the abducting eye	• Multiple sclerosis due to involvement of MLF (medial longitudinal fasciculus)
IV. Sea-saw nystagmus	• One eye moves down and other moves up	• Lesion around third ventricle
V. Optokinetic nystagmus	• It occurs when eyes attempt to follow a moving object. Slow phase occurs in the direction of movement of object and fast phase in opposite direction	• Normal reflex phenomenon

☞ *Test for the nystagmus*

The tests are done to detect the presence of nystagmus, determine the direction, rate, amplitude and its type so as to reach at definite conclusion.

I. **Spontaneous nystagmus at rest.** Nystagmus on forward gaze is detected with ease at rest. However, to detect the nystagmus on deviation of eyes, patient's head is held with left hand and patient is asked to look at a definite point, say the top of right index finger or ball pen which is first held in the midline and then moved to left, right, upwards and downwards. Remember deviation >30 in any direction should be avoided. *Note the direction of nystagmus* (fast component).

II. **Hallpike manoeuvre for positional vertigo and nystagmus.** Read this manoeuvre in testing of VIII nerve.

SYNCOPE

Syncope refers to loss of postural tone, inability to maintain erect posture followed by unconsciousness. It is a symptom of decreased cerebral perfusion. It occurs commonly in standing position due to postural drop in BP but it can occur in sitting position in cardiac conduction defects called *Stokes-Adam attacks*. The loss of consciousness is briefer than an epileptic fit (Table 5.3).

Causes of Syncope

1. **Syncope due to inadequate vasoconstrictive mechanisms**
   - Vasovagal (vasodepressor)
   - Postural hypotension (autonomic neuropathy)
   - Carotid sinus hypersensitivity
   - Antihypertensive drugs (hydralazine, alpha-methyl dopa)
2. **Syncope due to hypovolaemia**
   - Fluid or blood loss
   - Addison's disease
3. **Syncope due to reduction in venous return**
   - Cough and micturition syncope
   - Mediastinal compression
   - Straining during defaecation
   - Valsalva manoeuvre
4. **Syncope due to reduction in cardiac output**
   - *Left ventricular outflow tract obstruction*, e.g. valvular heart disease, hypertrophic cardiomyopathy.
   - *Right ventricular or pulmonary outflow obstruction*, e.g. pulmonary stenosis, pulmonary hypertension, pulmonary embolism.
   - *Myocardial disease* (infarction, inflammation)
   - *Cardiac tamponade* (pericardial effusion)
5. **Syncope induced by arrhythmias**
   - Sinoatrial and AV blocks
   - Supraventricular/ventricular arrhythmias
   - Ventricular asystole
6. **Syncope due to cerebrovascular disturbance**
   - TIAs
   - Vertebrobasilar insufficiency
   - Hypertensive encephalopathy
7. **Miscellaneous causes**
   - Hypoxia
   - Anaemia
   - Hypoglycaemia

TABLE 5.3: The Distinction between Syncope and an Epileptic Fit

Feature	Syncope	Epilepsy
Precipitating factors	Emotional, painful or stressful stimuli	Unusual or recognised
Position at occurrence	Upright	Any position
Diurnal pattern/timing	Daytime	Day and night
Onset	Subacute or gradual	Acute
Aura	Absent	Present
Motor symptoms and signs	Motionless, flaccid, may have a few clonic jerks	Often tonic or tonic-clonic, or clonic jerks
Colour of the skin	Pale or ashen-gray	Pale or flushed
Cyanosis	Absent	May be present
Breathing	Slow, shallow	Stertorous
Urinary and/or faecal incontinence	Rare	Usual
Tongue biting	Rare	Common
Injury	Rare	Common
Postictal phenomenon	Rare	Confusion, headache, drowsiness, sleep
Period of unconsciousness	Brief (a few seconds)	Short (a few minutes)

- Hyperventilation
- Prolonged bed rest

Symptom Analysis

Q. **Ask about age and sex.**
- Vasovagal syncope is common in young while postural and cerebral syncope is common in old.

Q. **Relation with posture.**
- Syncope occurs in erect posture except cardiac syncope (arrhythmias Stokes-Adam attacks) which can occur in any position.

Q. **What is the duration of unconsciousness?**
- It is a few seconds in syncope, i.e. briefer than an epileptic fit.

Q. **History of blood or fluid loss.**
- Postural hypotension due to hypovolaemia can lead to syncope.

Q. **Ask about cough (for cough syncope) straining at micturition (micturition syncope).**

Q. **Ask about pulmonary (asthma, COPD), cardiac disease (valvular obstructive lesions, MI, cardiomyopathy).**
- All the above diseases can lead to syncope.

Q. **Ask about diabetes, HT, hypoglycaemic attacks.**
- Diabetic autonomic neuropathy and hypoglycemia can lead to syncope.

Q. **Ask about prolonged bed rest.**
- Prolonged bed rest leads to syncope due to postural hypotension.

Q. **What are associated systemic symptoms?**
- Associated premonitory symptoms in common three types of syncope are given in Table 5.4.

> *Remember.* Sometimes one can confuse syncope with an epileptic fit. Certain differences (Table 5.3) can solve the problem in most of cases.

WEAKNESS OR PARALYSIS

Weakness means reduction in normal power of one or more muscles. Paralysis and the suffix *"plegia"* implies weakness that is severe and complete or nearly complete. On the other hand, *paresis* implies partial weakness. The *prefix "hemi"* refers to one half of the body, *"para"* to both the lower limbs and *"quadri"* to all the four limbs.

Causes

I. **Upper motor neuron weakness**
- *Cerebrovascular accident*, *tumour* (cerebrum, brain stem), *ischaemia* or *haemorrhage* of cerebrum/brain stem (hypertensive, subarachnoid, subdural), *demyelination* (multiple sclerosis), *infections* (encephalitis, meningitis), *trauma* and *congenital diplegia* or *cerebral palsy*, *cord compression* (tumour, abscess).

II. **Lower motor neuron type of weakness**
- Poliomyelitis, peripheral neuropathies, myasthenia, episodic paralysis and muscular dystrophies.

Symptom Analysis

Ask about the following

Q. **Ask about age.**
- Cerebral palsy leading to diplegia is common in children and adolescent, brain tumour in young and CVA in older persons.

Q. **Is there any inability to move the limb/part or side of the body?**
- Inability to move the limb/part or side of the indicate paralysis.

Q. **What is its onset?**
- Acute onset of weakness occurs commonly due to stroke, brain tumour while chronic progressive weakness occurs in muscular disorders.

Q. **Is it stationary or has progressed? if, yes, then how it progressed?**

TABLE 5.4: Analysis of Systemic Symptoms

Feature	Cardiac syncope	Vasovagal syncope	Neurogenic syncope
1. Premonitory symptoms	Light headedness, palpitation, chest discomfort, dyspnoea and convulsions	Nausea, perspiration, pallor, light-headedness	Headache, confusion, hyperexcitability, visual or auditory hallucinations and aura
2. Period of unconsciousness	Brief, death-like pallor present	Brief, pallor with ashen-gray skin	Prolonged unconsciousness (>1 min), motor-seizure activity, urinary incontinence, tongue biting
3. Recovery	Rapid or fast	Slow recovery with nausea and light-headedness	Recovery with prolonged headache or focal neurologic deficit

- Weakness in CVA is either stationary or may sometime progress but brain tumour, muscular dystrophies cause progressive weakness.

Q. Which area of the body is involved?
- It may be monoplegia, paraplegia, hemiplegia or quadriplegia.

Q. Does the weakness affect one or both sides?
- One side involvement indicates hemiplegia. Both sides involvement indicates quadriplegia or double hemiplegia.

Q. What movements are affected?
- Voluntary movements are affected in paralysis.

Q. Is there any difficulty in combing hair, trying to reach high shelf or difficulty in getting out of a chair, or taking a high step up?
- All these features suggest proximal myopathy due to any cause.

Q. Does the weakness increase with effort and improve after rest?
- Myasthenic weakness increases with effort and relieved on rest.

Q. Are there any associated sensory or other symptoms?
- Fever associated with weakness of limbs indicates Guillain-Barré syndrome or infective brain lesion.

Q. Is weakness episodic or persistent?
Read episodic weakness below:
- Episodic weakness following an epileptic fit indicates Todd's paralysis.
- Persistent headache, nausea and vomiting due to raised intracranial tension with weakness indicate brain haemorrhage, subdural haematoma, brain tumour.
- Sensory disturbance with weakness indicate sensorimotor neuropathies.

Q. Is there any difficulty in opening a jaw or combing or using hand tools (e.g. scissors, screw driver)?
- All these features suggest small muscle weakness due to any cause.

EPISODIC WEAKNESS

Episodic weakness means sudden onset of intermittent muscle weakness.

Causes

The common causes are:
I. *Electrolyte disturbances*
- Hypo- or hyperkalaemia due to any cause.
- Hypercalcaemia and hypocalcaemia (tetany).
- Hyponatraemia.

II. *Neuromuscular junction disorders*
- Myasthenia gravis.
- Myasthenia-myopathic syndrome. (Lambert-Eaton syndrome).

III. *Muscle diseases*
- Periodic paralysis, myotonias.
- Metabolic defects of muscles.

IV. *CNS disorders*
- Cataplexy and narcolepsy.
- Multiple sclerosis.
- TIAs.

V. *Miscellaneous*
- Hyperventilation (alkalosis).
- Hypoglycaemia/diabetes.
- Addison's disease, thyrotoxicosis.

Symptom Analysis

Ask about the following

Q. Does episodic weakness occur at rest? What does precipitate it?
- Hypokalaemic periodic paralysis occurs at rest immediately after cessation of exercise. Diarrhoea, high carbohydrate diet, diuretics, steroids, and hyperthyroidism are important precipitants.

Q. Ask about history of chronic renal disease, i.e (CRF), or Addison's disease.
- Hyperkalaemic period paralysis occurs in the setting of chronic renal disease (chronic renal failure) or Addison's disease. Ask about clinical features of these diseases.

Q. Ask about vomiting, diarrhoea for potassium loss.
- Potassium loss occurs from *GI tract* (diarrhoea, vomiting) burns, excessive sweating, pancreatitis or through *kidneys* (diuretics, salt wasting nephropathy, hypo-aldosteronism). Hypokalemia is a common cause of episodic weakness.

Q. History of carpopedal spasms.
- Carpopedal spasms due to tetany may be hypocalcaemic, alkalotic, hypokalaemic and hypomagnesaemic. In case of tetany, try to explore the underlying cause of electrolyte disturbance.

Q. History of thyrotoxicosis.
- Thyrotoxicosis can lead to episodic weakness.

Nervous System

Q. History of muscle disease or myasthenia.
- Episodic weakness may occur in metabolic muscle disorders or myasthenia gravis (autoimmune disorder).

Q. Is the patient anxious? Is he/she hyperventilating?
- Hyperventilation may produce recurrent attacks of weakness but these patients have normal strength when tested.

Q. History of diabetes/hypoglycaemia.
- Episodes of hypoglycaemia may produce transient subjective weakness.

Q. Is there any sleep disturbance?
- Patients with narcolepsy, cataplexy and sleep paralysis may have sudden loss of strength and tone during the attack.

MOTOR SYMPTOMS

Ask about the following motor symptoms

1. **Spasms:** It refers to brief, unsustained contractions of a muscle or muscles resulting in pain and rigidity of the muscles involved. It results from abnormal electrical activity of CNS, motor neurons or muscle(s) itself. Flexor or extensor spasms result from UMN lesions.

Symptom Analysis

Q. Ask about painful spasm/muscle cramps
- **Cramp:** It refers to paroxysmal, spontaneous, painful and prolonged contraction of a muscle or muscles (painful spasms). They occur in tetany.

Q. Is there any history of rigidity of limbs?
- **Stiffness:** It refers to rigidity (parkinsonism) or spasm (tetanus), causing difficulty in walking.

Q. History of injury or IM injection.
- Injury or IM injection may result in hematoma, pain and muscle spasm, rigidity.

2. **Myalgia.** It is a muscular pain in the absence of muscle weakness, is usually viral in origin (influenza, Coxsackie virus). *Fibrositis, fibromyalgia* and *fibromyositis* are synonyms for a disorder associated with muscle pain/ tenderness. Myalgia may be *polymyalgia rheumatica* (occurs over age 50 and is characterised by pain, stiffness in shoulders and hip muscles) or may be a symptom of other rheumatological disorders (rheumatoid arthritis, SLE, PAN, scleroderma and mixed connective tissue syndrome).

Symptom Analysis

Q. History of pain in muscle of around the joints, back, shoulders, legs, etc.
- Pain and stiffness of joint, back shoulders indicate polymyalgia or rheumatological disorders.

SENSORY SYMPTOMS (Read the Sensory System Examination)

THE GAIT

The normal gait and its abnormalities are discussed at the end.

HISTORY

The symptoms of neurological disorders are so vague that detailed history and elicitation of clinical signs will enable the physician to come to some definite diagnosis. The anatomy and physiology of nervous system help to localise the site of the lesion and to narrow down the differential diagnosis. In structural disease of the nervous system localising signs act as clues to the diagnosis. However, e.g. epilepsy, migraine may not produce abnormal signs on examination, hence, the history taking is of clinical significance.

PRESENT HISTORY

In the history, emphasis should be laid on:
i. *Time relationship of symptoms*, i.e. onset, progression or regression, frequency, duration, etc.
ii. *Localisation*, e.g. which part of the body is affected the most. Is involvement symmetrical or asymmetrical?
iii. *Precipitating factors*, e.g. Do the symptoms increase by any specific activity, e.g. exercise, sleep, posture, reading, eating, coughing, micturition, sexual activity or by external stimuli, e.g. sound, smell, heat or cold?
iv. *Associated symptoms:* Are there other associated or accompanying symptoms in addition to presenting, symptoms, i.e.
   - Numbness, tingling, paraesthesias, cold, or warmth (sensory disturbance).
   - Weakness, clumsiness, stiffness, unsteady gait (motor system disturbance).
   - Headache, nausea, vomiting, seizures (symptoms of raised intracranial pressure).
   - Visual disturbances, e.g. diminution of vision, diplopia, scintillating spots.
   - Disturbance in consciousness, e.g. confusion, delirium, stupor.

- Psychological disturbances, e.g. depression, euphoria, agitation, somnolence, appetite disturbance, change in libido.

PAST HISTORY
- Past history of diabetes, hypertension, renal disease or dialytic therapy, alcoholism, smoking, tuberculosis must be asked.
- Any past history of diarrhoea or malabsorption or acute respiratory infection.
- Some neurological disorders (e.g. epilepsy, hydrocephalus) may present many years after the causative event. It is, therefore, important to ask about:
  - Pregnancies (length of term, intrauterine problems).
  - Delivery (normal, assisted or operative).
  - Neonatal health (severe jaundice, respiratory difficulty, infections and convulsions).
  - Problems during infancy (e.g. convulsions, trauma, infection).
  - *Childhood and adulthood* (e.g. trauma to head or spine, infections such as meningitis, encephalitis, surgical operation).

DRUG HISTORY
- Ask about the drug being taken or has been taken in the past such as anti-tubercular, anti-epileptics, anticoagulants, anti-psychotics, oral contraceptives, nitrofurantoin, vincristine.
- History of intake of poison, e.g. organophosphorous compounds.
- History of vaccination, e.g. predisposition to AIDS, hepatitis and demyelinating disorders, etc.

FAMILY HISTORY
1. Many neurological disorders may be genetically transmitted in families, e.g. hereditary ataxias, muscular dystrophies, myotonias, Huntington's chorea and hereditary neuropathies.
2. In some neurological disorders, genetic factors play some roles, e.g. epilepsy, multiple sclerosis, migraine, stroke, dementia.

SOCIAL AND PERSONAL HISTORY

Ask about the following
1. **Occupation:** Patient's occupation may be causative or triggering factor for certain neurological disorders.
   - Exposure to toxic chemicals (toxic neuropathies or encephalopathies) such as lead, mercury, industrial solvents, OP compounds, etc.
   - Recurrent overuse of certain joints predisposing to entrapment neuropathy (e.g. carpal tunnel syndrome).
   - Prolonged visual work, i.e. watch makers, watch mechanics (tension headache, migraine).
   - History of recent travel.
   - Occupation requiring prolonged stay outside home, e.g. *sadhu or saint*, sailors, truck driver are predisposed to sexually transmitted disorders/AIDS.
2. **Diet**, e.g. vegetarian or non-vegetarian (neurocysticercosis), alcohol intake, quality of diet.
3. **Marital status:** Marriage, divorce, bereavement and change in occupation are important precipitating factors for tension headache, migraine, depression, may also trigger attacks of multiple sclerosis and epilepsy.
4. **Sexual contact:** History of contact with unknown partner must be asked to explore any possibility of sexually transmitted diseases.

EXAMINATION
A neurological examination requires to be systematic. It includes:
1. General physical examination
2. Proper neurological examination

GENERAL PHYSICAL EXAMINATION

☞ General Observation
Observe the *general posture*, *dressing* and *gait* as soon as patient walks into the room for examination.
- It gives valuable information regarding general and neurological status of a person.

☞ Head (Cranium)
Look for any abnormality of the skull
The abnormalities to be observed are:
- Large skull with protuding jaw and prominent furrows over forehead (*gigantism*).
- Hyperosteosis (*Paget's disease*)
- Microcephaly (congenital, zira virus infection is recently blamed)
- Irregularity of the skull, e.g. localised bony swelling, tumour or erosion, multiple myeloma, fractures.
- Tenderness of skull (polymyalgia rheumatica)
- Intracranial bruits to be heard with bell of stethoscope on frontal region, lateral occipital region and on each closed eyeball for angiomas, carotid cavernous fistula, tumours of glomus jugulare (best heard over mastoid or jugular vein).

☞ Skin

Following points are to be noted:
- *Cafe au lait* spots, subcutaneous and plexiform neurofibromas (*von Recklinghausen's disease*)
- *Cutaneous angiomas* (Portwine stain). They may occur in *Sturge-Weber syndrome*. *Telangiectasia of skin* may be associated with intracranial telangiectasia.
- *Adenoma sebaceum over face* may be present with *tuberous sclerosis*.
- *Herpes zoster lesions* infection (papulovesicular eruption) is associated with herpetic neuralgias.
- *Any rash*, e.g. exanthematous rash (measles, mumps, rubella) or *butterfly rash* over face in SLE.
- *Thick tight skin* over face and extremities occurs in systemic sclerosis.
- *Signs of nutritional deficiencies*, e.g. angular stomatitis, cheilosis, pellagerous skin, anaemia for nutritional neurological disorders.
- *Scar marks, injection marks*, may be present in drug addicts. *Burn marks* are seen in neuropathies. *Gangrene of the phalanges* or *painful fingertips* may be seen in embolic phenomenon. *Bed sores* indicate prolonged illness or unconsciousness or paraplegia.
- *Tuft of hair* over the spine may be seen in spina bifida.
- *Skin tumours*, e.g. melanoma.

☞ Eyes

Detailed examination of the eyes is discussed under cranial nerve examination. However, look for the following on general physical examination:

- Unilateral proptosis, conjunctivitis, chemosis, karatitis or corneal ulceration.
  Examine the iris with torch light for any *colour change* (discolouration).

- Normally the iris is black in colour with a circular hole in the centre called the *pupil*.
- **Heterochromia** refers to different colours of the iris, indicates intraocular disease or albinism. In inflammation (*iritis*), the iris looks muddy with a small pupil and there is ciliary flush (congestion).
- **Iritis** may be a manifestation of rheumatoid arthritis; connective tissue disease or a manifestation of other systemic disease such as sarcoidosis.

The Pupils

- Inspect the pupils for size, shape and symmetry. If the pupils are large (>5 mm), small (<3 mm) or unequal on two sides, measure them with a card with black holes of varying sizes. Pupillary inequality of less than 0.5 mm (anisocoria) is considered as normal.
- Assess the pupillary reactions to light (direct and consensual) and accommodation.

Various pupillary abnormalities and reaction to light are presented in Table 5.5.

Methods: Ask the patient to look at a distant object and shine a bright light or pin-torch obliquely into each pupil in turn. Note the pupillary reaction:

TABLE 5.5: Pupillary Abnormalities in Common Disorders

Disorder	Size of the pupil	Reaction
III cranial nerve paralysis or parasympatholytic agents use (dilated pupil)	A. Abnormal > normal side	• Efferent pupil defect • Light or accommodation reaction absent on the affected side • Normal side reacts consensually
Ciliary ganglion lesion (Adie's myotonic pupil): It is benign tonic pupils with absent tendon jerks, seen in young women	B. Abnormal > normal side	• Light reaction absent on the affected side • Accommodation reaction is slow and sustained
Retinal/optic nerve disease	Abnormal > normal side	• Afferent pupil defect • Poor direct light reflex, normal consensual reflex (reaction) and normal accommodation reaction on the affected side • Reduced consensual reflex on the normal side
Neurosyphilis (pretectal lesion), i.e. **Argyll Robertson pupil**	C. Small, irregular, unequal	• Light reflex absent • Accommodation reflex present
Sympathetic lesion (Horner's syndrome): It consists of meiosis, ptosis, enophthalmos, anhydrosis, loss of ciliospinal reflex)	D. Abnormal < normal side (small pupil)	• Reaction to light and accommodation present • Does not dilate with cocaine drops

- Pupillary constriction in the same eye indicates direct reaction.
- Pupillary constriction of the opposite pupil indicates consensual reaction.

The light reflex pathways and interpretation of direct and consensual light reflex are presented in Fig. 5.1.

Warning: Always darken the room and use a bright light before labelling that a light reflex is absent.

If reaction to light is impaired or questionable, then test *for near reaction or accommodation reaction* in normal room light.

Method: To test the reaction to accommodation, ask the patient first to look into the distance and then at an object (finger or pencil) held at 10 cm distance from the face. Watch for pupillary constriction with near object called *convergence (accommodation) reaction* (Fig. 5.2).

Bilateral pupillary constriction on convergence of the eyes to near object is called *accommodation reflex*.

Normal pupils are often described in the case notes by mnemonics **PERLA** (**P**upils **E**qual and **R**eactive to **L**ight and **A**ccommodation).

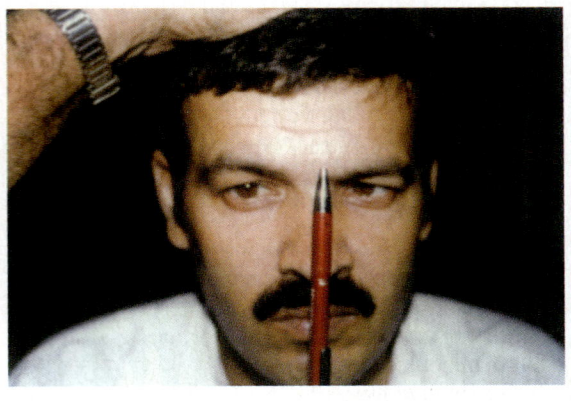

Fig. 5.2: Testing for convergence.

In *Argyll Robertson's pupil*, the light reflex is absent and accommodation reflex (near reaction) is retained (remember mnemonics AR pupil as accommodation retained).

In *Adie's pupil*, the light reflex is absent but accommodation reflex is slow.

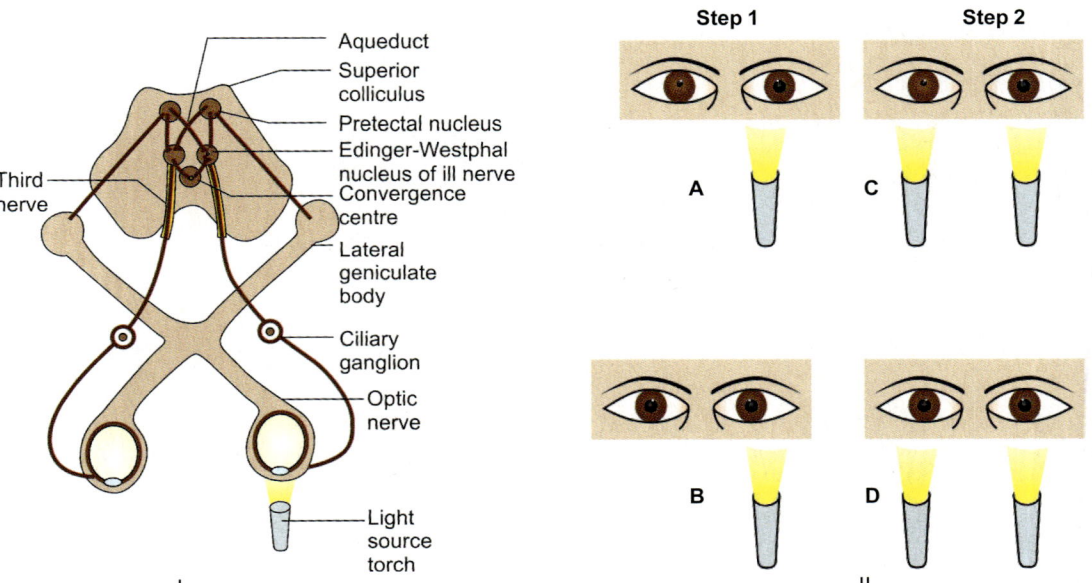

Fig. 5.1: The light reflex. I. Pathways, II. Direct and consensual light reflex and its interpretation.

I. Pupillary light reflex and its afferent and efferent pathways. Some fibres concerned with light reflex can bypass the lateral geniculate body to pretectal nucleus.

II. Direct and consensual constriction of pupils to light. Step 1: Shine a light source into that pupil in question. (A) No direct constriction, consensual reflex intact, indicates topical mydriatics or Argyll Robertson pupil. (B) No direct or consensual constriction indicates monocular blindness. Step 2 : After 5 seconds, shine the light into the contralateral pupil. (C) No direct constriction, but direct constriction of the contralateral pupil suggests topical mydriatics, Argyll Robertson pupil, or monocular blindness. D. No direct constriction of either pupil indicates death or profound brain stem damage.

Common Abnormalities of Pupil

I. Small (constricted) pupils
Sympathetic nerve fibres involved. Could also be due to local eye disease or drug induced.

Causes
i. Cervical sympathetic compression in lymphomas (*Horner's syndrome*).
ii. Brain stem involvement (*pontine haemorrhage*).
iii. Posterior inferior cerebellar artery infarction (*lateral medullary syndrome*).
iv. Neurosyphilis (*Argyll Robertson's pupil*)
v. Local ocular disease. e.g. *iritis, iridocyclitis*
vi. *Parasympathomimetic agents,* e.g. organophosphorous compounds, morphine, heroin, etc.

II. Large (dilated) pupil
3rd cranial nerve or ciliary ganglion is involved. It can also be due to local disease of the eye or drug induced.

Causes
- 3rd cranial nerve palsy in midbrain (nuclear) or outside it in cavernous sinus (*cavernous sinus thrombosis*)
- Parasympatholytic agents/drops (*atropine, scopolamine, hyoscine*)
- A tonic pupil (*Holmes-Adie pupil*)
- Ciliary ganglion lesions (*herpes infection, trauma, ischaemia due to diabetes*)
- Ocular diseases, e.g. acute glaucoma, retinal or optic nerve disease.

III. Unequal pupils (anisocoria)
Approximately 10–12% normal individuals have slight pupillary inequality. Such physiological unequal pupils react normally to light. *Pathological pupils* (variation >0.5 mm between two pupils) dilate and constricts abnormally. The causes of constriction (meiosis) and dilatation (mydriasis) of pupil have already been described.

Eye Movements

☞ Look for deviation of eyeball (squint)

Squint: Deviation of eyes from their normally conjugate position is termed as *strabismus* or *squint*.

Types
I. **Paralytic.** It is caused by weakness or paralysis of one or more extraocular muscles. It may be:
   Divergent: Due to paralysis of medical rectus.
   Convergent: Due to paralysis of lateral rectus.
II. **Non-paralytic (concomitant).** There is no paralysis of extraocular muscles. It is caused by an imbalance in ocular muscle tone. The differences between paralytic and non-paralytic squints are given in Table 5.6.

TABLE 5.6: Differentiation between Two Types of Squint

Feature	Paralytic	Non-paralytic
Cause	Paralysis of one or more extraocular muscles; may be convergent or divergent	• No paralysis of the muscles • It is due to imbalance in ocular muscle tone, hence, mostly hereditary
Onset	Acute, acquired in later life	Slow, present since childhood
Movements	Restricted in the direction of paralysed muscle	Good in all the directions
Diplopia	Present	Absent
Associated symptom and signs	Long-standing paralytic squint often results in abnormal head posture with the head turned or tilted to minimize diplopia	As diplopia is absent in this type of squint there is no abnormal head posture

Testing for Squint
- Test movement in all directions of gaze (read cranial nerves examination). Both eyes should move symmetrically with no diplopia. If diplopia is present, the most peripheral double vision is the one from the paretic eye.
- **The cover/uncover test.** The cover/uncover test is particularly useful in detecting small concomitant squints in children. It helps to differentiate between paralytic and non-paralytic squint.

Paralytic squint: In paralytic squint, the deviation of the eye in a direction opposite to the action of the muscle is called primary deviation of squint. If the unaffected (normal) eye is covered so that patient fixes the gaze with the affected eye (squinting eye), the covered normal eye will deviate still more than the primary deviation of the affected eye.

Non-paralytic squint: Here the squint is absent at rest and movements are equal for all positions of the eyes. The movements of the squinting eye are usually unimpaired when the fixing eye is covered. Diplopia is rare.

Method
- Ask the patient to look at a distant object.
- Cover one eye

- Closely observe uncovered eye for any movements. If it moves to take up fixation, that eye is squinting
- Repeat the sequence for the other eye
- Tests for paralytic squint. Determine the direction of gaze that maximizes the deviation.

The Ocular Fundus

Examination of the ocular fundus constitutes an important part of complete medical examination. Fundus is seen with the help of an ophthalmoscope. Valuable informations can be gathered about the state of the *optic disc*, and of the *arteries and veins of the retina*, in addition to the detection of local eye disorders.

To see the more peripheral structures, to evaluate the macula well or to investigate unexplained visual loss, ophthalmologists or internists dilate the pupil with some mydriatic drops unless contraindicated (head injury, narrow angle glaucoma).

☞ *Examine the fundus systematically for*
- *Optic disc (shape, colour, physiological cup, margins, etc).*
- *Retinal blood vessels, macula*
- *The periphery of the fundus.*

Steps of Examination

- The patient should be examined either sitting or lying down in a darkened room.
- Ask the patient to look straight at a distant object.
- Stand or sit on the side to be examined at an arm's length from the patient and keep your eyes level with that of the patient.
- To look at the right eye, hold the ophthalmoscope with lenses at zero in the right hand.
- Use your right eye to examine the patient's right eye and *vice versa* (left eye for patient's left eye).
- Switch on the instrument and shine it at pupil. The ophthalmoscope should then be brought as close as possible to the patient's eye and the light is directed slightly nasally.
- If the eye closes, open it gently.
- Demonstrate the red reflex of the fundus and note the nature of any opacities in the media.

The ocular media (cornea, lens and vitreous) are normally clear. Note any opacity while observing the red reflex. Dense opacities may completely obscure the reflex (e.g. cataract). The depth of the opacity can be determined by moving the ophthalmoscope.

Opacities in the media of the eye (cornea, anterior chamber, lens, vitreous) will appear as black specks or lines against the red glow.
- Corneal opacities move in opposite direction
- Lens opacity stay stationary
- Vitreous opacities move in the same direction of ophthalmoscope.

- Keeping the beam pointing in the above mentioned direction and the red reflex in view, move close to the patient, stopping just clear off the lashes.
- In this way, optic disc can be focussed. If, instead of disc, retinal vessels are in focus (seen), follow them to reach the fundus.
- If the optic disc is not in focus, the strength of the lenses of the ophthalmoscope should be gradually reduced until the disc becomes focussed.
- Note any abnormality considering the fundus as a clock with the disc at the centre. The disc diameter (1.5 mm) is used as a unit of measurement; for example you can say haemorrhage is seen at 3'o clock position at two discs diameter distance from the disc.

Characteristics of Normal Fundus

i. **The optic disc**
   Shape: Round or slightly oval (Fig. 5.3).
   Colour: Pink with slight temporal pallor.
   Physiological cup: A depression in the central part, is more pale than the surrounding disc and from it retinal vessels enter and leave the eye.
   Edge (margin) of the disc: The retinal blood vessels radiate from the disc, dividing dichoto-mously into many branches and pass towards the periphery. The arteries or arterioles have a smaller calibre than the veins, and have a bright red colour. Healthy vessel walls are not visible. Note the normal and abnormal pulsations.

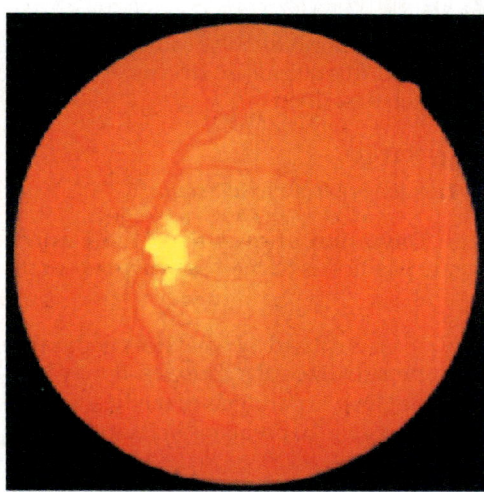

Fig. 5.3: Normal fundus.

Spontaneous retinal artery pulsations are abnormal and occur in glaucoma and aortic regurgitation.

Macular region. It is a portion of the posterior retina containing xanthophilic pigment (hence, macula lutea) and two or more layers of ganglion cells. The *fovea* (5.5 mm in diameter) lies at the centre of macula and is devoid of blood vessels. Macular involvement produces greater reduction of the vision.

The Abnormalities of the Fundus (Figs 5.4 to 5.7)

i. **Retinal atrophy**: Old injuries and inflammation may result in atrophic scars. White patches of atrophic retina occur in congenital coloboma, high myopia and retinal degeneration.

ii. **Abnormal pigmentation**: Macular degeneration occurs in old persons (age related process) in which retinal pigment epithelial changes cause hypopigmentation and pigment clumping at the macula. Central vision is poor.

Melanomas. Benign choroidal melanomas are flat dark lesions while malignant melanomas are raised, enlarge progressively and often metastasize.

Retinitis pigmentosa is associated with pigment deposits like bony spicules, seen in Laurence-Moon-Biedl syndrome.

iii. **Abnormal exudates** (Table 5.7)

iv. **Optic atrophy**: It is defined as atrophy of optic nerve fibres with reduction or loss of tiny blood vessels. In this condition, the disc is paler than normal, and may even be white (Fig. 5.4).

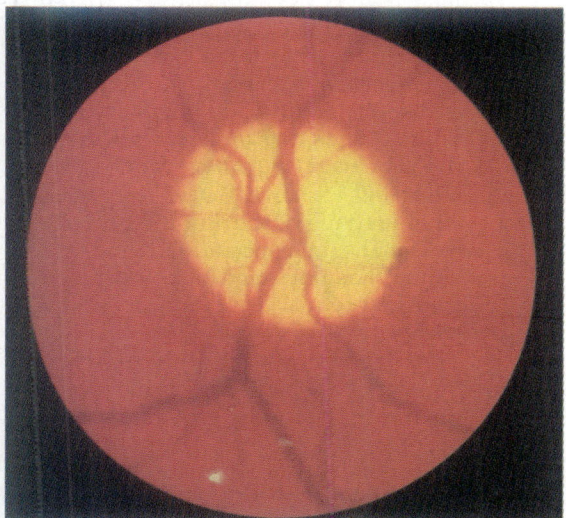

Fig. 5.4: Fundus photograph of a patient with optic atrophy.

In optic atrophy, the number of capillaries that cross the disc margin is reduced from normal 10 to 7 or less (*Kestenbaum's sign*).

TABLE 5.7: Abnormal Deposits on the Retina

Hard exudates	Soft exudates
They are deep	They are superficial
Well defined, deep seated (hence hard)	Irregular or ill-defined, superficial (hence soft)
They are often arranged in rings. At the macula, they may arrange in a star (macular star)	They look-like deposits of cotton wool
They are caused by leakage of proteins though an abnormal permeable blood vessel	They occur around areas of infarcted retina and may be associated with other features of retinal ischaemia (venous dilatation, haemorrhage, new blood vessels). They are due to swelling of optic nerve fibre layer
They are seen in hypertension, diabetes, and following retinal vascular occlusions	They are seen in retinal artery ischaemia or infarction due to hypertension, retinal vein occlusion. They are seen in raised ICP

The classification of optic atrophy into *primary* (disc is flat, chalky-white in colour with clear cut margins), *secondary* (atrophy follows papilloedema) and *consecutive* (glucomatous) is confusing, hence, avoided.

Causes
1. Inherited, e.g. Leber's optic atrophy (Fig. 5.4).
2. Toxic, e.g. ethambutol, methylalcohol, carbon monoxide and ethylene glycol (antifreeze).
3. Glaucoma.
4. Extensive retinal disease.
5. Ischaemic optic atrophy.
6. Demyelinating disease, e.g. multiple sclerosis, Devic's disease.
7. Trauma, e.g. avulsion of optic nerve.
8. Tumours, e.g. pituitary adenoma, craniopharyngioma.

v. **Papilloedema**: It is bilateral optic disc swelling from raised intracranial pressure. Disc changes in papilloedema (Fig. 5.5) are:
- The swollen disc is pink and hyperaemic
- Disc vessels clearly visible, more numerous, curve over the borders of the disc. There is venous dilatation and loss of venous pulsations.

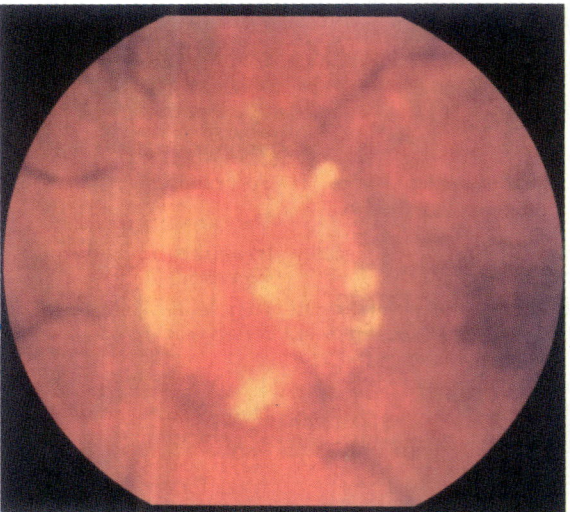

Fig. 5.5: Papilloedema. The fundus photograph was taken from a patient with raised intracranial pressure. Note the disc oedema, haemorrhage and cotton wool exudate.

- The margins are blurred
- The physiological cup is not visible, i.e. cup is lost and full.

Calculation of papilloedema in diopters: The elevated disc of papilloedema can be measured by noting the differences in diopters of the two lenses used to focus clearly on the disc and on univolved retina.

Causes
1. *Raised intracranial pressure* due to tumours, brain abscesses, meningitis, obstructive hydrocephalus, subdural haematoma, subarachnoid haemorrhages, dural sinus thrombosis and idiopathic.
2. *Cerebral oedema*
3. *Accelerated or malignant hypertension*
4. *Haematological disorders*, e.g. anaemia, leukaemia.
5. *Respiratory diseases*, e.g. emphysema, carbon dioxide narcosis.
6. *Vitamin A* deficiency or excess
7. *Hypoparathyroidism*
8. *Optic nerve tumour* (Foster-Kennedy syndrome) in which there is ipsilateral optic atrophy and contralateral papilloedema.
9. *Pseudopapilloedema* due to drusen (optic nerve drusen are refractile deposits within substance of the optic nerve head).
10. *Papillitis*

vi. **Optic neuritis:** It results from inflammatory, demyelinating or vascular disease leading to marked loss of vision. There may be retrobulbar involvement (retrobulbar neuritis) in which neither the doctor nor the patient sees anything, i.e. vision is lost. The differences between optic neuritis and papilloedema are summarised in Box 5.1. Optic neuritis is frequently followed by optic atrophy, residual reduction in visual acuity and scotomas (central or peripheral). It may occur unilaterally or bilaterally (Devic's disease, multiple sclerosis).

Box 5.1	Differentiation Between Optic Neuritis and Papilloedema
Optic neuritis	*Papilloedema*
• Eye movements are painful	• They are painless
• Ocular tenderness on compression of closed eye	• No such tenderness
• In papillitis, there is hyperaemia and some swelling of the disc	• Marked swelling of the disc with loss of cup (e.g. cup is full)
• Severe visual loss	• Minimal visual impairment
• There may be signs of inflammation, e.g. hazy vitreous and retinal exudates	• No signs of inflammation

vii. **Retinal haemorrhages**
a. *Superficial retinal haemorrhages* are flame-shaped horizontally arranged along the nerve fibres. They occur in hypertension.
b. *Deep haemorrhages* are round blotches and spots looking like microaneurysms. Both occur as dots (aneurysms) and blots (haemorrhage) in diabetic retinopathy.
c. *Subhyloid haemorrhages*, are large, round haemorrhage obscuring the underlying retina. They may occur following subarachnoid haemorrhage or follow bleeding from new retinal vessels in diabetic retinopathy.
d. *Vitreous haemorrhage.* The fundus is hidden by a dark haze of blood. The blood may be distributed diffusely through the vitreous gel or form clots which cause tadpole-like floaters. It is an important cause of sudden loss of vision.

Causes
1. Hypertension
2. Diabetes

3. Trauma
4. Blood disorders, e.g. anaemia, sickle cell disease, leukaemia, bleeding diathesis
5. Anticoagulants
6. Subarachnoid haemorrhage
7. Retinal vein occlusion
8. Age-related macular disease

viii. *Occlusion of central artery of retina*: It refers to sudden, and often total loss of vision. The fundus changes are:
  1. Pale and swollen optic disc and surrounding retina
  2. A cherry-red spot at the macula
  3. The retinal arteries are narrow and thread-like. It is due to embolic occlusion of retinal vessels from an atheromatous plaque.

ix. *Retinal vein occlusion:* In central vein occlusion a little vision is retained. The fundus changes are:
  1. Large flame-shaped haemorrhages and cottonwool spots or exudates splashed over the fundus.
  2. Swelling of the optic disc
  3. Gross venous dilatation.

x. *Hypertensive retinopathy* **(Fig. 5.6)**: The fundus changes are:
  1. Diffuse or segmental narrowing of arterioles/arteries and thickening of their walls. The thick-walled arterioles compress the veins at crossings (*venous nipping*) giving "*silver wiring*" appearance.
  2. Flame-shaped haemorrhages.
  3. Hard exudates. Sometimes star-shaped exudates around the macula (*macular star*).
  4. Papilloedema may occur especially in malignant hypertension.

xi. *Diabetic retinopathy* **(Fig. 5.7)**: The fundus changes are:

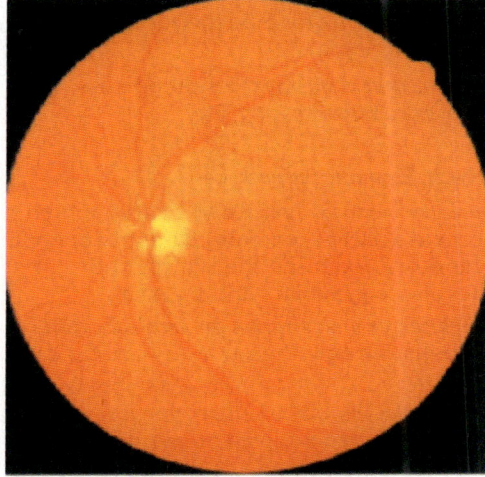

Fig. 5.7: Diabetic background retinopathy. Note the blot (haemorrhages), microaneurysm (dots) and a few hard exudates in the retina. This is a characteristic appearance of fundus in diabetic background retinopathy.

  1. *Microaneurysms.* Capillary microaneurysms are the earliest abnormality detected in background retinopathy.
  2. Dots and blots haemorrhage.
  3. Both hard and soft exudates (cotton-wool).
  4. Neovascularisation—new vessels extend into vitreous and may bleed, are seen in proliferative diabetic retinopathy.
  5. Pre-retinal and vitreous haemorrhage.
  6. Fibrosis, retinitis proliferans and retinal detachment.

☞ **Ear, Nose and Throat**

Look at the ear for

- Otitis externa.

Look for ear discharges

- Chronic suppurative otitis media can lead to 7th cranial nerve palsy and meningitis.

Elicit mastoid tenderness

- Mastoid tenderness suggests mastoiditis which can lead to jugular foramen syndrome.

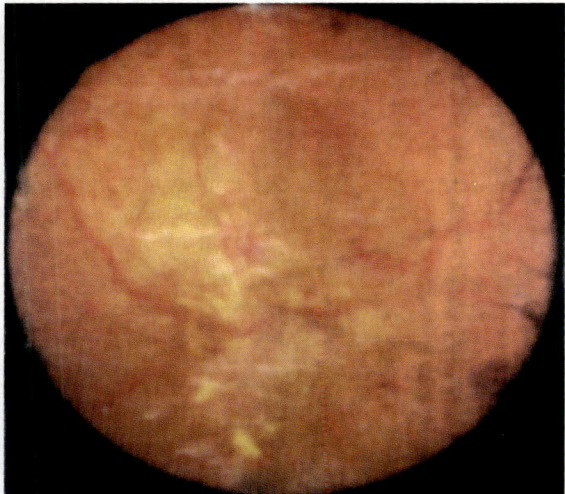

Fig. 5.6: Hypertensive retinopathy with macular star. Note the punctate hard exudates forming a macular star. Note also the flame-shaped haemorrhage and two small soft exudates.

Look at the nose and nasal septum for

- Depressed bridge of the nose may occur in tertiary syphilis, relapsing polychondritis, leprosy and Wegener's granulomatosis, gummatous lesion may be present on nasal septum.

Look at nasopharynx for evidence of any malignancy (nasopharyngioma).

Look at the oral cavity for dental abscess, tonsillar abscess, gum hypertrophy, etc.

☞ **Neck.** *Examine the neck, i.e.*
- *Look for cervical lymphadenopathy* which may occur as a part of generalised lymphadenopathy. Therefore, examine the lymph nodes at other sites also, e.g. axillary and inguinal.
- *Palpation or auscultation for cervical carotid bruit:* Embolism from atheromatous carotid can lead to stroke.
- *Look at the thyroid for enlargement.* Look for the signs of thyrotoxicosis or hypothyroidism, if present (these signs are discussed in unit on endocrine system examination).
- *Examine neck stiffness* and *signs of meningitis*.

☞ **Breasts.** *Examine the breast for any lump.*

- Carcinoma of the breast is a common source of distant metastasis including brain.

☞ **Examine vitals,** e.g. pulse, BP, temperature and respiration.
- *Slow pulse and heart rate (bradycardia)* may occur in raised intracranial pressure, tumour, Stokes-Adams attack and hypothyroidism. *Rapid heart rate (tachycardia)* may indicate an infection, arrhythmias (atrial fibrillation) or thyrotoxicosis. Arrhythmias in valvular heart disease predispose to cerebral embolisation (stroke).
- *Blood pressure*: Hypertension can lead to encephalopathy, lacunar infarct, atherothrombogenesis and brain haemorrhage.
- *Temperature*: Fever indicates infective or inflammatory brain disorders. Both *hyperthermia* and *hypothermia* are associated with neurological symptoms.
- *Respiration*: Respiratory irregularities (e.g. Cheyne-Stokes respiration, irregular slow respiration) may occur in raised intracranial pressure and brain stem disorders.

SYSTEMIC NEUROLOGICAL EXAMINATION

It includes examination of:
- Higher mental functions
- Speech and language
- Gait and cerebellar functions
- Cranial nerves
- Motor system
- Sensory system
- Other associated/involved system.

MENTAL STATUS/HIGHER MENTAL FUNCTIONS

The essential elements of mental status examination are:
1. Consciousness, appearance, behaviour and communication.
2. Mood/emotional status.
3. Thoughts and perceptions (delusions and hallucinations).
4. Cognitive functions, e.g. memory, intelligence, attention, information, vocabulary, calculations, and abstract thinking and constructional ability.
5. Release of primitive reflexes.

☞ **Consciousness:** *Assess the level of consciousness by talking*
Level of consciousness primarily reflects the patient's capacity for arousal or wakefulness. It is determined by the level of voice (normal or loud) shaking or applying a stimulus to arouse the patient to perform in response to escalating stimuli (Table 5.8). For categorisation of level of consciousness, use Glasgo Coma Scale (it is discussed in Unit on examination of unconscious patient).

☞ **Appearance or facial expression.** Observe the patient at rest and while interacting with others. *Is patient anxious, depressed or apathetic?*

Facial immobility or expressionless face in neurology is seen in parkinsonism, dementia.

☞ **Posture and motor behaviour:** *Look for any unusual posture or features in the behaviour, e.g. facial tics, fidgetiness of anxiety, crying, handswinging of agitated depression, slowed movements of parkinsonism, singing and dancing movements of chorea.*

There may be abnormal posture in encephalitis and cerebral palsy (Figs 5.8A and B).

☞ **Mood or emotional state:** *Evaluate the patient mood during the interview. Note as follows*
   i. Does the patient appear happier than normal (*elated* or *euphoric*) or filled with despair or dismay (*depression*) or angry?

TABLE 5.8: Assessment of Level of Consciousness

Level	Technique	Abnormal response
Alertness	Speak to the patient in normal voice. An alert patient responds, i.e. opens the eyes, looks at you and answers the questions appropriately (arousal intact)	Inattentive patient or patient with disturbed consciousness may not respond to command or questions
Lethargy	Speak to the patient in a loud voice. Ask "How are you?" "What is your name?"	A lethargic patient appears drowsy but opens the eyes and looks at you/responds to the questions and then falls asleep
	Shake the patient gently as if awakening a sleeper	An obtunded patient opens the eyes and looks at you, but responds slowly and is some-what confused. Alertness and interest in the surroundings are less
Stupor	Apply a painful stimulus: For example; *pinch a tendon, rub the sternum or roll a pencil across a nail bed*. No stronger stimulus needed	A stuporous patient arouses from sleep only after painful stimuli. Verbal responses are slow or even absent. The patient lapses into an unresponsive state when the stimulus ceases. There is minimal awareness of self or environment
Coma	Apply repeated painful stimuli	A comatosed patient remains unarousable with eyes closed. There is no evident response to any stimuli

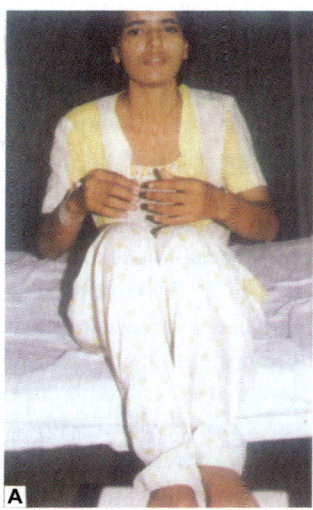

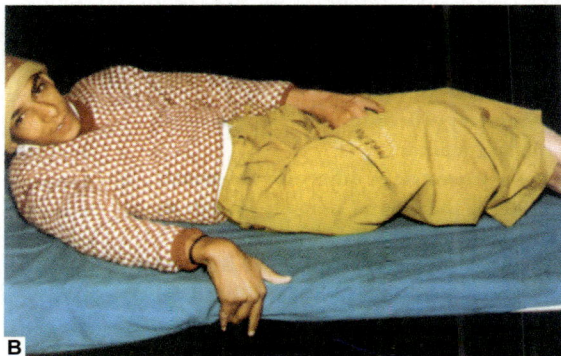

Figs 5.8A and B: (A) Catatonic posture following encephalitis (postencephalitic); (B) Dystonic posture in a patient with cerebral palsy.

☞**Thought and perceptions:** *Is there any delusion? Does the patient perceive hallucinations of any type?*

Delusions are false beliefs which continue to be held despite an evidence to contrary. Examples include; *delusions of persecution* (someone wants to prosecute him/her), *grandiose delusions* (he/she thinks himself/herself as President of India or a big man), *delusional jealousy* (someone is jealous of him/her) and *delusions of reference* (someone pay special attention to him/her).

Delusions are most often associated with psychotic disorders, may occur in delirium and dementia.

Hallucinations are false subjective sensory perceptions in the absence of relevant external stimuli. Hallucinations may be *auditory, visual, olfactory, gustatory, tactile* or *somatic*.

ii. Is there any blunting of emotion during talking, e.g. family or financial success is described without pleasure or patient laughs after relating a misfortune or breaks into tears after narrating a pleasant news?
iii. Does the patient enjoy life or fed up with life?
iv. Is there any suicidal intent or tendency?
v. Is there any sense of *depersonalisation or derealisation* by asking whether things seem as real as they should be or whether they seem changed in some mysterious way?

- Mood or emotional disturbance occurs in psychotic disorders.
- *De Jevu* and *De Jamaiu* phenomenon occur in temporal lobe lesion.

- Hallucinations of taste and smell are characteristic of temporal lobe epilepsy (partial seizures).
- Hallucinations of small animals or insects crawling through the room, or on the walls, or bed are particularly associated with delirium tremens (alcohol withdrawl syndrome).
- In occipital lobe lesions, visual hallucinations may occur.
- Hallucinations may occur in post-traumatic stress disorders and schizophrenia.

☞ **Insight or Awareness about Surroundings and Judgement**

One should assess whether the insight into the illness is intact or not by asking *"What brings you to the hospital?" "What seems to be your trouble"? "What do you think is wrong?"* Note whether the patient is aware of himself/herself and the surroundings.

Patients with psychotic disorders often lack insight into their illness. Denial of impairment may accompany some neurological disorders.

Judgement can be assessed by noting the patient's response to family situations, jobs, use of money or interpersonal conflicts. *Who will look after your financial affair while you are in the hospital? "If your husband starts abusing you again, what will you do"?*

Poor judgement is seen in dementia, delirium, mental retardation and psychotic states.

☞ **Cognitive functions.** *Assess them as follows*

i. **Orientation to time, place, person.** Assess patient's ability to recognise place, time or person by asking the following questions:
   - *Time* (you can ask about the time of day, day of the week, month, season, date and year, duration of hospital stay).
   - *Place* (ask about patient's residence, names of the hospital, city and state).
   - *Person.* (you can ask the patient's own name, and the names of the relatives and friends).

Disorientation occurs especially when the memory or attention is impaired as in delirium or organic brain disorders.

ii. **Memory:** Memory consists of the ability to grasp and retain the new information, requires adequate input, registration and recall. To test the recent memory, inquire about the events of the day including the day's weather, today's appointments and medications or diet taken today. *Ask the patient to recall what have you taken in the breakfast or dinner? What have you read in the paper or seen on the television?* In framing questions, one should keep in mind the patient's educational qualification, background and their likely personal interests.

Recent memory is impaired both in delirium and dementia. Amnestic disorders such as Korsakoff psychosis also impairs memory.

N.B. *To test remote or long-term memory* inquire about birth days, anniversaries, numbers, name of the schools attended, jobs held, or past historical events such as wars.

For short-term memory, you can ask for the events happened a few seconds or minutes ago.

- Loss of memory is called *amnesia*. Short-term memory loss is characteristically impaired in Wernicke-Korsakoff syndrome and in many patients with Alzheimer-type dementia.

iii. **Intelligence:** It is a higher cognitive function. Assess it during the history-taking. *Inquire about person's work or hobbies, reading, favourite television programmes* or *current events*, which give a rough and ready estimate of intelligence.

Frequent changes of work or employment after an accident or a serious illness in patients with a previously good work record suggests brain damage.

iv. **Calculating ability** is another cognitive function and tests the memory and reasoning, indicates more serious and specific defect. Ask the patients simple, arithmetic questions i.e. (*"what is 4 + 3? - - -*), "*what is 5 6? - -* . The task can be made more difficult by asking to *subtract 7 from 100* (i.e. 93, 86, 79 - - -). You can ask to spell a five-letter word "W-O-R-L-D" backwards.

Poor calculating ability may be a sign of dementia or may accompany aphasia (encephalitis).

v. **Constructional ability.** Patient is asked to copy figures of increasing complexity onto a piece of blank paper. Show each figure one at a time and ask the patient to copy it (Fig. 5.9).

If vision and motor ability are intact, poor constructional ability or apraxia suggests dementia or parietal lobe damage (hepatic encephalopathy).

SPEECH AND LANGUAGE

Speech is a mean of communications, expressing or understanding thoughts and ideas through symbols in the form of spoken or written words. Speech disorders are mainly of two types:

Nervous System

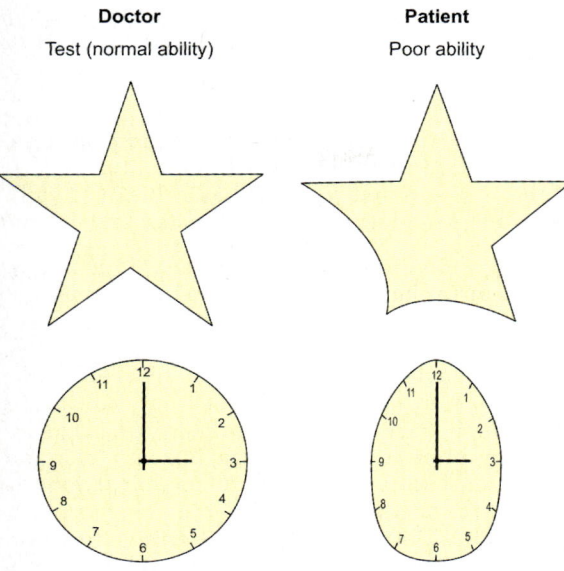

Fig. 5.9: Constructional apraxia.

1. *Disorders of articulation (dysarthria) and phonation (dysphonia)*. These are disorders of peripheral nervous system involving the organs (i.e. lips, tongue, palate, mouth, etc.) taking part in articulation and phonation.
2. *Disorders of the structure and language (dysphasia)*. These are disorders of CNS. The language areas are situated in the dominant hemisphere. The dominance of hemisphere is decided by handedness of a person. In the vast majority of right-handed persons the left hemisphere is dominant. About a third of left-handers have a dominant right hemisphere; the others have either left-sided or bilateral language representation. The main language areas and their association fibres are:
   a. **Broca's area** (*motor speech area*): It is situated in the inferior frontal gyrus of the dominant hemisphere. It is concerned with generation of spoken speech. The motor commands generated in the Broca's area reach the lips, tongue, palate, pharynx, larynx and respiratory muscles via the facial nerve and cranial nerves 9th, 10th and 12th. It co-ordinates the movements of lips, tongue, mouth and larynx to produce words (spoken speech).
   b. **Wernicke's area**: In right-handed person. It lies in the temporal lobe and the adjoining parietal region and is concerned with the understanding of spoken speech and comprehension of language and the selection of words to convey meaning. The visual speech area (Wernicke's area) represents the reception or understanding of written speech. It is situated in temporal lobe. A special area (centre for writing) is situated in frontal lobe (cortical area for movement of fingers and hand).

The mechanism of speech: The Broca's and Wernicke's areas are connected by an arcuate fasciculus. The language information generated in the Wernicke's area to the spoken speech is passed anteriorly via the arcute fasciculus to Broca's area for motor commands.

From the Broca's area, the motor commands pass to parts concerned with articulation and phonation (e.g. lips, tongue, pharynx, palate, larynx and respiratory muscles) via the cranial nerves 7th, 9th, 10th and 12th for production of sounds known as spoken speech.

The decoding of spoken speech, expression of ideas and concepts (speech comprehension) is the function of Wernicke's area. Injury to this area leads to auditory sensory aphasia, word deafness or difficulty in comprehension of spoken speech.

DISORDERS OF SPEECH

1. Disorders of language called *aphasia/dysphasia*
2. Disorders of articulation called *dysarthria*
3. Disorders of phonation called *dysphonia*

Dysphasia or Aphasia

Dysphasia or aphasia is a disorder of language content of speech. It can occur with lesions over a wide area of the dominant hemisphere. The term *dysphasia* is defined as loss or impairment of spoken language Dysphasia is detected by the patient's inability to produce the correct word (*anomia*) at appropriate time. When a patient is asked to name objects or parts of objects, if *dysphasia* is present either no word will be produced or the wrong word or a nonsense word will be produced (*paraphasia*). Aphasia means complete abolition of speech.

Types of Aphasia

1. **Broca's (anterior) aphasia:** The characteristics are:
   1. Nonfluent aphasia in which speech is just hesitant with reduced verbal output.
   2. Word comprehension is intact
   Site of lesion is in Broca's area (frontal gyrus)
   Causes include CVA, head injuries and brain tumour/space occupying lesion.
2. **Wernicke's (posterior) aphasia**
   - Fluent, rapid and effortless speech.
   - Articulation is good

- Word and reading comprehension is impaired. Sentences/words are malformed (paraphasias) or invented (neologisms).
  Site of the lesion. Wernicke's area (temporal gyrus). **Causes** include CVA, head injury and brain tumour.
3. **Conduction dysphasia** is produced by lesions involving the association fibres (*arcuate fasciculus*) between Broca's and Wernicke's areas. In this disorder, the patient is unable to repeat phrases or chords spoken by the examiner. Speech is nonsense with neologisms. Comprehension is normal.
4. **Global aphasia:** Patients with large lesions in middle cerebral artery territory over which speech areas are situated or there are elements of both anterior (Broca) and posterior (Wernicke) dysphasias are said to have "*global aphasia*". Such patients have impaired flow of language production, i.e. nonfluent speech with impared comprehension. It is often associated with hemiplegia, hemianaesthesia and visual defects.

☞ *Examination sequence for speech testing*

Spoken speech is assessed by *fluency* (rate, flow and the content of speech and use of words) during conversations. The area of fluency of speech lies posterior to central fissure. The *nonfluent aphasia* means verbal output is reduced. The lesion lies anterior to central sulcus. **Paraphasias** means the words are either malformed ("*I write with a den*"), wrong or inappropriate ("*I write with a bar*"), or invented ("*I write with a dar*"). If the patient speech lacks fluency, proceed with further testing as outlined in Table 5.9.

Alexia and dyslexia. Alexia is defined as the loss or impairment of the ability to read. It is an acquired speech defect. Dyslexia is a developmental abnormality in which person is unable to learn to read.

In temporoparietal alexia due to lesion in the left dominant hemisphere (temporoparietal region) there is alexia (disturbance in reading) and agraphia. Patient may produce some letters or their combinations which do not have meaning. The patient may be considered as illiterate for written and printed language symbols. The associated features include (i) right hemiparesis, right sensory loss, right homonymous hemianopia, etc.

Grestman syndrome (involvement of watershed area) with right/left disorientation, finger agnosia, agraphia and acalculia is present.

Occipital alexia. In this type of alexia, there is inability to read but writing ability is present. It is called *alexia without agraphia*. Right homonymous hemianopia is present in most of the cases. The lesion lies in the occipital lobe (posterior cerebral artery lesion).

Frontal alexia. In this type, patient can read some words but cannot name or spell individual letters. There is associated motor aphasia (Broca's), right hemphegia and sensory loss and visual field defects.

Nominal aphasia (anomic aphasia). It is a non-localising aphasia, occurs due to involvement of either hemisphere. The characteristic feature is word finding difficulty (read Table 5.9). These patients have associated findings of hemiplegia, hemianaesthesia, visual field defect. The *causes* include; SAH, raised intracranial pressure, concussion (brain trauma), encephalitis and toxic and metabolic encephalopathies. The nominal aphasia may be the only residual deficit following recovery from aphasia of any origin.

Aphemia. It is aphasia of acute onset in which patient is mute initially but able to express his/her ideas in

TABLE 5.9: Testing for Aphasia

Word comprehension	Ask the patient to follow a one-stage command, such as "point to your nose". Try a two-stage command "Point to your mouth, then your knee"
Repetition of words This tests the integrity of arcuate fibres	Ask the patient to repeat a phrase of one syllable words i.e. "Today is Tuesday". Repetition failure occurs in conduction aphasia
Naming an object. Anomia is difficulty in finding words. Anomic aphasia is seen in SAH, raised ICP, encephalitis, toxic and metabolic encephalopathies	Ask the patient to name a shown object, e.g. a comb or pen. The test can be made difficult by asking the patient to name the components of a watch. Inability to name is called *anomic aphasia*
Reading comprehension (read alexia and dyslexia)	Ask the patient to read a paragraph loudly. This may reveal an associated dyslexia
Writing This tests the centre for writing situated in cortical area meant for movements of hands and fingers	Ask the patient to write a sentence. This cannot be assessed if the patient has a motor deficit of writing hand. Errors of form, grammar and sentence indicate *dysphasia*. A person who can write a correct sentence does not have *aphasia*.

writing. With return of verbalisation, the speech ouput is slow and hypophonic. Patient is able to comprehend spoken speech. Right hemiplegia is often present. Patient has difficulty in performing on command such acts as whistling, coughing, blowing, sucking, etc, but there is no difficulty in performing limb activities such as making a fist, waving good bye, etc.

Apraxia. The term *'apraxia'* means inability to perform certain acts or movements when asked to do so. Before testing apraxia, make sure that there is no sensory or motor deficit or ataxia. This can be tested by asking the patient to use objects to make or initiate certain movements. For instance, when given a pen and asked to write with it, the aparaxic patient may fail to open the pen or to write with it or may show an inability to recognise the end to be used for writing. It is important to be sure that patient understands the command.

Apraxia results from damage to either the dominant hemisphere (left parietal cortex) or to both hemispheres, or association fibres through the corpus callosum. When corpus callosum is involved, apraxia is limited to left side or both sides.

Agnosia. It is failure to recognise sensory imposition in the absence of any sensory impairment. It may be visual agnosia, i.e. failure to recognise an object by the patient on visual presentation but he/she recognises it easily and even name it, if allowed to feel or hear the sound of the object.

Auditory agnosia means unable to recognise non-verbal sound even though these can be heard such as whistling, dog barking, etc. It suggests right temporal lobe involvement. Amnesia is frequently present.

Dysarthria

If *dysarthria* is suspected ask the patient to repeat a phrase which requires precise articulation, e.g. *British Constitution*. The causes of dysarthria and their characteristics are given in Table 5.10.

Dysarthria may be caused by mechanical factors such as ill-fitted dentures, but invariably occurs due to weakness or impaired co-ordination of the muscles of speech (orolingual muscles).

Dysarthric speech is indistinct and difficult for listener to understand. However, in dysarthria, the grammatical construction of speech is normal and the patient's comprehension of spoken speech and written language is preserved. Normally elevation of soft palate is used to close off the nasopharynx for production of explosive consonants gutturals (k and g). Weakness of palate (bulbar palsy) or anatomical defects in palate (X nerve lesion) cause 'nasal' speech with failure to produce the nasal gutturals consonants correctly. For example, such a patient will pronounce *'egg'* as *'eng'*. Paralysis of tongue (XII nerve lesion) produces lingual dysarthria in which there is difficulty in pronouncing lingual guttarls, i.e. t, s, d. In facial palsy, there is *labial dysarthria* with difficulty in pronouncing b, p, m, etc.

TABLE 5.10: Types of Dysarthria and their Characteristics

Type	Mechanism	Characteristic
Myopathic type	Weakness of muscles of face and tongue	Indistinct speech with poor articulation
Myasthenic type	Motor end plate involvement leading to LMN type of weakness	Indistinct speech with fatigue and dysphonia, fluctuating severity. This can be tested by asking the patient to count up to 50; speech becomes indistinct due to fatigue after sometime
Bulbar (flaccid) paralysis	Lower motor neuron lesion of brain stem	Indistinct, slurred, often nasal speech. Ask the patient to speak *"egg"*, he/she will pronounce it as *"eng"*
Scanning or staccato speech	Cerebellum	Slurring, impaired timing and cadence, sing-song quality of speech. This can be tested by asking the patient to say "artillery"; it will be pronounced as "ar-til-ler-y" meaning thereby each word is scanned. Staccato speech is explosive with slurring of words
Spastic dysarthria	Bilateral pyramidal tracts above the pons (pseudobulbar palsy, hemiplegia)	Indistinct, slurred, imprecise pronunciation, breathy, mumbling speech. This can be tested by asking the patient to pronounce "British Constitution; it will be pronounced as "Brizf Conshishushon"
Parkinsonism	Basal ganglia	Indistinct, rapid, stammering, quiet speech
Hyperkinetic dysarthria	Chorea	Rapid output with articulation

Dysphonia

It is defined as disturbed phonation. The production of tones in speech is achieved by movements of expired air through the larynx. Vibrations of the vocal cords generate frequency changes used in speech and singing. Poor vocal cord movements and poor respiratory function may cause dysphonia, characteristically seen in laryngeal involvement such as recurrent laryngeal nerve palsy or laryngitis.

- Vocal cord paralysis (unilateral) produces hoarse, low-pitched and rasping voice.
- In paralysis of respiratory muscles (GB syndrome, polio) patient does not speak loud, talks in whispers.

OTHER SPEECH DISORDERS

Agraphia: Spelling and grammar are impaired in written language.
Echolalia: Spoken words by someone is repeated without meaning. It is seen in temporoparietal lesion (Alzheimer's disease).
Palilalia: Involuntary repetitions of same words and phrases.
Lalling speech (baby speech). Patient speaks in 'baby fashion' with a dropping out of difficult consonant. It is inborn inability to understand the meaning of sounds.

EXAMINATION OF CRANIAL NERVES

THE OLFACTORY (FIRST) CRANIAL NERVE

It is concerned with sense of *smell*. It carries sensory fibres from the nose and reach the olfactory bulb through the cribriform plates. Sensory fibres from the nose are subsequently relayed in the olfactory area of the cerebral cortex, the uncus and parahippocampal gyrus (temporal lobe). Thus, in temporal lobe epilepsy (uncinate fits), hallucinations of smell constitute an *aura*.

> Olfactory hallucinations are characteristic of temporal lobe epilepsy, are often associated with involuntary smacking movements of lips and unusual feelings in the epigastrium.

☞ *Testing for the sense of smell* (Fig. 5.10)
- First of all, make sure that nasal passages are clear and patient is not having cold.
- Each nostril is to be tested separately.
- Occlude each nostril by gentle/finger pressure.
- Ask the patient with eyes closed to sniff and identify the odour of each test substance placed before each nostril.

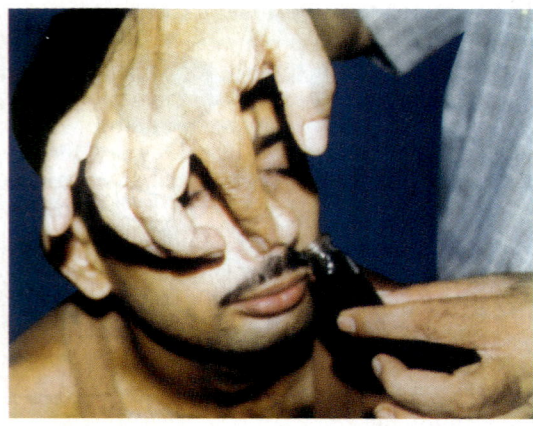

Fig. 5.10: Testing for the sense of smell.

- The test substances include vials of peppermint, vanila, coffee, almond oil. Common bedside substances such as soap, fruit or scent can be used.

A normal person perceives odour on each side, and can identify it.

Disorders of Smell

Anosmia: Anosmia refers to loss of sense of smell, while hyposmia means diminished sense of smell, can occur normally due to obstruction of nasal passage (e.g. catarrh), hence, must be excluded before labelling.

The **causes** of anosmia are:
- Smoking, ageing and use of cocaine.
- Local trauma or head injury causing damage to cribriform plate and the olfactory tract
- Nasopharyngeal tumour and meningioma of olfactory nerve.
- Carcinoma of paranasal air sinus.
- *Kallmann's syndrome* (hypogonadotrophic hypogonadism).

Parosmia refers to perversion/alteration of sense of smell, i.e. pleasant odours seem offensive. It is sometimes of psychological origin but may occur following partial recovery of olfactory nerve from trauma. Certain drugs and sinus infection can also cause it.

Hallucination of smell. They occur due to irritative lesion of olfactory apparatus and constitute an aura of temporal lobe epilepsy (uncinate fits).

THE OPTIC (SECOND) CRANIAL NERVE

Anatomy of Visual Pathways

Each optic nerve arises as axons of retinal cells, at the back of eye and passes through the optic canal

Nervous System

of the sphenoid bone to meet the opposite optic nerve to form *optic chiasma*. In the optic chiasma, the fibres from the medial half (nasal half) of each retina representing the temporal field cross; while those from the lateral (outer) half representing the nasal field remain on the same side. In this way, an *optic tract* consisting of fibres from outer half of the retina on the same side and inner half of the retina of opposite side is formed. Each optic tract then relays into the *lateral geniculate bodies* of the same side. Now *optic radiation* starts from the lateral geniculate bodies and reach the ipsilateral thalamus, now passes through the posterior limb of the internal capsule and relay *in visual cortex (calcarine cortex)* in the occipital lobe. The fibres representing the upper visual fields fan out through the temporal lobe; whilst those representing the lower field fan out through the parietal lobe. In this way, the left half of the field of vision is represented in the cortex of right hemisphere and *vice versa* (Fig. 5.11).

Visual Field Defects (Table 5.11)

Homonymous field defect means involvement of same part of visual field in both the eyes. The lesion lies distal to optic chiasma.

Hemianopia means one half of the visual field is lost. It may be *homonymous hemianopia* (lesion in optic tract), *bitemporal hemianopia* (lesion in optic chiasma) or *quadrantic hemianopia* in which one quadrant of visual field is lost (upper quadrantanopia in temporal lobe lesion and lower quadrantanopia in parietal lobe lesion are shown in Table 5.11).

Incongruous type of field defect means visual field defects are not identical in both eyes, occurs in lesion of the optic tract.

Macular sparing means sparing of ocular vision in homonymous hemianopia due to occipital lobe.

Visual sensory inattention. When sensory inattention is present, the patient will be able to detect single stimulus on both sides but will ignore stimulus when two fields are stimulated simultaneously on one side.

Testing of Second Nerve

The visual acuity and visual fields must always be tested. Other aspects of visual perception inclu-ding *colour vision, visual localisation* and *visual recognition* may also be tested if appropriate. It is hereby stressed that while testing the second nerve for vision, any refractory error if present must be corrected and there should not be any evidence of an ocular disease that might impair vision. Each eye must be separately.

- Visual acuity
- Colour vision
- Field of vision

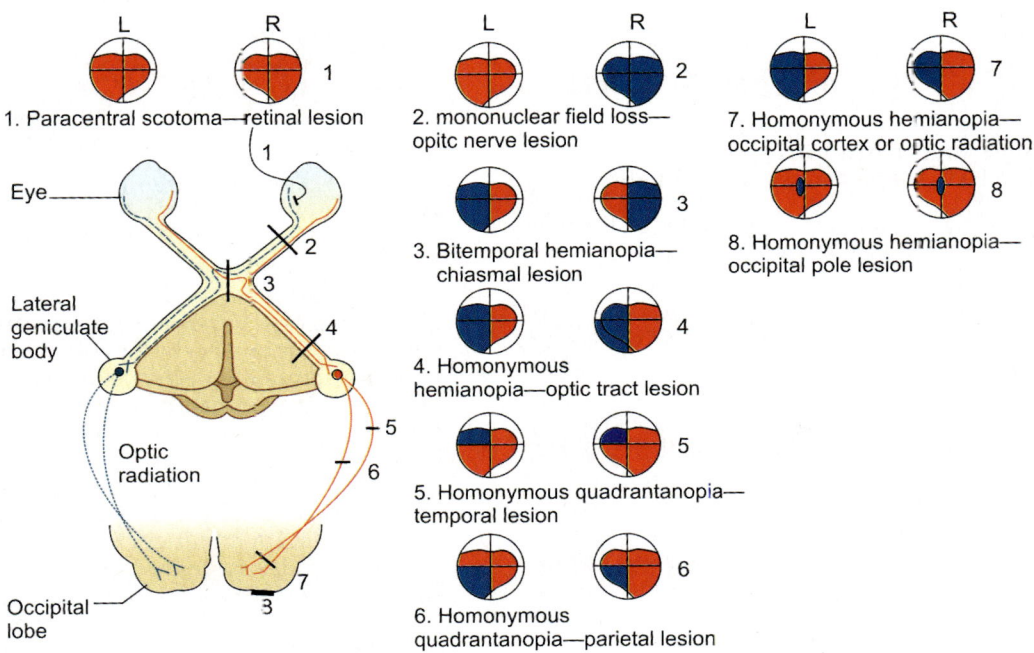

Fig. 5.11: The visual pathway and various sites of lesions (*see* Table 5.11, 1 to 8).

TABLE 5.11: Clinical Manifestations of Visual Field Defects

Site	Causes	Symptoms	Visual field loss	Associated physical signs
Optic disc, retinal lesion (1)	• Vascular disease vasculitis) • Glaucoma • Inflammation	• Partial or complete loss of vision depending on site	• Altitudinal field defect • Arcuate or paracentral scotoma	• Reduced acuity • Visual distortion • Abnormal retinal appearance
Optic nerve (2)	• Optic neuritis • Sarcoidosis • Tumour • Leber's optic atrophy	• Partial or complete visual loss in one eye • Often painful eye • Central vision particularly affected	• Central scotoma • Paracentral scotoma • Uniocular blindness • Optic atrophy may be seen	• Reduced acuity • Reduced colour vision • Loss of direct light reflex
Optic chiasma (3)	• Pituitary tumours • Craniopharyngioma • Sarcoidosis	• May be none • Rarely diplopia	• Bitemporal hemianopia	• Pituitary function abnormalities
Optic tract (4)	• Tumour • Inflammatory disease	• Disturbed vision to one side of midline	• Incongruous contralateral homonymous hemianopia	
Temporal lobe (5)	• Stroke • Tumour • Inflammatory disease	• Disturbed vision to one side of midline	• Contralateral homonymous upper quadrantanopia	• Memory/language defect
Parietal lobe (6)	• Stroke • Tumour • Inflammatory disease	• Disturbed vision to one side of midline. Bumping into things	• Contralateral homonymous lower quadrantanopia	• Contralateral sensory disturbance • Optokinetic nystagmus
Occipital lobe (7) (optic radiation)	• Stroke • Tumour • Inflammatory disease	• Disturbed vision to one side of midline. Bumping into things • Reading difficulty	• Homonymous hemianopia with macular sparing	• Damage to other structures supplied by posterior cerebral circulation
Occipital pole (8)	-do-	-do-	• Homonymous hemianopia with macular sparing	-do-

- Pupillary reflexes (read examination of eye in the General Physical Examination of this unit).

A. Testing for Acquity of Vison. It is tested for each eye separately for distant and near vision

I. For near vision
1. *Perception of light.* This method is used when visual activity is markedly reduced to perception of light only. This is tested by the light from a torch which is turned on and off intermittently and patient is asked to perceive it. Each eye is tested separately by covering the other eye.
2. *Finger counting and hand movements.* Different numbers of fingers are brought before patient's eye at varying distance and patient is asked to count them. Hand movement method is used when patient is not able to count the fingers placed before each eye, but can perceive hand movements in front of eyes.

II. Distant vision
3. *Jaeger test chart.* It is used for testing near vision. The chart is held about 14 inches from the eyes.
4. *Snellen's test chart.* It is used for minor dearrangements of visual acquity. The chart is placed 6 meters away on level with the eyes of the patient. The number by the side of each line indicates the numbers of feet/meters at which the letters can be read by one with normal vision. The acquity of vision is expressed as a fraction, the numerator corresponding to the distance at which smallest row of letters read by the patient should be read by normal eye. For example, if patient eye sight is normal called 6/6 which means he/she will read the smallest letters at 6 meters distance. Similarly with marked diminution of vison, patient will read the row of letters at 6 meters distance which a normal person can read at 60 meters distance called 6/60 vision.

Abnormal Visual Acquity

1. **Amblyopia** means defective visual acquity in both eyes. It is caused by *drugs, toxins (tobacco, alcohol), diabetes, uraemia, migraine* and lesion of *visual cortex*.
2. **Amaurosis.** It means complete blindness. It may be gradual (*optic atrophy, glaucoma*) or rapid onset (*retinal detachment, occlusion of central artery or vein of retina, vitreous haemorrhage, toxins-induced, migraine, uraemia,* etc.)
3. **Night blindness** called *nyctalopia* is due to Vit A *deficiency, retinitis pigmentosa* and *quinine poisoning toxicity*.
4. **Hemeralopia**—it means day blindness, is due to fatigue and pupillary constriction. It is common symptom of alcoholism and tobacco smoking.
5. **Teichopsias** (distorted figures). The figures appear distorted, i.e. smaller or large; zigzag or glittering in ophthalmoplegic migraine.

B. Testing for Colour Vison

Colour Vision is tested for colour blindness. Specially coloured cards, *skins of wool (Halmgren's wool)* or a series of designated colour plates. *Ishihara's test plates* are used to test colour blindness. Most common congenital colour blindness is *red-green blindness*. Colour vision is affected in the *lesions of cortex* as well as in *hysteria*.

C. Testing for the Field of Vision:
The visual field means the extent of the vision when we look at an object. The extent of field of vision varies as follows:
1. Larger the stimulus used the larger is the field of vision and *vice versa*.
2. Bright illuminated objects have larger field than dim object.
3. Moving objects used for field of vision are better than stationary objects.

Confrontation method: The visual field can be assessed by many methods but the simplest and the best confrontation method (hand movements and finger counting test, Fig. 5.12).

This method tests the field of vision of the patient with that of examiner, hence the field of vision of the examiner should be normal. Both eyes are tested together for binocular vision and test each eye separately for monocular vision so as to exclude a field defect involving a part of the visual field of one eye only. A moving finger or an object is brought from the periphery towards centre.

Method (Fig. 5.12)
- Sit in front of the patient at one metre distance.
- To test the right eye of the patient, ask him/her to cover his/her left eye with the left hand, and look steadily at your left eye.

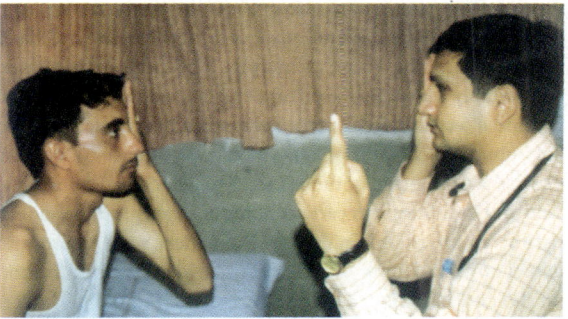

Fig. 5.12: Testing of visual field (cor frontation methods).

- Cover your right eye with your right hand and look steadily at patient's right eye.
- Hold your left hand to your left side at an arm's length in a plane midway between patient and yourself.
- Bring moving index finger of left hand from periphery to the centre until you yourself can see its movements. Now ask the patient whether he/she also sees the movements, making sure that patient is steadily fixing the gaze on your eye.
- If the patient is unable to see the finger, keep bringing it nearer and nearer until he/she does see it.
- Test the field in this way in all the directions, i.e. upwards, downwards and sidewards (right and left) using the extent of your own field as a reference for comparison.
- Map out peripheral fields in every direction roughly. This gives a rough estimate of the field of vision.

Screening visual fields for major field defect.
Hold both hands at shoulder width apart about one meter in front of the patient with three fingers raised on one hand and two on the other hand. Now ask how many fingers are up; if answer is five then screeing test is passed. An answer of three or two indicates that one or other field is missing. Now use red pin method discussed below for all field of vision.

Red pin test: This outlines the central field. This test can be performed by using a red pin instead of finger held up in the field of vision of the patient in the same manner as described above. A central scotoma (central area of impaired vision) can be recognised by this method because the red or white pinhead cannot be perceived in the area of impaired vision (scotoma).

The Normal and Abnormal Field of Vision
1. The normal binocular visual field extends 160° horizontally and 130° vertically with a blind spot 15° from fixation in the temporal field.

2. The *physiological blind spot* (a scotoma) is situated on the temporal side of the central point of the visual field. It is the point of entry of optic nerve into the retina (*optic disc*) situated slightly to nasal side of the macula when seen with ophthalmoscope. The *blind spot* sometimes may not be visible in an uncooperative patient or if the patient is attempting to mislead the examiner.
3. *Visual field defects*. They are central or peripheral. Peripheral constrictions of visual field is seen in optic atrophy, hysteria, bilateral involvement of visual centre and retinal disease. Concentric constricted field of vision occurs in glaucoma, papilloedema. A *scotoma* is a localised field defect surrounded by a seeing area. The patient notices a 'hole' in his vision. The scotoma may be central, peripheral, unilateral, bilateral, positive or negative.
   - Central scotomas involve fixation, occurs due to involvement of macula or optic nerve lesion or poisons (tobacco, alcohol) or visual cortex lesion.
4. *Positive and negative scotomas*: The term *positive scotoma* is used when the patient sees a dark spot in visual field which does not correspond to any real object outside the eye. The *negative scotoma* (scotoma proper) referes to an abnormal blind area/defect in the visual field in which patient is unable to see an external object.
   - **Ring scotomos** are characteristics of retinitis pigmentosa (*Laurence-Moon-Biedl syndrome*)
   - **Arcuate scotomos** are diagnostic of glaucoma.
   - **Tubular vision** is seen in multiple sclerosis optic neuropathy (toxic, ischaemic), retinal haemorrhage/infarct
   - **Altitudinal defect** (defect confined to upper or lower half of field of vision) occurs in optic neuropathy and retinal infarct.

Causes of Visual Field Defects

The causes of visual field defects include; glaucoma, retinitis pigmentosa, the age related macular disease, cerebrovascular disease, carotid vascular disease, brain tumours and trauma.

Perimetery (Recording the Field of Vision)

It means mapping out of field of vision by perimeter as a permanent record. The patient is seated comfortably with chin placed on a chin rest adjusted in such a way that the eye to be tested is oriented at the centre of hemispherical, lighted field upon which spots of lights of varying intensities, colours or sizes are projected or moved so as to detect the limits of the field and its intensity in various parts.

Perimetery charts out the limits of perception, hence, surveys the monocular field of vision. The central point on the chart corresponds to the point of fixation (Fig. 5.13). Around this point are arranged a series of more or less concentric lines each of which denotes equal visual acquity—an isopor.

Since the fixation point is not exactly central, hence the outer and inner fields are unequal. With an object of 5 mm diameter, the extent of average field of vision is 100° laterally, 60° superiorly and medially and 75° inferiorly. The field chart is depicted in Fig. 5.13.

The visual pathways and their field defects have already been depicted in Fig. 5.11.

Fundoscopy

Read the fundus examination in the general physical examination of eye in this unit.

THE OCULOMOTOR (III), THE TROCHLEAR (IV) AND THE ABDUCENS (VI) CRANIAL NERVES

The 3rd, 4th and 6th cranial nerves are called motor nerves for eye movements and also control the size of the pupils.

THE THIRD (OCULOMOTOR) NERVE

The oculomotor (III) nerve nucleus lies in the midbrain near the preaqueductal gray matter. The nerve passes between the cerebral penduncles, then comes closer to posterior communicating artery and enters the cavernous sinus. Further It enters the orbital fossa through the *superior oblique fissure* where it subdivides into its terminal branches to

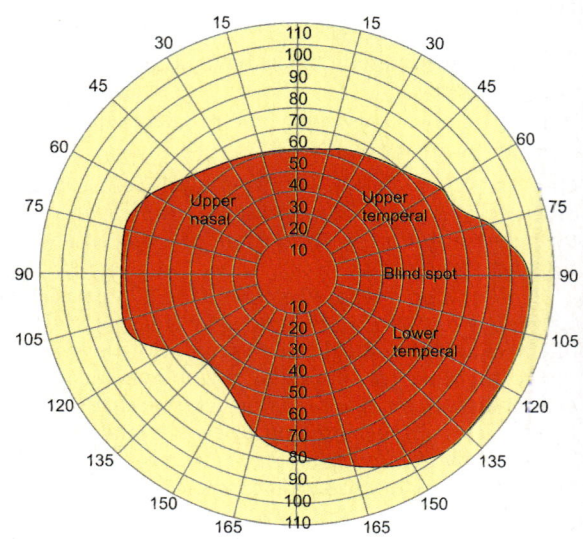

Fig. 5.13: The normal right field of vision using a white object of 5 mm diameter. The field is mapped out on a perimeter at a distance of 330 mm. Note the restriction of lower nasal field by the bridge of nose.

innervate the *superior rectus* (SR), *medial rectus* (MR), *inferior rectus* (IR), *the inferior oblique* (IO) and *levator palpebral superioris muscles* (LPS). These muscles open the upper lid (LPS), move the eyeball upwards (SR, IO), downwards (IR) and medially (MR).

The parasympathetic fibres of the 3rd nerve arise from the *Edinger-Westphal nucleus* and supply the sphincter muscles of the iris which cause constriction of pupil, and the ciliary muscle, which is responsible for focussing the lens for near vision

It supplies all the eye muscles except *lateral rectus* and *superior oblique*.

THE FOURTH NERVE

The trochlear (4th) nerve arises from its nucleus in the mibrain. The fibres decussate before leaving the mibrain just below the inferior colliculus. The nerve passes forward and laterally in relation to the rostral pons. It comes out of the free edge of tentorium and enters the cavernous sinus and then pass forwards to superior oblique fissure to enter the eye where it innervates the superior oblique (SO) muscle, contraction of which causes downward movement of the eyeball when the eye is adducted.

It is motor nerve to superior oblique.

THE SIXTH NERVE

The abducens (6th) nerve originates from the nucleus situated in the midline of the pons. It hooks around the facial nerve nucleus and comes out between medulla and pons. It has a long intracranial course, hence, is liable to get compressed under the effect of raised intracranial pressure producing diplopia on lateral gaze. After exit from the pons, it enters the cavernous sinus and lies in direct relation to the internal carotid artery. Now it enters the eye through superior oblique fissure to supply the Lateral Rectus (LR) muscle, the contraction of which causes abduction of the eye.

It is motor nerve to lateral rectus.

☞ Testing of Ocular Movements

The six external ocular muscles move the eyeball in different directions (Fig. 5.14). The movements tested include *adduction, abduction, elevation, depression* and *rotation around an imaginary anteroposterior axis passing through centre of pupil.*

Method (Follow Movements)

- Inspect the eye for any abnormality.

Narrowing of the palpebral fissure occurs due to ptosis (3rd nerve palsy or Horner's syndrome) or due to local lid disorders.

Widening of fissures occur in Graves' disease or exophthalmos due to any cause.

- Hold the head of the patient in neutral position and test for ocular movements with both the eyes open.
- Look for squint and nystagmus.

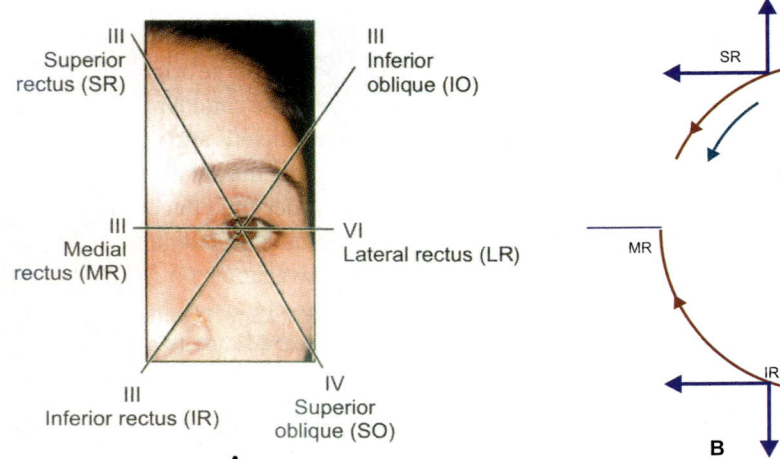

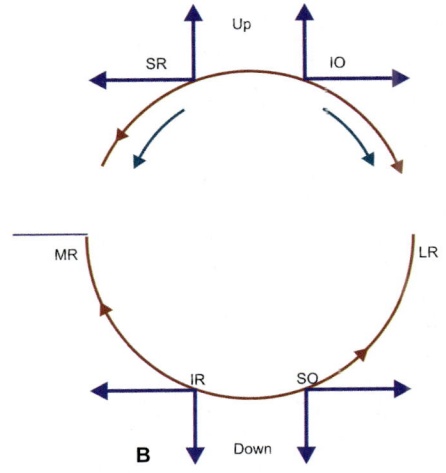

Figs 5.14A and B: Functions of external ocular muscles (left eye). The superior rectus and inferior rectus act as elevator and depressor alone respectively when eye is in abduction; and inferior oblique and superior oblique act in similar way when the eye is in adduction
- Superior rectus in addition to elevator is also adductor and internal rotator.
- Inferior rectus is depressor, adductor and external rotator.
- Superior oblique is a depressor abductor and internal rotator.
- Inferior oblique is an elevator, external rotator and abductor

- Test the movement by asking the patient to look up and down and to the right and left from the mid-position of gaze. Test the up and down movements in full adduction and in full abduction also.

The eyes normally move 50° medially, 30° upwards and 50° downwards.

- Now ask the patient to fix gaze on the examiner's finger and to report if double vision occurs while following the movement of the finger held at 60 cm away.

Diplopia indicates 3rd, 4th and 6th cranial nerve palsy (LMN lesion).

- Move the finger up and down, then to the right and up and down, and then to the left and up and down. If necessary, repeat the examination, one eye at a time to distinguish muscle paralysis and gaze paralysis.
- Record the direction of diplopia if present and where maximal separation of the images occurs.
- If diplopia is present, ask the patient to close one eye at a time to identify which eye is producing the false image.
- To test convergence, bring the finger from a distance towards the tip of the nose and ask the patient to focus on it.
- Look for nystagmus while testing the ocular movements.
- Record the direction of nystagmus (vertical, horizontal, rotatory) and the direction of gaze in which it is most marked.
- Note the direction of fast component of nystagmus, whether it changes direction with direction of gaze and whether the degree of nystagmus is different in each eye.

Common Abnormalities

1. Involuntary Deviation
- Conjugated deviation to one or the other side or upwards or downwards occurs in hemispherical lesion.
- In cerebral lesion, there may be *skew deviation* (one eye is directed upwards and other is directed downwards)

2. Exophthalmos (Proptosis).
It is defined as forward protrusion of one or both the eyes with the result a portion of white sclera is clearly visible above and below the cornea.

It can be unilateral or bilateral (common)

☞ *Methods of testing*

i. Stand in front of the patient and ask him/her to look straight forward. Observe the visibility of upper and lower sclera.

Both upper and lower sclera are clearly visible in moderate to severe proptosis (Fig. 5.15).

ii. Another method is to stand behind the patient. Tilt the patient's head backwards. Look vertically down the slanting forehead in

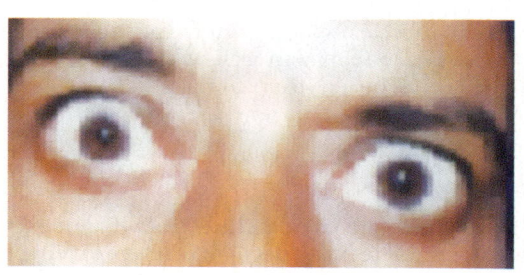

Fig. 5.15: Exophthalmos. Note the wide palpebral fissures and visibility of both upper and lower sclera with staring look.

the plane of superciliary ridges. Protrusion/visibility of the eye globe indicates proptosis.

iii. Hertel exophthalmometer—a handheld instrument is used to record it.

Causes: The causes of unilateral and bilateral exopthalmos are given in Table 5.12. Exophthalmos is a common sign of Graves' ophthalmopathy.

TABLE 5.12: Common Causes of Exophthalmos

Unilateral	Bilateral
1. Early thyrotoxicosis (i.e. eyes are not necessarily involved)	1. Thyrotoxicosis (Fig. 5.15).
2. Retrobular tumour (painless, progressive exophthalmos)	2. Superior vena cava syndrome (raised JVP, congestion, chemosis and proptosis)
3. Cavernous sinus thrombosis (Proptosis, chemosis, 3rd, 4th, 6th cranial nerves palsy)	3. Craniostenosis
4. Orbital pseudotumour (pain, limited eye movements and proptosis)	4. Bilateral cavernous sinus thrombosis
5. Orbital cellulitis (i.e. pain, lid erythema, proptosis and conjunctival chemosis.	5. Cushing's syndrome
6. Carotid cavernous fistula (i.e. proptosis, diplopia, glaucoma, redness of eye and a bruit may be heard on ausculation of head or orbit. It is called pulsating exophthalmos	

Consequences of exophthalmos

Exophthalmic ophthalmoplegia. It refers to weakness of extraocular muscles due to increase in interstitial fluid volume and increase in retrobulbar pressure.

Malignant exophthalmos. It is defined as progressive bulging of the eyeballs, conjunctival oedema, corneal ulceration and visual loss.

3. **Enophthalmos.** It refers to retraction of the eyeball within orbit.

   Causes: They include trauma, paralysis of cervial sympathetic (Horner's syndrome), following surgical removal of orbital contents, facial hemiatrophy (a cogenital abnormility)

4. **Ptosis.** Drooping of the upper eyelid is called *ptosis*.

   Types: It can be congenital or acquired, complete or partial (sight dropping of the lid), unilateral or bilateral. In complete ptosis, palpebral fissure is obliterated (Fig. 5.16).

   Causes: Congenital ptosis may be unilateral or bilateral, results from dysgenesis of the levator palpebral superioris or from its abnormal insertion into the lid. *Acquired ptosis* is unilateral in 3rd nerve palsy and Horner's syndrome but is usually bilateral in tabes dorsalis, myasthenia gravis, snakebite, periodic paralysis, etc. The common causes of ptosis are:

   I. Causes of unilateral ptosis
   - 3rd nerve palsy (Fig. 5.16).
   - Horner's syndrome (partial or pseudoptosis; Fig. 5.17).
   - Mechanical ptosis (enlargement or deformity of upper lid due to infection, trauma, swelling on it).

   II. Causes of bilateral ptosis
   - Tabes dorsalis.
   - Myasthenia gravis.
   - Chronic progressive external ophthalmoplegia (due to mutations of mitochondrial genes).
   - Myotonia dystrophica
   - Oculopharyngeal myopathy
   - Congenital (uncommon)
   - Snakebite
   - Botulism
   - Periodic paralysis
   - Senile ptosis (seen in old persons)

☞ *Testing for ptosis*
- Stand in front to the patient (face to face).
- Ask the patient to look upwards or elevate the upper eyelid voluntarily.

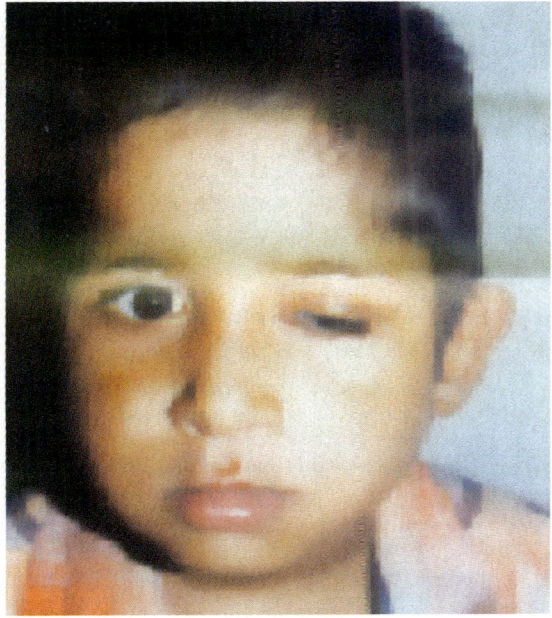

Fig. 5.16: Ptosis due to 3rd cranial nerve paralysis on left side (true ptosis).

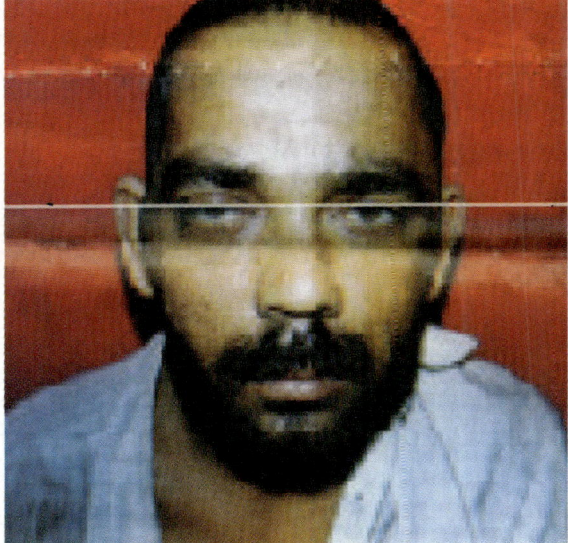

Fig. 5.17: Ptosis of right eye (Horner's syndrome).

In ptosis, patient cannot elevate the eyelid voluntarily but sometimes he elevates the lid by exerting the frontal belly of occipitofrontalis, therefore, to rule it out, now push down the frontal belly of occipitofrontalis by your left hand and ask the patient to look upwards. Now if he/she cannot do so, ptosis is present.

5. Pseudoptosis

It refers to partial drooping of the upper lid. It is seen in Horner's syndrome (Fig. 5.17). Eyelid can be lifted completely in pseudoptosis but not in true ptosis (Fig. 5.16).

The differences between ptosis (3rd nerve palsy) and pseudoptosis or partial ptosis due to sympathetic involvement (Horner's syndrome) are summarised in Table 5.13.

TABLE 5.13: Ptosis in 3rd Nerve Palsy and Horner's Syndrome

3rd cranial nerve palsy	Horner's syndrome
• Usually complete ptosis (palpebral fissure is obliterated)	• Partial or pseudoptosis (palpebral fissure is narrowed)
• Pupil dilated on involved side	• Pupil constricted
• Squint (paralytic, horizontal and vertical)	• No squint
• No enophthalmos	• Enophthalmos present
• Ciliospinal reflex present	• Ciliospinal reflex absent
• Extraocular muscle palsy present	• Extraocular muscles are normal but there is paralysis of Müller's muscles
• No loss of sweating on the side involved	• Anhidrosis (loss of sweating) on affected side present

DISORDERS OF OCULAR MOVEMENTS

Disordered eye movements occur due to involvement of extraocular muscles in ocular myopathies and diseases of myoneural junction (myasthenia gravis), metabolic encephalopathies and drug toxicity (toxicity of phenytoin and carbamazepine). The classification of disorders of ocular movements based on the type of neurological involvement, i.e. nuclear, infranuclear and supranuclear is given in Table 15.14 and causes of 3rd, 4th and 6th cranial nerves involvement are depicted in Table 5.15.

Third Nerve Palsy (Fig. 5.16)

It produces following
Signs on the side involved.
- Unilateral ptosis on the side involved.
- Dilated and fixed pupil.
- Squint (paralytic) and diplopia on lateral gaze.
- Paralysis of accommodation.
- Position of eyeball down and out due to squint.
- Paralysis of the eye movements due to weakness of muscles supplied by 3rd nerve.

TABLE 5.14: Classification of Disorders of Eye Movements based on the Site of Lesion

1. **Nuclear and infranuclear lesions (individual nerve paralysis)** they cause diplopia.
   - 3rd nerve palsy
   - 4th nerve palsy
   - 6th nerve palsy
2. **Supranuclear lesions (above the brain stem or cerebellum or basal ganglia)** cause gaze palsy, nystagmus.

A. *Conjugate gaze palsy*
   - Lateral gaze palsy
   - Upward gaze palsy
   - Downward gaze palsy
   - Internuclear gaze palsy

B. *Complex supranuclear gaze palsies*
   - Cerebellar diseases producing nystagmus.
   - Basal ganglia disorders producing pursuit movements

Causes: The common causes of an isolated 3rd nerve palsy include:
i. Diabetes.
ii. Posterior communicating artery aneurysm.
iii. Pituitary or other tumours.
iv. Trauma and vascular disease.

> **N.B.** Lesions due to diabetes or vascular disease tend not to involve the pupil, in contrast to compressive lesions (e.g. aneurysm).
>
> The **causes** of painful third nerve palsy include diabetes, intracranial aneurysm and ophthalmologic neuralgia.

Fourth (Trochlear) Nerve Palsy

It produces:
- *Impaired downwards movement.* On attempting to look downwards in mid-position of gaze the eyeball is rotated outwards by the unopposed action of inferior rectus.
- Diplopia is the main complaint particularly on looking down and during reading. There is rarely a visible squint. The patient will often adopt a compensatory head tilt away from the side of the lesion.

Causes: Isolated lesions of 4th nerve palsy are uncommon and include *diabetes, hypertension,* and *head trauma.* Damage to the nerve may occur in superior oblique tendon through which it passes following *head injury, ENT surgery* and in patients with *rheumatoid arthritis.*

Sixth (Abducens) Nerve Palsy (Fig. 5.18)

It produces:
- *Inability to move the eye outwards* (laterally) and diplopia (double vision) occurs on attempting to look laterally (Fig. 5.18).
- *Convergent squint* (eyeball is rotated medially) due to unopposed action of the medial rectus innervated by 3rd nerve.

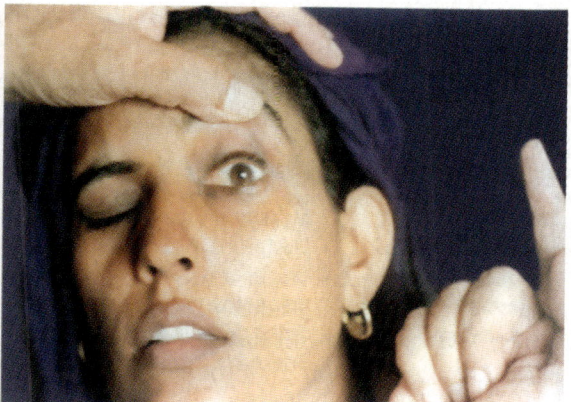

Fig. 5.18: Abducens nerve (VI CN) palsy on left side. Note that left eye cannot be abducted beyond midline.

Causes: Isolated 6th nerve palsy is common in *raised ICP* due to its long intracranial course (a false localising sign, i.e. the nerve is displaced or compressed without actual involvement). The common **causes** include, *head injury, diabetes, chronic SOM (Gradenigo's syndrome)*.

The 6th nerve palsy may be a false localising sign in raised intracranial pressure due to any cause.

As already discussed, in addition to isolated lesions, the 3rd, 4th and 6th cranial nerves may be involved in combinations (Table 5.15) and are usually associated with other features.

Supranuclear 3rd, 4th and 6th Nerves Lesions

Paralysis of supranuclear 3rd, 4th and 6th nerves palsy produces gaze paralysis.

A. **Conjugate gaze paralysis.** Normally the movements of the two eyes are symmetrical, called *conjugate ocular movements*. Supranuclear (upper motor neuron) lesions lead to paralysis of conjugate movement of the eyes. The causes of gaze palsy are given in Box 5.2.

B. **Other saccadic and pursuit gaze movements.** The saccadic (rapid, programmed conjugate fixation movements) and pursuit (following) gaze movements can be tested separately by

---

Box 5.2 Common Causes of Gaze Palsy

Gaze palsy	Causes
• Upwards and downwards gaze	• Space occupying lesions around the pineal gland and tectal region. • Aqueductal stenosis • Hydrocephalus
• Failure of upward gaze with loss of light reflex but preservation of accommodation reflex	• Steele-Richardson-Olzewski syndrome • Parinaud's syndrome (e.g. lesion of pineal gland or ventral midbrain)
• Lateral gaze	Lesions of frontal eye field (FEF) in pons. • Destructive lesions (haemorrhage) cause conjugate eye deviation towards the side of lesion (patient looks towards his lesion). • Irritative lesions (e.g. epileptic fit) cause deviation of eyes and head opposite to the side involved (healthy side)
• Internuclear ophthalmoplegia (Fig. 5.20)	• Lesion of the *medial longitudinal fasciculus (MLF)* in the midbrain or upper pons. On attempting lateral gaze, there is weakness of adducting eye and nystagmus of abducting eye. **Causes** include multiple sclerosis, vascular disorders and tumours of the brain stem
• One-and-half syndrome	A lesion involving the PPRF (parapontine reticular formation) and the MLF on the same side. There is failure of lateral conjugate deviation in one eye and adduction of the same eye on the side of the lesion. There is nystagmus on abduction (lateral movement) of the opposite eye. Thus, as the name indicates one eye will not move at all horizontally and the other eye move only in abduction, i.e. one-and-half movements are paralysed.

TABLE 5.15: The Site, Pathology and Associated Features of 3rd, 4th and 6th Nerves Palsy (External Ophthalmoplegia)

Site	Lesion/Cause	Nerve(s) involved	Associated features
Brain stem	Infarction (midbrain)	3rd (midbrain)—Weber's syndrome	Contralateral pyramidal signs
	Haemorrhage (pontine)	6th (ponto-medullary junction)	Ipsilateral lower motor neuron 7th palsy
	Demyelination (pons)	Millard-Gubler-Fovoulli syndrome	-do-
	Intrinsic tumour (brain stem)		Other brain stem/cerebellar signs
Intramenin-geal course	Meningitis (infective/malignant)	3rd, 4th and/or 6th	Signs of meningitis
	Raised intracranial pressure	3rd (uncal herniation)	Signs of raised ICT
	Aneurysms	3rd (posterior communicating artery)	Pain head and neck
		6th (basilar artery)	Features of subarachnoid haemorrhage
	Cerebellopontine angle tumour	6th	• 8th, 7th, 5th nerves involvement • Ipsilateral cerebellar signs
	Trauma	3rd, 4th and/or 6th	Other features of trauma
Cavernous sinus	Infection	3rd, 4th and/or 6th	May be 5th cranial nerve involvement also
	Thrombosis (Fig. 5.19)	3rd, 4th and/or 6th	Chemosis, conjunctival suffusion
	Carotid artery aneurysm Caroticocavernous fistula	3rd, 4th and/or 6th	Pupil may be fixed, mid-position (sympathetic plexus on carotid may also be affected)
Superior orbital fissure	Tumour (e.g. sphenoid wing meningioma), granuloma	3rd, 4th and/or 6th	May be proptosis, chemosis
Orbit	Vascular (e.g. diabetes, vasculitis) Infections Tumour Granuloma Trauma	3rd, 4th and/or 6th	Pain Pupil often spared in vascular 3rd nerve palsy

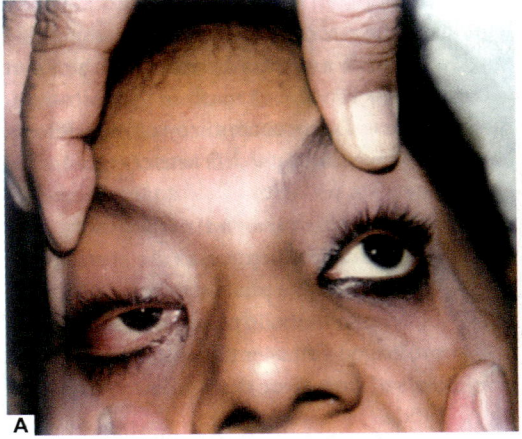 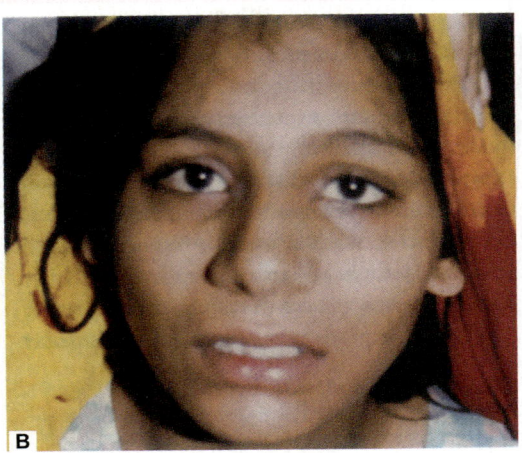

Figs 5.19A and B: Right cavernous sinus thrombosis in a postpartal female. (A) There is chemosis, lid oedema, conjunctival congestion and external ophthalmoplegia (immobile right eye) due to 3rd, 4th and 6th nerves palsy; (B) The same female patient after recovery.

asking the patient to move his/her eyes rapidly from fixation on one finger to another held about 30° away in horizontal plane and by asking him/her to follow a slowly moving finger across visual space in the same or in the vertical plane. In Huntington's chorea and Parkinsonism, pursuit movements are slowed or interrupted by slowed saccades.

C. Nystagmus: It has been discussed in the beginning.

D. Squint (strabismus): It has been discussed in the beginning.

Ophthalmoplegia

It is defined as loss or abnormality of ocular movements. It can be due to:

1. *Supranuclear palsies* of 3rd, 4th and 6th cranial nerves. It produces weakness or loss of conjugate movements.

2. *Internuclear ophthalmoplegia.* There is nystagmus and dissociated conjugate movements (read Box 5.2 and Fig. 5.20).

3. *Individual nerve palsy and ocular myopathies.* They produce diplopia, squint and defective ocular movements.

External ophthalmoplegia. It means paralysis of extraocular muscles due to involvement of 3rd, 4th and 6 nerves (nuclear and infranuclear involvement). The causes are listed in Table 5.15.

THE FIFTH (TRIGEMINAL) CRANIAL NERVE

The trigeminal nerve is a mixed nerve. It arises from the side of pons by two roots, i.e. **sensory** and **motor**.

The **sensory root** takes origin from the nerve cells in the *trigeminal ganglion (Gasserian ganglion)* and enters the side of the pons at its middle. The *principal*

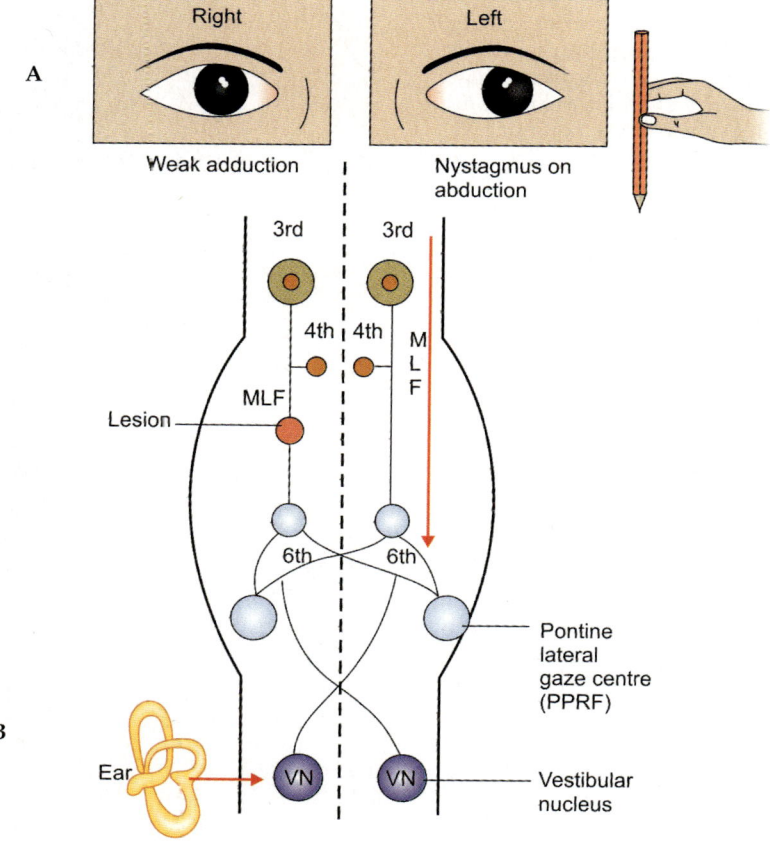

Figs 5.20A and B: Right internuclear ophthalmoplegia (diagrammatic illustration). (A) On attempted lateral gaze to the left produces weak adduction of right eye and left abducting eye shows nystagmus. Convergence to rear stimulus is preserved indicating that right eye can adduct normally and there is no paralysis of medical rectus. The lesion lies in right medial longitudinal fasciculus (MLF). A lesion in or near to the PPRF causes impaired conjugate lateral gaze to the same side. (B) Interconnection of 3rd, 4th and 6th cranial nerves with the PPRF via MLF.

sensory nucleus and the *motor nucleus* of the fifth nerve lie in the pons near the floor of the 4th ventricle; the sensory nucleus is lateral to motor and receives fibres for the sensations of touch, joint position sense and two-point discrimination sense. An another sensory nucleus (*bulbospinal nucleus or tract*) extends from the pons through the medulla to second cervical segment (C_2) of the spinal cord before ascending in the medial leminscus. This nucleus receives fibres for pain and thermal sensation. Owing to inversion of the fibres going through this nucleus, the upper part of the face is represented in the caudal part of nucleus (*upside—down representation*). The sensory root expands to form ganglion from which three divisions of Vth nerve (*ophthalmic, maxillary* and *mandibular*) arise.

The **motor root** arise from the *motor nucleus* in the pons and join the mandibular division to supply the muscles of mastication (*masseter* and *pterygoid muscles*).

The first (ophthalmic) division (V1) after arising from *Gasserian ganglion* passes through the cavernous sinus and superior orbital fissure, supplies sensations to the skin of upper nose and eyelid, forehead and scalp (Fig. 5.21) as well as the cornea, conjunctiva, lacrimal gland, parts of mucosa of the frontal, sphenoidal and ethmoidal sinuses and upper part of nasal cavity. The lesion of the ophthalmic branch results in loss of sensations from the areas described above. There is loss of corneal sensation and corneal reflex. Trophic changes in the cornea may develop called *neuropathic keratitis*.

The second (maxillary) division (V2) arising from the *Gasserian ganglion* comes out of the base of skull through foramen rotundum to supply the cheek, skin of temple, the side of nose, upper lip, mucous membrane of mouth, roof of pharynx, gums, teeth and palate of the upper jaw on same side. The lesion of this division leads to loss of sensations from the areas described above as well as loss of palatal reflex.

The third (mandibular) division (V3) after arising from the Gasserian ganglion comes out of the skull through foramen ovale and supplies sensations to teeth and gums of the lower jaw, mucosa of cheek, floor of the mouth, anterior two-thirds of the tongue, temporomandibular joint, external and internal ear, and the skin of lower lip and jaw on the same side. It supplies the parasympathetic fibres to the salivary glands through its lingual branch to chorda tympani of VII nerve.

The motor branch of the 5th nerve passes through the mandibular division (V3) and innervates muscles of mastication (the masseters, temporalis, medial and lateral pterygoids, the anterior belly of digastric) on same side. It also supplies the mylohoid, tensor palatini and tensor tympani muscles.

☞ **Testing of the 5th Nerve**

The Sensations

The sensations are tested in the usual way:
- Test light touch and pain by using wisp of cotton wool and pin-prick respectively. The temperature sensation can be tested by using test tube containing warm and cold water.
- Two-point discrimination on the upper and lower lips is tested by using calipers. Normally a separation of 3–4 mm can be detected.
- Test the sensations in each divisions of the nerve separately comparing both the sides, i.e. the right with the left.
- Look for trophic skin changes over the face.

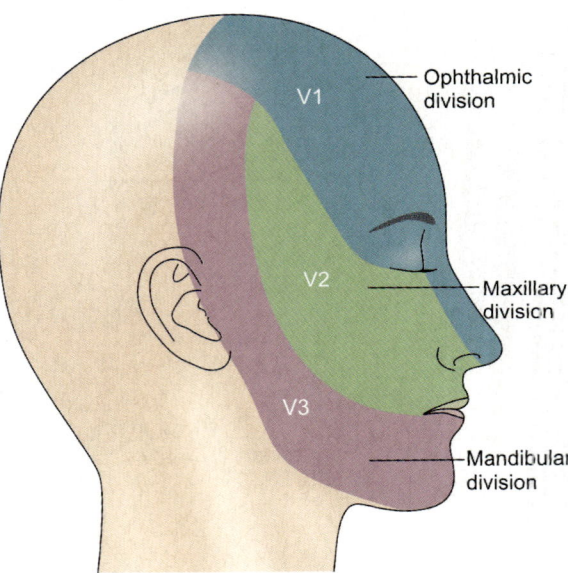

Fig. 5.21: Fifth cranial nerve. Three peripheral distribution of Vth nerve to the face.

☞ **Testing for the Motor Function**
- *Inspect the muscles of mastication* for wasting above zygomatic arch for temporalis and below for masseters.

The hollow above and below the zygomatic arch indicates paralysis of temporalis and masseters respectively.

- *Palpate the masseters* (Fig. 5.22A) and *temporalis* (Fig. 5.22B) for tone, bulk and symmetry as the patient clenches the teeth. There is hypotonia of these muscles in Vth nerve palsy.

Nervous System

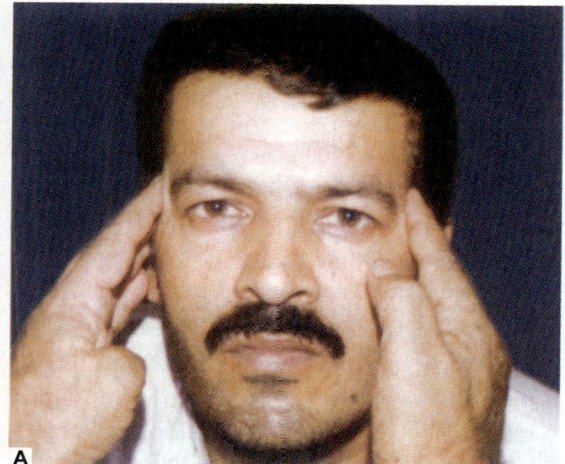

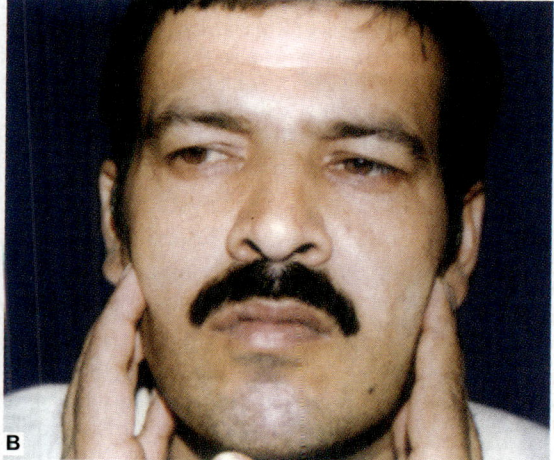

Figs 5.22A and B: Testing the motor part of Vth cranial nerve. (A) Palpation of both temporalis muscles for tone; (B) Palpation of both masseters for tone. Tone is tested during contraction of these muscles during clenching of teeth.

- Ask the patient to open the jaw against resistance (hand is placed below the jaw to resist opening). Difficulty in opening the jaw indicates weakness of pterygoids, mylohyoid and anterior belly of digastric.
- *Alternatively* patient may be asked to move the lower jaw against resistance from side to side. In Vth nerve palsy, there is diminished or absent movement of the jaw to the side opposite the paralysis.

In bilateral paralysis of the muscles of mastication, the lower jaw drops and active movements cannot be performed.

☞ **Testing the Reflexes**

1. Corneal Reflex (Fig. 5.23)
- Afferent is 5th nerve and the efferent is VII nerve.
- Make the patient to sit comfortably. Ask him to look at the ceiling or into the distance or to the opposite side.
- Twist a light wisp of cotton into a fine hair and lightly touch the lateral margin of the cornea.
- Observe the presence of direct and consensual corneal reflex. If the reflex is present, the patient blinks.

Touching of the cornea in a normal person produces brisk contraction of the orbicularis oculi (e.g. blinking). A unilateral stimulus produces bilateral reflex blinking, i.e. the direct and consensual responses due to bilateral innervation of the reflex through Vth nerve.

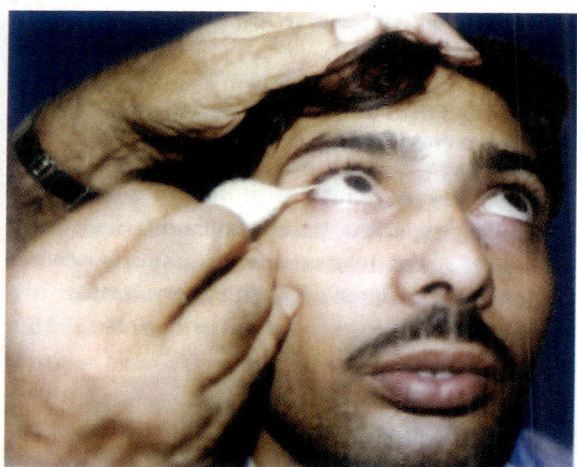

Fig. 5.23: A unilateral stimulus to cornea produces bilateral blinking.

2. The Jaw Jerk
The jaw jerk being a deep tendon jerk, is elicited by tapping the jaw with percussion hammer.
- Ask the patient to hold the half-open mouth.
- Put your left index finger over the lower jaw.
- Tap the finger with percussion hammer and observe for the closure of the jaw. This is often not elicitable in young persons.

The positive response means is brisk contraction of the jaw muscles producing closure of the jaw (normal response is either absent or minimal elicitable jaw jerk). Both afferent and efferent pathways are subserved by the Vth nerve. A brisk jaw jerk indicates bilateral UMN lesion above the level of pons (e.g. multiple sclerosis, motor neuron disease).

Causes of Vth Nerve Palsy (Table 5.16)

Common Abnormalities

The signs of trigeminal nerve lesion

i. Diminution of the corneal reflex may often be the first sign of a fifth nerve lesion.
ii. A complete fifth nerve lesion produces; following signs on the side involved.
   - Unilateral sensory loss on the face, tongue and buccal mucosa.
   - The jaw deviates to the side of the lesion when the mouth is opened due to unilateral pterygoid weakness. When patient tries to move the jaw from side to side there is difficulty in moving it to contralateral side.

TABLE 5.16: Causes of Trigeminal Nerve Palsy

1. **Brain stem (nuclear or infranuclear) lesion:**
   - Multiple sclerosis, glioma, stroke, syringobulbia
2. **Cerebellopontine angle lesion** (VII and VIII nerves also involved)
   - Acoustic neuroma, brain secondaries, meningioma
3. **Gasserian ganglion** lesions at petrous temporal bone
   - Trigeminal neuroma, herpes zoster and chronic SOM (Gradenigo's syndrome)
4. **Cavernous sinus lesion** in addition, the 3rd, 4th and 6th cranial nerves are also involved
   - Aneurysm of internal carotid artery
   - Extension of a pituitary neoplasm
   - Cavernous sinus thrombosis
5. **Peripheral nerve lesions**
   - Nasopharyngeal carcinoma
   - Trauma
   - Leprosy
   - Sarcoidosis
   - Guillain-Barré syndrome
   - Collagen vascular diseases
   - Idiopathic trigeminal neuropathy

Note: Facial asymmetry resulting from V nerve palsy may give rise to apparent deviation of jaw which is differentiated from 7th nerve lesion by preservation of side to side movement of the jaw.

iii. *Central (brain stem) lesion of the lower trigeminal nerve* nuclei produces a characteristic circumoral sensory loss with other signs of brain stem involvement.
iv. *When spinal nucleus of the Vth nerve alone is involved*, the sensory loss is limited to pain and temperature on the side of the face involved but touch is preserved (dissociated sensory loss).

TRIGEMINAL NEURALGIA (TIC DOULOUREUX)

It is common in middle aged and elderly:
Facial pain is the hallmark of the disease which occurs in bouts or paroxysms, is sharp or lancinating in character and radiates to territory of one or more sensory divisions of a trigeminal nerve or may be limited to a branch of a division such as infraorbital branch, etc. (*branch trigeminal neuralgia*). The pain disturbs routine activity, is triggered by touching, washing of face, brushing of teeth, shaving, cold breeze, eating, talking and application of lotions and cosmetics. Paroxysms of the pain are transitory and last for a few seconds. The disease runs a course of relapses and remissions which become less frequent as the disease advances.

The cause of the pain remains unknown. In some cases, an aberrant loop or artery may press the rootlets of trigeminal nerve as they emerge from the pons.

The second and third divisions are affected most followed by first: There is no sensory loss.

If there is sensory loss or motor symptoms or signs accompanying trigeminal neuralgia, then it is secondary to certain neurological diseases such as multiple sclerosis or meningoma of trigeminal nerve. The differential diagnosis of facial pain (trigeminal neuralgia) is discussed in Table 5.17.

THE SEVENTH (FACIAL) CRANIAL NERVE

The facial nerve is a *mixed nerve*:
- It innervates the muscles of face concerned with expression.
- It forms an efferent limb of corneal reflex (afferent being the Vth nerve) and also the palmomental reflex (primitive reflex), the nasopalpebral reflex (glabellar tap) and the efferent limb of stapedius reflex.
- It supplies secretory motor fibres (parasympathetic fibres) to the lacrimal glands (producing tears) and submandibular glands (producing saliva)
- It carries taste sensation from the anterior two-thirds of the tongue through the chorda tympani branch.

The *motor nucleus* of the 7th nerve lies in the pons, its fibres hook around the 6th nerve nucleus in the

Nervous System

pons, and then comes out of lateral pontomedullary junction, and joins the sensory nervus intermedius.

The *nervus intermedius* contains parasympathetic fibres (secretomotor) from the superior salivary nucleus and taste fibres which have their cell bodies in geniculate ganglion and synapse centrally with *nucleus solitarius* (*gustatory nucleus*). It comes out of pons along with 7th nerve, travels in between 7th and 8th nerves to internal auditory meatus. The facial nerve along with nervus intermedius pass through the facial canal of the temporal bone in the middle ear, emerges from the skull at stylomastoid foramen.

In the middle ear, it gives off a branch to the stapedius muscle (which dampens all tympanic vibrations, hence its involvement produces hyperacusis). After leaving the skull, the 7th nerve supplies fibres for the corneal reflex and the other reflexes. The scretomotor branch passes to the pterygopalatine ganglion and supplies the lacrimal gland through the greater petrosal nerve and tongue through the chorda tympani.

Causes of VIIth Nerve Palsy

Read the differential diagnosis depending on the cause of VII nerve involvement (Table 5.18).

Symptoms and Signs of Facial Nerve Palsy

These are summarised in Table 5.19.

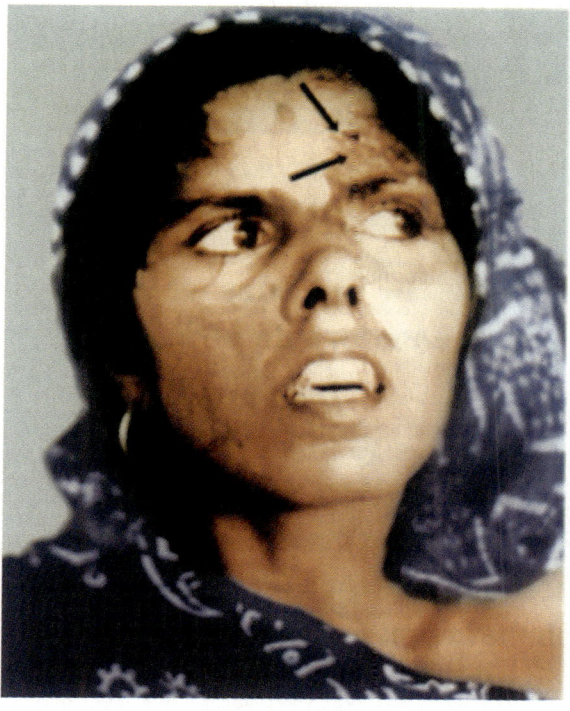

Fig. 5.24: Post-zoster neuralgia. Note the typical lesion (arrow) that was associated with severe pain.

TABLE 5.17: Differential Diagnosis of Trigeminal Neuralgia

Cause of facial pain	Characteristics
• Trigeminal neuralgia	• Already discussed
• Migrainous neuralgia (cluster headache)	• Unilateral bouts of pain around one eye, cheek or forehead. The pain is throbbing, severe, and disturbing, and may show nocturnal frequency. It is common in males of middle age • Lacrimation and nasal congestion, red conjunctiva on the affected side • The neuralgia occurs in clusters (repeated for a number of weeks, followed by a respite for a number of months before another cluster occurs)
• Atypical facial pain	• Dull, boring ache or pain over the face which is ill-defined and non-localised • May be unilateral or bilateral • Occurs either in too anxious or too depressed patients
• Temporomandibular arthritis (Costen's syndrome)	• Common in elderly females • Pain is severe, aching, gets intensified by chewing or movements of the jaw • Mostly unilateral and limited to temporomandibular joint. It is due to rheumatoid arthritis.
• Malocclusion of teeth	• Pain over the face and jaw, may be referred to other areas • Intensified by chewing or movements of the jaw • Dental examination will reveal malocclusion
• Post-zoster neuralgia (Fig. 5.24)	• History of severe facial pain or burning of the face. The pain is increased by contact or movement • History of herpes zoster infection over the face with typical vesiculo-papular eruptions • Dermal scars of herpetic lesions may be present • It is unilateral, may involve any division of the Vth nerve • Sensory disturbances such as paraesthesias or slight sensory loss may be present

TABLE 5.18: Differential Diagnosis of Facial Nerve

I. Palsy due to pontine lesion (*causes*: tumour, vascular lesion, demyelination)

Clinical features are:
- 6th and 7th cranial nerves with contralateral hemiplegia (*Millard-Gubler syndrome*)
- Pin-point pupil on the side involved
- Ataxic nystagmus
- Internuclear ophthalmoplegia

II. Palsy due to cerebellopontine angle lesion (*causes*: Acoustic neuroma, meningioma)

Clinical features are:
- 7th and 8th nerve palsies on the side involved
- Loss of sensation over anterior two-thirds of tongue due to involvement of nervus intermedius

III. Palsy due to lesion at internal acoustic meatus, i.e. Bell's palsy, trauma, otitis media, Ramsay Hunt syndrome, tumour

Clinical features are:
- 7th nerve palsy
- 8th nerve palsy
- Hyperacusis (e.g. sounds appear louder than normal) due to involvement of stapedius muscle
- Loss of taste from anterior two-thirds of tongue

IV. Palsy due to lesion at stylomastoid foramen (*causes*: Mumps, tumour of parotid gland, sarcoidosis, Bell's palsy, trauma, Guillain-Barré syndrome)
- Paralysis of all the muscles of the face
- Taste and lacrimation is preserved

TABLE 5.19: Symptoms and Signs of Facial Nerve Paralysis

Symptoms	Signs
Dribbling or drooling of saliva from the angle of the mouth on the affected side	Angle of the mouth droops on the affected side on clenching the teeth. Facial asymmetry present due to paresis of facial muscles
Creases of face or skin folds are effaced or blunted on affected side	Nasolabial fold gets effaced on the affected side when patient is asked to show his/her teeth
Forehead is unfurrowed (expressionless), face is immobile	Patient is unable to make furrows on the affected side on looking upwards.
Palpebral fissure on affected side is wide.	Cornea is visible on affected side. Difficulty in closing the affected eye as patient is asked to close the eyes, hence, is liable to exposure keratitis
Food collects between teeth and cheeks on the side involved	Patient has difficulty to blow out the cheeks

Examination of VIIth Nerve

The VIIth nerve can only be tested at the face (testing of facial muscles only, Table 5.20 and Fig. 5.25). The taste sensation is tested from anterior two-thirds of the tongue.

☞ *Testing of taste sensation*
- Instruct the patient not to speak or retract the tongue during examination as this will dissipate the liquid substance onto the opposite side of the tongue as well as to its posterior one-third.
- Now gently hold the protuded tongue with a swab. Put a drop of testing substance (e.g. sweet, salt, bitter or sour) on the anterior two-thirds of each side of the tongue in turn.
- Ask the patient to identify the substance by pointing to the appropriate word written on a piece of paper or card.

☞ *Testing for lacrimation (Schirmer's test)*
Put a piece of special blotting paper under the lower eyelid and remove it after 5 minutes. Normally at least 10 mm of blotting paper will be dampened (wet) by evoked tear secretion.

> In facial nerve palsy, there is diminished or absence of tear secretion. In facial nerve palsy, there is loss of taste sensation over anterior two-thirds of tongue.

Common Abnormalities

Paralysis of VIIth Nerve: It could be *supranuclear* (lesion alove the pons), *nuclear* (lesion in the pons) or *infranuclear* (lesion below the pons).

Upper motor neuron *vs* **lower motor neuron lesions** of 7th nerve are discussed in Table 5.21.

Facial weakness: It could be due to upper motor neuron involvement or 7th nerve paralysis or diseases of myoneural junction or facial muscles (myopathy). It may be unilateral or bilateral. The causes of facial weakness (both UMN and LMN causes) are given in Box 5.3.

Idiopathic (Bell) Palsy (Fig. 5.26)

It is the most commonly seen in patients of all age groups and both the sexes. It is commonly unilateral, rarely bilateral. The cause is unknown. The site of the lesion is compression of facial nerve within facial canal or at stylomastoid foramen due to oedema or swelling of the nerve or nerve sheath at these sites. The *precipitating factors* include *ischaemia, viral infections, trauma* or *cold exposure*.

Nervous System

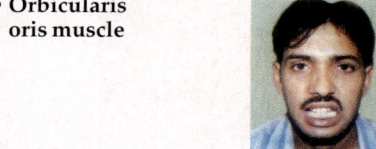

TABLE 5.20: Testing of the Facial Nerve (Figs 5.25A to E)

Test for	Figure (normal response)	Method
• Orbicularis oris muscle	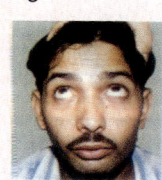 **Fig. 5.25A:** Normal person can clench the teeth without any abnormality of angles	☞ Ask the patient to clench the teeth • In facial nerve palsy, the angle of the mouth droops on the affected side
• Frontalis muscle	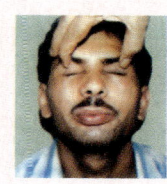 **Fig. 5.25B:** A normal person can make furrows	☞ Ask the patient to look upwards (e.g. make furrows over the forehead) while you hold the head in neutral position • A patient with facial paralaysis cannot make furrows over the forehead on the affected side
• Orbicularis oculi	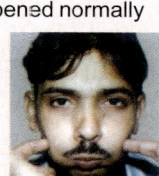 **Fig. 5.25C:** Normal closure of the eyes against resistance. Eyes can not be opened normally	☞ Ask the patient to close both the eyes as tightly as possible • In facial palsy, the eyelids on the affected side do not cover the eyeball properly and firmly ☞ Now try to open the closed eyes with the fingers (Fig. 5.25C) • In facial nerve palsy, the eye on the affected side can be opened without any resistance or remain partially open as compared to healthy side. The eyeball on the involved side rolls slightly upon aris and outwards (Bell's phenomenon)
• Buccinator	**Fig. 5.25D:** Normal person can blow out the cheeks. Air does not leak on pressure applied with fingers on both the sides	☞ Ask the patient to blow out his/her cheeks by tightly closing the lips • In facial palsy, the affected side will not blow out due to leakage of air through the angle of the mouth on the involved side or he/she incompletely blows out the affected cheek as compared to healthy side ☞ Now ask the patient to hold the cheeks in fully blown out position. Press both the cheeks between index fingers and thumbs of your both hands (Fig. 5.25D) • In facial palsy, air leaks out on pressure applied on the involved side due to weak cheek muscles
	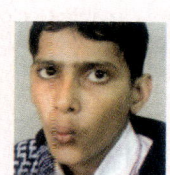 **Fig. 5.25E:** A normal person can whistle	☞ Ask the patient to whistle (Fig. 5.25E) • In facial palsy, patient is not able to whistle
• Platysma		☞ Ask the patient to wrinkle up the skin of neck • In facial nerve palsy, patient is unable to do this

Box 5.3: Common Causes of Facial Weakness

I. Upper motor neuron weakness

Unilateral
- Usually vascular (CVA)
- Cerebral tumour
- Multiple sclerosis

Bilateral
- Often vascular (CVA)
- Motor neuron disease

II. Lower motor neuron weakness
- Bell's palsy
- Parotid tumour
- Head injury
- Tumour at the base of skull
- Sarcoidosis
- Myasthenia gravis
- Guillain-Barré syndrome or polyneuropathies
- Myopathies (e.g. myotonic dystrophy)

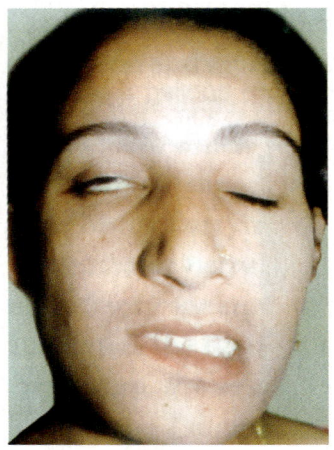

Fig. 5.26: Bell's palsy (right side). The right eye remains partially open when asked to close the eyes. The eyeball on involved side rolls upwards and outwards called *Bell's phenomenon* present.

Symptoms and signs include acute or subacute onset of pain behind a ear or on one side of the face followed by flaccid (LMN) paralysis of all the muscles of face leading to asymmetry of the face. Patient may complain of paraesthesias over the face but there is no objective sensory loss. Occasionally, taste sensation may be involved. Hyperacusis occurs if nerve to stapedius is involved. Severe lesion may cause loss of salivation and tears formation.

Taste and lacrimation will be preserved if the lesion is distal to or at the stylomastoid foramen.

Hemifacial spasms: Hemifacial spasms occur commonly in middle aged women, are characterised by intermittent narrowing of the palpebral fissure on the affected side, and the facial muscles contract to pull the angle of the mouth upwards. The cause is unknown but compression of 7th nerve by loops of cerebellar arteries or by AVM (AV malformation) or cerebellopontine tumour is implicated.

TABLE 5.21: Differences between Upper Motor Neuron and Lower Motor Neuron Facial Paralysis/Palsy

Upper motor neuron	Lower motor neuron
• Lesion is above the pons	Lesion is in the pons or below the pons
• Corticonuclear fibres (pyramidal tract fibres) are involved	7th nerve itself or its nucleus is involved
• Facial palsy/paralysis is limited to lower part of the face on one side, the upper part is spared due to its bilateral innervation	Facial paralysis involves all the muscles of the face on one side (complete facial paralysis)
• Patient can make furrows on forehead on looking upwards	• Furrows are lost on the affected side on forehead (flat forhead)
• The eye closure is well preserved while corner of the mouth will droop, saliva may dribble and the nasolabial fold is flattened on the affected side of the face	• The patient is unable to close the eye; and impaired blinking, loss of nasolabial folds and drooling of saliva from the mouth is present
• Smiling is preserved	• Smiling is involved because of involvement of emotional facial movements
• Taste is normal	• Taste to anterior two-thirds of tongue is impaired if the chorda tympani branch is damaged
• It is invariably associated with uncrossed haemiplegia (supranuclear 7th palsy and haemiplegia are on the same side) due to involvement of contralateral cortical or subcortical pathways	• Associated with crossed hemiplegia (*Millard-Gubler's syndrome*) in which 7th nerve palsy is opposite to the side of hemiplegia
• Usually secondary to some cause, e.g. CVA, multiple sclerosis, tumour, etc.	• Usually idiopathic (cause unknown)

THE VESTIBULOCOCHLEAR (VIII) NERVE

The vestibulocochlear nerve, as its name suggests has two branches; *vestibular* and *cochlear*.

The *cochlear* branch is concerned with hearing. The *vestibular* branch is concerned with maintenance of correct posture, eye coordination and movement.

The *vestibular* nerve carry impulses from three semicircular canals, the *utricle* which senses the tilting of the head; and the *saccule* which senses the angular acceleration of the head.

The *vestibular* nerve (division) joins the *cochlear* nerve (division) to form *vestibulocochlear nerve*. The nerve enters the cranium through the internal auditory meatus, traverses the cerebellopontine angle and enters the brain stem at pontomedullary junction. In the brain stem, the vestibular fibres terminate in the four vestibular nuclei (superior, inferior, lateral and medial). Through fibres in the medial *longitudinal fasciculus (MLF)* in the brain stem, it is interconnected with the III, IV and VI cranial nerves. Most fibres project to the cerebellum, while some descend to the spinal cord to form vestibulospinal tracts. Ascending fibres from the brain stem relay through the medial geniculate body to the posterior temporal lobe.

The vestibular part of VIII nerve forms the afferent limb of both the *oculocephalic (doll's eye reflex)* and *oculovestibular (caloric) reflexes*.

The oculocephalic reflex involves conjugated movements of the eyes in response to changes in head position.
The oculovestibular reflex (caloric test) involves elicitation of eye movements following irrigation of external ear canal by either cold or warm water.

The cochlear nerve originates from the *organ of corti* which is a spiral tube containing receptor hair cells and a cavity filled with fluid. Sound waves are transmitted through the fluid to the hair cells which are further transmitted through the fibres of cochlear nerve in the internal auditory meatus to the brain stem. The fibres then synapse in the cochlear nuclei. From the cochlear nuclei, second order fibres ascend to the superior olivary and trapezoid nuclei. Central fibres then ascend up the lateral leminscus, and synapse in the *inferior colliculus* and *medial geniculate body* before entering the auditory cortex in the superior temporal gyrus (areas 41 and 42). The ascending auditory pathways decussate at several places so that each cortical region receives impulses from both the ears.

☞ **Testing of VIII Nerve**

Hearing (Cochlear Functions)

Auditory acquity. It is possible to make a preliminary assessment of hearing by asking the patient whether he/she can hear the doorbell or telephone (sound outputs around 60 dB) and whether conversation in a quiet environment can be heard (normal levels about 40 dB).

If the patient prefers a loud voice in a quiet environment, this implies a hearing loss of 70–80 dB is present.

Clinical testing (free-field voice testing). It can be performed by asking the patient to repeat word spoken at varying intensities. This testing employs phonetically balanced words (e.g. baseball), number combinations (e.g. 9-4) and combinations of number and letters (9-M-4). In such testing, one ear is tested at a time. The examiner stands to the side of the ear to be tested and occludes the other ear.

Rinne's test (Fig. 5.27). It determines whether air conduction is better than bone conduction or *vice versa*. Normally and in sensorineural deafness; air conduction (AC) is better than bone conduction (BC). In middle ear deafness or conductive deafness BC > AC (bone conduction is better than air conduction).

Weber's test (Fig. 5.28). It is a lateralising hearing test. It provides additional information about the type of deafness. Normally, sound arises in the midline and heard equally in both the ears when a vibrating tuning fork (256 or 512 H_2) is placed over the vertex or forehead. In *sensorineural deafness*, fork is heard better on healthy side (Rinne –ve) and in *conductive deafness* on the diseased side (Rinne +ve, Box 5.4).

Box 5.4	Tunning Fork Tests		
Test	Normal	Conductive deafness	Sensori-neural deafness
Rinne	AC > BC	BC > AC (Rinne +ve)	AC > BC
Weber	No lateralisation	Lateralsed to diseased side	Lateralised to healthy side (Rinne –ve)

In conductive deafness, Rinne is said to be positive.

Audiometry and evoked potentials: In clinical practice, deafness or impaired hearing is best studied using audiometry and brain stem evoked potentials to determine the precise aetiology.

Testing for the Vestibular Function

Balance and orientation of body in space depends on the sensory inputs from:
- Vestibular system.
- The eyes
- Muscles, joints and skin receptors (somatosensory system)

Ataxia: *Imbalance or unsteadiness* is defined as impaired ability to maintain postures in the intended orientation of the body in space. It generally manifests as ataxia while standing or walking. The ataxia results from disorder of *spinocerebellar* or *vestibular* or *sensory inputs*.

☞ *Perform the Romberg's sign for ataxia*

In labrinthine disease, patient falls to the side involved on standing with eyes open (Romberg's negative). The vertiginous ataxia of labrinthine disease is differentiated from sensory ataxia by negative Romberg's sign (read Romberg's sign under testing for gait and stance).

Nystagmus (Read it as a symptom also)

It is voluntary conjugate ocular movements with rhythmical oscillations of the eye. The direction of quickest movement decides the side of nystagmus. Nystagmus is either induced or spontaneous.

Generally, in *vestibular disturbance*, nystagmus is enhanced by movement of the eyes in the direction of fast phase and diminished movement in the opposite direction. In the *destructive vestibular lesion*, the contralateral vestibular system dominates being intact and drives the eyes to the side of the lesion. This movement to the side of the lesion will be slow phase and opposite to the lesion will be the fast phase. The nystagmus will be maximal when looking in the direction opposite to lesion.

In vestibular destructive lesion, nystagmus will be on the side opposite to the lesion.

1. **Visual fixation.** Vestibular nystagmus is enhanced without visual fixation, i.e. visual fixation attenuates or inhibits nystagmus and vertigo. Nystagmus should also be assessed by using Frenzel's glasses which have a 20 dioptre lens and, therefore, abolishes fixation.

Persistent positional nystagmus occurring with ocular fixation implies central lesion (brain stem disease and lesions in the region of fourth ventricle).

2. **Electronystagmography** is a graphic recording of eye movements which can be measured. As

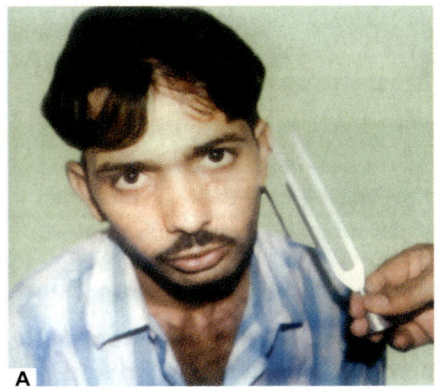

A

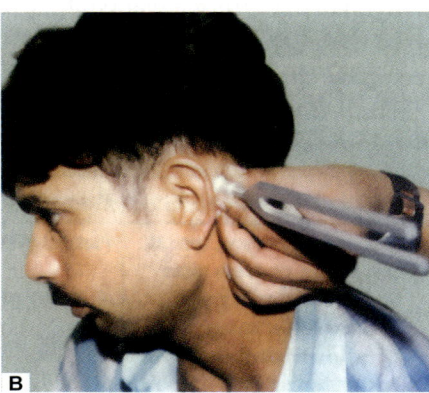

B

Figs 5.27A and B: Rinne's test: (A) Bring the vibrating tuning fork in front of ear (say left). Ask the patient to report as soon as vibrations stop. When patient notices that the vibrations have stopped, put the tuning fork on the mastoid process on same side (B). Ask whether now vibrations are audible or not, to decide whether air conduction is better than bone conduction or *vice versa*.

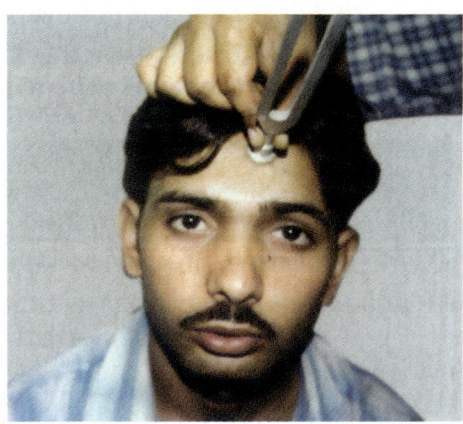

Fig. 5.28: Weber's test. Put the vibrating tuning fork over the middle of forehead. Ask the patient on which side the vibrations are best audible to decide on which side bone conduction is better (Rinne +ve).

the eye acts as a dipole (the cornea as a positive and retina as a negative), eye movement results in an altered potential difference between the two electrodes on a moving paper strip. In this way, one can measure the velocity, amplitude and frequency of eye movements or nystagmus and permanent record can be obtained.

3. **Dix and Hallpike method (Fig. 5.29). Positional vertigo** is precipitated by a recumbent head position either to the left or to the right. Positional vertigo is elicited by making the patient to sit on a couch and fix the eyes on the centre of the forehead of the examiner. The patient's head is turned 45° to the left (Fig. 5.29A) or right and then is rapidly lowered to 30° below the horizontal (Fig. 5.29B). The patient has to keep the eyes open during this procedure so that examiner can observe the nystagmus. The patient is instructed to report vertigo or dizziness during this procedure. The nystagmus is induced within the latent period of 2–5 seconds and disappears within a few seconds.

This is most important sign of benign paroxysmal positional vertigo (BPPV). The nystagmus has fast component directed towards the lower most ear.

The repetition of the test will produce a little abnormality (adaptation). Whatever may be the cause, the benign nature of this syndrome is characterised by disappearance of the symptoms with time in most of the cases. Alcohol abuse and psychotropics may induce transient positional vertigo.

Testing for Gait and Stance

In VIII nerve paralysis, the patient may get imbalance of gait (vertiginous ataxia). Patients tend to fall to the side of the lesion. This is tested by *Romberg's sign* (negative)

Romberg's sign (positive for sensory ataxia). This is a sign of proprioception. Patients with uncompensated unilateral labyrinthine or cerebellar lesion (vertiginous ataxia) show instability to the side of the lesion with their eyes closed which becomes more marked when their eyes are open (Romberg's sign is negative). Patients with posterior column disease (*sensory ataxia*), will sway or fall with the eyes closed but will stand normally with the eyes open (Romberg's positive). Patients with central lesions sway to both sides with eyes open or shut.

Romberg's sign differentiates sensory ataxia from other ataxias (cerebellar, vertiginous and hysterical)

☞ Reflex Eye Movements

They should be tested to detect brain stem lesions. The test includes:

I. **Doll's eye movement** (*oculocephalic reflex*). Rotate the patient's head from side to side (Fig. 5.30) and observe the eyes movements:

- *In coma with intact brain stem* produces conjugate deviation of eyes opposite to the head movement. This is normal response.

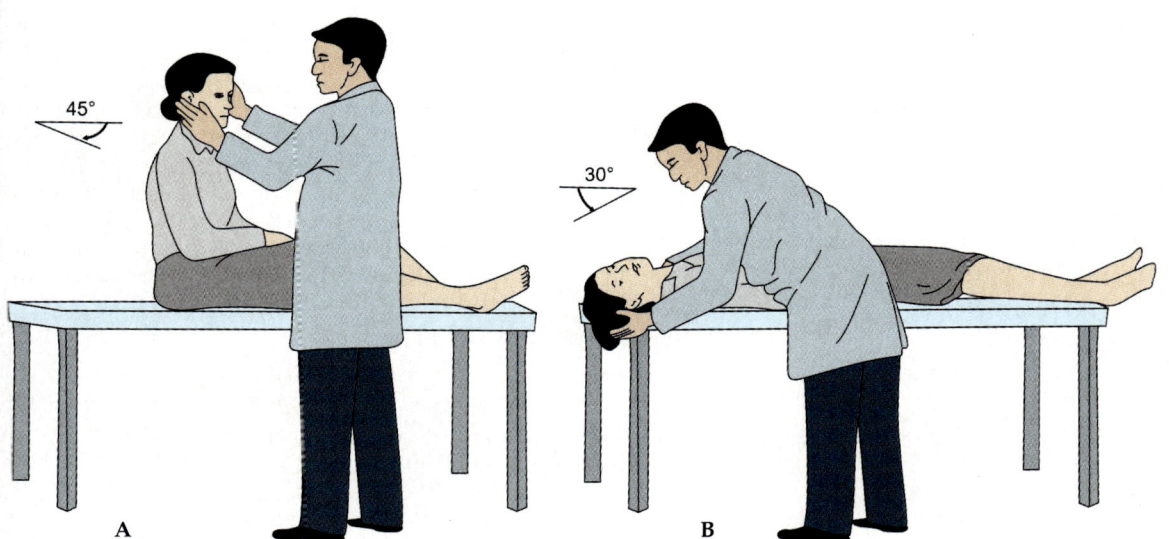

Figs 5.29A and B: Dix and Hallpike manoeuvre to elicit nystagmus in a patient with positional vertigo.

- *In brain stem lesion*, the eyes move to one side not to the other (lateral gaze palsy).

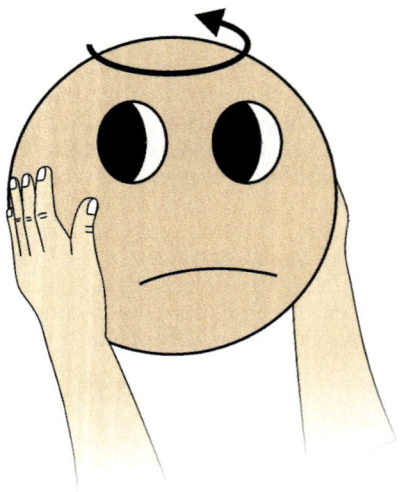

Fig. 5.30: Doll's head manoeuvres. It is used to assess the eye movements in comatosed patient. Rolling of the head to one side causes counter-rolling of the eyes to opposite side in coma.

II. Caloric test. This is most frequently employed test to assess the performance of vestibular end-organ. The test is performed by making the patient in recumbent position (lying down) and head is flexed at 30° in order to bring the lateral semicircular canal in horizonal position. Each external auditory meatus is irrigated, in turn with water at 30° and 40°C. The thermal gradient induces nystagmus by stimulating vestibular system.

In caloric test, irrigation of 1 ml of warm water produces nystagmus away from involved side while cold water irrigation produces nystagmus towards involved side. The test is useful in unconscious patients (read unit on examination of unconscious patient).

Common Abnormalities of VIII Nerve

Deafness (Hearing Loss): A loss of hearing can result from lesions in the external auditory canal, middle ear, inner ear or central auditory pathways. Lesions of external auditory canal, middle ear or tympanic membrane cause *conductive type* of deafness, while lesions of the inner ear or eight nerve (cochlear division) or central auditory pathways cause *perceptive or sensorineural type* of deafness. The two types of deafness are compared in Table 5.22 and causes of deafness are listed in Box 5.5.

Box 5.5 Causes of Deafness

Conductive deafness
I. **Obstruction of external auditory canal**
   - Wax, debris and foreign body
   - Otitis externa (swelling of lining of the ear canal)
   - Canal stenosis
   - Neoplasm
II. **Middle ear or tympanic membrane**
   - Chronic otitis media (perforation of tympanic membrane)
   - Disruption of ear ossicles by trauma or infection
   - Otosclerosis (fixation of ear oscicles)

Sensorineural deafness
- **Ageing**
- **Noise-induced deafness** (occupational, loudspeakers, personal stereo)
- **Viral infections** e.g. mumps, intrauterine rubella
- **Ototoxic drugs** e.g. aminoglycosides, (gentamicin), frusemide, cytotoxic (cisplatin), beta blockers, aspirin and quinine
- **Trauma** (fracture of temporal bone)
- **Meningitis**
- **Cochlear otosclerosis**
- **Meniere's disease**
- **Acoustic neuroma** or other cerebellopontine angle tumour

Normally, a tone is heard louder by air conduction than by bone conduction. With a *conductive* deafness the bone conduction stimulus is perceived louder than the air conduction stimulus (BC > AC). With perceptive or sensorineural deafness, both air and bone conduction perceptions are reduced but

TABLE 5.22: Comparison of Two Types of Deafness

Type	Site of lesion	Conductive tests	Auditory acquity	Speech discrimination
1. Conductive deafness	External ear, middle ear or tympanic membrane	Air conduction is impaired (thresholds for air conduction elevated) but bone conduction is normal (i.e BC > AC)	Retained	Normal
2. Perceptive or sensorineural deafness	Inner ear, cochlear nerve, central neural pathway	Both air and bone conduction are impaired (thresholds for both conduc-tion elevated) but air conduction (AC) is still better than bone conduction (BC), i.e. AC > BC	Impaired or fluctuates	Impaired

the air conduction stimulus is perceived louder as in normal hearing (AC > BC).

Tinnitus: It is defined as the perception of a sound when there is no sound in the environment. It is associated with a conductive or sensorineural (perceptive) deafness. The causes of tinnitus are more or less same as the causes of deafness. Most cases of tinnitus complain of a *ringing, rushing* or *hissing sound in the ear*. Tinnitus must be distinguished from *autophony*—an abnormal perception of patient's own voice as well as the breath sounds. Autophony is similar to the sensation experienced when holding a sea shell to the ear. The commonest cause is patulous eustachian tube.

THE GLOSSOPHARYNGEAL (IX), VAGUS (X) AND ACCESSORY (XI) NERVES

These nerves are considered together, being related anatomically, functionally and in terms of clinical examination.

The *glossopharyngeal, vagus* and *accessory nerves* arise as a series of rootlets in an order from above downwards from the posterolateral sulcus of medulla.

The spinal part of the XI (*accessory*) nerve emerges from the cervical cord, perhaps beginning as low as the sixth cervical root. It ascends up through the foramen magnum to meet its second medullary part to form the accessory nerve. All the three nerves (IX, X, XI) pass through the jugular foramen. The medullary part of the XI nerve separate and join the *vagus* (X) nerve to supply motor fibres to the larynx and pharynx. The spinal portion of XIth nerve supplies *sternomastoid* and upper portion of the *trapezius* muscles.

The parasympathetic fibres of IX nerve arise from the inferior salivary nucleus and relay in the otic ganglion. They supply parotid glands. The parasympathetic fibres of X nerve supply all the viscera.

The sensory, motor and parasympathetic innervations of *glossopharyngeal, vagus* and accessory are given in Table 5.23.

Symptoms of IX and X Nerves Palsy

- *Nasal regurgitation of fluids during swallowing.* This is common symptom due to paralysis of soft palate resulting in defective elevation of the palate during swallowing.
- *The voice may have nasal quality (nasal speech)* due to inability to pronounce certain words which require complete closure of nasopharynx. Thus, egg is pronounced as 'eng', "rub" becomes "rum" and so on.
- *Dysphagia, dysphonia, hoarseness* and *loss of gag reflex.*

Physical Signs of IX Nerve Palsy

1. Unilateral loss of palatal, tonsillar or pharyngeal sensation on the side involved.
2. Absent or depressed gag reflex (afferent limb of the reflex is involved) on side involved.

Glossopharyngeal neuralgia is idiopathic like trigeminal neuralgia where brief attacks of lancinating pain occur over the side of throat radiating down to the neck and back of jaw. These attacks are precipitated by swallowing or protuding the tongue. There is no paralysis of the nerve.

Physical Signs of X Nerve Palsy

1. The voice may sound hoarse or may have nasal quality. The patient can not cough clearly (*bovine cough*) due to recurrent laryngeal nerve paralysis.
2. Bilateral paralysis may produce stridor or even respiratory obstruction because the paralysed cords partially blocking the airway.

TABLE 5.23: Sensory and Motor Innervation of IX, X and XI Cranial Nerves

Nerve	Motor innervation	Sensory innervation	Parasympathetic innervation	Reflex
IX (glosso-pharyngeal)	Stylopharyngeus muscle	Mucosa of pharynx, tonsils, soft palate, conveys taste fibres to posterior third of the tongue, lining of tympanic cavity and eustachian tube	Parotid gland	It constitutes an afferent limb of the *gag reflex*
X (vagus)	Muscles of upper pharynx, soft palate, all the intrinsic muscles of larynx and crico-thyroid muscle	Dura mater of posterior cranial fossa, some part of skin of external auditory meatus	All the abdominal and thoracic viscera	It is involved in oculocardiac and carotid sinus reflexes
XI (accessory)	Sternomastoid and trapezius muscles	Nil	Nil	Nil

☞ Testing of IX and X Nerves

- Observe the movements of the palate by asking the patient to open the mouth as wide as he/she can. Depress the tongue with a tongue depressor while torching the light at uvula. Note the position of uvula at rest. Now ask the patient to say 'aah' and note whether both sides of the palate arch upwards (Fig. 5.31).

In unilateral paralysis, the involved side remains flat and immobile and the median raphe will be pulled to the healthy side (Fig. 15.38).

In bilateral paralysis the palate does not move at all.

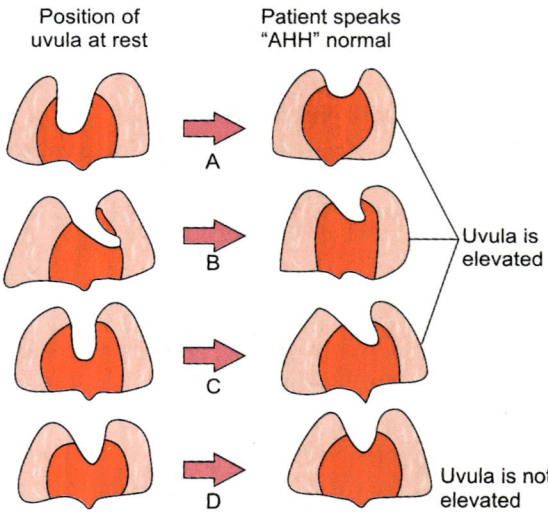

Fig. 5.31: Testing of cranial nerves IX and X. (A) Normal uvula is in the midline at rest, and elevated in the midline with "AHH..."; (B) Right CN IX and X paralysis: Uvula is deviated to nondiseased (left) side at rest and elevated and deviated to the left with "AHH..."; (C) Right CN IX and X paralysis: Uvula is in the midline at rest, get elevated and deviated to the nondiseased (left) side with "AHH..."; (D) Bilateral CN IX and X paralysis: Uvula is in the midline at rest and there is no-movement with "AHH..."

N.B. Remember that minor degree of asymmetry of palate and of tongue can occur in hemiplegia with UMN VII nerve palsy. It differs from palatal palsy which is LMN type of paralysis.

- Assess the tonsillar, palatal and pharyngeal tactile sensation using a dampened swab stick and tongue depressor. Test the taste sensation over posterior third of the tongue as described under 7th nerve.

Sensations are lost over these regions in IX nerve palsy.

- The gag reflex may be elicited by touching either the tonsil or pharynx with a tongue depressor or spatula. There will be contraction of pharyngeal muscles. Test each side separately. It is unpleasant and difficult to test the gag reflex, hence, to be performed only when there is other evidence of IX or X nerve palsy.

Gag reflex is absent or diminished in IX (afferent limb) and X (efferent limb) or both nerve palsy.

- Assess the volume and quality of the patient's speech, noting if the voice is hoarse or has a bleating or nasal character.

In unilateral X nerve palsy, the speech is blurred, hoarse and ineffectual. Bilateral palsy produces stridor or respiratory obstruction.

- Ask the patient (cough reflex) to determine whether this is more nasal or bovine than normal.

Bovine cough is a characteristic feature of recurrent laryngeal nerve palsy.

- To test the palatal closure of nasopharynx ask the patient to puff out the cheeks.

Normally, both sides of palate elevate in a symmetric fashion and the uvula remains in the midline. In order to puff out the cheeks, the palate must elevate and occlude nasopharynx. If palatal movement is weak, air will escape audibly through the nose.

Causes of IX and X Nerves Palsy

The causes of unilateral and bilateral palsy are as follows:

I. Unilateral IX and X cranial nerves palsy
- Fracture of base of skull
- Neoplasm of base of skull (meningioma)
- Recurrent laryngeal nerve (branch of X nerve) palsy is due to;
  - Bronchial carcinoma
  - Mediastinal tumour (lymphoma)
  - Aortic arch aneurysm
  - Dilated left atrium in mitral stenosis

II. Bilateral Xth nerve palsy
- Progressive bulbar palsy (motor neuron disease).
- Pseudobulbar palsy (bilateral UMN lesion in CVA or multiple sclerosis).

☞ Testing of accessory (XI) nerve

It is a pure motor nerve.

- Inspect the trapezius muscle from behind and sternomastoid from the front for any wasting or atrophy. Palpate these muscles to assess tone and bulk.

In XI nerve palsy, the shoulder will appear drooped and the arm will appear lower than the healthy side. In bilateral sternomastoid paralysis head will droop forwards (neck flexion).

☞ *Testing of trapezius and sternomastoid*
- To test the trapezius, ask the patient to shrug his/her shoulder while the examiner presses downward on them (Fig. 5.32A) or ask the patient to shrug the shoulder and maintain them elevated, then apply pressure downward on the shoulder.

Normally, a person can shrug the shoulder against resistance, but can not do so if XI nerve is paralysed.

- To test the right sternomastoid, ask the patient to rotate the head to the left side while a hand is placed against the left side of the chin to stop rotation of the chin (Fig. 5.32B). Normally, the muscle stands out prominently during the manoeuvre.

Paralysis of sternomastoid (XI nerve palsy), causes weakness of rotation of the chin to the opposite side.

- You can examine the left sternomastoid by placing left hand on right side of chin of the patient.
- You can test both sternomastoids simultaneously by asking the patient to depress the examiner's hand placed below the chin while examiner try to resist it.

Common Abnormalities
- In the cervical region, the spinal component of XI nerve may be involved in *syringomyelia, poliomyelitis, motor neuron disease* and spinal *cord tumours.*
- In the intracranial course, it may be a part of jugular foramen syndrome (*glomus jugulare tumour* producing IX, X and XI nerves plasy).

THE HYPOGLOSSAL (XII) NERVE

It is a pure motor nerve.
The fibres of XII nerve originate from the hypoglossal nucleus in the lower medulla. The nerve travels the medulla and comes out from its ventral aspect. It runs a short course in posterior cranial

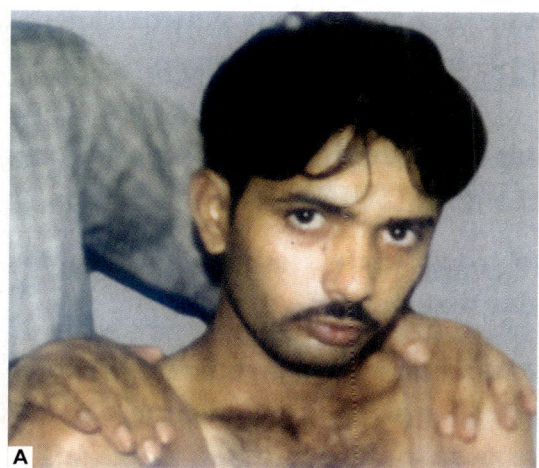

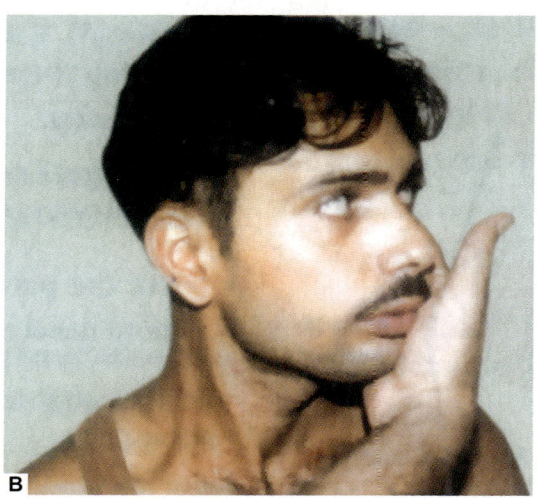

Figs 5.32A and B: Testing for the accessory (XIth cranial) nerve. (A) Testing of both the trapezius muscles; (B) Testing of right sternomastoid.

fossa. It leaves the skull through hypoglossal canal or foramen. Through its branches, it innervates the muscles of the tongue (e.g. *genioglossus, styloglossus* and the *hypoglossus*).

☞ *Testing of XII nerve*

A. Testing for deviation of tongue
- Ask the patient to protude the tongue; observe any deviation of tongue.

In XII nerve palsy, the tongue is deviated to the paralysed side instead of being protuding straight. The medial raphe is convex towards healthy side (Fig. 5.33).

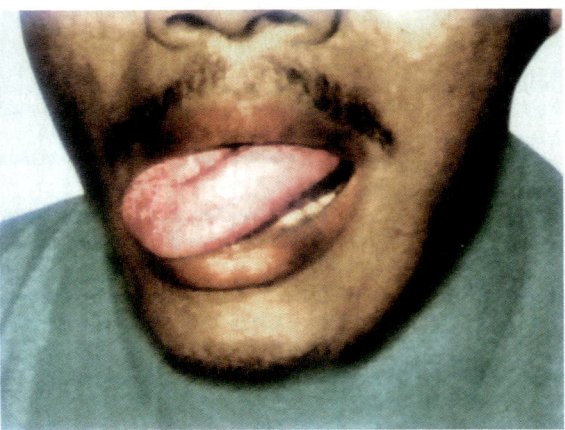

Fig. 5.33: Right hypoglossal (XII cranial nerve) palsy. Tongue deviates to right on protrusion indicating an ipsilateral LMN lesion.

N.B. Apparent deviation of the tongue occurs in facial palsy and loss of teeth on one side which is distinguished from true deviation (XII nerve palsy) by twisting of the tongue as well as deviation of angle of the mouth to the paralysed side while the median raphe is normal. This is called *pseudodeviation* of the tongue.

B. Atrophy and fasciculations.
- Look for wasting and fasciculations in the resting position of the tongue (tongue lying inside the mouth). Palpate the tongue between thumb and fingers for tone.

C. Testing for the lateral movements of tongue
- Assess the movements from side to side; observe whether this can be done freely.
- Ask the patient to lick each cheek with the tongue; feel the strength with a finger as the patient protrudes the tongue into each cheek in turn.
- Assess the hypokinesia of tongue movements by asking the patient to say *"ah, ah, ah"* as quickly as possible, and to make rapid-in and rapid-out and side-to-side movements of the tongue.

I. Signs of Unilateral XII Nerve Palsy

A. Lower motor neuron type (nuclear or infranuclear)
- *There is atrophy or wasting of the tongue* on the side involved. Fasciculations may be present which are best seen when the tongue lies in the mouth in resting position.
- The tongue tends to deviate on the side of the lesion.
- The tongue cannot be moved freely from side-to-side
- The bulk of the muscle mass is reduced on palpation of the protuded tongue on the side involved.

B. Upper motor neuron (supranuclear) paralysis
- Unilateral UMN lesion of XII nerve produces (spastic tongue) deviation of the protuded tongue to paralysed side without atrophy or fasciculations. This is a feature of pseudobulbar palsy (CVA) involving the XIIth nerve.

II. Bilateral XII Nerve Palsy

In LMN (bulbar) paralysis, the tongue is flat, atrophic lying listless in the mouth with loss of movements. In UMN lesion (pseudobulbar palsy) the tongue is spastic and shrivelled up.

Common Abnormalities

- Tremors of the tongue are seen in Parkinson's disease, either when the tongue is at rest or protuded.
- The lower cranial nerves IX, X, XI and XII are frequently affected bilaterally producing dysphagia, dysarthria and nasal regurgitation (a characteristic triad). The lower cranial nerves may be affected unilaterally in the *jugular foramen* (IX, X and XI) or at the base of skull along with XII nerve and sympathetic innervation to the eye (*Horner's syndrome*).

Jugular Foramen Syndrome

It is a syndrome of involveent of IX, X and XI cranial nerves in Jugular foramen inside the skull (*vernet syndrome*) and outside the skull (*collet-siccard*). The causes are:
1. Carcinoma of nasopharynx.
2. Fracture of the base of skull.
3. Jugular foramen neoplasm/carotid body neoplasm
4. Basal meningitis
5. Metastases at the base of brain.
6. Jugular vein thrombosis.
7. Neurofibromatosis
8. Paget's disease

Bulbar Palsy

It involves the lower cranial nerves either from lesion in the medulla or outside the brain stem. Pharyngeal, palatal and tongue muscles are weak, resulting in difficulty in swallowing, nasal regurgitation, the slurred and unintelligible speech and difficulties pronouncing the labials and dentals. Tongue is toneless, listless and immobile.

The **causes** of bulbar palsy include *genetic*, i.e. Kennedy's disease (X-linked bulbospinal neuronopathy), *vascular* (infarction of medulla), *degenerative* (motor neuron disease, syringobulbia), *inflammatory* and *infective* (myasthenia, Guillain-Barré, poliomyelitis, lyme disease, vasculitis) and *neoplastic lesion* (brain stem glioma and neoplastic meningitis). The differences between bulbar and pseudobulbar palsy are summarised at the end of Unit (read brief synopsis of neurological disorders, Table 5.36).

Pseudobulbar Palsy

It results from an upper motor neuron lesion of the bulbar muscles involving the corticobulbar tracts. Face is expressionless, tongue is spastic and there is emotional blunting leading to frequent involuntary laughing.

The **causes** are: (i) *Bilateral cerebral lacunar infarcts*, (ii) *motor neuron disease*, (iii) *multiple sclerosis and brain stem tumour*.

THE MOTOR SYSTEM EXAMINATION

It includes:
- *Inspection and palpation* of muscle groups for atrophy/wasting; hypertrophy or bulk of the muscles or contractures.
- *Assessment of tone* (increased/decreased).
- *Testing of muscle strength or power and grade it.*
- *Elicitation of reflexes* (e.g. deep tendon, superficial and visceral) for presence/absence/exaggeration.
- *Testing of co-ordination and gait.*
- *Involuntary movements* (spontaneous or induced).

Symptoms of Motor System

The symptoms of motor system involvement are varied and include;
1. Paralysis or weakness (UMN or LMN).
2. Impairment of co-ordination (ataxia).
3. Changes in tone and posture (hypo or hypertonia, dystonia).
4. Involuntary movements (dyskinesia or hyperkinesia)
5. Slowness of movements and activity (hypokinesia and bradykinesia).
6. Loss of learned movement patterns (dyspraxia).

Pathways of Motor System

Upper Motor Neuron Pathway

The motor system pathways (corticospinal tracts) are outlined in Fig. 5.34. The pyramidal tracts (corticospinal fibres) extend from motor cortex (precentral gyrus) to the spinal cord. The decussation of fibres occur at the level of junction of medulla and spinal cord. Some of the fibres crossing to the opposite side constitute *lateral corticospinal tract* and remaining uncrossed fibres constitute *anterior corticospinal tract* and end in spinal cord.

☞ **Inspection and Palpation**

The patient should be examined in underwear only so as to observe the limbs and muscles clearly in a good light. The muscle bulk and power is noted.

In health, normally the lower limb muscles are symmetrical and well developed. In the upper limbs, the musculature on the dominant side (the limb used more) is often well developed, as in the racquet arm of tennis player.

The change in bulk of muscles may be either *atrophy* (loss of bulk) or *hypertrophy* (e.g. occupational, muscular dystrophy—Duchenne type)

The causes of muscle weakness according to site of lesion are described in Table 5.24.

In order to determine the anatomical cause of atrophy, it is necessary to know the distribution of weakness, whether *focal* or *diffuse*, primarily *proximal* or *distal* and whether it involves a *peripheral nerve* or a *spinal segment*. Assessment of weakness is determined in a *group of muscles* (muscular dystrophy), or a *limb or limbs* (monoplegia, paraplegia, diplegia) or *one half of the body* (hemiplegia) or *all the four limbs* (quadriplegia) by assessment of tone. When muscle wasting is accompanied by fibrosis, the muscles become hard, inelastic and shortened due to contractures. Contractures develop due to prolonged hypertonia.

- **Proximal *vs* distal type of weakness.** Also determined whether muscle weakness is proximal or distal. The causes are given in Table 5.25.

Lower Motor Neuron Pathway

Lower motor neuron pathway extends from the anterior horn cells in the spinal cord (Fig. 5.34B) to the muscle spindles. The pathways passes from anterior horn cells through the motor root, peripheral nerve, myoneural junction and the muscles. The lower motor neuron thus act through the local reflex arc the afferent pathway is motor and efferent pathway is sensory containing posterior root ganglion. The lower motor neuron paralysis produces hypotonia (flaccidity), trophic changes (Table 5.24).

TABLE 5.24: Causes of Muscle Weakness

Anatomical site and type	Clinical features	Common causes
Upper motor neuron (spasticity)	• No muscle wasting • Weakness of a group of muscles or a limb or limbs or one side of the body • Hypertonia (spastic paralysis) • Hyperreflexia (exaggerated deep tendon jerks) and loss of superficial reflexes • Hypokinesia of movements	• CVA (e.g. hemiplegia), spinal cord disease or injury (paraplegia or quadriplegia) and multiple sclerosis
Lower motor neuron (flaccidity)	• Muscle atrophy • Loss of movements and muscle weakness • Hypotonia (flaccid paralysis) • Fasciculations • Absent reflexes (deep tendons as well as superficial) • Contractures of muscles • Trophic changes	• Peripheral neuropathies, radiculopathies, anterior horn cell damage (e.g. poliomyelitis), motor neuron disease (Fig. 5.35 B)
• *Peripheral neuropathy* (Fig. 5.35A)	• Symmetrical distal weakness and wasting • Symmetrical peripheral distal sensory (glove and stocking types) • Loss of peripheral tendon reflexes • Trophic changes	• *Genetic* (hereditary, motor, sensory), *metabolic* (diabetes, renal failure), *toxic* (alcohol, drugs), *inflammatory* (G.B. syndrome, leprosy), *deficiency*, e.g. B_1 and B_{12}, *other*, e.g. paramalignant
• *Myopathies*	• Muscle wasting usually proximal • Hypotonia with diminished/absent reflexes • Pseudohypertrophy of calves (Fig. 5.36) in Duchenne's muscular dystrophy • Tenderness (polymyositis)	• *Hereditary* (e.g. various muscular dystrophies), *alcohol and other toxins, collagen vascular disorder* (polymyositis)
• *Myasthenic* (Fig. 5.37)	• Abnormal fatiguability of muscles • The extraocular muscles, proximal muscles, muscles of mastication, speech and facial expression are commonly affected • Movements initially are strong but weakens with exercise or continued action • Worsening of symptoms towards the end of the day • The reflexes are preserved initially, may be lost later on • No sensory loss	1. Thymic dysplasia or tumour associated with other autoimmune disorders 2. Drug-induced, e.g. D-penicillamine, lithium, propranolol 3. Paraneoplastic-myasthenic myopathic syndrome (*Lambert-Eaton syndrome*) due to oat cell carcinoma 4. Snakebite
• *Psychogenic*	• Inconsistent weakness • No associated feature	• Stress or anxiety • Compensation claims
• *Myotonic* (inherited or acquired)	• Continued muscle contraction after cessation of voluntary effort, e.g. relaxation is impaired after muscular contraction (persistent hand grip after relaxation) • Myotonia is accentuated by rest and cold, is best demonstrated in hands, tongue and other muscles • The patient has well-developed muscles inspite of weakness • The jerks are preserved	1. Myotonia congenita 2. Paramyotonia 3. Acquired myotonia

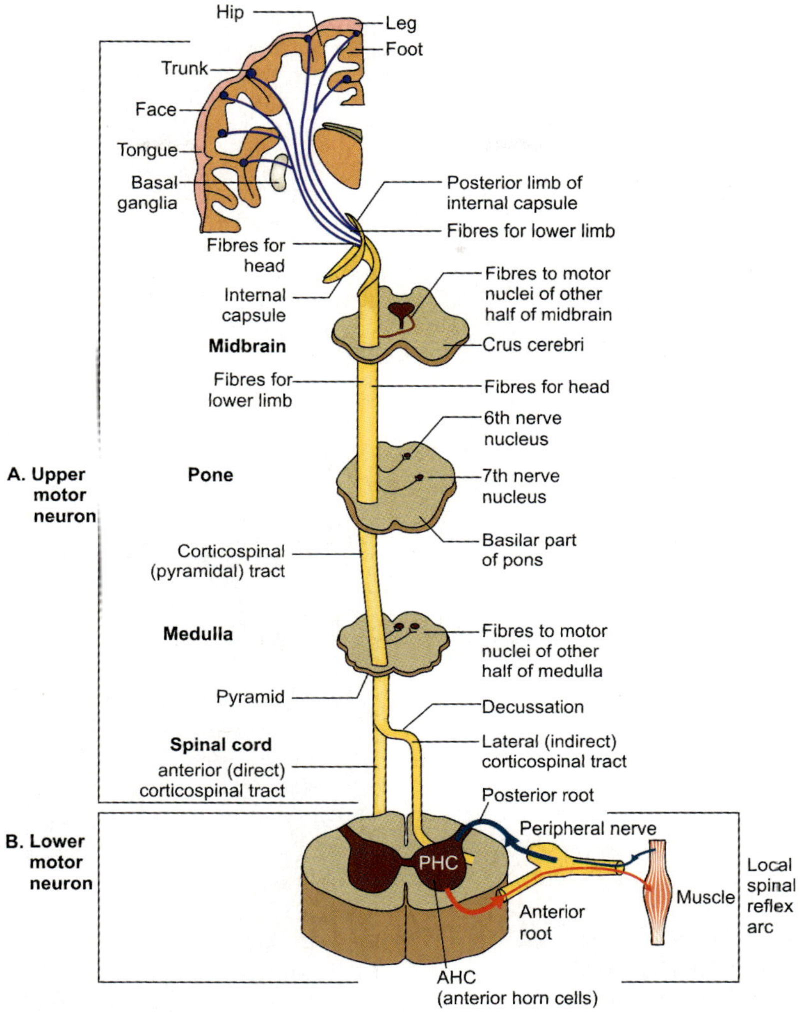

Nervous System

Fig. 5.34: (A) Diagrammatic representation of UMN and LMN. The UMNs have inhibitory control over LMN; (B) Spinal reflex arc.

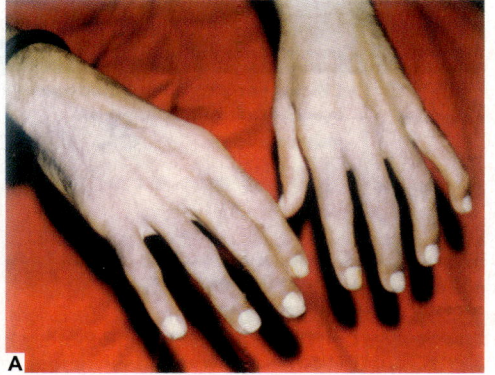
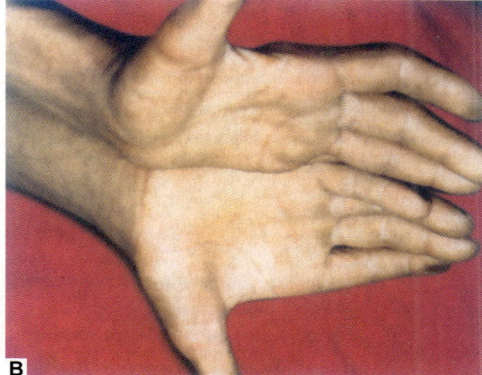

Figs 5.35A and B: Wasting of small muscles of hands. (A) In peripheral neuropathy. Note the bilateral wrist drop; (B) Motor neuron disease. Note wasting of the thenar and hypothenar muscles.

Assessment of Tone of Muscles

Tone is governed by local reflex arc (LMN) and its higher control (UMN).

Local (spinal) reflex arc (Fig. 5.34B) consists of anterior horn cells, afferent fibres (*motor root*), peripheral nerves, muscle spindles, skin and subcutaneous tissue, efferent fibres (*sensory root*) and posterior horn cells. The anterior and posterior horn cells are interconnected by internuncial neuron, e.g. *gamma* and *alpha*. Gamma neurons which are excitatory, are under control of exrapyramidal fibres and alpha neurons (inhibitory neurons) are controlled by pyramidal fibres.

Muscular tone is a state of contraction or tension. It is judged by the resistance felt when a joint is moved passively through its range of movement.

In normal person, there is slight 'elastic' type of resistance from the adjacent muscles.

☞ *Testing for the tone* (**resistance to passive movements**)

- Ask the patient to relax. Patient's attention may be diverted by talking during the test, if patient is unable to relax.

TABLE 5.25: Causes of Proximal and Distal Weakness

Proximal muscle weakness	Distal muscle weakness
(Difficulty in climbing upstairs, standing from sitting position, Gower's sign positive, Fig. 5.38) • Muscular dystrophy (Fig. 5.36) • Polymyositis • GB syndrome • Limb girdle myopathy (Fig. 5.38B) • Porphyria • Thyrotoxic or other endocrinal (Cushing) myopathies • Metabolic myopathies, e.g. diabetic amyotrophy • Periodic paralysis (e.g hypokalaemia) • Steroid-induced • Malignancy-paraneoplastic	• Polyneuropathy • Distal myopathy • Myotonic dystrophy • Charcoat-Marie-Tooth disease

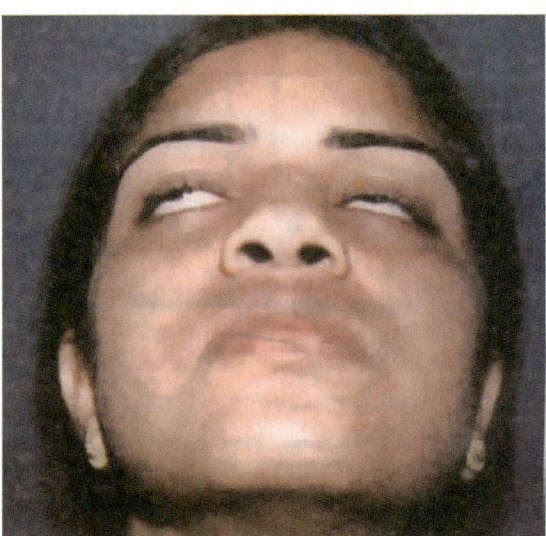

Fig. 5.37: Myasthenia gravis. A young female with myasthenia gravis developed bilateral ptosis while talking.

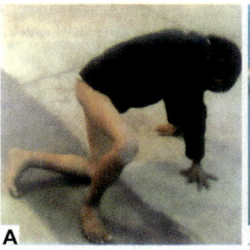 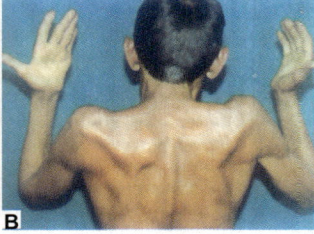

Figs 5.38A and B: (A) Positive Gower's sign in Duchenne's muscular dystrophy; (B) Fascioscapulohumeral (limb girdle) myopathy. Note the weakness/wasting of the shoulder girdle muscles and winging of the scapulae. Winging is more pronounced when patient attempts to push against a resistance, e.g. a wall or otherwise.

Fig. 5.36: Muscular dystrophy. Duchenne's muscular dystrophy with pseudohypertrophy of calf muscles.

- Passively flex and extend each joint in turn to get a feel of muscle resistance. The resistance offered by the muscles during passive movements represents the degree of tone, i.e. *normal*, *decreased* or *increased*.
- In the upper limbs, tone is tested at bigger joints, i.e. shoulder, elbow and wrist.

Remember. Spasticity in upper limbs is more obvious during attempted extension and in the lower limbs during attempted flexion.

- In the lower limbs, test the tone at the hip by internally and externally rotating the resting leg and by briskly raising the patient's knee off the bed and observing whether the ankle is also raised off the bed. Test the tone in knee muscles by flexing and extending the knee (Fig. 5.39). Similarly test the tone at ankle by dorsiflexion and plantarflexion of foot against resistance.

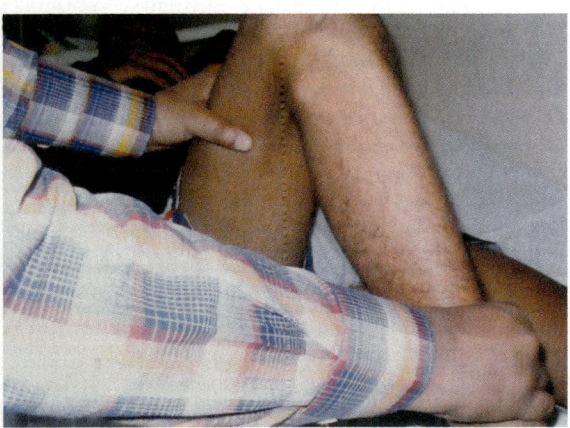

Fig. 5.39: Testing the tone of muscles at knee.

Remember. Tone is tested in the muscles acting at various joints.

Muscle contour and feel: Tone can also be tested by direct palpation of the muscles at rest. The muscles are *firm* to feel if tone is increased and *soft* to feel (flabby) if tone is decreased. Tone can be judged by shaking or swinging a normal limb or extremity passively. This is particularly useful in hypotonia when the limb will show irregular pendular movements.

Common Abnormalities

Tone is maintained by the spinal reflex arc (Fig. 5.34B) modulated by cerebellum and basal ganglia. Tone may be increased (*hypertonia*) or decreased (*hypotonia*).

Hypotonia. It refers to decreased tone, is demonstrated by loss of resistance when a limb is moved passively or when a upper limb is released from a distance falls on the bed without any resistance or when a leg is shaken, the foot moves without resistance. It occurs due to involvement of afferent or efferent limb of spinal reflex arc. Hypotonic muscles are soft on palpation. Due to hypotonia, the upper limb may assume a characteristic *Rag-doll posture* on outstretching, i.e. hyperextension at elbow with over-pronation of forearm, wrist flexed and fingers hyperextended at metacarpophalangeal joints.

Causes
- Lower motor neuron lesion, e.g. tabes, poliomyelitis (Fig. 5.40), peripheral neuropathy.
- Cerebellar disorders
- Chorea
- Tone is reduced during sleep.
- Certain drugs.
- Neuronal shock in upper motor lesion.

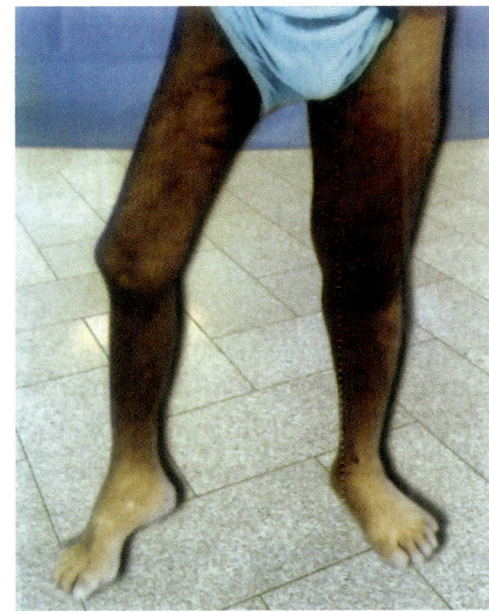

Fig. 5.40: Postpolio paralysis of right lower limb with contracture at the ankle. Patient walks on the toes due to contracture of Achilles.

Hypertonia. It manifests either as spasticity or rigidity. The *spasticity* is characterised by building-up of resistance during the early part of the passive movement, then there is sudden lessening of the resistance. It may be *clasp-knife* type where the resistance is encountered either in the beginning or at the end of a passive movement. It is seen in pyramidal lesions, e.g. hemiplegia, paraplegia, quadriplegia. Spasticity in the upper limb is infrequently more obvious on attempting extension; whereas in the lower limb it is more obvious with attempted flexion. It is associated with other signs suggestive of pyramidal lesion *(UMN signs)*.

Clonus. It is defined as rhythmic series of muscle contractions in response to sudden stretch, indicates increased tone.
- If there is hypertonia, elicit the clonus at knee *(patellar clonus)* and ankle *(ankle clonus)*. It is discussed along with deep tendon jerks.

Causes

It is seen in:
- Pyramidal lesion due to any cause (e.g. *CVA, multiple sclerosis, spinal cord injury* or *disease and degenerative spondylitic myelopathy*).

Rigidity means sustained resistance encountered throughout the range of passive movement. It may be *lead-pipe type* in which resistance is uniform throughout the passive movement due to contractions of agonists and antogonists (seen in parkinsonism) or *cog-wheel type* in which continuous resistance is broken by rhythmic jerks due to alternate contractions of agonists and antagonists regularly (jerky feel), hence, denotes rigidity with interspersed tremors. It can be enhanced by asking the patient to clinch the fists *(Jendrassik's manoeuvre)*. It is also seen in parkinsonism where tremors regularly interrupt the rigidity.

The types of rigidity are:
1. *Decerebrate rigidity (cerebral or brain stem lesions)* is characterised by typical posture in which the limbs are stiff, extended, head is erect and jaw is closed. The righting reflexes are abolished but tonic neck and labrinthine reflexes remain intact and the deep tendon jerks are exaggerated. It is due to release of vestibular nuclei from the higher pyramidal control.
2. *Hysterical rigidity* means the resistance increases proportionately with increasing force during passive movement of the limb. It is usually of long duration, precipitated by alarm, excitement or fatigue.
3. *Reflex rigidity* refers to muscle spasm in response to pain, e.g. board-like rigidity of abdomen in peritonitis, neck rigidity in meningitis.
4. *Paratonic rigidity (gegenhalten phenomenon)* refers to stiffening of a limb in response to contact and a resistance to passive changes in posture or position. The strength of antagonists increases as one increases the force to change the position of the limb. It is seen in catatonic states and in patients with clouded or confused consciousness due to any cause especially dementia.

Differences between spasticity and rigidity are enumerated in Box 5.6.

Myotonia (Fig. 5.41). It means prolonged increased tone of affected muscles which persists even after the voluntary movement has ceased and is followed by slow relaxation. Sudden movement may be followed by marked spasm and inability to relax. Repetition of movement brings about loss or decrease in hypertonicity. It is tested by *"shaking the hand with the patient and then let it go"*—produces persistence of the grip that relaxes slowly (Fig. 5.41). Similarly forcible closure of the eyes followed by sudden opening results in slow opening of the eyes. Similarly making a tight fist and holding it for few seconds and then sudden opening the fist produces slow opening of the fingers and fist and even the wrist involuntarily flexes because of sustained after contractions and delayed relaxation of the fingers. The **causes** of myotonic rigidity are *myotonic dystrophy, congenital myotonia* and *paramyotonia*.

Percussion myotonia. It can be elicited by sudden tapping the thenar eminence with a percussion hammer which is followed by apposition of the thumb that stays for several seconds before relaxation begins. It can also be elicited by tapping on the extended tongue, deltoid or other muscles where a 'dimple' is produced that relaxes slowly.

Box 5.6	Differentiation Between Spasticity and Rigidity	
Spasticity		**Rigidity**
• Seen in pyramidal lesions		• Seen in extrapyramidal lesions
• Resistance is encountered either in the beginning or at the end of passive movement		• Resistance is continuous throughout passive movement either uniform or intermittent
• It is stretch sensitive phenomenon. It is proportional to the speed of the applied stretch		• It is stretch-uniform, remains constant with application of varying stretch
• Involves only anti-gravity muscles e.g. extensors of the upper limbs and flexors of the lower limbs		• Involves all groups of muscles (agonists and antagonists) to equal extent
• Deep tendon jerks are exaggerated		• Deep tendon jerks are either normal or diminished

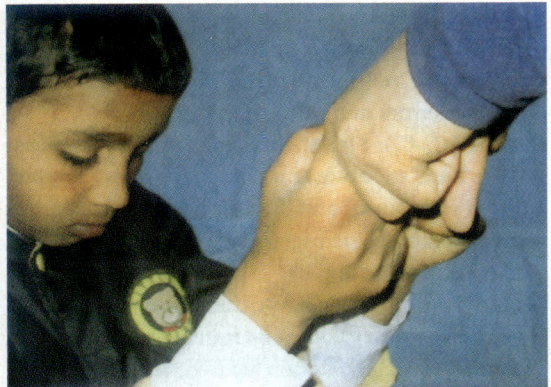

Fig. 5.41: Myotonia (persistent handgrip).

☞ *Testing of muscle strength and power*

Watching the gait and activity: Strength and muscle power can be judged quickly by watching the patient walking, standing from lying down or sitting position, during dressing and undressing and while jumping or hoping. These movements require proximal and distal strength and co-ordination of various movements and much can be learnt by observing them carefully.

There are two methods by which muscle power can be determined, *isometric* and *isotonic*. **Isometric testing** is more sensitive in detecting degree of weakness. The muscle power grading by Medical Research Council (UK) is given in Box 5.7. Using this system which is clinically based, paresis/paralysis occurs within the grade 5 range; this can be subdivided into 4+ (movement against moderate resistance) and 4− (movement against slightest resistance) to give greater precision of muscle strength.

The muscle power is tested in a group of muscles acting on a joint (Box 5.8) in case of paralysis and in individual muscle in case of myopathy, mononeuritis or compression of motor root(s). The testing of individual muscle is described separately (Table 5.26).

Box 5.7	Medical Research Council (UK) Grading of Muscle Power
Grade 0 :	No muscle contraction visible (no power)
Grade 1 :	Flicker or trace of muscle contraction but no movement of joint.
Grade 2 :	Active movement with gravity eliminated
Grade 3 :	Active movement against gravity
Grade 4 :	Movement against resistance, i.e. against moderate resistance (4+) and against slightest resistance (4−)
Grade 5 :	Normal power (active movement against full resistance)

Box 5.8	Testing of Muscle Power in a Group of Muscles Acting on a Joint

Test muscle power in proximodistal direction
A. Upper limb muscles. Test power in:
- Abductors and adductors of shoulder
- Flexors and extensors of shoulder
- Flexors and extensors of elbow
- Flexors and extensors of wrist
- Spinators and pronators of forearm
- Extensors of fingers at both the metacarpo-phalangeal and interphalangeal joints
- Finger and thumb flexors, extensors, adductors and abductors

B. Test the strength of the **abdominal muscles** as a whole by asking the supine patient to raise the head against resistance.

C. Lower limb muscles. Test power in:
- Hip flexors and extensors, adductors and abductors
- Knee flexors and extensors
- Foot dorsiflexors, plantar flexors, inverters and everters

☞ *Method of testing*
- Explain the nature and object of examination to gain full cooperation of the patient.
- Examine individual muscle groups in both limbs alternatively, or in some instances simultaneously, so that the strength of right and left can be compared.

Isometric testing: Either ask the patient to contract a group of muscles as possible and then to maintain the contracted position while the examiner tries to overpower the muscle group being tested. This is called *isometric testing*. It is more sensitive in detecting the degree of paresis.

Or

Isotonic testing: Ask the patient to move the joint while examiner attempting to halt the movement. This is called *isotonic testing* of strength.

> **N.B.** Remember that false findings will be recorded during pain, loss of proprioceptive sensations and muscle fatigue (myasthenia gravis). Therefore, it is advisable to feel or palpate the contraction of the muscle, wherever accessible.

Common Abnormalities

By testing a group of muscle, one can identify the type of weakness in a group of muscle or muscles, or a limb or one-half side of the body. The causes of such weakness have already been discussed in Table 5.24. If such a weakness is found, a more detailed examination of muscles, peripheral nerve or spinal segment should be undertaken.

☞ *Testing for the individual muscles of upper and lower limbs (Table 5.26 and Fig. 5.43)*

It is useful to test the individual muscle(s) in myopathy and radiculopathy.

THE REFLEXES

I. Primitive Reflexes Testing

In organic brain disorders (diffuse degenerative disorders) certain reflexes released from the control of higher centre may be elicitable. All these primitive reflexes appear during infancy, disappear during childhood and adulthood, reappear or released during damage to higher centres by diffuse organic disease. Some reflexes such as *grasp reflex* may be elicitable even in focal lesions in frontal lobe disease. The important higher level reflexes are:

- *Grasp and avoiding reflexes*
- *Palmomental reflex*
- *Snout and sucking reflexes*
- *Glabellar tap reflex*

All these reflexes are under higher control, get released when the higher control centres, e.g. frontal lobe(s) is diseased or damaged.

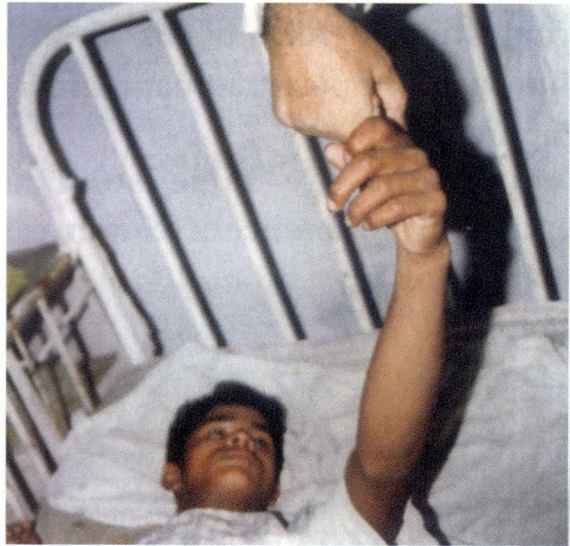

Fig. 5.42: Grasp reflex. The patient tries to grasp the finger of examiner hand.

A. Grasping and avoiding reflexes: Grasp reflex is elicited by stroking the lateral aspect of palm of the patient's hand by firmly moving a stimulus (pencil or examiner's finger) distally between the patient's thumb and forefinger (Fig. 5.42). The patient's hand tries to grasp the object or move towards it to grasp it. This grasp reflex is not inhibited even if the patient's attention is diverted. If observer tries to pull the object or his/her finger (used as a stimulus)

The avoiding response (reflex). It is usually elicited by applying the stimulus on the ulnar side of the hand. Patient tries to move away or withdraws his/her hand away from stimulus.

Both grasping and avoiding reflexes or responses are elicited in patients with contralateral frontal lobe disease, e.g. Alzheimer's disease.

B. The palmomental reflex: Stroke the skin of the palm near the thenar eminence, there is contraction of ipsilateral mental muscle (a subcutaneous muscle) causing puckering of the chin.

C. Snout and sucking reflexes: Apply gentle pressure by your knuckles against the patient's lips, there is puckering of the orbicularis oris (forming a snout). Similarly, the reflex can be elicited by tapping the finger placed on the lips with a tendon hammer or with a finger of other hand, there is contraction of facial musculature.

Sucking reflex is just an anticipatory opening of the mouth in response to visual stimuli, e.g. shining the metal end of a tunning fork or just touching cheeks near the corner of the mouth.

D. Glabellar tap reflexes (Fig. 5.44): A series of finger tap at the glabella normally produces two or three blinks and then response is inhibited, but in *Parkinsonism* or *diffuse degenerative disorders*, the response is not inhibited, i.e. each glabellar tap is followed by a blink.

II. Tendon Reflexes (Jerks)

These are phasic, monosynaptic stretch reflexes involving only two neurons and a particular spinal segment. They are based on the principle that a sudden stretch of a tendon excites a valley of impulses that travel along the sensory (afferent) side of spinal reflex arc and reach the muscle via the efferent (motor) side of the arc and causes it to contract briefly which can be seen and felt. Thus, it tests the integrity of afferent, efferent pathways and their interconnections in the anterior horn cells in the spinal segment supply of that muscle.

Method of Elicitation

- Always use same type of hammer.
- Always examine these reflexes in the same manner.

Nervous System

TABLE 5.26: Testing of the Muscles (Figs 5.43A to CC)

Figure	Root value	Muscle testing
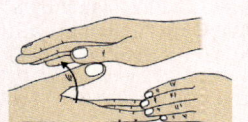 **Fig. 5.43A:** Testing the abductor pollicis brevis.	C_6, C_7	*Abductor pollicis brevis.* The patient is asked to abduct the thumb at right angle to the palmar surface of the index finger (Fig. 5.43A) against resistance of the examiner's thumb. The muscle normally is seen and felt to contract during this manoeuvre but fails to do so if median nerve is involved (e.g. carpal tunnel syndrome) or there is atrophy of the small muscles of the hand.
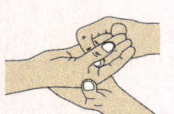 **Fig. 5.43B:** Testing the opponens pollicis.	C_6, C_7	*Opponens pollicis:* Instruct the patient to touch the top of the little finger with the top of the thumb. Oppose this movement with your thumb or index finger (Fig. 5.43B). Feel for the resistance; failure to do so indicates paralysis.
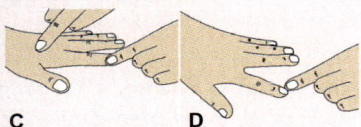 **Figs 5.43C and D:** (C) Testing the first dorsal interosseous muscle; (D) Testing the first palmar interosseous muscle.		*Testing the interossei muscles* (First dorsal interrosseous, Fig. 5.43C). Instruct the patient to separate the thumb from the fingers. Now ask him/her to abduct the index finger against your resistance failure to do so indicates paralysis of ulnar nerve or atrophy of small muscles of hand. *First palmar interosseous* (Fig. 5.43D). Ask the patient to adduct the index finger of pronated hand against resistance.
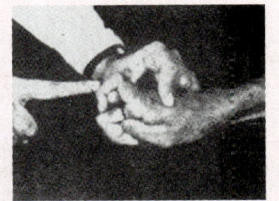 **Fig. 5.43E:** Testing for interossei and lumbricals.	C_8-T_1	*Testing of other interossei and lumbricals* Test the ability of the patient to flex their metacarpophalangeal joint and extend the distal interphalangeal joints (Fig. 5.43E). The interossei are adductors (palmar interossei) and abductors (dorsal interrosei) of fingers. A clawhand deformity is produced if they are paralysed such as ulnar nerve palsy. This is due to retention of power in the long flexors and extensors of the two fingers. The first phalanges are overextened and the distal two are flexed. There is separation of the fingers.
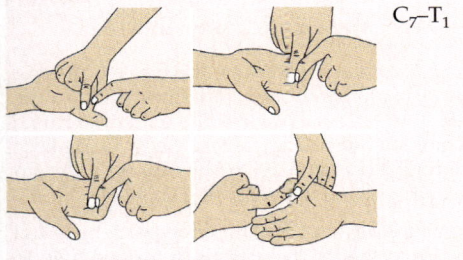 **Fig. 5.43F:** Testing the long flexors of the fingers.	C_7-T_1	*Testing of long flexors* of fingers (e.g. flexor digitorum profundus I, II and III (C_7-T_1) and flexor digitorum sublimis (C_7, C_8)). The long flexors are individually tested by flexion at the interphalangeal joints as demonstrated in Fig. 5.43F. The long flexors are simultaneously tested by asking the patient to squeeze your fingers. Allow the patient to squeeze only your index and middle fingers; this is sufficient to assess strength of hand grip (Fig. 5.43G). 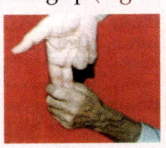 **Fig. 5.43G:** Testing the power of the small muscles of the hand
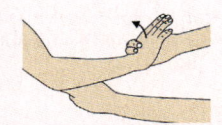 **Fig. 5.43H:** Testing the extensor carpi radialis longus C6, C7.	C_6, C_7	*Flexors and extensors of the wrist.* Ask the patient to make the fist. This results in forcible contraction of both the flexors and extensors of the wrist. To test the extensors of the wrist (Fig. 5.43H), ask the patient to extend the wrist against resistence. If the extensors are weak, then he/she can not do so. If extensors are weak, the wrist becomes flexed leading to wrist drop as occurs in radial nerve paralysis.

Contd.

Figure	Root value	Muscle testing
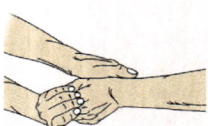 Fig. 5.43I: Testing the flexor carpi radialis.		To test the flexors of wrist, ask the patient to squeeze your fingers. The grip will be weak, if flexors are weak. Now ask the patient to make the fist and try to overcome the wrist-flexion by your hand (Fig. 5.43I). Failure to do so indicate paralysis of wrist flexion
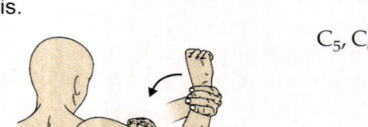 Fig. 5.43J: Testing the biceps.	C_5, C_6 C_5, C_6	*Flexors of the elbow* **Biceps:** It is tested by asking the patient to bend the supine forearm against resistance. The muscle contracts and stands out prominently (Fig. 5.43J). **Brachioradialis:** Place the forearm midway between prone and supine positions. Now direct the patient to flex the forearm against resistance. The muscle is seen to contract and stands out prominently at the upper part of forearm.
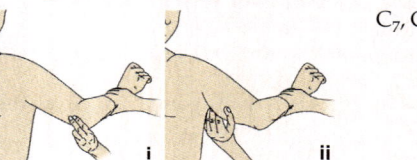 Fig. 5.43K: Testing the triceps: (i) Long head; (ii) The whole muscle.	C_7, C_8	*Extensor of the elbow.* **Triceps:** It is tested by asking the patient to extend the forearm against resistance (Fig. 5.43K (i) and (ii)). The muscle is seen to contract and stands out prominently at the back of arm.
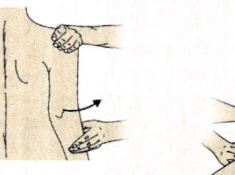 Fig. 5.43L: Testing the supraspinatus (e.g. abduction between 0 and 30°). 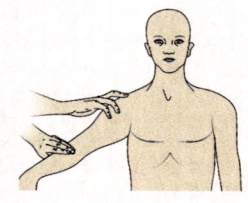 Fig. 5.43M: Testing the deltoid (e.g. abduction between 30° and 90°).		*Abductors of the shoulder.* *Supraspinatus and deltoid:* These are abductors of shoulder. The first 30° movement (0–30°) is carried out by the supraspinatus and rest 60° (30° to 90°) is carried out by deltoid. *Method:* Ask the patient to abduct the forearm against resistance. The first 30° is tested for supraspinatus (Fig. 5.43L). Now ask the patient to abduct the arm to 30° and now further abduct the arm against resistance. The deltoid contracts and is seen and felt (Fig. 5.25M) Abduction becomes weak if these muscles are paralysed.
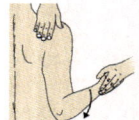 Fig. 5.43N: Testing the infraspinatus.		*Infraspinatus* is an external rotator at shoulder. It is tested by asking the patient to keep the arm along the side of the chest and flex the forearm at right angle (Fig. 5.43N). Now ask the patient to rotate the limb externally against your resistance, the elbow being kept along the side throughout the manoeuvre. The muscle belly can be seen and felt by keeping your hand below the spine of scapula. *Pectorals:* Pectoralis major is flexor of the shoulder. It can be tested by asking the patient to outstretch the arms in front and then to clap the hands together while you resist the movement and try to hold them apart (Fig. 5.43O). The muscle is seen and felt to contract and stands out prominently in front of chest. *Serratus anterior:* This is the scapular muscle which keeps the scapula tight to the chest, hence, its paralysis produces separation of the scapula from the vertebral column called "winging of the scapula", and patient is unable to lift the arm above a right angle.
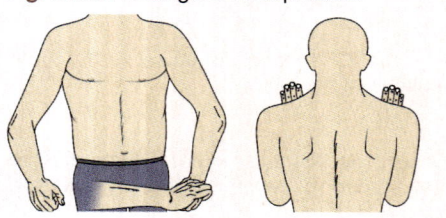 Fig. 5.43O: Testing the pectoralis major. Fig. 5.43P: Testing the serratus anterior.		Serratus anterior The muscle is tested by asking the patient to push against a wall, the muscle contracts and keeps the scapula bound to chest (Fig. 5.43P), paralysis produces winging of scapula.

Contd.

Nervous System

Figure	Root value	Muscle testing

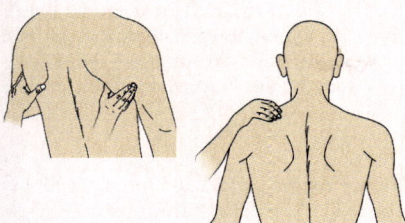

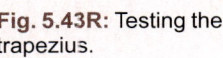

Fig. 5.43Q: Testing the latissimus dorsi.

Fig. 5.43R: Testing the trapezius.

Latissimus dorsi: Stand behind the patient. Ask the patient to clasp the hands behind their back. Offer resistance to the backward and outward movement. The muscle bellies stand are prominently as the posterior axillary folds which can be seen and felt (Fig. 5.43Q). Alternately the muscles can be tested by asking the patient to cough forcibly. The muscles contract and make the posterior axillary fold prominent.

Trapezius: Ask the patient to shrug his or her shoulder while the examiner opposes this movement. (Fig. 5.43R), or ask the patient to place the shoulder backwards. Trapezius stands out prominently during this manoeuvre.

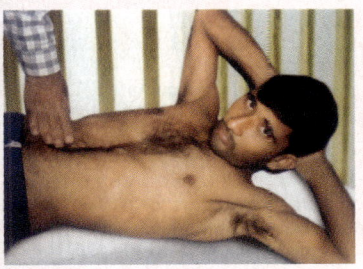

Fig. 5.43S: Testing of rectus abdominis.

Muscles of the trunk

Abdominal muscles: Rectus abdominis is the muscle supplied by ventral rami of T_7–T_{12}. The upper portion (above the umbilicus) is supplied from T_7 to T_9 and lower portion from T_{10}–T_{12}. The main action of the muscle is flexion of the spine testing. Ask the patient to lie supine and elevate his/her body from the pillow without support or against resistance. You can see and feel the contractions of rectus abdominis on both the sides (Fig. 5.43S) and umbilicus is central. In case of paralysis on one side, the umbilicus will be pulled to the other side by the unopposed action of nonparalysed muscle. Paralysis of a portion of anterior abdominal muscle will displace the umbilicus either upwards (lower abdominal muscles paralysis) or downwards (upper abdominal muscle-paralysis). This is called *Beevor's sign*, helps to localise the lesion in spinal cord disease.

Muscles of the lower limbs

1. *Testing the small muscles of the foot.* The small muscles of the foot are tested for *adduction*, *abduction* of toes and great toe similar to the small muscles of the hand. Interossei are again adductors and abductors in the foot. Paralysis of the interosseous produces foot deformity. Similarly foot deformity occurs in a, patient with hemiplegia. Pes cavus is hollowing of the sole, occurs in familial peripheral neuropathy.

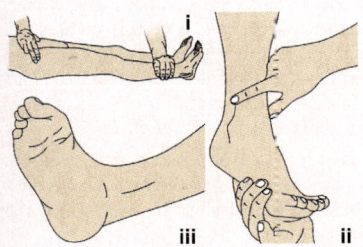

Fig. 5.43T: Testing the muscles of foot: (i) Tibialis posterior (e.g. invertor of foot); (ii) Peroneus longus and peroneus brevis (main evertors of the foot); (iii) Wasting of small muscles of the sole produce foot deformity.

2. *Dorsiflexion and plantar flexion of toes and the feet* are tested by asking the patient to elevate or depress the part against resistance. The inverters and evertors are tested as given in the Fig. 5.43T.

3. *Extensors and flexors of knee:* The extensor (quadriceps) of the knee is tested by bending the knee of the patient with your hand and then asking the patient to extend it against your resistance. Contraction of this muscle can be seen and felt in the thigh (Fig. 5.43U).

   Flexors of the knee (biceps femoris, semitendinosus, semi membranosus) are tested by asking the patient to lie prone. Now flex the knee against resistance. The muscles can be seen and felt on lateral side (biceps) and medial side (semimembranosus) respectively (Fig. 5.43V).

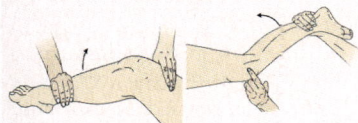

Fig. 5.43U: Testing the quadriceps femoris.

Fig. 5.43V: Testing the hamstring muscles.

4. *Extensors of the hip:* (e.g. gluteus maximus and hamstrings). Ask the patient to lie supine with knees extended. Lift the foot off the bed and keep the palm of your hand below the foot. Ask him/her to push it down against your resistance (Fig. 5.43W). Judge the power in the extensors of the hip by estimating the resistance.

Contd.

Figure	Root value	Muscle testing

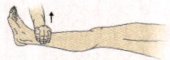

Fig. 5.43W: Testing the extensors of hip.   Fig. 5.43X: Testing the flexors of hip.

5. *Flexors of the hip* (e.g. Iliacus, psoas major and psoas minor). Ask the patient to lie supine with legs extended. Ask the patient to raise the leg (flex the leg) off the bed against resistance (Fig. 5.43X). Assess the resistance to decide power in the muscles.

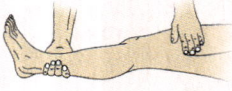

Fig. 5.43Y: Testing the adductors of hip.

Adductors of hip (e.g. *adductor longus, adductor brevis, adductor magnus,* gracilis and pectineus). Adductors are flexor of thigh also. Ask the patient to lie supine with legs separated but straight. Now ask the patient to move the limb towards midline against resistance (Fig. 5.43Y). Assess the power in the muscles from the resistance offered.

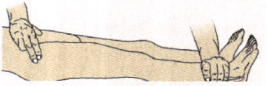

Fig. 5.43Z: Testing the abductors of the thigh (hip).

Abductors of the hip (e.g. gluteus medius and gluteus minimus). Place the patient's legs together while the patient is supine. Ask him/her to separate them against resistance (Fig. 5.43Z). Assess the power in the muscles.

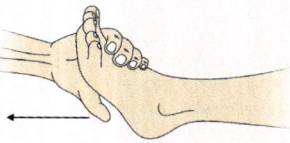

Fig. 5.43AA: Testing the medial (internal) rotation of hip.

Rotators of the hip: Lateral or external rotators (e.g. obturator internus, quadriceps femoris). *Medial rotators* (e.g. obturator externus): To test the rotators, ask the patient to lie supine with limbs extended. Now ask him/her to roll the limb outwards (lateral rotation) or inwards (medial rotation) against resistance (Fig. 5.43AA).

"*Babinski's rising up sign*". In the abdominal muscles weakness, patient is not able to rise from the bed with out support. Babinski's rising up sign is elicited by asking the patient to lie supine with legs extended and rise up without support. Normally the legs do not rise. In spastic paralysis (UMN paralysis) of a leg such as in hemiplegia, the affected limb will rise first, but in hysterical paralysis or malingering, this does not occur, hence, this sign differentiates hysterical weakness from spastic weakness.

Erector spinae: The erector spinae and back extensors are tested by asking the patient to lie prone and lift the head from the bed by extending the neck and back. Normally, they can be seen standing out and prominently during manoeuvre.

Neck muscles

Neck flexors (e.g. *longus collis* C_2, C_6, *longus capitis* C_1 to C_3; *rectus capitis anterior* C_1 to C_2, *sternomastoid* C_2, C_3, and XI cranial nerve, *scalenus anterior*; C_4–C_6) are tested by asking the patient to flex the neck while you resist this movement by placing your hand at the forehead. Note the amount of resistance which you have to apply for this.

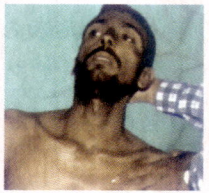

Fig. 5.43BB: Testing the neck extensors.

Neck extensors (e.g. *semispinalis capitis, longissimus capitis, rectus capitis posterior major and minor*) are tested similarly as flexors. Ask the patient to extend neck against your resistance (Fig. 5.43BB). Assess the amount of resistance used. Neck rotator (e.g. sternomastoid) testing has been discussed in examination of XI cranial nerve.

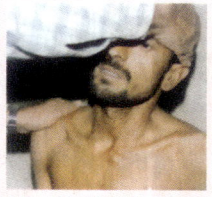

Fig. 5.43CC: Testing the lateral bending.

Lateral bending of the neck (e.g. *sternomastoid, scalenus anterior, splenius cervicalis, rectus capitis lateralis*) is tested by asking the patient to bend the neck laterally against resistance (Fig. 5.43CC) or first bend the neck laterally and then try to counteract this bending to assess the power to be used.

Nervous System

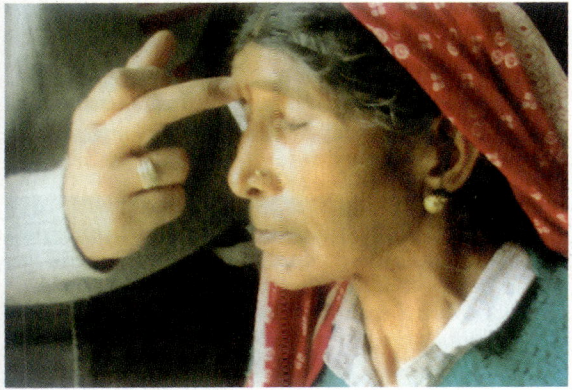

Fig. 5.44: Elicitation of glabellar sign.

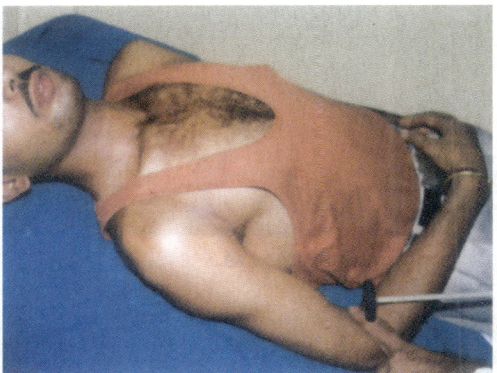

Fig. 5.45: Biceps jerk.

- Always stand on the side of the bed.
- Always make sure that patient is warm and comfortable.
- Reassure the patient that hammer is soft, will not cause any harm. Let the patient should feel it or examine it.
- The patient should be asked to be relaxed, i.e. "let the muscles go to sleep".
- Expose the part to be examined properly by putting off the clothes. In the lower limb examination, the genitalia to be properly covered and protected.
- The reflexes can easily be tested with the patient supine on a couch/bed, but some neurologists prefer to elicit the jerks with the patient sitting on the edge of the couch facing the examiner.
- Strike the tendon to stimulate stretch receptors in muscles by a sharp blow struck with percussion hammer at 90° to the direction of pull. Strike the tendon not the muscle. Since mechanical stimulation of a muscle belly may produce contraction of that muscle which is not dependant on that reflex arc.
- Grade the response observed (read the grading).

A. Upper Limb Reflexes

1. **Biceps (C_5–C_6):** Flex the elbow to right angle and place the forearm in midprone position. Place your thumb or index finger on the biceps tendon in anticubital fossa and tap the tendon with the hammer. The biceps contracts and flexes the elbow (Fig. 5.45).
   - **Inversion of biceps and supinator.** This means brisk finger flexion following elicitation of biceps or supinator jerks. It indicates C_5–C_6 lesion with loss of biceps and supinator reflexes. This is due to hypertonicity of finger flexors muscles.

2. **Supinator (C_5–C_6):** Place the forearm in midprone position. Tap the styloid process of the radius. The supinator contracts followed by flexion and supination of forearm (Fig. 5.46).

3. **Triceps (C_6–C_7):** Flex the elbow and allow the forearm and the hand to rest over the patient's chest. Support the forearm with your hand and tap the triceps tendon just below olecranon.

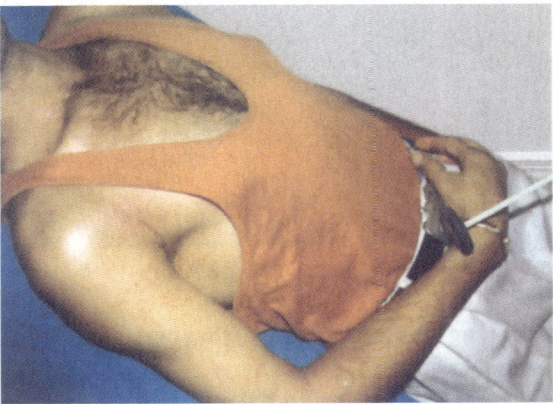

Fig. 5.46: Supinator jerk.

The triceps contracts which can be seen or felt (Fig. 5.47).
   - **Inversion of triceps:** On tapping the tendon at olecranon, there is flexion of the forearm with flexion of fingers. It signifies the cord lesion at C_8.

4. **Finger flexion (C_7–C_8):** Ask the patient to semiflex the fingers. Place your middle and index fingers on the palmar surface of the hand. Sudden tap over the fingers will cause flexion of the fingers and the thumb (Fig. 5.48).

5. **Hoffmann's sign (Fig. 5.49):** The patient's hand is pronated and observer holds the index or middle

finger of the patient between his/her thumb and index finger of left hand. Briskly flick down the patient's finger tip with the right thumb and release it suddenly. Observe the movement of the thumb.

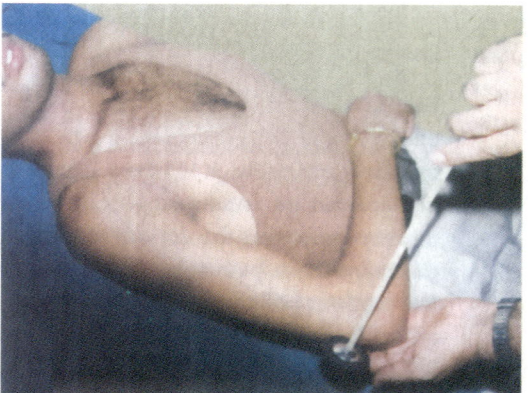

Fig. 5.47: Elicitation of triceps jerk during lying down. The some reflex can be elicited in the sitting position also.

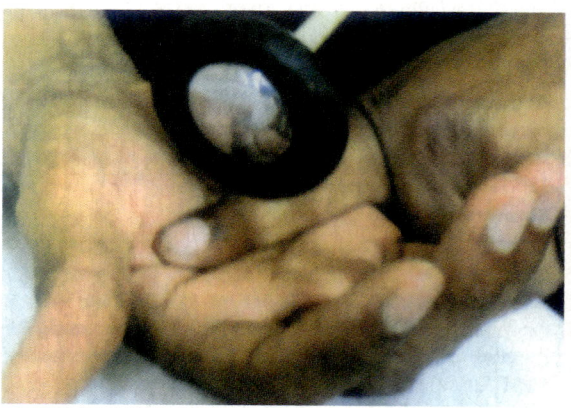

Fig. 5.48: Finger flexion jerk.

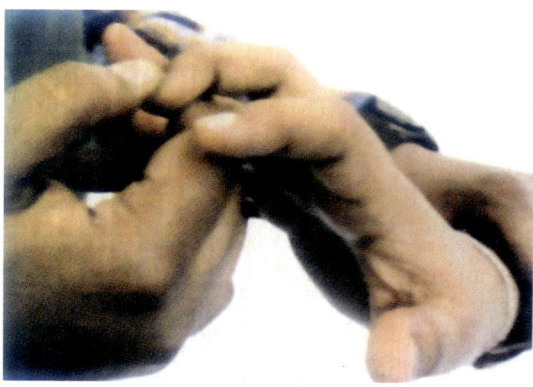

Fig. 5.49: Hoffmann's sign.

The sign is elicited when the upper limb jerks are exaggerated. It has significance similar to clonus in lower limbs. A positive response results in adduction and flexion of the thumb and flexion of fingers.

6. **Wartenberg's sign (Fig. 5.50):** Hook the patient's fingers except the thumb of right hand with your right hand. Try to pull the fingers with your hand. Observe the movement of the thumb. Normally, the thumb adducts with this manoeuvre, but flexion of the thumb indicates positive response. It carries same significance as the Hoffmann's sign.
7. **Jaw jerk (Vth cranial nerve).** It has been discussed under examination of Vth cranial nerve.
8. **Pectoral reflex (C_7):** This reflex may sometime be useful in localisation of the lesion. It is usually not elicited but can be employed if needed. Place the extended index and middle fingers on the lateral border of the pectoralis muscle and tap it with percussion hammer. The muscle contracts.

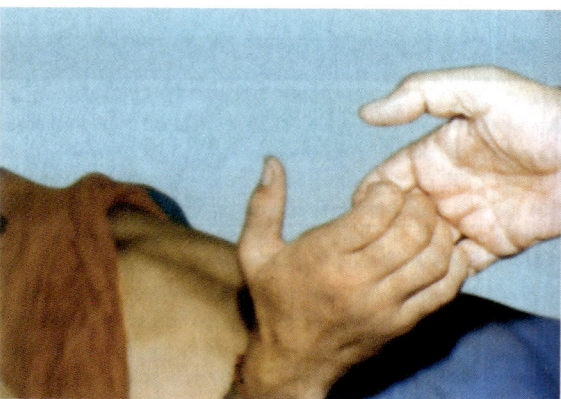

Fig. 5.50: Wartenberg's sign.

9. **Deltoid reflex (C_5):** The upper fibres of deltoid are supplied by XI cranial nerve and lower fibres by C_5. Place the finger across the tip of shoulder and tap it. The deltoid contracts.

B. Lower Limb Reflexes

1. **Knee jerk (L_2, L_3, L_4):** It is tested with patient supine. Place your hand or forearm under the knee (Fig. 5.51) to be tested and may be crossed on the opposite knee so that legs do not come in contact with each other and knee rests on the observer's hand or forearm. Strike the tendon just below the patella and observe for the contraction of quadriceps muscle in the thigh as well as extension of the knee. Both the knee jerks can be elicited simultaneously by this method by putting the arm under both the knees

and tapping them below the patella. *Alternatively*, the reflex can sometimes be tested easily with the patient sitting up, the legs hanging freely over the edge of the bed. The patient may then cross one knee over the other.

Inverted knee jerk: On eliciting the knee jerk. Instead of extension of the knee (normal knee jerk), there is flexion of the knee due to strong contraction of hamstrong muscles. This indicates a lesion at L_2, L_3 and L_4 segments.

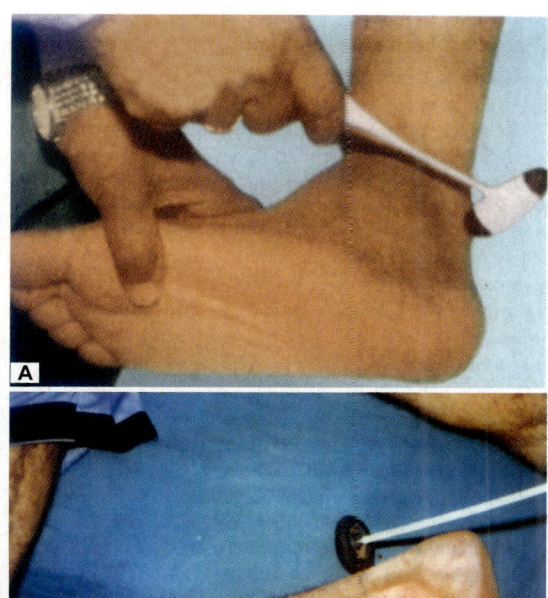

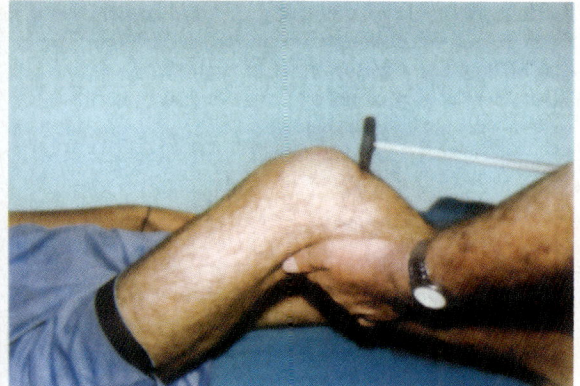

Fig. 5.51: Knee jerk.

Figs 5.52A and B: Elicitation of the ankle jerk. (A) Conventional method; (B) Alternative method.

Pendular knee jerk: While eliciting a knee jerk there will be *to and fro movements* of legs several times (more than 3 times) before coming to rest. It indicaes cerebellar disease. It is tested in sitting position, the legs haning freely over the edge of the bed.

2. Ankle jerk (S_r, S_2): Place the lower limb on the bed so that it lies everted and slightly flexed. Stretch the Achilles tendon slightly by dorsiflexing the foot (Fig. 5.52A) with the other hand. Now, tap the tendon on its posterior surface of the ankle. Observe the contraction of the calf muscles as well as plantar-flexion of ankle.

Alternatively, the reflex can be elicited when the patient is kneeling on a chair or stool with his/her feet hanging over the edge (Fig. 5.52B). The ankle is dorsifixed sufficiently and blow is delivered.

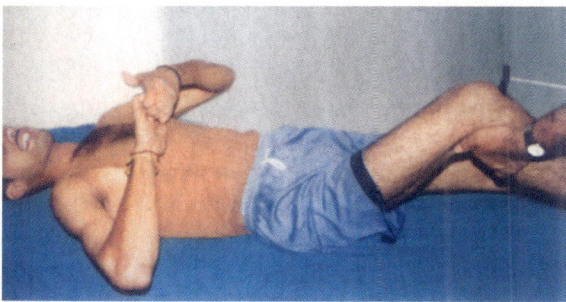

Fig. 5.53: Reinforcement phenomenon (Jendrassik's manoeuvre).

Reinforcement or Jendrassik's manoeuvre (Fig. 5.53). It is a manoeuvre used to elicit the tendon reflexes when either they are not elicitable or barely elicitable. It is based on the principle that motor activity can be enhanced by contracting another muscle thereby increasing the activity of gamma efferent system. In this manoeuvre, patient is asked to clench the teeth or clench the fist of ipsilateral hand or pull the flexed fingers of two hands against each other.

CLONUS

Remember. Once the deep tendon reflexes are found to be exaggerated, then proceed to elicit the clonus.

Knee clonus (patellar clonus). Patient lies supine with knees extended. Give sudden jerk to the patella initially, followed by sustained pressure with the thumb and index finger in a downward direction on the patella (Fig. 5.54). Feel for the intermittent jerky movements due to muscle contractions.

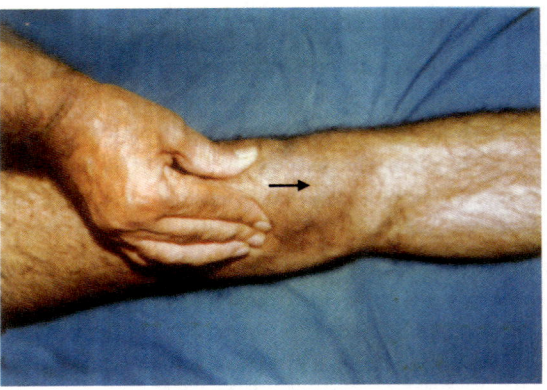

Fig. 5.54: Patellar clonus (→)

Ankle clonus (Fig. 5.55). Support the flexed knee with one hand in the popliteal fossa so that ankle rests gently off the bed. Dorsiflex the foot briskly with the other hand and sustain the pressure. Inspect and feel for sustained movements of foot due to involuntary muscle contractions of hypertonic muscles.

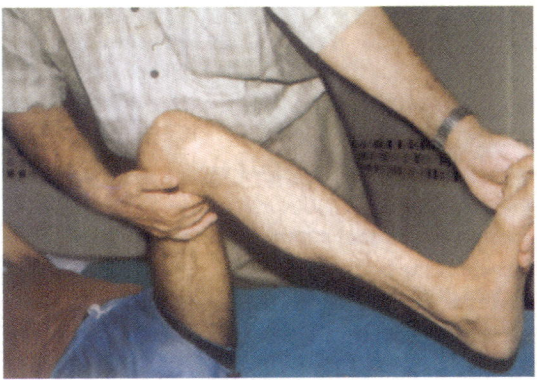

Fig. 5.55: Ankle clonus.

Wrist clonus. Make the patient lie supine and rest. Grasp the hand and passively flex/extend at the wrist joint 3 times, the last time in full extension for several seconds. Feel for any involuntary movements of hand.

Movements of hands >2 times in the extended posture indicates clonus.

N.B. A few beats of clonus are present in a normal person particularly tense or anxious persons having normal plantar response, hence called *ill-sustained clonus* or *unsustained clonus*.
- Presence of clonus indicated grade IV status of reflexes (read grading below)

Grading of Reflexes

The tendon reflexes are graded as below:
Grade 0 : Absent
Grade I : Present (a normal jerk)
Grade II : Brisker than normal.
Grade III : Very brisk (exaggerated).
Grade IV : Associated with clonus in case of knee or ankle jerk.

Abnormalities of Tendon Jerks

The tendon reflexes may be *increased*, *decreased* or *absent*, and sometimes may have *pendular quality*. Normal jerk is defined as sudden contraction followed by sudden relaxation. The abnormal jerks are discussed below.

I. Increased reflexes (hyper-reflexia): It means the jerks are brisk or exaggerated as compared to normal and/or if one side is involved, then brisker than the other side.

Causes

A. Generalised exaggeration of reflexes
- Upper motor neuron lesion of brain and spinal cord. In spinal cord compression, the jerks are increased below the level of compression.
- Anxiety or nervousness due to sympathetic overactivity.
- Thyrotoxicosis due to sympathetic overactivity.
- Tetanus due to spasms of muscles.
- Hysteria (voluntary hypertonicity).
- Strychnine poisoning (hypertonicity).
- Fright (sympathetic overactivity).
- Tetany (excessive muscular excitability).

B. Unilateral exaggeration of reflexes
- Hemiplegia (jerks are exaggerated on the side involved)
- Unilateral spinal cord lesion (hemisection of spinal cord)

II. Decreased reflexes (hyporeflexia) or absent reflexes (areflexia)

Causes

A. Bilateral/generalised decreased/absent reflexes
- Lower motor neuron lesion involving the local reflex arc, i.e. polio, neuropathy, myasthenia and myopathy.
- Neuronal/spinal shock in UMN lesion.
- Muscle contractures due to marked spasticity/rigidity.

- Normal individual who are unable to relax.

B. Unilateral decreased/absent reflexes
- Paresis of single nerve or a few nerve roots subserving the reflex or reflexes, i.e. radiculopathy and a group or groups of muscles paralysis.

III. Pendular jerks
- Cerebellar disease. This is due to combination of ataxia and hypotonia in cerebellar disease.
- Chorea.

IV. Myotonic jerks (hung-up reflex): In this type of jerks, contraction and the relaxation phase of the jerks is prolonged (slightly hung), i.e. the jerks are slower than normal with prolonged relaxation. Myotonic jerk can be elicited in the same way as the pendular jerk. Here the jerk remain in prolonged contracted phase (called hung up), the slow relaxation.

Causes
- Myxoedema (delayed relaxation is typical)
- Hypothermia

THE SUPERFICIAL REFLEXES

Pathway
The superficial reflexes have, in addition to a local *spinal reflex arc*, a superimposed cortical pathway—a *cerebral arc*. Impulses ascend through the spinal cord and brain stem to the sensory parietal cortex, jump to the motor cortex through cerebral connections. The efferent impulses from the motor cortex pass down the pyramidal tracts to the anterior horn cells of the brain stem and spinal cord at each level. Hence, a lesion of the reflex arc or a upper motor neuron lesion involving pyramidal tract will abolish these superficial reflexes.

Remember: There is a paradox in the UMN lesion where the deep tendon jerks are exaggerated but the superficial reflexes are absent. While in LMN lesion, both (deep and superficial reflexes) are absent.

Alteration of Superficial Reflexes

Loss of Reflexes
- Unilateral loss of reflexes occur in UMN lesion on that side.
- Unilateral loss of reflexes also occur due to involvement of dermatomes of spinal arc (LMN). This loss of reflex(es) has clinical significance in localisation of the lesion.

Exaggeration of Reflexes
The superficial reflexes are exaggerated in *chorea, parkinsonism* and *amyotrophic lateral sclerosis, anxiety* or *hysteria* (as a part of general hyperreflexia). It has been believed that lesion involving the red nucleus is associated with increased superficial reflexes.

Elicitation of Superficial Reflexes
1. **The superficial abdominal reflex [(T_6–T_{12}): Upper T_6–T_9 and lower T_{10}–T_{12})]**
   - Position the patient supine with relaxed upper limbs by the side of the body. Ask the patient to relax the abdomen.
   - Stroke the upper and lower quadrants of the abdominal wall on each side lightly with a key or a wooden stick from outside inwards (Fig. 5.56). It does not matter much whether you stroke from outside inwards or inwards to outwards.
   - Observe any muscle contraction.

Normally, following a stimulus there is reflex homolateral contraction of the anterior abdominal muscles, retraction of linea alba and the umbilicus towards the quadrant stimulated.

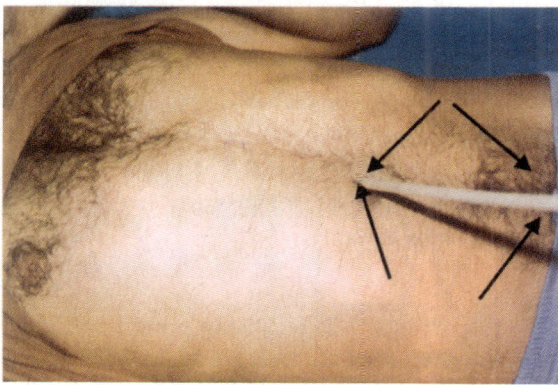

Fig. 5.56: Abdominal reflexes.

The causes of absent abdominal reflexes are
a. Unilateral loss
   - Lesions of the reflex spinal arc involving segmental innervation of these reflexes on that side
   - UMN lesion above the spinal level T_6–T_{12} on that side.
b. Bilateral loss
   - Marked obesity or overdistended abdomen such as ascites (bilateral loss).
   - Multiparous women with lax abdomen (bilateral loss).
   - In anxious and elderly patients.

2. **Cremasteric reflex (L_r–L_2)**
   - Position the patient with thigh externally rotated and legs separated (abducted)
   - Stroke the skin of inner upper thigh with a stick (Fig. 5.57) from below upwards.
   - Observe the upwards movement of the ipsilateral testicle.

Normal response is the contraction of the cremasteric muscle with elevation of ipsilateral testicle.

The causes of absent cremasteric reflex are
- Lesions involving the spinal dermatome L_1 – L_2.
- Pyramidal lesion.
- Hydrocoele.
- Hernia.
- Older persons

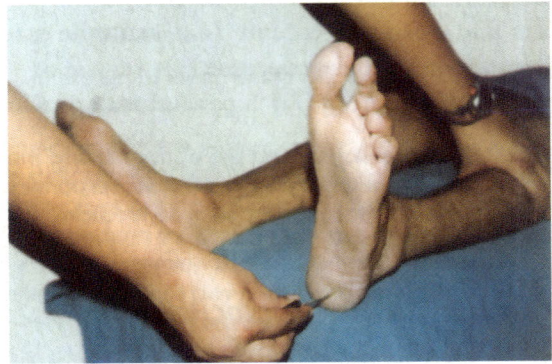

Fig. 5.58: Methods of eliciting plantar response.

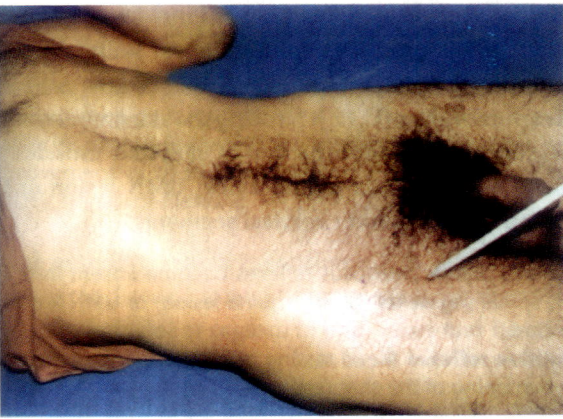

Fig. 5.57: Cremasteric reflex.

The absent reflex has a localising value. Its absence indicates either the lower motor neuron lesion involving L_1–L_2 segments or UMN lesion of the cord above this level.

3. **The plantar reflex (Fig. 5.58)**
It is also a superficial reflex
- Place the patient supine in relaxed position with knees extended. If patient is not sufficiently relaxed, engage him/her in conversation so as to distract his/her attention.
- Just hold the ankle with left hand above the foot or over the knee so as to prevent withdrawl of the foot.
- Gently stroke the outer edge of the sole of the foot by a key or a stick from the heel towards little toe and then medially across the metatarsus. Note the response.

Normal plantar reflex response is flexion of great toe, flexion and adduction of other toes, plantar flexion of foot. This is called *Babinski's sign negative* (normal).

Abnormalities of Plantar Response

Plantar withdrawl responses: The plantar reflex is never completely absent in the healthy subjects. However, a stronger stimulus or an irritating stimulus in an hypersensitive patient may evoke withdrawl of the limb (e.g. initial flexor response is quickly followed by extension of toes and withdrawl of leg).

Abnormal (Babinski's) response (*an extensor plantar response*). Positive Babinki's sign indicates always an upper motor neuron lesion and is considered pathognomonic of it when present.

A positive Babinski's sign means dorsiflexion (extension) of the big toe and fanning of the other toes with slight dorsiflexion of the ankle and flexion of knee and hip. It is actually considered as generalised flexor response of the lower limb.

Note: There is confusion regarding the use of plantar extensor responses when only one of the components is present. Most of the physician take the response positive when only great toe is dorsified.

Not elicitable: If plantar reflex is not elicit by any method, the reinforcement (*Jandrassik's manoeuvre*) method (*clinch the fists*) may be employed to evoke a response. Other means employed to evoke a response in such a case are:
- Application of warmth to the cold skin or rubbing the sole of the foot to make the skin sensitive.
- Turn the patient's head to opposite side to divert the attention of the patient.
- A different stimulus may be used.

☞ **How to elicit plantar reflex when great toe or foot is amputated**

In case of *amputated* great toe, the fanning of lateral four toes, dorsiflexion (extension of the ankle) and eversion of the foot is taken as a *positive response*, while if the foot is amputated, then strong contraction of fascia lata and flexion of knee and hip, is taken as positive response on scratching the stump with a key or a stick *(Brissaud's reflex)*.

The causes of plantar extensor response (Babinski's positive) are:
1. **Physiological**
   - In infants below one year of age.
   - Deep sleep.
2. **Pathological**
   - Pyramidal (corticospinal tract) lesions.
   - Deep coma or following anaesthesia.
   - Hypoglycaemia.
   - Following an epileptic fit (post-seizures)
   - Metabolic encephalopathy.
   - Neuroleptics.

The causes of absent plantar response are:
- Loss of sensation over the foot (L_5–S_1), e.g. prolapsed disc or peripheral neuropathy.
- Paralysis of extensor hallucis.
- Thickened (hyperkeratotic) skin.
- Cauda equina lesions.

Other Methods to Elicit Plantar Reflex

In extensive corticospinal tract damage, the area from which the extensor plantar reflex can be elicited (receptive field) enlarges, spreading first inwards and over the whole sole and then upwards along the leg to the knee and even higher, therefore, other tests are based on this enlargement of receptive area, also called *plantar equivalence* (Box 5.9).

4. **Corneal reflex.** Read examination of V Cranial nerve.
5. **Palatal reflex.** Read examination of cranial nerves IX and X.
6. **Anal reflex (S_3–S_4).** Stroking or scratching the skin around the anus in a circular manner produces contraction of anal sphincter.
7. **Bulbocavernous reflex (S_3–S_4).** Pinching dorsum of the glans penis produces contraction of bulbocavernous muscle.
8. **Scapular reflex (C_5–T_2).** Stroking the skin in interscapular region produces contraction of scapular muscles. This becomes absent in high cervical UMN lesion or LMN lesion involving lower cervical segments.

> Anal and bulbocavernous reflexes become absent involving S3–S4 spinal segments (cauda equina lesion) or UMN lesions of the cord.

Box 5.9 Plantar Equivalence

- *Oppenheim sign.* Stroking with heavy pressure by the thumb and index finger from above downwards along the shin (anterior surface of tibia) evokes an extensor response.
- *Gordon's reflex* (Schaefer's sign). Pinching the Achilles tendon evokes plantar extensor response.
- *Chaddock's sign.* Stroking the skin around the lateral malleolus in a circular fashion evokes plantar extensor response.
- *Stransky's sign.* Passive abduction of the 5th digit evokes a response.
- Other signs such as *Bing sign, Gonde sign, Moniz sign* are just similar to the above 4 signs, are not practised usually.
- *Rossolimo's sign.* It is similar to Hoffmann's sign in UMN lesion where there is flexion of all the five toes (the greater toe is plantar flexed rather than dorsiflexed).

---

9. **Mass reflex.** Positive reflex indicates severe cord lesion. Stroking any portion below the level of spinal cord lesion, i.e. thigh or foot in the midline, produces
   - Flexion of the lower limbs.
   - Plantars become extensors
   - Sweating below the level of lesion
   - Evacuation of bowel/bladder.

☞ VISCERAL REFLEXES TESTING

These reflexes pertain to visceral functions such as *swallowing, defaecation, micturition* and *sexual activity*.

Swallowing (deglutition) reflex. Ask the patient about any nasal regurgitation of food through the nose. Also ascertain whether there is any difficulty in swallowing (dysphagia).

Ask the patient to drink water. Note any nasal regurgitation or cough during swallowing.

> Dysphagia in neurological disorders (motor dysphagia) pertains to liquids more than solids, whereas mechanical dysphagia (obstruction in the oesophagus or pharynx) is limited to solids only.

Defaecation. Ask the patient about any difficulty with defaecation or continence. Ask also about any abnormal anorectal sensations.

Tone of the voluntary anal sphincter can be tested by introducing the lubricated gloved finger into the anus and noting any laxity or paralysis (toneless) or spasm of the sphincter. The degree of tension of anal sphincter during a voluntary squeeze by asking—*"tighten on my finger"*—should be noted. It can be further tested by anal reflex and cough reflex (anal sphincter contracts briskly in response to sudden cough).

Damage to innervation of pelvic floor musculature produces relaxation of anal sphincter leading to incontinence of urine and faeces during stress (stress incontinence).

Micturition. Ask about any difficulty in controlling or initiating micturition and whether bladder and urethral sensations are normal. Retention, incontinence or urgency of micturition should be noted.

Neurological disorders with atonic distended urinary bladder produce overflow incontinence due to loss of bladder sensation. This is associated with distended bladder in the suprapubic region. Urge incontinence (incontinence occurs at regular intervals reflexly as it fills, in response to sudden noise, to movement or to exposure to cold), is an early feature of intrinsic spinal cord lesions.

Sexual activity. When incontinence is associated with neurological disease, sexual functions (e.g. penile erection, ejaculation in male) or orgasm in both sexes may be affected, hence, may be asked.

SPASMS (EXTENSOR AND FLEXOR)

Extensor spasms refer to involuntary extension of the whole limb during plantar extensor response, indicate severe corticospinal tract lesion without posterior column involvement.

Flexor spasms refer to involuntary sudden flexion of the whole lower limb (withdrawl response) during plantar extensor response. Flexor spasms of limbs in spinal cord disease indicate severe disease. The **causes** of flexor spasms are:
1. Spinal cord disease/compression.
2. Bilateral UMN lesions at higher level.
3. More common in combined involvement of corticospinal tracts and posterior column (e.g. multiple sclerosis, subacute combined degeneration)
4. Presence of bedsore or UTI in patients with cord lesion.

Both flexor and extensor spasms are abnormal involuntary responses, indicate nothing but an exaggerated plantar extensor response (read paraplegia—a case discussion in 258 Clinical Cases in Medicine by Dr. SN Chugh).

☞ TESTING FOR THE CEREBELLAR FUNCTIONS

Co-ordination and Gait

Co-ordination means smooth recruitment, interaction and co-operation of separate muscles or a group of muscles during a movement (motor act). The co-ordination depends on:
- Afferent impulses from the muscles and joints subserving postural sense.
- *Cerebellar function:* Cerebellum is main organ for coordination.
- *Vestibular system:* It orients the position of body in space.

Testing of co-ordination indirectly refers to testing of the cerebellar function provided tone of the muscles is normal. The cerebellum plays an important role in the co-ordination of voluntary, automatic, and reflex movements. The cerebellum has a central vermis which is concerned with maintenance of the body posture, and two lateral cerebellar hemispheres which control the limb movement on its own side.

Clinical Features

Patient with cerebellar disease complains of difficulty in threading a needle, buttoning and unbuttoning the shirt, difficulty in holding a glass full of water and ataxia.

Ataxia means instability or staggering due to incoordination of the muscles.

Causes of ataxia
1. Cerebellar disease (cerebellar ataxia)
2. Vestibular disease (vertiginous ataxia)
3. Sensory system involvement (posterior column, peripheral nerves, called sensory ataxia)
4. Hysterical (psychogenic, astasia abasia)

Note: Sensory ataxia is Romberg's sign positive while other ataxia, i.e. cerebellar, vertiginous, hysterical are Romberg's sign negative (read Romberg's test).

Tests for Co-ordination

A. Testing for Upper Limbs Ataxia
i. *Clinical observation:* A useful method is to watch the patient dressing or undressing, handling a book or picking of pins or a glass of water, since these movements are more complex and practised daily, the disturbance of these movements indicates disturbed co-ordination.
ii. *Outstretched arms test:* It is a screening test for co-ordination. Ask the patient to hold the out

stretched arms with wrists slightly dorsiflexed in front of him/her. Observe (i) Whether patient has difficulty in maintaining this posture. The drift of one arm indicates pyramidal lesion, called *arm drift sign*.

Now ask the patient to close the eyes and observe if the hands remain at the same level. **In cerebellar disease**, one hand may rise up and oscillate. Now tap the each arm sharply. If it tends to fall it suggests hypotonia of cerebellar disease, affected side tends to oscillate and returns to the original position after several bounces.

iii. *Finger-nose test*: Ask the patient to hold one arm outstretched, and then with the tip of the index finger, alternately touch the tip of the nose and the examiner's finger (Fig. 5.59).

- *Nose-finger-nose test*: To make the finger nose test more complex perform "nose-finger-nose" test by asking the patient touch his/her nose, then moving examiner's finger tip in space so that the patient has to adjust 'aim' and lastly his/her nose again.
- To test sensory ataxia, repeat the procedure with the eyes closed.

In sensory ataxia, the patient may carry out the act (finger nose test) without much difficulty with eyes open, but becomes unstable (ataxic) when the eyes are closed.

In cerebellar ataxia, the patient is unable to perform the act with the eyes open. The finger moves to the nose in wavering fashion and ultimately brought to the nose fairly accurately. In addition, there may be *intention tremors, dysmetria* and *dyssynergia*. In *dysmetria* the patient is unable to stop at the nose, instead finger is pushed beyond the nose to the cheek (he has metered the distance wrongly hence, dysmetria). In *dyssynergia*, the act or movement is not carried out smoothly but is broken into its constituent parts, which can be seen, for example, in finger nose test, he/she first flexes the elbow, then the wrist and then finger which is now moved. All these comonents can be seen. Intention tremors mean tremors appear, become more marked and coarse as the finger approaches the nose.

Finger to finger test (pointing and past pointing test). The patient is asked to outstretch both the arms to a horizontal level and then bring in the tips of index fingers in a wide circle to approximate them exactly in the midline with eyes open and then closed (Fig. 5.60).

In the unilateral cerebellar lesion, the finger on the side involved is ataxic, will either undershoot or overshoot the finger on the normal side. There may be past pointing of the fingers.

Rapid alternating movement (adiadochokinesis): The patient is asked to perform alternately pronation and supination in a rapid fashion (Fig. 5.61, pronation and supination test).

In cerebellar lesion, there is slowness and irregularity in performing the movement on the side involved as a result of incoordination called *dysdiadochokinesis*.

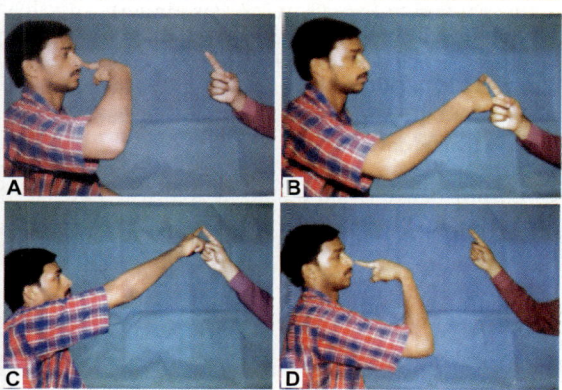

Figs 5.59A to D: Finger nose test for coordination. (A) Ask the patient to touch the tip of nose while you hold your finger in front of him/her; (B) Ask the patient to touch your (e.g. examinee) finger; (C) Move finger from one position to another and ask the patient to touch it every time; (D) The patient touches the finger alternatively while the examiner moves the finger backwards and side-to-side. The patient touches the examiner's finger first and his/her tip of the nose later alternatively.

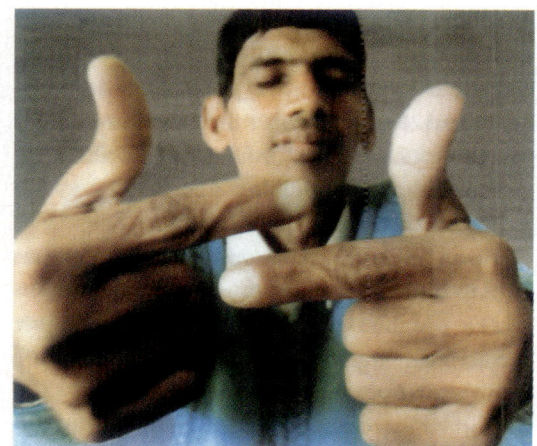

Fig. 5.60: Finger to finger test in cerebellar ataxia, Note the past-pointing with eyes open which becomes marked with eyes closed.

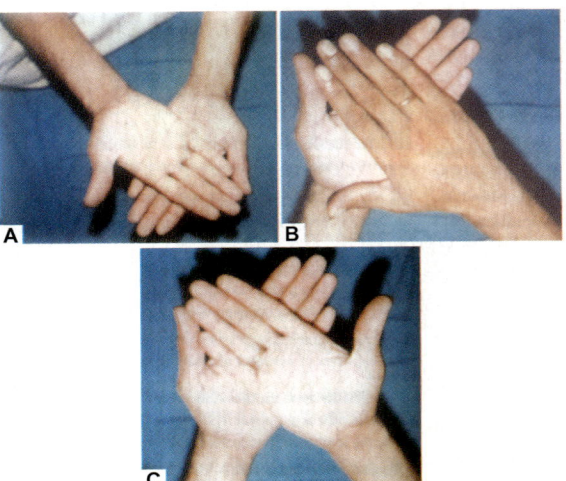

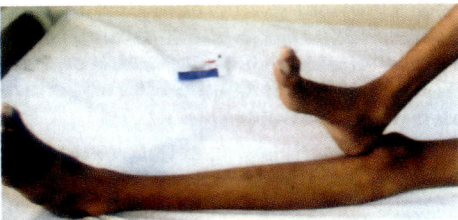

Fig. 5.62: Knee-heel test (the heel-shin test).

- Ask the patient to raise one leg at the hip and place the heel of the flexed leg on the opposite knee and slide the heel down along the shin (anterior surface of the tibia) towards the ankle and then lift it again and repeat the process again.

Figs 5.61A to C: Testing the rapid alternating movement, i.e. pronation and supination test (adiadochokinesis). Patient is explained the test by the examiner performing the movement himself/herself. Now patient is asked to perform supination (A) and pronation (B) and again supination (C) quickly as far as possible. Note any slowness of movement or its irregularity.

In cerebellar disease the heel overshoots the knee while placement (*intention tremor*). As the heal is carried downwards it begins to execute *action tremors*.

In posterior column disease (*sensory ataxia*), the patient may miss the knee and when he/she moves it downwards, it sways to one side or the other or may slide off the leg entirely.

Similarly you can ask the patient to close and open the fist on both sides as rapidly as patient can or pat his knees with palms and dorsas of the hands (*rapid hand tapping*). The slowness of movements indicate cerebellar disease.

Rebound phenomenon/test: Normally, contraction of antagonistic muscles is followed by the relaxation of the agonists due to co-ordination between antagonist and agonists; the loss of co-ordination leads to rebound test/phenomenon. The test is performed as follows.

"The patient is asked to flex the upper limb at shoulder and elbow with clenched fist. The examiner pulls the wrist against resistance offered by the patient and then suddenly releases it. Normally, the contraction of triceps against resistance will stop the tendency towards flexion, but in cerebellar disease, this tendency is lost leading to exaggeration of flexion and overshooting of the forearm due to unopposed flexion".

☞ **B. Testing for the Truncal Ataxia**

In cerebellar disease, the patient is unable to maintain balance when sitting. The patient sways to one side or the other, or may fall forwards or backwards when sits on bed/chair or when asked to rise from lying down position without using his/her hands.

C. Testing for Lower Limb Ataxia

Knee-heel test (the heel-shin test, Fig. 5.62)

"*Finger-toe test*" ask the patient first to raise the leg and touch the examiner's finger held in a suitable position in space with the great toe before placing the heel on the knee. Still to make it more complex, the finger can be moved from one place to another.

- The test is repeated with eyes open and closed.

In cerebellar lesion characteristic irregular side-to-side-side movements (*action tremors* or *intention tremors*) occur with eyes open as soon as toe reaches the finger. In addition, there may be overshooting of finger called *dysmetria*.

Writing in the air. Alternate test is to draw or write something in air. Ask the patient to draw circle in the air with toes or forefinger. Normally, the circle will be drawn smoothly and accurately but irregularity will be noted in the cerebellar disease due to ataxia.

Pendular knee jerks. Elicit the knee jerk while leg is hanging freely. In patients with cerebellar disease there will be swinging movements of foot like a pendulum of clock (to and fro movements) several times (> 3 times) before coming to rest. Pendular knee jerk is a manifestation of hypotonia and incoordination in patients with cerebellar disease.

Tandem walking (the heal-toe test of gait, Fig. 5.63): The patient is asked to walk in a straight line on the floor either bare-footed or wearing fleet-shoes, placing one heel directly in front and above the opposite toes. Observe the gait in general, and in particular note any tendency to stagger and the side to which the patient preferentially falls.

Repeat the process with eyes open and with eyes closed.

In hysteria, there may be a false positive Romberg's sign. There is marked unsteadiness both with eyes open and closed with swaying at the hip not at the ankle.

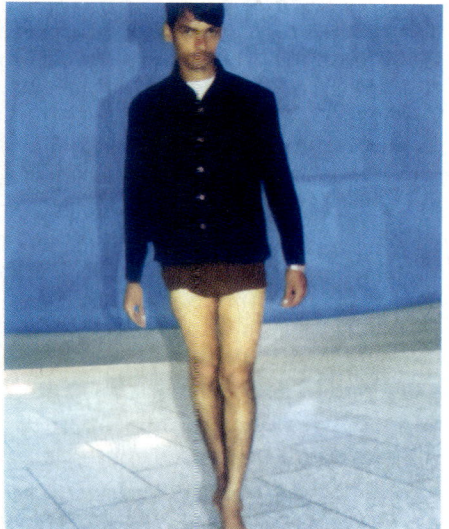

Fig. 5.63: Tandem walking.

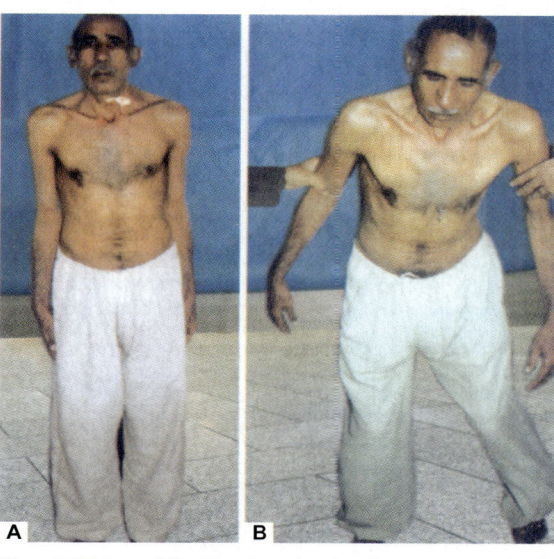

Figs 5.64A and B: Romberg's sign for sensory ataxia. (A) Patient does not deviate during standing with feet close together and the eyes open; (B) Tends to fall (becomes ataxic) when asked to close the eyes.

In unilateral cerebellar lesion, patient tries to deviate towards the side of lesion. In *lesion of the vermis*, patient tries to fall forwards or backwards. In *sensory ataxia*, patient may walk fairly well with eyes open, but on closing his eyes he sways and staggers.

Romberg's test (Fig. 5.64): It is a test for loss of position sense (*sensory ataxia*) in the legs. It is not a test of cerebellar function.

The patient is asked to stand with feet close together, and if this can be done then to stand in this posture with the eyes closed. Observe for any swaying or tendency to fall, if does not sway, now ask the patient to close the eyes and observe for swaying.

In sensory ataxia, the Romberg's sign is positive (i.e. the patient is able to maintain the upright posture when the eyes are open, but tends to sway or fall when the eyes are closed, called Rombergerism). It patient who is ataxic with eyes open but becomes more ataxic with eyes closed is also positive for Romberg's sign.

Patients with cerebellar or labrinthine lesions tend to sway or fall towards the side of lesion with the eyes open which does not increase or increases a little when the eyes are closed (Romberg's sign is negative).

Gait: The gait in cerebellar disease is unsteady, staggering and wide based, called *drunken or reeling or ataxic gait*.

The signs of unilateral cerebellar disease are
1. *Abnormal finger-nose, dysdiadochokinesis,* and *abnormal heel-shin test* on the side of lesion.
2. *Horizontal phasic nystagmus* towards the side of lesion.
3. *Intention tremors* with *pastpointing, dysmetria* and *dyssnergia*.
4. *Truncal ataxia* (patient has difficulty in maintaining balance while sitting and unassisted walking).
5. *Gait ataxia* (wide-based unsteady gait).
6. *Pendular knee jerks.*
7. *Hypotonia*

GAIT

Gait being an important element of assessing the disability, can be rewarding for neurological diagnosis. Patterns of weakness, loss of co-ordination, and proprioceptive (posterior column) sensory loss produce a range of abnormal neurological gaits. Neurogenic gait disorders need to be distinguished from those due to skeletal abnormalities, which are characterised by pain producing an *analgic gait*, or limb. Gaits that do not fit either pattern may be due to "functional" or nonorganic disorders and are usually incompatible with any anatomical and physiological deficit.

☞ EXAMINATION OF GAIT

The patient is asked to walk away from the observer, to turn round at a given point and then to come back. Note the following points:

- Is the patient able to walk or not?
- If unable, how much help does he/she need? If the patient is able to walk without help, then ask him to walk along a straight line (*tandem walking*), and note whether he/she sways or tends to fall on any side.
- To decide whether the gait fits into any of the well-recognised gait disorder, note the *posture, tone* and *arms swinging during walking* (for *parkinsonism*), *the base* on which patient walks (narrow, or broad), *movements of the foot (high-steps* or *circumduction*), etc. The various abnormal gaits are:

  1. **Spastic gait (hemiplegic gait).** It is seen in patients with stroke (e.g. hemiplegia).

     - In this type, one arm is held immobile and close to the side with elbow, wrist and phalangeal joints flexed. The leg is extended with plantar flexion of the foot. During walking, patient either drags the foot, often scraping the toe or move the leg outward and forward in an arc (*circumducting gait*, Fig. 5.65A).

  2. **Scissors gait** (Fig. 5.65B): It is seen in paraplegia/quadriplegia with bilateral spastic lower limbs.

     - The limbs are stiff. Each leg is advanced slowly and the legs (thighs) tend to cross forward on each other at each step like a scissor. This is due to spasticity of adductors of hips. The steps are short.

  3. **High-steppage or slapping gait** (Fig. 5.65C): It is seen in sensory neuropathy or foot drop (LMN lesion) or dorsal column lesion.

     - These patients either drag their feet along the ground or lift them too high to clear the ground and then bring them down with a slap on the floor. They are unable to walk on their heels. The high-steppage gait may be unilateral or bilateral.

  4. **Fascinante or short shuffling gait:** It is seen in parkinsonism (Fig. 5.65D).

     - In this gait, patient stands in a stooped posture, with head and neck forward and hips and knees flexed. The patient walks with short, rapid steps in shuffling manner so as to appear as if the patient is trying to catch the centre of gravity. Arms swinging is decreased. Axial tone is increased and patient turns around stiffly "all in one piece". Postural instability is evident on anteropulsion/retropulsion. In some cases, if the patient is suddenly

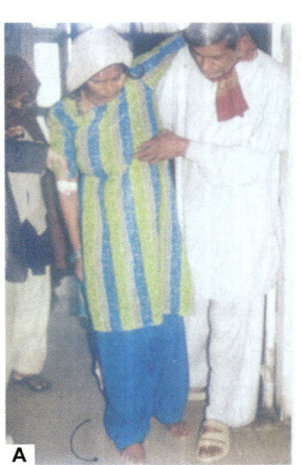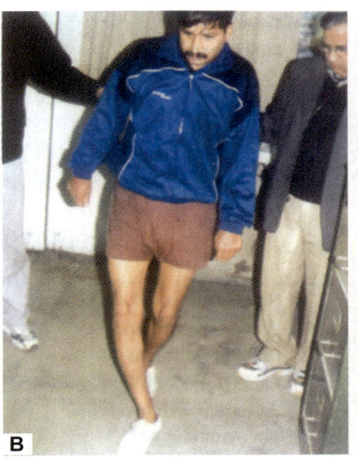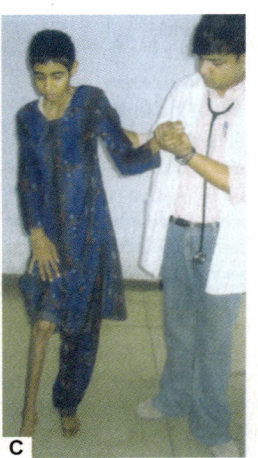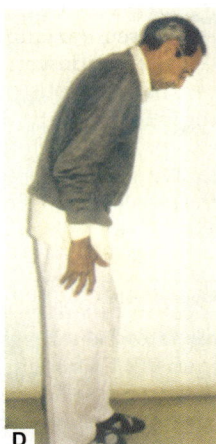

Figs 5.65A to D: Abnormal gaits. (A) Hemiplegic (arc-shaped or circumducting). The patient makes an arc while putting the hemiplegic lower limb forward. (B) Paraplegic gait (scissoring gait). The lower limbs cross when patient walks. This is due to adductor spasm of lower limbs, indicates paraplegia in flexion. (C) High-steppage gait. A patient with peripheral neuropathy demonstrating the high steppage gait. Note the foot drop while the patient is lifting the foot-off the ground. (D) Parkinsonism. Note the characteristic gait (e.g. short-shuffling or fascinating) and stooped posture.

pulled backwards (retropulsion) or pushed forwards, he walks in that direction and is unable to stop.

5. **Cerebellar gait (drunken or reeling gait):** It is seen in patients with a cerebellar disease.

   - The gait is ataxic (staggering), unsteady, and wide-based find greater difficulty on the turns. These patients cannot stand steadily with feet together, whether their eyes are open or closed.

6. **Rapid tapping gait (magnetic gait):** It is seen in bilateral corticospinal lesions deep in the cerebral hemisphere (*frontal lobe lesion*) due to cerebrovascular disease.

   - The gait is wide-based, short-stepped but rapid tapping is *called marche a petits pas*) resembling the rapid steps of a ballet dancer on her points. There are usually other UMNs signs, i.e. bilateral plantar extensor response and exaggerated jaw jerk.

7. **The waddling gait (gait of duck):** It is seen in proximal myopathy, muscular dystrophy and osteomalacia.

   - The gait is like the gait of a duck. The body is tilted backwards with an increase in lumbar lordosis; the base is wide and the body sways from side to side with each step.

   Note: Bilateral hip disease produces a similar gait (*Trendelenburg's gait*)

8. **Hysterical gait (astasia-abasia):** Bizarre or irregular gait which does not fit into any of the above described patterns. It is seen in hysteria. Miraculously, the patient does not fall.

   - *Astasia-abasia* is a typical hysterical gait disorder in which patient has normal co-ordination of leg movements in bed while sitting, but is unable to stand or walk without assistance. If attention is diverted, stationary balance is sometimes maintained and several steps are taken normally followed by a dramatic demonstration of imbalance, and tendency to fall towards examiner's arm or a nearby bed.

9. **Gait apraxia:** In an apraxic gait, there is normal power in legs with no abnormal cerebellar signs or proprioception loss, yet the patient can not walk. This is a higher cerebral dysfunction in which feet appear to be glued (stuck) to the ground and patient can not walk inspite of normal movements in bed.

INVOLUNTARY MOVEMENTS

These are unintended extra-movements that occur either at rest or during voluntary act or movement, mostly are due to diseases of the basal ganglia. (extrapyramidal system).

Involuntary movements may be rhythmical or regular (*tremors*) and non-rhythmical or irregular (*chorea, athetosis, dystonia, hemiballismus, tics* and *myoclonus*). They may be generalised or focal/local.

A. Generalised Involuntary Movements

Tremors

These are regular, rhythmical, repetitive oscillatory movements of a part of body around a fixed point resulting from alternate contractions and relaxation of groups of muscles along with their antagonists. They may involve hands (fingers), tongue, head, lips or eyelids.

They are classified in two ways, i.e. depending on the position or posture of a limb and according to amplitude, i.e.

I. According to posture
- Static tremors
- Intention tremors/action tremors
- Flapping tremors

II. According to amplitude
- *Fine*, i.e. more frequency (7–10/sec) less amplitude.
- *Coarse*, i.e. less frequency (4–5/sec) more amplitude.

Static or resting tremors: These are present at rest become less marked when hands are outstretched. They may be fine or coarse.

Causes. These include parkinsonism, anxiety, thyrotoxicosis, alcoholism, drug induced, mercury poisoning, benign essential (familial) tremors.

Action tremors/intention tremors: They are absent at rest, brought out by voluntary movement, get intensified at the end of movement. They are usually coarse tremors.

Causes: Cerebellar disease, multiple sclerosis.

Flapping tremors (asterixis). They are present on outstretched hands in the form of flaps of finger is (up and down movements) in conscious patients. In unconscious patients, flaps can be demonstrated by holding the patient's hand and passively dorsiflexing it. The fingers move like flaps (flexion and extension movements). This is a characteristic sign of *hepatic encephalopathy* indicating brain stem reticular formation dysfunction.

Differential Diagnosis of Tremors (Table 5.27)

Chorea

These are brief, rapid, jerky, irregular, non-repetitive, quasi-purposive movements involving the face, head, and limbs (Fig. 5.66). They occur at rest, become less obvious during voluntary movement and are increased by nervousness or anxiety.

> Chorea literally means 'a dance', hence, choreiform movements are dancing movements occurring at various joints.

Causes: The causes of chorea are:
1. *Hereditary,* e.g. Huntington's chorea, Wilson's disease, cerebellar degeneration, multisystem atrophy.

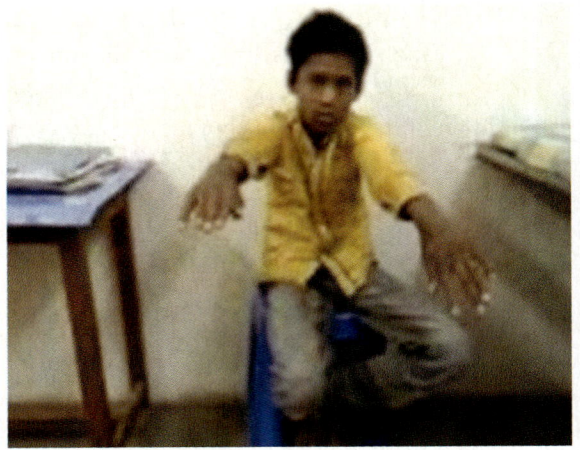

Fig. 5.66: Sydenham's chorea. Note the dancing movements of chorea.

TABLE 5.27: Differential Diagnosis of Tremors

Type	Characteristics	Causes	Associated features
Postural	Fine (8–10/sec) Absent at rest Present during posture and movement	• Physiological • Familial (essential) • Anxiety • Thyrotoxicosis • Post-alcoholic • Drug induced	Fatigue and stressed persons Present in other members of the family Anxious looking "patients with tachycardia • Signs of thyrotoxicosis may be present • History of alcoholism and its abstinence • Drugs (salbutamol, terbutaline) • History of asthma with intake of beta-agonists
Intention	Coarse (4–5/sec) Absent at rest Present during action increased by movement. Head may be affected.	• Cerebellar • Multiple sclerosis	Other signs of cerebellar disease Paralysis, diplopia, nystagmus, slurred speech, internuclear ophthalmoplegia
Resting	Coarse (<5/sec) Present at rest Reduced by action, voluntary movement. Sometimes, a pin-rolling character may be noticed in which thumb moves across the tips of all fingers	• Parkinsonism • Senile • Wilson's disease	• Other features of parkinsonism • Old age • Keyser-Fleischer's ring, cirrhosis of liver
Flapping (asterixis) (dysfunction of brains stem reticular formation)	Fine (7–10/sec) Present in outstretched hands or during action in conscious patient. In unconscious, it is demonstrated by passively dorsiflexing the hand of the patient. Hold the one hand of the patient with your left hand above the wrist, dorsiflex it with your right hand and maintain the same posture for seconds. Movements of the hand of the patient indicate asterixis	• Hepatic encephalopathy • Uraemia • Respiratory failure • Raised intracranial pressure • Poisoning with hypnotics	• Other signs of hepatic encephalopathy • Other features of CRF (anaemia, HT, foul breath) • Features of COPD and CO_2 narcosis • Headache, vomitting, papill oedema and features of CNS disease • History of intake and other features of poisoning

2. *Birth injury* (e.g. kernicterus).
3. *Cerebral trauma.*
4. *Infective/inflammatory*, e.g. rheumatic fever (Sydenham's chorea), postencephalitic chorea, Creutzfeldt-Jakob disease.
5. *Endocrinal/metabolic*, e.g. pregnancy (chorea gravidarum), hypoglycaemia, hypoparathyroidism, chronic liver disease.
6. *Drug-induced*, e.g. levodopa, tricyclics antidepressants, dopamine agonists, phenothiazines, oral contraceptives.
7. *Vascular*, e.g. lacunar (small vessesl) infarct.
   - Hemiplegia with chorea (chorea mollis), atherosclerotic.
8. *Degenerative*, e.g. senile (old age).

☞ *Method of demonstration*

Inability to maintain posture (Fig. 5.67A). Ask the patient to outstretch the upper limbs in front of him/her and maintain this posture. If chorea is present, the patient will start to have rapid jerkings of the upper limbs and can no longer hold the limbs for sometime, i.e. there is instability to maintain a posture.

The other characteristics of chorea are:
- Hypotonia
- *Pendular jerks* (hung-up reflex). It is due to hypotonia and choreiform movement superimposition.
- *Pronator sign* (Fig. 5.67B). There is tendency towards pronation of the forearms when the upper limbs are raised above the head with hands opposing each other (Fig. 5.67B). Similarly when patient is asked to outstretch the arms and hands in front of him/her, horizontally with arms supinated, thumb and fingers extended and eyes closed, there is unilateral pronation of forearm and partial downward drifting of the hand with partial flexion of the elbow and internal rotation of shoulder. This is called pronator drift sign. The sign is positive both in pyramidal lesion (hypertonicity in hemiplegia), chorea and unilateral cerebellar lesion (hypotonia).
  Milking sign (waxing and waning of the grip). Ask the patient to grip or squeeze the examiner's finger or hand, there is waxing and waning of the grip.
- *Reptile tongue.* Ask the patient to protude the tongue and keep it in that position. The patient protudes it momentarily and takes it back into the oral cavity with a reptile speed.
- *Dinner-fork deformity.* The patient is asked to outstretch the hands and spread the fingers. He/she adopts a characteristic posture, i.e. hyperextended limb with hyperpronation of forearm, flexion of wrist, extension of metacarpophalangeal joints with separation of fingers, i.e. dinner-fork deformity.

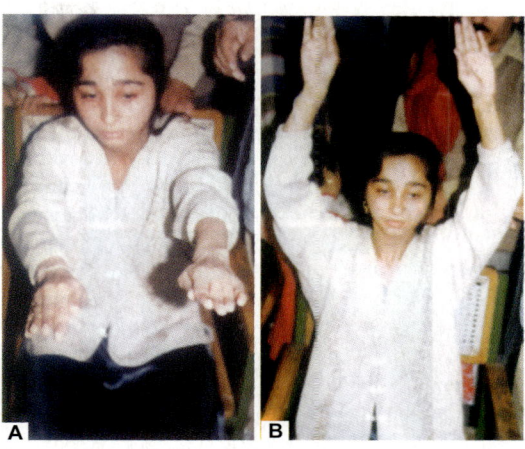

Figs 5.67A and B: (A) Inability to maintain the posture. Pronator sign in chorea; (B) Note the pronation of forearm when patient outstretches her supinated forearms or raises her arms above the head.

Differential Diagnosis of Chorea

The differences between two types of chorea are tabulated in Table 5.28.

TABLE 5.28: Differentiation between Two Common Types of Chorea

Huntington's chorea	Sydenham's chorea
1. Occurs in middle age (4th or 5th decade)	Occurs in early age (5–15 years)
2. Hereditary (inherited as autosomal dominant) or familial	It is infective (rheumatic) in origin
3. Mental features (e.g. mental retardation) present	No mental features
4. Other associated features e.g. ocular movements	Other components of John's criteria may or may not be present
5. Progressive disorder	Non-progressive, gradually resolves spontaneously
6. Non-recurrent	Recurrences are common. Chorea gravidarum is an example
7. Generalised chorea	Usually generalised, but hemichorea may occur
8. Positive family history	Family history negative

Athetosis

Athetoid movements are slow, rhythmic, twisting and writhing movements having a large amplitude and involve face and distal extremities. Athetosis is usually associated with hypertonia. The differences between chorea and athetosis are tabulated (Table 5.29).

TABLE 5.29: Differentiation between Chorea and Athetosis

Chorea	Athetosis
1. Caudate nucleus is involved	Putamen is involved
2. Tone is decreased (hypotonia)	Tone is increased (hypertonia)
3. Rapid, jerky, quasi-purposive movements of limbs with abnormal respiratory movements	Slow movements, extension and supination of the arm (twisting, writhing movements) with alternating flexion and extension of the fingers
4. Often increased with excitement	No effect of excitement
5. Proximal parts involved	Usually distal parts involved
6. Pendular jerks	Normal jerks

Causes
- Congenital.
- Birth injuries.
- Toxic, e.g. phenothiazines, manganese, carbon monoxide poisoning, Wilson's disease.
- Metabolic, e.g. phenylketonuria.
- Cerebral palsy.
- Drugs, e.g. L-dopa.
- Encephalitis.
- Atherosclerosis.
- Cerebral anoxia.

Hemiballismus 'Ballism'

The name is derived from the Greek word meaning "*to throw*". These movements are wide and flinging in character and confined to one side of the body, hence referred to as *hemiballism*. These movements are absent during sleep. If patient is at rest, these movements are minimal, but any attempt to move is followed by wide flinging movements. They occur due to involvement of contralateral subthalamic nucleus of *Luys*.

Causes include; birth injury, tumour and vascular lesion of basal ganglia. They can be congenital.

Myoclonus

It is a brief, shock-like muscular contractions that may involve the whole muscle or a small number of muscle fibres. Soft palate may be involved (*palatal myoclonus*). The contractions may be too weak to cause any movement or may be too strong to cause violent movements. It usually disappears during sleep but often occurs in response to extraneous stimuli such as loud noise, light, pinprick or touch. It can occur spontaneously. The site of the lesion is either olivodentate system or cerebral cortex. The causes of myoclonus are given in Table 5.30.

TABLE 5.30: Causes of Myoclonus

I. **Physiological**
- Sleep jerks, hic cup
- Benign infantile myoclonus

II. **Pathological**

a. *Essential myoclonus*
- Hereditary, sporadic

b. *Epileptic myoclonus*
- Epilepsia partialis continua
- Photosensitive myoclonus
- Infantile spasms
- Juvenile myoclonic epilepsy

c. *Baltic myoclonus, symptomatic myoclonus*
 1. Lafora body disease.
 2. Wilson's disease.
 3. Subacute sclerosing panencephalitis
 4. Mitochondrial disease
 5. Creutzfeldt-Jakob disease
 6. Metabolic encephalopathy
 7. Toxic, e.g. bismuth, heavy metals
 8. Drugs, e.g. L-dopa, tricyclic antidepressants
 9. Post-hypoxic myoclonus
 10. Focal CNS damage, e.g. tumour, trauma, stroke

Dystonia

It is defined as syndrome of sustained muscular contractions of trunk and limbs muscles, resulting in fixed abnormal posturing or shifting postures. The term *dystonia* is used to include all repetitive and twisting, intermittent task-specific or action involunatry movements accompanied by increased tone and abnormal postures. Dystonia is due to extrapyramidal dysfunction usually involving the basal ganglia. It may be *focal, segmental, generalised* or *hemidystonia*.

Causes: The causes are:

A. Focal Dystonia
 i. *Primary such as torsion dystonia* (Fig. 5.68)
 ii. *Secondary focal dystonia*
 - Spasmodic torticollis (wry neck), i.e. turning of neck to one side.
 - Writer's cramp/violionist cramp/barbar cramps, etc.
 - Spastic dystonia.
 - Blepharospasm (frequent opening and closing of eyes).

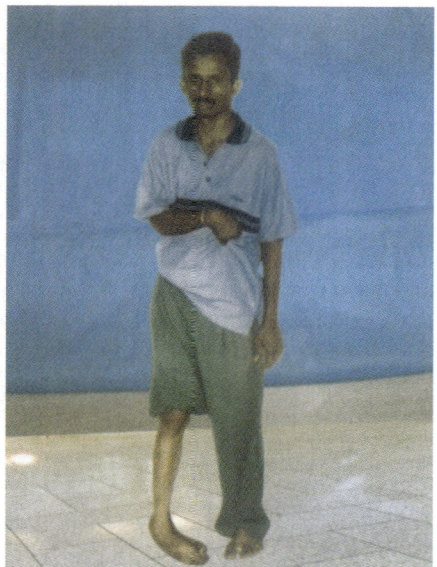

Fig. 5.68: Torsion dystonia. Note the increased tone and fixed posture of right upper and lower limb. There is inversion and plantar flexion of right foot. Patient walks on toes on right side.

- Metabolic disorders, e.g. homocysteinuria
- Oromandibular dystonia (involuntary opening and closing of mouth, Fig. 5.69) pouting, snouting, frequent licking of lips, etc.
- *Opisthotonus* (there is arching of spine like a bow, i.e. head and toes touch the bed).

B. Generalised Dystonia
Secondary generalised dystonia
- Cerebral anoxia, kernicterus.
- Trauma, tumour, vascular lesions.
- Encephalitis.
- Drugs (phenothiazines), toxic (copper).

B. Localised Involuntary Movements

Fasciculations and fibrillations (Box 5.10).
Fibrillations are intermittent, irregular contractions of a single muscle fibre or a group of muscle fibres, hence, are not seen usually except in the tongue. They are recorded on EMG.

Fasiculations are subcutaneous twitches or flickers of the muscle bellies when the muscles are at rest, result from intermittent and irregular contractions of a group of muscle fibres or a fascicle (muscle bundle), i.e. the whole motor unit. They may be absent at rest, but can be induced by percussion of muscle, mechanical stimulation, fatigue and cold. Fasciculations are seen in actively degenerating muscles but not in degenerated muscles, hence, disappears when the muscles are totally degenerated. They are attributed to Wallerian degeneration of the motor axon.

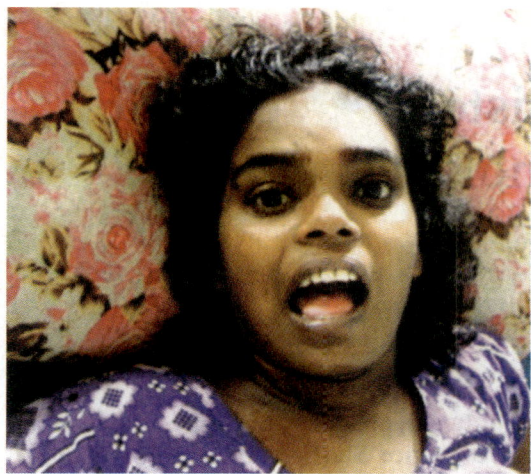

Fig. 5.69: Oromandibular dystonia. There is forced facial opening and closing of the mouth.

Box 5.10	Differences between Fibrillations and Fasciculations	
	Fibrillations	*Fasciculations*
	They are due to contraction of a single muscle fibre	They are due to contraction of a group of muscle fibres, i.e. fascicle.
	They are too weak to be seen	They can be seen as ripples within the muscle
	They cannot be provoked but recorded on EMG	They can be provoked by physically tapping the muscle bellies

☞ *Method of examination/elicitation.*
They spontaneously appear over the muscle underneath the skin as ripples. They can be induced by tapping the muscle belly with tips of the fingers such as thigh and calf muscles. They signify the involvement of anterior horn cells. The *causes* are:
- Motor neuron disease
- Spinomuscular dystrophy (peroneal muscular atrophy)
- Syringomyelia/syringobulbia
- Poliomyelitis (recovery phase)
- Intramedullary tumours.
- Peripheral neuropathy (early or recovery phase).
- Hypoxia, hypoglycaemia, thyrotoxic myopathy
- Cervical spondylosis, neuralgic amyotrophy (limited to upper limbs)

- Diabetic amyotrophy (limited to lower limbs).
- Benign, e.g. fasciculations are present without muscle wasting, seen in anxiety and fatigue states. They are common among students.

Myokymia

They are transient or persistent quivering or flickering movements which affect a few muscle bundles within a single muscle but are not sufficient to cause a movement of a joint. Thus, they are larger and widespread flickers than fasciculations. They are not associated with weakness and wasting. Myokymia commonly involves orbicularis oculi. The *causes* are:
- It may occur as a benign phenomenon in fatigued or stressed muscles in anxious patients.
- Facial myokymia may be due to lesion of the facial nerve or its nucleus.
- It may occurs as a generalised myokymia (*Isaac's syndrome*).

> Myokymia are wide flickers than fasciculation due to involvement of many fascicles than a single fascical in fasciculation.

Tics and Habit Spasms

They are brief, repetitive, stereotyped, co-ordinated movements occurring at irregular intervals. Example includes *motor tics*, i.e. repetitive blinking, facial grimacing and shoulder shrugging tics may be *vocal* (simple or complex).

The *causes* are:
- Gille de la tourette's syndrome.
- Drugs, e.g. phenothiazines and amphetamines.

Dyskinesia

These are involuntaly movements of face **(Fig. 5.70)** oral, buccal, lingual and masticatory muscles of choreiform nature produced by antipsychotic medication.

Muscle Spasm

Spasm, refers to involunatry muscular contractions resulting in a movement. It can be protective also. They are of several types.

i. **Tetanic spasms** are characterised by sudden intermittent forceful involuntary contractions of small muscles of hands and feet (*carpopedal spasm*). The hands in carpopedal spasm adopt a peculiar posture in which the fingers and thumbs are adducted and there is flexion at metacarpophalangeal joints and extension at interphalangeal joints and there is apposition of thumb (*main d' accoucheur hand—Fig. 1.18*). Pedal spasms are less frequent. Tetany is due to neuromuscular excitability resulting from hypocalcaemia or alkalosis or both. Tetany can be latent or manifest. In latent tetany, these spasms can be provoked by certain manoeuvres:
   a. *Trousseau's sign*. Raising the blood pressure above systolic level produces characteristic carpal spasm within 3 to 5 minutes (Fig. 5.71).
   b. *Chvostek's sign*. A tap at facial nerve at angle of jaw produces twitchings of facial muscles.

ii. **Tetanus spasms:** They are sudden violent sustained contraction of both agonists and antagonists muscles due to loss of central inhibition. In tetanus, there are generalised spasms of skeletal muscles involving the jaw (*lock jaw* or *trismus*), neck and shoulder muscles producing pain and stiffness, face (*risus sardonicus, Fig. 5.72A*), back muscles (*opisthotonus, Fig. 5.72B*) and smooth muscles

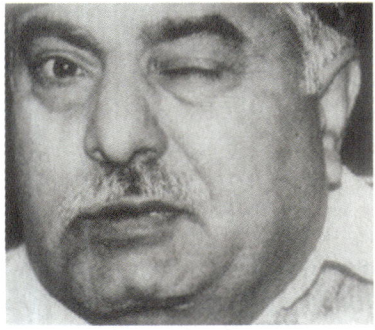

Fig. 5.70: Facial dyskinesia/facial dystonia.

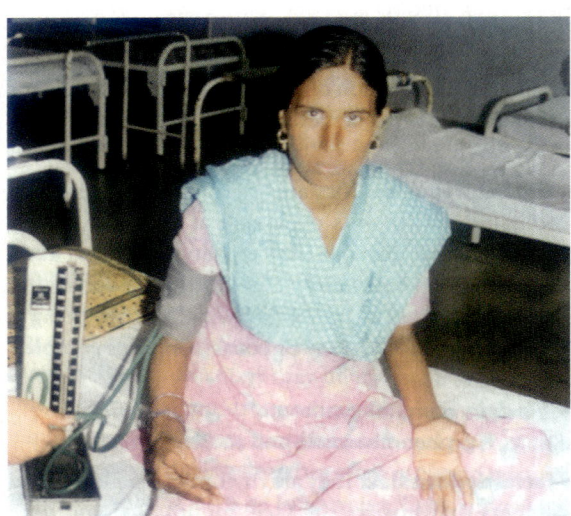

Fig. 5.71: Trousseau's sign.

Nervous System

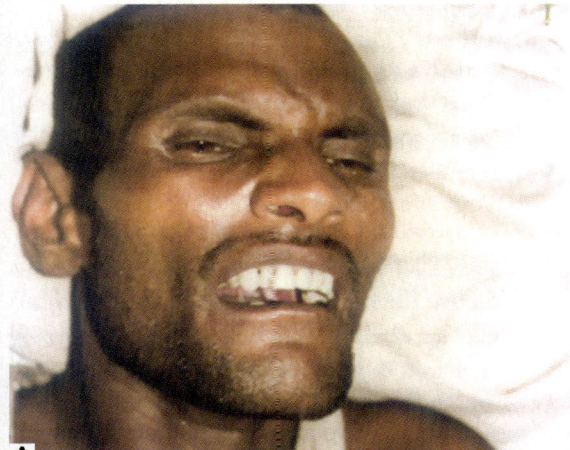

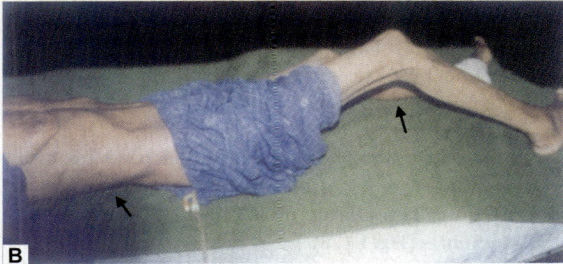

Figs 5.72A and B. Risus sardonicus (A) and opisthotonus; (B) in tetanus.

involving the laryngeal, oesophageal and respiratory muscles. The muscles of hands and feet are spared. Rigidity occurs along with spasms. Autonomic disturbances may also occur in tetanus. In tetanus, spasms may occur spontaneously or provoked by noise, light and handling of the patient, i.e. just putting the hand over the abdomen may induce abdominal spasm.

iii. **Occupational spasms.** These spasms are common in those persons whose occupation require the use of their hands persistently in certain types of movements. These spasms may sometimes may be painful enough to prevent the individual from continuing the job. Examples include *writer's*, *typist*, *telegraphist's* and *piano-players cramps*. Most of these spasms are psychogenic.

iv. **Hemifacial spasms.** These are unilateral, brief irregular spasmodic contractions of facial muscles, commonly follows a Bell's palsy. In most cases, there is no apparent cause.

v. **Blephrospams** (read dystonia).

vi. **Oculogyric spasms.** They are characterised by tonic spasms of extraocular muscles, the eyes being turned upwards for seconds or minutes or hours, commonly seen in postencephalitic or drug induced parkinsonism called *oculogyric crisis*.

Muscle Cramp (Fig. 5.73)

They are painful spasm of a part or whole of the muscle, especially of the calf muscles, is common in normal people. It is common in *electrolyte disturbances*, i.e. hyponatraemia, hypokalaemia, hypomagnesaemia. It is due to hypercontraction of muscle fibres and is relieved by passive stretch of the affected muscle. They can be produced by *fatigue, overuse of muscles, calcium and vitamin* (B1 and C) *deficiency*.

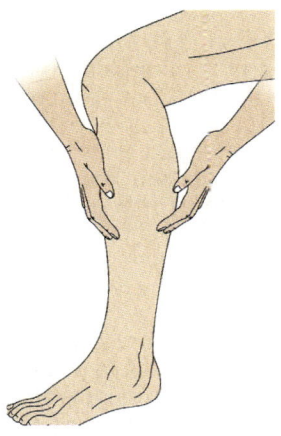

Fig. 5.73: Muscle cramp. Person is trying to relieve it.

Neck Muscle Spasms (Neck Rigidity)

Neck muscle spasms may occur due to cervical spine disease or meningitis.

☞ *Examination for Signs of Meningeal Irritation*

In patients suspected of meningitis (e.g. fever, disturbed consciousness, neck stiffness), the following signs may be elicited.
- Neck stiffness (rigidity)
- Kernig's sign
- Brudzinski's sign

Neck stiffness. It is not specific to meningitis, indicates spasm of the paravertebral muscles, hence, may be seen in cervical spine disease or meningitis and meningeal irritation by blood in subarachnoid haemorrhage. Neck stiffness is a protective mechanism to reduce pain during neck flexion in conscious patients, therefore, lost in patients with deep coma. The neck stiffness occurs both in meningitis and meningism (Box 5.11).

The Kernig's and Brudzinski's signs are also protective muscular spasms, have same clinical significance as neck stiffing.

> **Box 5.11** Difference between Meningism and Meningitis

Meningitis	Meningism
• Neck pain and rigidity both present	• Only neck rigidity
• Kernig's sign more prounced	• Less pronounced
• Convulsions and coma common	• Rare
• Cranial nerve palsies common	• Rare
• Turbid CSF with cellular changes	• Clear CSF with no cellular change

Method

1. **Neck stiffness:** Ask the patient to lie supine and support the occiput with both hands and gently flex the neck until chin touches the chest (Fig. 5.74).
   Neck rigidity is said to be present if bending of neck produces pain and spasm of the neck muscles or it may be difficult to bend the neck due to resistance and bending of neck lifts the whole body like a log of wood.
2. **Brudzinski's sign:** During testing for neck stiffness, if the hips and knees get flexed, the sign is said to be positive. Normally they remain relaxed and motionless. In meningitis, there will be reflex flexion of hip or knee on one side or both sides. Similarly while flexing one thigh (*leg sign*) there is reflex flexon of other thigh to overcome pain in meningitis.
3. **Kernig's sign** (Fig. 5.75)
   • Ask the patient to lie supine with legs straight.

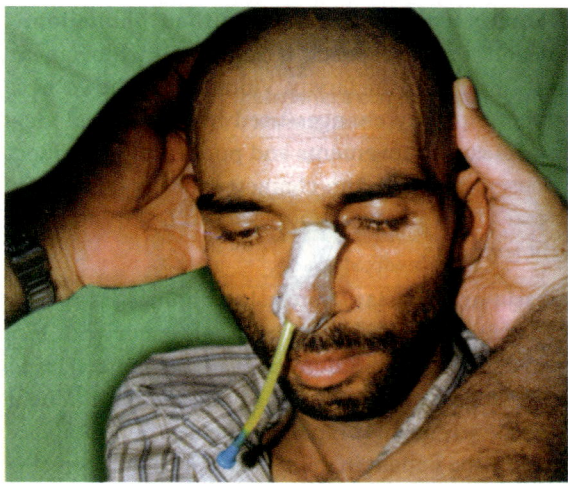

Fig. 5.74: Method to test the neck stiffness.

• Passively flex one leg at the hip and the knee, and now extend the knee slowly while keeping the hip in flexion (Fig. 5.75A). Observe the other limb for reflex flexion.

> Reflex flexion of opposite limb indicates positive Kernig's sign.
> Pain and increased resistance to extending the knee or flexion of the opposite limb indicate meningeal irritation.

• If conventional Kernig's sign described above is negative, you can further augment it by dorsiflexing the foot (Fig. 5.75B) and observing for the similar response. In some cases, this manoeuvre may cause positive Kernig's sign.

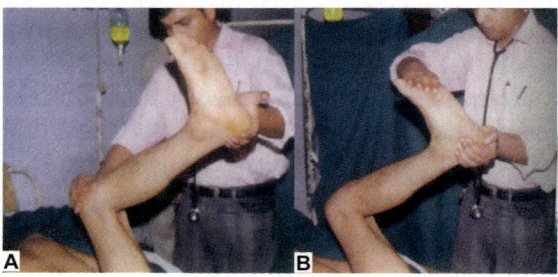

Figs 5.75A and B: Testing for Kernig's sign.

THE SENSORY SYSTEM

It consists of

I. Peripheral Sensory System (Spinal Cord)

i. *Sensory receptors.* Sensory receptors relays impulses from the skin, subcutaneous tissue, mucous membranes, deeper structures (muscles, tendons, joints) and viscera.

ii. *Sensory pathways.* They carry cutaneous and proprioceptive sensory impulses to thalamus and sensory cortex. Sensory fibres carrying the sensation of touch, pain, temperature, position, joint and vibration pass through the peripheral nerves and posterior (dorsal) roots and enter the spinal cord (Fig. 5.76A) and ascend to reach the sensory cortex.

Diseases of the first order neuron, i.e. peripheral nerves, posterior roots involve all modalities of sensation.

Sensory Pathways (Fig. 5.76)

After they have entered the spinal cord, sensory impulses reach the sensory cortex via one of the two pathways; the spinothalamic tracts or posterior columns.

Nervous System

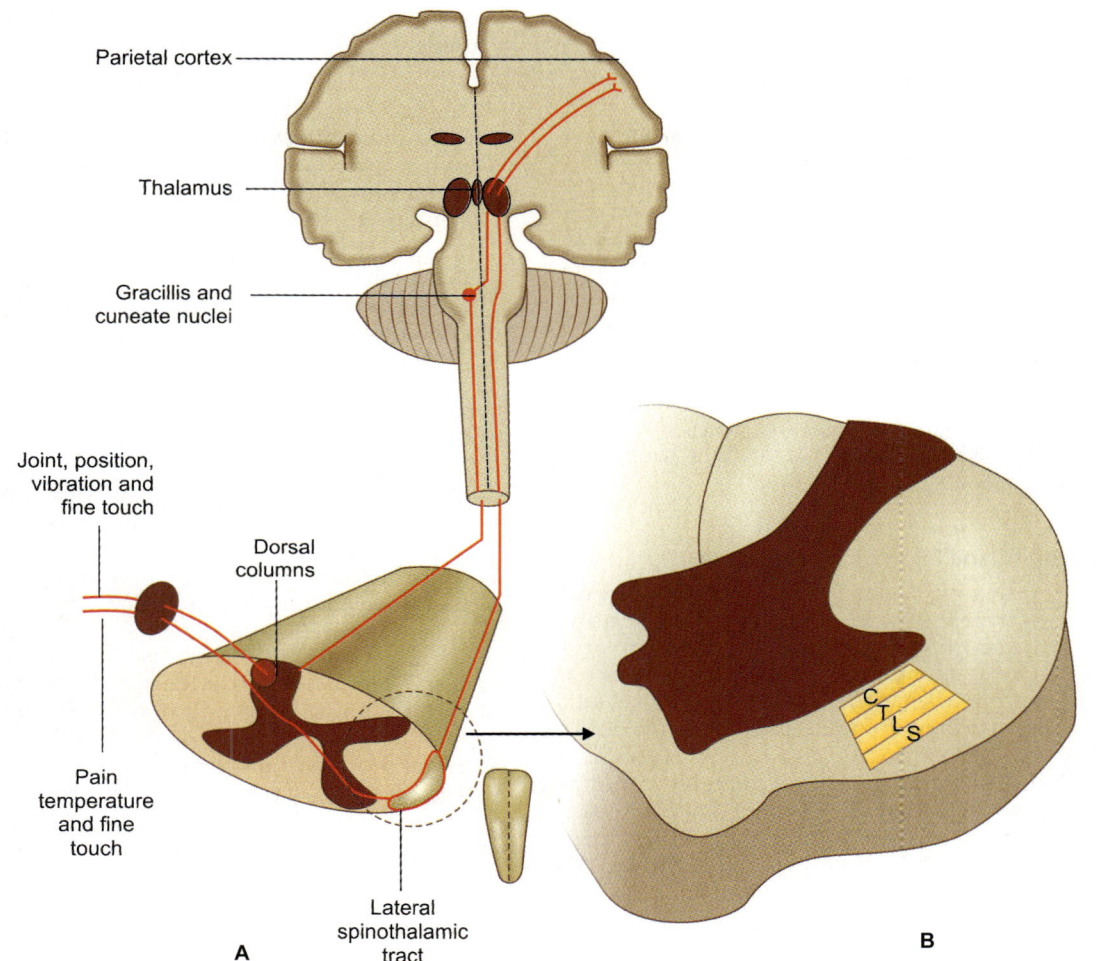

Figs 5.76A and B: The sensory pathways—spinothalamic tract and posterior column. (A) The main sensory pathways; (B) Spinothalamic tract to show its layering in the cervical region, i.e. C represents fibres from cervical region, T from thoracic, L from lumbar and S from sacral region.

1. **The spinothalamic tracts (lateral and anterior):** A group of smaller, slower-conducting first neuron fibres carrying the sensation of *pain, crude, touch* and *temperature* from peripheral parts pass through the dorsal root (root ganglion) into the posterior horn of spinal cord and synapse with secondary neurons. The secondary (*second order*) neuron fibres then cross to the opposite side either immediately or within a few segments up and continue into the lateral and anterior columns of the cord and ascend to the brain stem as the *lateral* and *anterior spinothalamic tracts* to reach the thalamus where they relay. The fibres from the lower parts are arranged laterally while those from the upper part move medially in these tracts. The *third order neuron* carry the impulse from the thalamus to the cortex as thalamocortical fibres.

2. **Posterior columns:** It is other group of different large-fast conducting fibres carrying the sensations of *fine touch, position, pressure, joint* and *vibration* that do not relay in spinal cord but pass directly into the posterior columns (*tract of gracilis* or *cuneate*) of the cord and travel upwards to the medulla. The fibres synapse in the *gracile* and *cuneate nuclei and then second order neuron* fibres arise and cross to the opposite side at the medullary level and continue on to the thalamus as *medial lemniscus*. Higher in the brain stem, the spinothalamic tracts and medial leminsci are joined by second neuron fibres from cranial nerve nuclei on each side. A new relay of fibres

(*third order neuron*) carry these impulses from the thalamus to the sensory cortex in parietal lobe called *thalamocortical fibres*.

> *Remember.* At any level of spinal cord, there are two groups of sensory fibres, i.e. *spinothalamic tract* carrying sensation of pain, crude touch and temperature from the opposite side, and *posterior column* carrying sensation of position, fine touch, vibration, and other discriminatory sensation from the same side, therefore, a unilateral lesion of the spinal cord (*Brown-Séquard syndrome*) will therefore cause loss of pain and thermal sensibility below the level of the lesion on the opposite side of the body—while on the side of the lesion (ipsilateral), there is, disturbance of sense of position, movement, vibration, stereognosis and tactile localisation and discrimination.

Symptoms and Signs of Sensory System

1. **Hypoaesthesia (decreased sensation).** It means sensations of pain, touch and temperature are diminished as compared to normal. **Anaesthesia** means loss of sensation, manifests as burn marks as these patients inadvertently may burn the extremiteis or fingers.
2. **Paraesthesias and dysaesthesias.** *Paraesthesia* denotes altered sensation perceived spontaneously (without an apparent object). *Dysaesthesia* refers to altered sensation elicited by touch or other stimuli. These may be in the form of pins and needles, feeling of tingling or crawling of ants and feeling of warmth or coldness.
3. **Numbness.** The word 'numbness' can have many meanings; when a patient says that a limb is numb, he or she may mean that the sensation in that part is abnormal.
4. **Analgesia** refers to loss of pain sensation.
5. **Thermoanaesthesia** means loss of thermal sensation.
6. **Hyperaesthesia** means exaggerated perception of a sensation in response to mild stimuli (touch or pinprick).
7. **Hyperalgesia** denotes an exaggerated pain response to a noxious stimulus.
8. **Hyperpathia** is an inappropriate perception of sensation where a mild painful stimulus evokes intense pain and touch sensation may be perceived as pain sensation. In thalamic infarct (*a thalamic syndrome*), the pain often perceived is either intense or inappropriately (e.g. touch felt as pain) felt.
9. **Allodynia** describes a phenomenon in which an ordinary nonpainful stimulus is perceived as painful stimulus. An example is painful sensation felt during an application of vibrating tuning fork.
10. **Romberg's sign.** It has already been discussed.
11. **Lhermitte's sign** (*Barbar chair sign*). In a lesion of posterior column in the cervical cord, sudden flexion or extension of the neck sends an 'electric-shock' like sensation down the trunk to lower limbs. This is seen in multiple sclerosis.
12. **Root pain.** Pain resulting from inflammation or compression of any root is called *nerve root pain*. In some diseases such as *trigeminal neuralgia* (V nerve distribution), *glossopharyngeal neuralgia* (IX nerve distribution) *postherpetic neuralgia* and *discogenic radiculopathies* (compression of nerve root by disc prolapse), the description of pain and its distribution is diagnostic.

> In radiculopathy, the root pain corresponds to the dermatome involved, increases with manoeuvres that increase intra-abdominal or intraspinal pressure such as coughing, sneezing, straining at stool, etc.

13. **Spurling's sign:** In cervical disc disease, external and lateral rotation of the neck narrows the neural foramina and produces radicular pain.

II. Cortical (Postcentral Gyrus) and Subcortical (Thalami) Sensory Centres

They receive the peripheral impulses and integrate them.

At the thalamus (*subcortical level*), the general quality of sensation is perceived (e.g. pain, cold, touch, pleasant, unpleasant) but fine distinctions are not made. It also receives sensations, from the lateral and medial geniculate bodies that are concerned with vision and hearing respectively. It also receives visceral sensations via autonomic fibres that pass along the posterior columns. For full perception, a third group of sensory neurons (*third order neuron*) sends impulses from the thalamus to the sensory cortex (postcentral gyrus) as thalamocortical fibres.

The somatosensory centre in the postcentral gyrus of the cerebral cortex is concerned with *perception, localisation, recognisation of the nature of stimuli applied* and can *discriminate between two simultaneously applied stimuli.* Representation of the body parts in the sensory cortex corresponds topographically to that in the motor cortex.

> A lesion involving the sensory pathway below thalamus or in the thalamus will impair all the sensory modalities with hyperpathia (*thalamic syndromes*) on the opposite side.

A cortical lesion will cause contralateral loss of cortical sensations such as *sense of position*, *vibration*, *tactile localisation* and *discrimination* and *stereogonosis*.

Sensory impulses not only participate in reflex activity but also give rise to conscious sensation, calibrate body position in space and help regulate internal autonomic functions like blood pressure, heart rate and respiration.

Sensory System Examination

Examination of the sensory system need to be approached with caution since lesions at different sites in the sensory pathways produce different kind of sensory loss. Pattern of sensory loss combined with associated motor findings help to localise the site of lesion, for example,

1. A lesion in the sensory cortex may not impair the perception of pain, touch and position but does impair tactile localisation and discrimination. A person so affected cannot appreciate the size, shape or texture of an object by feeling it (*astereognosis*) and therefore cannot identify it.
2. Loss of sensation of position, vibration and movement (joint) with preservation of other sensations localise the disease to posterior columns.
3. The loss of all sensations from the waist down, in a patient with spastic paraplegia indicates spinal cord transection.

Spinal Dermatomes

A knowledge of *dermatomes* also helps in localising lesion. A *dermatome* is defined as a band or an area of the skin innervated by the sensory root of a single spinal segment. The spinal cord is organised in segments from each of which a pair of anterior (motor) and posterior (sensory) nerve roots arise. Dermatomes have been mapped out in Fig. 5.77. The distribution of a few main peripheral nerves is also depicted in the same figure on the left. Their levels are considerably more variable because there is overlapping among dermatomes. The sensory nerves from each side of the body also overlap slightly across the midline.

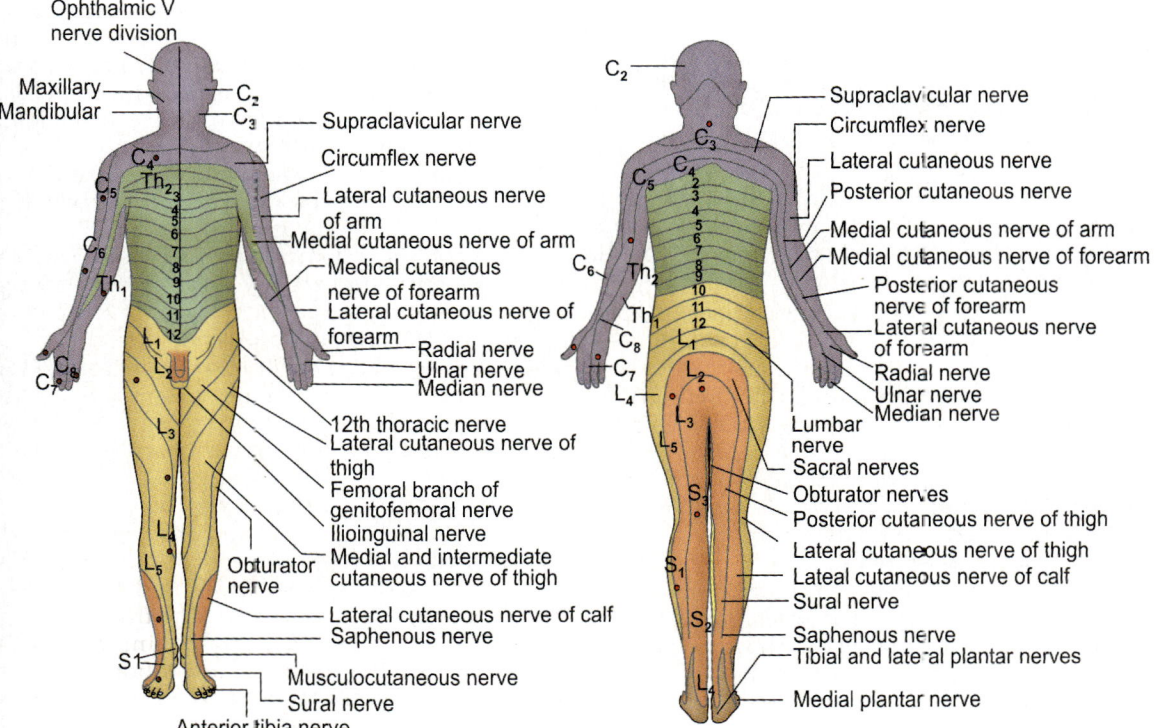

Figs 5.77A and B: Dermatomal mapping and peripheral nerve innervation of the body. The points for testing the sensations are indicated by red dots (•). By testing the sensations at these marked points you can calculate the dermatomal and peripheral nerve involvement.

The spinal cord extends from the foramen magnum to end at L_1; the meninges continue down as far as the body of S_2 vertebra creating a space called *cul de sac*. This is the space containing CSF where lumbar puncture is usually done. There is also a cervical enlargement extending from C_5 to C_7. The lumbar segments lie opposite to the T_{10} and T_{12} spine and the next interspace.

The spinal segments do not correspond exactly with the vertebral bodies overlying them. This is clinically important while assessing the level of compression in a patient suffering from spinal cord disease. To determine which spinal segment is related to which vertebral body, the applied formula is as follows:
- For cervical vertebrae, add 1 (1+) to get spinal segment.
- For T_1 to T_6, add 2 (2+) to get spinal segment.
- For T_7–T_9 vertebrae, add 3 (3+) to get spinal segment.
- T_{10} vertebra overlies L_1 and L_2 segments.
- T_{11} vertebra overlies L_3 and L_4 segments.
- T_{12} vertebra overlies L_5 segment.
- L_1 vertebra overlies sacral and segments.

Remember. If vertebral level is known, then addition is done for calculation of spinal segment level as described above. If spinal segment has been calculated from the sensory loss or loss of jerk, then subtraction is done to calculate the vertebra for radiological purpose.

How to count the vertebra?
1. The spine of C_7 vertebra is prominent at the level of shoulder from which you can palpate the upper dorsal vertebrae down.
2. On the front of the body, there is a line of demarcation between the T_2 and C_4 at the level of clavicle.
3. The nipple lies at the level of T_6; the xiphisternum at T_8, the umbilicus at T_{10} and inguinal ligament at T_{12}.
4. However, in the lower dorsal region on the back the tip of a spinous process marks the level of the body of the vertebra below hence, you can count them from the spine of C_7.
5. Similarly, the line between anterior iliac spines passes in the interspace between L_I and L_2. The spinous process above this line is L_I vertebra and below it is L_2 vertebra. This also constitute a land mark to count the diseased vertebra.

Remember. The vertebra involved or diseased is decided clinically by deformity/gibbus/tenderness and radiologically by destruction and/or reduction of interspace, then correlation is made.

Clinically in the spinal cord compression/disease, after determining the segments involved, radiology/imaging of the vertebrae is ordered keeping the approximately calculated vertebral level in the centre and including one or two vertebrae above and one to two vertebrae below. For example, if segments involved are T_1 to T_6 (loss of upper abdominal reflexes), then vertebral body will be T_6 minus 2 = T_4 level, which means upper thoracic vertebrae are to be X-rayed or scanned. Similarly, you can calculate other vertebral level.

Sensory Tracts
I. **Spinothalamic tracts:** They carry the sensation of touch, pain and temperature from superfacial structures, hence, called superficial sensations.
II. **Posterior columns** (tracts of gracilis and caneatus). They carry sensation of position (joint sense), vibration, tactile localisation and two-point discrimination, stereognosis, graphaesthesia and sensory inattention.

Rules of Examination
1. For sensory system examination patient must be alert, motivated and intelligent enough to respond promptly to the stimulus. The procedure of testing must be explained to the patient and explain what the patient has to do for response. In an unconscious patient, it is not possible to test the sensations. In obtunded (semiconscious) patients, sensory examination is reduced to observing the briskness of withdrawl or wincing or facial grimacing to painful stimuli. In the alert but uncooperative patient, some idea of proprioceptive sensations can be made by noting the patient's best performance of movements requiring balance and precision.
2. Sensory examination should not be imposed if the patient is fatigued. Sensory examination such as pain, touch and vibration testing in the hands and the feet plus examination of stance and gait including the Romberg's sign will be suffice in a patient who has no neurological deficit.
3. Patient's eyes must be closed or covered during examination to ensure accuracy procedure. First explain the procedure of testing the sensation with the eyes open remembering that a sudden pinprick may evoke a frightening response and may shatter the patient's confidence. Once patient has known the procedure and has accustomed to pinprick and other modes of testing, then the sensations may be tested with eyes closed.
4. Patient is instructed to respond quickly to the stimulus applied by saying *'yes'*. The patient

under no circumstance should be asked "*Do you feel that?*" When a stimulus is applied.
5. Compare the findings on the two sides or with the abnormalities, if any, described by the patient in neurological history. Most persons are usually aware of sensory abnormality and may even complain except perhaps in the case of temperature sense which may be lost without patient being aware of it especially if area affected is around the shoulders (as in syringomyelia) rather than hands and feet.

☞ *Testing for the primary sensations*

Testing for the primary sensations and their pathways are given in Table 5.31.

Recording the sensory examination. The results of each sensory examination are mapped out on the skin with a skin pencil and then transferred to charts, meant for recording sensory changes (Table 5.31).

A. Exteroceptive (Superficial) Sensation

Touch (Fig. 5.78A)
- Ask the patient to close the eyes and to respond verbally as "*yes*" to each touch.
- Touch the skin with a wisp of cotton wool. The tissue paper and fine hair brush are alternative stimuli used.
- Avoid repeated timed stimuli so that patient does not anticipate or adapt to the stimulus.
- The stimulus for touch should be applied on non-hairy part of skin.
- Examine the spinal segments of neck and each limb sequentially, for example; in the upper limb start on the outer border of the arm (C_5), then proceed downwards to lateral border of forearm and thumb (C_6), then fingers (C_7), etc. For neck, start above (C_1) to the nape (C_3).
- Compare the sensation on each side of neck, each limb for symmetry. Touch the exactly similar parts on each limb exactly similarly for comparison.
- Mark the abnormal area of sensation by testing from the hypoaesthetic area towards normal. If the patient complains of dysaesthesia (an abnormal feeling) then map from the normal to the abnormal area.

TABLE 5.31: Testing of Primary Sensations

Sensation	Test device	Nerve endings	Pathways
Pain	Pinprick (Fig. 5.78B)	Cutaneous naked nerve endings (nociceptors)	Smaller, slower conducting axons and spinothalamic tracts
Temperature (heat)	Test tube filled with warm water (Fig. 5.78C)	Cutaneous thermoreceptors for heat	— do —
Temperature (cold)	Test tube filled with cold water (Fig. 5.78C)	Cutaneous thermoreceptors for cold	— do —
Crude touch	Cotton wisp, fine brush (Fig. 5.78A), pulp of finger	Cutaneous mechano-receptors with naked nerve endings	— do —
Fine touch	Blunt object, clip	Cutaneous mechanoreceptors	Large fast-conducting axons, dorsal (posterior) column, medial leminscus
Joint position sense (JPS)	Passive movements of joints (Fig. 5.79A)	Joint capsule, muscle spindles, and tendons	— do —
Vibration	Tunning fork 128 Hz (Fig. 5.79B)	Mechanoreceptor (Pacinian corpuscles)	— do —
Stereognosis	Palpation of objects with hand (Fig. 5.81)	Mechanoreceptors	Large fast conducting axons, posterior columns, medial leminscus and thalamocortical projections to the cortex
Tactile localisation and two-point discrimination	Two-point discriminator (cliper) or an opened up clip (Fig. 5.83)	Mechanoreceptors	— do —
Graphaesthesia (letter or number identification)	To draw letters or numbers on various parts of the body with a blunt object or finger tip (Fig. 5.82)	Mechanoreceptors	— do —

Pain (Fig. 5.78B)

- The point of a pin should be used as the stimulus. It is applied superficially not hard enough to evoke an unpleasant sensation.
- Use a new dress making or sterlised ordinary domestic pin or a disposable pin to avoid the risk of transmission of hepatitis and HIV. Avoid the use of a sharp hypodermic needle.
- Establish the baseline for sharpness (e.g. sternal area) before examining the limb.
- Test pinprick sensation from hypoaesthetic area towards normal on each side of neck, each limb and over the trunk.
- Ask the patient to report if there is change in the degree of sensation (hypoalgesia) or feeling sharper or more painful and patient winces (hyperalgesia).
- Touch each dermatome in turn.
- If any area of abnormal sensation found, map out its outlines.

Temperature Warm and Cold (Fig. 5.78C)

- It is tested with two test tubes containing warm and cold water.
- Ask the patient to close the eyes.
- Touch the patient's skin with a test tube filled with water of desired temperature (i.e. at 35 or 36° for warm sensation; and 28° to 32° for cold sensation). Patient should be asked to say whether the stimulus is hot or cold.
- Both cold and warm sensations should be tested separately as each stimulates different receptors in the skin.
- Sensation can be tested in each dermatome in turn similar to pain. For accurate comparison, only symmerical areas of skin should be tested.
- For improved discrimination, fill the two test tubes (or serum bottles or vials); one with warm and the other with cold water with a difference of temperature by 1° or 2°. Ask the patient to close the eyes and to distinguish between warm and cold while applying the container to the skin in a random sequence.

> Most of normal persons can distinguish temperature difference by 1°C.
> Inability to differentiate hot and cold or confusion of one with other is not uncommin in syringomyelia.

Dissociated Anaesthesia

It means loss of pain and temperature sense with preservation of touch and other sensory modalities. It is always due to lesion below the pons because here the lateral spinothalamic tract joins the medial laminscus.

> Dissociation between pain and temperature sensation on one hand and touch on the other hand is called dissociated anaesthesia.

Causes

1. Central cord lesion (syringomyelia, intramedullary tumours, haematomyelia)
2. Hemisection of spinal cord (dissociated anaesthesia in contralateral lower limbs or trunk).
3. Anterior spinal artery syndrome.
4. Lateral medullary syndrome, syringobulbia.

B. Proprioceptive Sensations

Joint Position Sense (JPS)

- Start testing sensation from the distal parts to the proximal part of the limb. In the upper limb, start test at the distal interphalangeal joint of the index finger. In the lower limb, test the joint sensation in the great toe first.
- Explain the patient with eye open the intended movements of the joint and name them (e.g. "that is up" and "that is down").

A. Testing of JPS in upper limb

- Hold the middle phalanx of a finger (e.g. index finger) with one hand (left hand) while holding the distal phalanx of the same finger between your thumb and index finger of other hand (right hand).
- Ask the patient to shut the eyes so as to avoid guessing.
- Move the distal phalanx up and down first to large extent then to smallest possible movement detectable in a random sequence and ask the

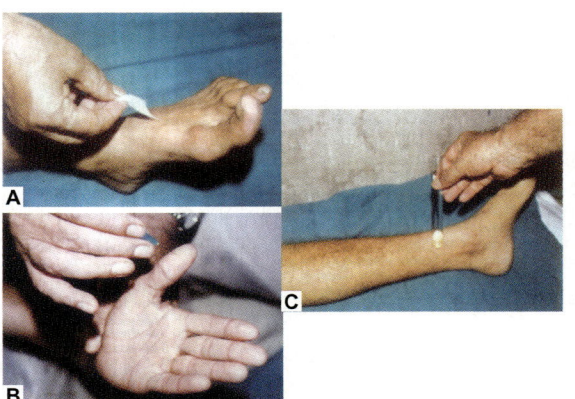

Figs 5.78A to C: Testing for the superficial sensations. (A) Touch; (B) Pain (pinprick); (C) Temperature.

patient to identify the direction of movement (Fig. 5.79A).
- Then test the other upper limb in similar fashion.
- If there is any abnormality of joint position sense (JPS) at the distal small joints, move to the proximal joints and progressing to wrist and elbow if joint position remained impaired.

B. *Testing of JPS in lower limbs*
- In the lower limb, start testing at the interphalangeal joint of the big toe.
- Hold the big toe with left hand between the thumb and index finger; and grasp the proximal phalanx in the other hand (right hand). Move the distal phalanx up and down as described above.
- Ensure that the examiner's fingers do not rub against the patient's other toes.
- If there is impaired sensation, proceed to examine the metatarsophalangeal joint and, if necessary, the ankle and knee.

Vibration Sense
Show the patient the tuning fork and make him/her acquainted with vibrations. Explain the whole procedure to the patient with the eyes open.
- Now ask the patient to close the eyes.
- To set the tuning fork into vibrations, strike it against the palm or any other soft object.
- First hold the vibrating tuning fork (128 Hz) over the sternum so that the patient identifies the sensation.
- Start testing over the base of thumb, then proceed over the bony prominences at wrist, elbow and shoulder.

Most normal persons can identify the slightest movement at the joint. Remember a patient with loss of position sense in the part being tested will have a 50% error rate because only two choices (yes or no) are available. Answers greater than 50% errors should be taken indicative of the absence of position sense.

In the lower limbs
- Start testing from the big toe (Fig. 5.79B). If necessary, next move proximally in turn to the medial or lateral malleolus (ankle joint), tibial shaft and ischial tuberosity and the anterior iliac crest (i.e. put the tuning fork at bony prominences from below upwards).

Deep Pressure Pain (Fig. 5.80). Superficial pain is carried by spinothalamic tracts while deep pressure path is carried through posterior column.

It can be elicited by either applying strong pressure or by pinching the muscle of forearm or calf or the tendo-Achilles. Note the wincing or grimacing of face due to pain. Deep pressure pain is abolished in peripheral neuropathy, tabes dorsalis while it is exaggerated in peripheral neuritis.

C. Cortical Sensations

1. Stereognosis. This is sense of ability to recognise the object by feel when placed in the hand (Fig. 5.81). This cortical sensation depends on the superficial sensation (i.e. feeling) and sense of position and movements (posterior column sensation), hence this sensation tests the integrity of spinothalamic tract, posterior column and sensory cortex where this sensation is interpreted. Therefore, one can use the term *"combined sensibility testing for stereognosis"*.
- Patient is asked to close the eyes. Various familiar objects such as *coins* or *keys* are placed in each hand. Patient is asked to feel them with hand and name them (Fig. 5.81). If he/she is not able to name then, he may be asked to describe the *size*,

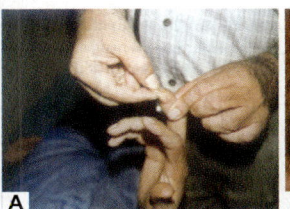
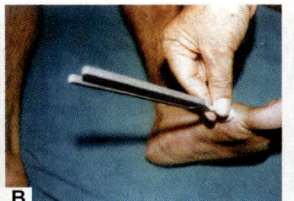

Figs 5.79A and B: Testing the sensations carried by posterior column. (A) Testing for position sense in middle finger; (B) Testing the sensation of vibration by tuning fork 128 Hz in the lower limb.

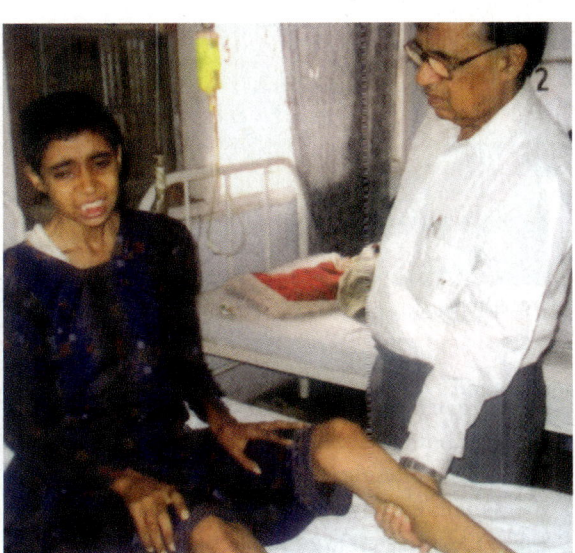

Fig. 5.80: Deep pressure pain testing.

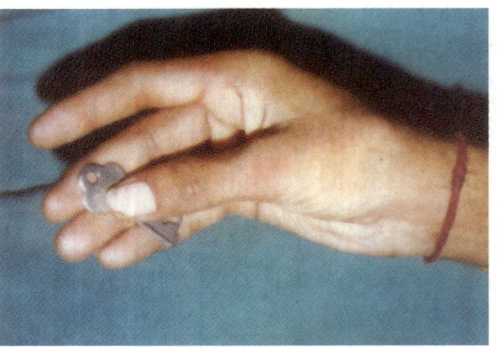

Fig. 5.81: Testing for object identification (stereognosis).

shape and *texture* of the object. Patient with loss of sense of touch (spinothalamic tract), loss of sense of position/movement (posterior column) and sensory parietal lobe lesion is either not able to recognise it (astereognosis) or may hesitate to answer (dysstereognosis).

> *Remember.* For testing stereognosis as a cortical sensation, peripheral sensation of touch and position sense should be intact.

> *Note.* Please do not use a bunch of keys because rattling sounds of keys will betray its nature.

Figure identification (graphaesthesia). This is tested in similar way as described above. Person is asked to recognise the figure or numbers inscribed in the palm of each hand (Fig. 5.82) provided they are of sufficient size. The loss of this sensation carry the same significance as stereognosis.

Tactile localisation and two-point discrimination. Tactile localisation is the ability to localise the site of stimulus applied to parts of the body with eyes closed. This is tested in similar way as sense of touch.

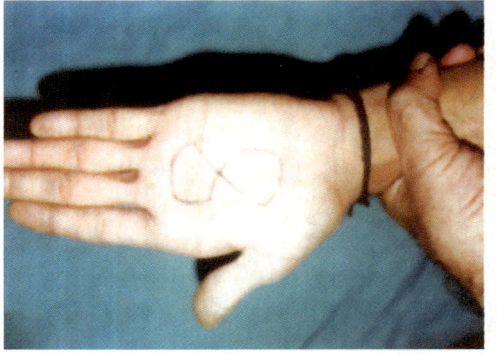

Fig. 5.82: Graphaesthesia (figure or number identification).

Two-point discrimination. The centre for discrimination sense lies in sensory cortex. This is tested by simultaneously touching areas of the skin at two-point by ordinary compass or divider (Fig. 5.83) or hairpins or heads of two ordinary pins. The points are first touched sufficiently apart to be recognised with the eyes closed as two point contact (double contact) and then slowly brought together until patient reports being touched at a single point only. The minimum distance between the two points that is appreciated is noted. Sites of sensation to be tested are the palms and soles, dorsal surface of hands and feet, the fingers tips and the shin.

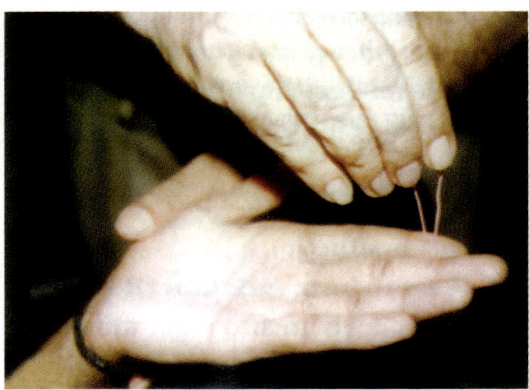

Fig. 5.83: Testing for two-point discrimination with the help of divider.

Normal person can recognise two points at a distance of 1–1.5 cm apart. Loss of sense indicates parietal lobe lesion.

Sensory inattention (extinction). When two stimuli with cotton wool or fingertips are applied simultaneously at two identical points on either side of the body, a patient with parietal lobe lesion will fail to appreciate individual touch on the affected side of a phenomenon, called *sensory inattention or extinction*.

Abnormalities of Sensations

Common patterns of sensory abnormalities are depicted in Table 5.33 and Figs 5.85A to H.

NERVE LESION (ENTRAPMENT NEUROPATHY)

SINGLE NERVE LESION (MONONEURITIS)

The identification of the sensory abnormalities resulting from peripheral nerve lesions or from the lesions of the brachial and lumbosacral plexuses can easily be done from a knowledge of cutaneous distribution of various peripheral nerves and components of the plexuses.

Common entrapment neuropathy, i.e. single nerve lesion and their features are given in Table 5.32.

Thickening of Nerves (Palpability of Nerves)

The nerve trunk or the peripheral nerves may be thickened and palpable. The causes are:
1. Leprosy.
2. Acromegaly, diabetes, amyloidosis.
3. Sarcoidosis.
4. Relapsing neuropathies, neurofibromatosis
5. Hereditary Charcot-Marie-Tooth disease. Dejerine-Sottas disease, Refsum syndrome.

AUTONOMIC NERVOUS SYSTEM (ANS)

APPLIED ANATOMY AND PHYSIOLOGY

The autonomic nervous system consists of afferent and efferent postganglionic sympathetic and parasympathetic neurons in the periphery and preganglionic components of these systems lie in the spinal cord, brain stem and cerebral hemispheres. This system is autonomous, is concerned with:
- Modulation of CVS and GI tract system.
- Temperature regulation.
- Sexual reflexes.
- Bladder and bowel reflexes
- Pupillary and respiratory reflex control

TABLE 5.32: Symptoms and Signs of Single Nerve Lesion (Entrapment Neuropathy)

Nerve involved	Symptoms	Signs	
Median at wrist (carpal tunnel syndrome)	Distressing pain and paraesthesia on the palmar aspect of the palm, waking the patient at night	*Motor:* Muscle weakness, wasting of abductor pollicis brevis (Fig. 5.84A)	*Sensory* loss over palmar aspects of three and half fingers, i.e. thumb, index middle and half ring fingers
Ulnar at elbow	Paraesthesia on medial border of hand. Weakness of hand muscles	Wasting and weakness of all hand muscles except abductor pollicis brevis	Palmar aspect of one and half fingers, i.e. little finger and half ring finger
Radial	Weakness of extension of wrist (wrist drop, Fig. 5.84B) and fingers, often precipitated by sleeping in chair with arms above the back of chair	Wrist and finger extensors, (Fig. 5.84B), supinator are affected (weak)	Base of the dorsum of thumb shows sensory loss
Peroneal	Foot drop, trauma to head of fibula	Dorsiflexion and evertor of foot are weak	Nil or dorsum of foot may show sensory loss
Meralgia prosthetica	Tingling and paraesthesia on the lateral border of thigh	Nil	Lateral border of thigh shows sensory loss

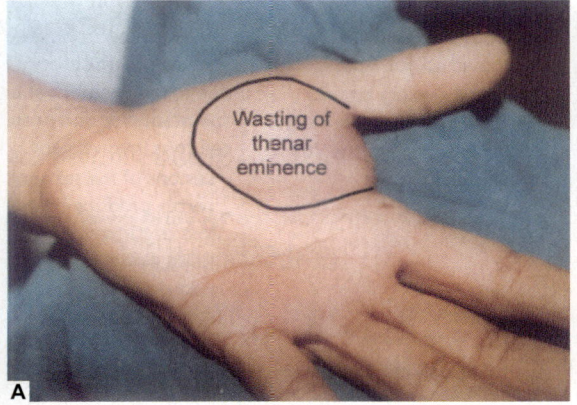
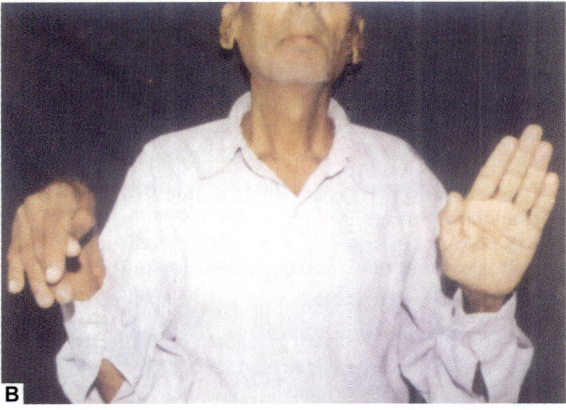

Figs 5.84 A and B: Single nerve lesions. (A) Carpal tunnel syndrome; (B) Wrist drop due to radial nerve palsy.

TABLE 5.33: Sensory Abnormalities at Various Level (Figs 5.85A to H)

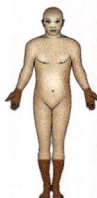 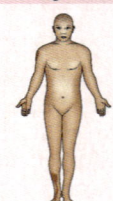 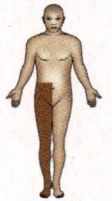 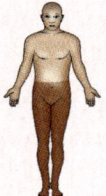

A. Generalised peripheral neuropathy

- Longest fibres being affected first, the sensory loss occurs in *"glove and stocking"* pattern (Fig. 5.85A)
- If the smaller nerve fibres are preferentially affected (e.g. in alcoholic polyneuropathy), pain, temperature sensations are lost whilst modalities served by large fibres (joint position, vibration) may be spared. On the other hand, the latter are particularly affected in demyelinating (e.g. G.B. syndrome) neuropathy. Calf tenderness may be present

B. Single dorsal root lesion (radiculopathy)

- Root pain in the distribution of a nerve root is a characteristic feature.
- Dermatomal pattern of sensory loss occurs (Fig. 5.85B) although this is often smaller than expec-ted because of the overlap of sensory territories
- Cauda equina lesion (multiple sacral roots involvement) produces saddle analgesia/anaesthesia

C. Posterior column lesion

- Dissociated anaesthesia, i.e. loss of proprioceptive sensations (joint position sense, vibration, two-point discrimination, stereogonosis, etc.) while pinprick pain and temperature sensations are preserved (Fig. 5.85C) on the side involved
- Dorsal (posterior) columns alone are affected in multiple sclerosis
- Unpleasant tight feeling over the limb involved

D. Transverse thoracic cord lesion (myelitis or compression)

- Loss of all sensory modalities below a clear cut segmental level on the trunk (Fig. 5.85D) although the level obtained clinically will vary by two or three segments because spinothalamic fibres do not cross at the same level but cross 2–3 segments below or above the level
- Very often at the top of the area of sensory loss, there is a zone of paraesthesia or hyperasthesia

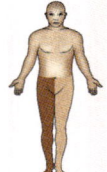 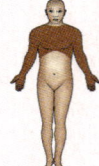 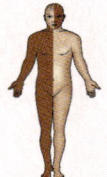 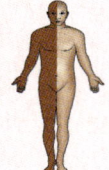

E. Unilateral cord lesion (Brown-Sequard)

Lesion damaging one side of the cord (hemisection, Fig. 5.85E) produces
- Contralateral loss of pain and temperature sensation (crossed spinothalamic tract involvement)
- Ipsilateral (same side) loss of joint position and vibration sense due to posterior columns involvement
- One the side of the lesion there is a bond of analgesia at the highest level due to root involvement (root entry zone)

F. Central cord lesion (syringomyelia)

- Dissociated sensory loss
- Lesion in the centre of the cord (syringomyelia) produces cape distribution of loss of pain and temperature by involving the spino-thalamic fibres crossing the cord (Fig. 5.85F).
- Posterior column sensations are spared, hence, the sensory loss is dissociated called dissociated anaesthesia

G. Midbrain stem lesion (lateral medullary syndrome)

- Thrombosis of posteriror inferior cerebellar atery—lateral medullary syndrome
- Sensory loss affecting all the modalities occur on the contralateral (opposite) side of the body due to involvement of crossed spinothalamic tract
- Ipsilateral sensory loss on the face due to involvement of spinal nucleus of the Vth cranial (facial anaesthesia)

H. Hemisphere (thalamic) lesion

Lesions in the cerebral hemisphere or thalamus produce loss of all forms of sensations on opposite side of the body (hemisensory loss, Fig. 5.85 H)
- Lesions of the sensory parietal cortex produce contralateral loss of cortical sensations (joint position, vibration, two-point discrimination and stereognosis) while pain and temperature may or may not be involved

Causes of autonomic dysfunction (Table 5.34)

TABLE 5.34: Causes of Autonomic Dysfunction

I. Central causes
- Shy-Drager syndrome
- Olivopontocerebellar degeneration
- Parkinsonism
- Huntington's chorea
- Hypothalamic disorders
- Chronic idiopathic anhydrosis
- Raynaud's syndrome
- Familial dysautonomia (Riley-Day syndrome)
- Tetanus (occasional)

II. Peripheral causes
- Diabetes mellitus
- Spinal cord disorders
- Peripheral neuropathies (amyloid, porphyria, alcoholism)
- Guillain-Barré syndrome
- Tabes dorsalis
- Lambert-Eaton syndrome

III. Focal causes
- Shoulder-hand syndrome
- Horner's syndrome
- Innervation anomalies (e.g. crocodile tears)

Symptoms of Autonomic Dysfunctions

1. **Cardiovascular**, e.g. postural hypotension, resting tachycardia, supine hypertension, fixed heart rate, arrhythmias and cardiac arrest.
2. **Gastrointestinal**, e.g. dysphagia, abdominal distension, nocturnal diarrhoea, constipation.
3. **Genitourinary**, e.g. hesitancy, retention and incontinence of urine and sexual impotence.
4. **Sudomotor**, e.g. gustatory sweating, anhydrosis.
5. **Vasomotor**, e.g. cold extremities, dependent oedema.
6. **CNS**, e.g. syncope, light headedness, diminished vision, diaphoresis, pallor.
7. **Pupillary**, e.g. miosis (constricted pupil), resistance to mediatrics.

TESTING FOR THE AUTONOMIC FUNCTIONS

1. Tests for Cardiovascular Functions

A. Parasympathetic

☞ *Beat to beat variation (R-R intervals on ECG).* Subject takes deep breaths 6 per minute and one of the limb lead on ECG is recorded. The difference between mean of the shortest and longest R-R intervals on ECG lead is calculated for heart rate variations.

Normal differences = 15 bpm
Abnormal = 10 or less bpm.

☞ *Valsalva manoeuvre (heart rate response).* Subject blows into an anaeroid BP instrument to maintain uniform BP of 40 mm for 15 secs. The ECG lead is recorded and measured for R-R interval immediately during manoeuvre and 15 seconds after release. The ratio of longest R-R interval (following release) and shortest (during manoeuvre) is calculated.

Normal = 1.21
Abnormal = < 1.00

☞ *Immediate heart rate response to standing.* Subject lies supine. The ECG leads are placed and machine is kept on running. The subject gets up quickly unaided to standing position. The R-R interval at 15 and 30 seconds is measured and heart rate calculated as ratio of 30:15.

Normal = 1.4
Abnormal = ≤ 1.0

B. Sympathetic

☞ *BP response to standing.* Blood pressure (BP) is recorded while supine and then on standing for at least 1 minute. Fall in systolic BP is noted.

Normal = Up to 10 mmHg
Abnormal = > 30 mmHg

☞ *BP response to sustained hand grip.* Hand grip maintained at 30% of maximal capacity up to 5 min. BP measured once every minute. Increase in diastolic BP is noted.

Normal = 16 mmHg
Abnormal = <10 mmHg

☞ *BP response to cold pressure test.* One hand of the subject immersed in ice water (1–4°C) and BP measured at 30 second and 1 minute. The rise in BP is noted.

Normal = 10–20 mmHg
Abnormal = < 10 mmHg

Sudomotor Function

- *The quantitative sudomotor axon reflex test for acetylcholine-induced sweating*: A reduced or absent response indicates a lesion of the post-ganglionic sudomotor axon.
- *Thermoregulatory sweat test (regional sweat response to elevation of temperature).* An indicator powder placed on the anterior chest on both sides changes its colour with sweat production during temperature elevation. The pattern of

colour changes is a measure of regional sweat abnormality, may suggest a peripheral or central lesion.

A unilateral decrease over half of the body suggests a central lesion.

NERVOUS SYSTEM AT A GLANCE

The signs of lesion in different parts of the brain and the paths involved are summarised in Table 5.35. The students must remember them at the time of examination.

TABLE 5.35: Signs of Lesions in Different Parts and the Paths Involved

I. Upper motor neuron lesion
- Weakness or paralysis of movement
- No wasting or atrophy
- Hypertonia—clasp-knife spasticity
- Exaggerated tendon jerks
- A plantar extensor response (Babinski's sign positive)
- Loss of superficial reflexes

II. Lower motor neuron lesion
- Weakness and paralysis of muscles
- Wasting and atrophy of muscles
- Fasciculations may be present
- Hypotonia
- Diminution or loss of tendon and superficial reflexes
- Trophic skin changes, i.e. burn marks, etc.

III. Basal ganglia (extrapyramidal lesion)
- Resting tremors of hands, especially pin-rolling movements.
- Rigidity—cogwheel or lead pipe.
- Bradykinesia or akinesia (slowness of movements)
- Expressionless (mask-like) face
- Festinant gait.

IV. Cerebellar lesions
- Ataxia (truncal and limb)
- Intention tremors of hands (limbs)
- Jerky nystagmus
- Stoccato or scanning speech
- Dysmetria—past-pointing, dysysnergia, dysdiodochokinesis
- Hypotonia and pendular jerks
- Smooth movements are replaced by jerky movements

V. Peripheral neuropathies
- Loss of all sensory modalities affecting the distal parts of the limbs in "*glove-stocking fashion*"

Contd.

Contd.
- Loss of peripheral tendon jerks (ankle, knee, supinator, finger flexion)
- Hypotonia of distal muscles
- Trophic skin changes (ulcer, burn mask)

VI. Lesion of lateral spinothalamic tract
- Impaired or loss of pain, crude touch and temperature sensation

VII. Posterior column involvement
- Sensory ataxia (Romberg's sign positive)
- Impaired joint sense position, deep pressure sense
- Diminished or loss of vibration sensation and asterognosis

VIII. Muscle disorders (myopathy)
- Wasting and weakness of muscles (may be proximal or distal)
- Hypotonia and loss of tendon jerks
- Pseudohypertrophy (Duchenne's type of myopathy)
- Gower's sign positive (difficulty in rising from sitting position)

IX. Parietal lobe dysfunction
- Dysphasia and dyscalculia
- Right and left disorientation
- Astereognosis, sensory inattention (extinction)
- Apraxia
- Amnesia and cognitive disorders
- Homonymous visual field defect
- Hemiparesis, monoparesis

X. Frontal lobe lesion
- Personality change
- Emotional change
- Antisocial behaviour
- Impaired memory
- Expressive dysphasia
- Incontinence
- Impaired smell
- Centralateral hemiparesis
- Primitive release reflexes
- Seizures

QUICK NEUROLOGICAL EXAMINATION

A detailed neurological examination may not be necessary in each and every case. The symptoms in neurology may pertain to specific area of involvement. Detailed examination in a patient who is not suffering from a neurological disease is time-consuming, boring and unwanted. Otherwise also, a short-cut neurological examination is performed by the physician in patients not suspected of neurological disease in order to exclude major neurological disability.

GENERAL PHYSICAL EXAMINATION
- Examine the skull, posture and spinal movements.
- Look for cutaneous naevi or burn mark, pigmentation or depigmentation.
- Listen for bruits in the neck and palpate the carotids.
1. **Mini-mental state examination.** Screening for the cognitive functions or dementia can be done during history taking and physical examination. No specific questions need usually be asked. Observe the patient while patient is giving the history or talking to the examiner. Assess mental function quickly as follows:
   - Is the history given by the patient accurate, concise and with insight? Or is the patient vague or concrete?
   - Is patient's behaviour and memory normal?
   - Is the patient well-dressed or cared for? Note the dress, hair-style, shoes, etc.
   - Is the patient aphasic or dysarthric?
   - Is the patient fully conscious or confused?

GAIT
Observe the patient while walking towards examiner and note:
- Is there any abnormality of gait? If yes, is it spastic, hemiparetic, ataxic or parkinsonian or hysterical?
- Is there any neurological deficit? Weakness of a part of the body or half side of the body should be looked for. Is there any foot drop?

CRANIAL NERVES
- Test the ocular movements and look for squint or nystagmus.
- Test for facial movements.
- Test movements of tongue and soft palate.
- Test for visual fields. Is there a hemianopia? If yes, is it homonymous, bitemporal or unilateral? Is central vision normal? Can patient read news paper or small prints with or without glasses?
- Look at the optic fundi for papilloedema or optic atrophy. Are there any changes in the fundus such as hypertensive, uraemic, diabetic or bleeding disorder?

MOTOR FUNCTION
- Have a hurried look for the tone of the muscle (normal, spastic or rigid or flaccid).
- Look for any weakness, wasting of the distal or proximal muscles.
- Look for ataxia in the limbs. If present, decide whether Romberg's sign is positive or negative.

Then proceed further for detailed cerebellar or sensory functions.
- Elicit one or two tendon reflexes such as biceps in the upper limb and knee jerk in the lower limb. Note whether present or absent, normal or exaggerated. Elicit the plantar response.
- Can the patient get up from the floor normally? Is there any difficulty in getting up from the low chair and climbing the stairs?

SENSORY
- Test the pinprick and light touch in all the four limbs from the periphery to the centre. Test sensations over the face also.
- Test one or two posterior column sensations especially the joint position sense in the upper and lower limbs. If necessary vibration sense may also be tested.

Note: After having the quick assessment of nervous system, one can proceed further for detailed neurological examination depending on the neurological complaints/deficit.

BRIEF SYNOPSIS OF THE NEUROLOGICAL DISORDERS

HYDROCEPHALUS AND RAISED INTRACRANIAL TENSION
Definition: *Hydrocephalus* implies dilatation of the ventricles of the brain. *Raised intracranial pressure* is defined as pressure more than 15 mm Hg (normal is 5–10 mm) meaured by devices implanted in the lateral ventricle or intraparenchymal placement.

Causes
I. *Congenital*, e.g. aqueductal stenosis, Dandy-Walker syndrome, Arnold-Chiari malformation, etc.
II. *Acquired*, e.g. encephalitis, meningitis, haemorrhage (subarachnoid, hypertensive) brain tumour, neurocysticercosis, dural sinus thrombosis
III. Benign or idiopathic

Clinical Signs and Symptoms
- *Triad of raised ICP is vomiting, headache and papilloedema*
- True localising signs depending on the cause
- False localising signs, e.g.
  - Bilateral/unilateral 6th nerve (common) or 3rd nerve (uncommon) palsy
  - Bilateral plantar extensor response
  - Bilateral mild cerebellar signs
  - Mild endocrinal dysfunction

Consequence of Raised ICP
- Herniation syndrome, i.e.
  Uncus herniation and/or cerebellar tonsillar herniation.
  and/or
  Transtentorial herniation
  Diagnosis is confirmed by CT scan/MRI and/or measurement of ICP.

PARKINSONISM

Definition: It is a movement disorder due to involvement of extrapyramidal system and is characterised by a *triad of rigidity, tremors* and *akinesia* or *bradykinesia*.

Parkinsonism plus syndrome refer to parkinsonism plus bulbar palsy, Shy-Drager syndrome or multiple system atrophies.

Causes
I. *Idiopathic* (primary)
II. *Secondary parkinsonism*
   - Viral infection (encephalitis, post-encephalitis)
   - Drug-induced and toxin-induced
   - Hypoxia, anoxia
   - Vascular involvement (atherosclerotic)

Clinical Features

General
- *Expressionless (mask-like) face, greasy skin* and *slow slurred speech*
- *Hypokinesia*, e.g. slow movements, impaired fine movements of fingers (hand), glabellar tap positive
- *Gait and posture*, i.e. stooped (bent) posture, fesinant gait, propulsion/retropulsion phenomenon positive, loss of balance on turning, slow turning movements.
- *Rigidity*: It is either cog-wheel or lead-pipe.
- *Tremors* (resting) of fingers/hands (pin-rolling, decreased by action, increased by emotion, intermittent)
- *Miscellaneous* (others): Normal tendon reflexes with plantar flexor response, micrographia, emotional lability and autonomic dysfuntion.

ATAXIA
It is defined as inability to sustain erect posture.

Causes
1. Cerebellar ataxia (spinocerebellar).
2. Friedreich's ataxia (heredofamilial).
3. Sensory ataxia.
4. Vertiginous (labyrinthine) ataxia.
5. Ataxia-telangiectasia.
6. Ataxia due to proximal myopathy.
7. Hysterical.

Diagnostic criteria for Friedreich's ataxia (hereditary ataxia)
1. Progressive ataxia of young (age at onset less than 25 years).
2. Plantars (bilateral) extensor with loss of ankle and knee jerks.
3. Dysarthria, nystagmus.
4. Pyramidal signs in lower limbs with loss of joint position and vibration sense (posterior column involvement).
5. Scoliosis/pes cavus.
6. Abnormal ECG (cardiomyopathy).
7. Deafness or diabetes may be associated.

Differential Diagnosis: Two common ataxias encountered are differentiated in Table 5.36.

TABLE 5.36: Distinction between Sensory and Cerebellar Ataxia

Feature	Sensory ataxia	Cerebellar ataxia
Muscle power	Diminished	Normal
Tone	Diminished	Diminished or normal
Deep tendon reflexes	Lost	Present (pendular)
Cerebellar signs	Absent	Present
Posterior column sensation	Lost	Preserved
Plantar reflex	Lost	Normal
Charcot's joint and trophic changes	Present	Absent
Romberg's sign	Positive	Negative
Gait	High steppage, Stamping	Broad-based
Common causes	• Tabes dorsalis	• Cerebillar Infarct
	• Peripheral neuropathy	• Friedreich's ataxia
	• Syringomyelia	• Multiple sclerosis

BULBAR AND PSEUDOBULBAR PALSIES

Read Lower Cranial Nerve Palsies (IX, X, XI and XII)

Bulbar palsy: The involvement of motor nuclei of lower cranial nerves (IX to XII) in the medulla is called *bulbar palsy*.

Pseudobular palsy is upper motor type of paralysis of lower cranial nerve (IX to XII) above the medulla.

Causes and clinical features (read the differences in Table 5.37): These patients present with speech disturbance, nasal regurgitation, dysphagia, etc.

TABLE 5.37: Differences between Bulbar and Pseudobulbar Palsies

Bulbar palsy	Pseudobulbar palsy
1. Rare	1. Common
2. Lower motor neuron type of paralysis of palatal, pharyngeal and tongue muscles	2. Upper motor neuron paralysis leading to spasticity of palatal, pharyngeal and tongue muscles
3. The muscles are atrophic or hypotonic	3. The muscles are spastic (tone is increased)
4. Gag and palatal reflex are lost	4. They are preserved
5. Tongue is atrophic and lies motionless	5. Tongue is spastic
6. Dysphonia, dysphagia and dysarthria present	6. Spastic dysarthria with indistinct speech present
7. Nasal regurgitation prominent	7. Not prominent
8. Jaw Jerk is absent	8. Jaw Jerk is exaggerated
9. No emotional change	9. Emotional lability (crying, laughing) present
10. Site of lession is medulla	10. Site of lesion is in both hemispheres (above the medulla).
Causes: Medulla oblongata infarction, MND, syringobulbia, GB syndrome poliomyelitis, vasculitis, brain stem glioma or meningitis	**Causes** include bilateral hemiphlegia, MND, multiple screlosis, brain tumour

MYOTONIA

Definition: Myotonia is defined as a state of continued muscle contractions with poor relaxation after the cessation of voluntary effort. Myotonic disorders are mostly inherited (autosomal dominant) or may be acquired.

Types of myotonias are:
I. Myotonia dystrophica
II. Myotonia congenita
III. Paramyotonia

Clinical Signs
- Increased tone
- Poor relaxation of hand-grip during shaking hand with the patient
- *Percussion sign* is positive, i.e. percussion over the thenar eminence or tongue produces a dimple
- Slow relaxation of eyes after closure.

Other features: These are usually present in dystrophic myotonia, i.e.
- Frontal baldness
- Cataract
- Mental retardation
- Cardiomyopathy or conduction defects
- Glucose intolerance
- Hypogonadism
- Repeated respiratory infections (low serum IgG)
- Somnolence

Diagnosis is confirmed on EMG

MUSCULAR DYSTROPHIES/MYOPATHIES

Definition: Myopathies are defined as genetically determined primary degeneration of muscle fibres without an evidence of involvement of central or peripheral nerves.

Classifications

I. X-linked
- *Duchenne* (severe) and *Becker* (mild) types.

II. Autosomal dominant
- Limb girdle (scapulohumeral and pelvifemoral)
- Congenital

III Autosomal recessive
- Fascioscapulohumeral
- Scapuloperoneal
- Oculopharyngeal or ocular
- Distal

Clinical Features (Table 5.38)

Diagnosis. The diagnosis is confirmed by EMG, muscle enzymes and muscle biopsy.

Differential Diagnosis (Table 5.38)

HEMIPLEGIA

Definition: Weakness of one-half of the body is called *hemiplegia* (hemi means *half*, plegia means *paralysis*). Partial weakness of one half of the body is called *hemiparesis*.

Causes

1. *Cerebrovascular disease*, e.g.
   - Transient ischaemic attacks (TIA).
   - Cerebral thrombosis, embolism, haemorrhage.
   - Internal carotid artery aneurysm or vascular malformation.
   - Sagittal sinus thrombosis.
   - Migrainous hemiplegia (transient hemiplegia).
   - Subdural haematoma/head injury.
2. *Brain tumour*.
3. *CNS infections*, e.g. encephalitis, meningitis, syphilis.
4. *Demyelination*, e.g. multiple sclerosis, demyelinating encephalitis.
5. Spinal hemiplegia, i.e. Brown-sequard syndrome.
6. *Functional*, e.g. hysterical.

Symptoms and Signs

UMN signs will be present on the side involved. They may be absent in the beginning due to acute neuronal shock but after a few days they appear after recovery from shock, i.e.

1. Spasticity of the limbs (tone is increased).
2. Exaggerated tendon reflexes, ankle and patellar clonus may or may not be present.
3. Superficial reflexes (abdominal) and cremasteric (in males) are absent.
4. Plantar response is extensor (positive, Babinski's sign).
5. Hoffmann's and Wartenberg's signs may be positive in the upper limb.
6. Hemiplegic (circumducting gait (Fig. 5.64A).
7. No muscle atrophy. No trophic changes.

Diagnosis and Differential Diagnosis

The diagnosis of hemiplegia rests on history, clinical examination and investigations. The differential diagnosis lies to find out its cause and to localise the site of the lesion. Functional disorders such as hysterical hemiplegia should be differentiated from organic one (Hoover's sign). Most of the cases belong to CVA, hence its three common causes are differentiated in Table 5.39.

Hoover's sign: It is useful sign to detect weakness in pyramidal lesion, hence, differentiates between

TABLE 5.38: Diagnostic Diagnosis of Muscular Dystrophies

Dystrophy	Mode of inheritance	Age at onset (year)	Clinical features	Other associated features
Duchenne	X-linked recessive	3–10	• Progressive weakness of girdle muslces • Inability to walk after age of 12 years • Kyphoscoliosis	• Cardiomyopathy • Mental retardation
Becker	X-linked recessive	Early (5–15 years) to late (30–40 years)	• Progressive weakness of girdle muscles • Still able to walk at the age of 15 years	• Cardiomyopathy
Limb girdle	Autosomal recessive	10–30	• Slowly progressive weakness of shoulder and hip girdle muscles	• Cardiomyopathy
Fascioscapulo-humeral	Autosomal dominant	10–40	• Slowly progressive weakness of face, shoulder girdle, foot dorsiflexion	• Hypertension • Deafness
Congenital	• Autosomal	• At birth or in first few months	• Hypotonia • Contractures • Delayed motor milestones • Progression to respiratory failure in some cases	• CNS abnormalities • Eye abnormalities
Oculo-pharyngeal	Autosomal dominant	50–60	• Slowly progressive weakness of extraocular, pharyngeal and limb muscles	—
Myotonic	• Autosomal	• 20–60 years (but in infancy if born to affected mother)	• Cardiac conduction defects • Cataract • Mental retardation • Frontal baldness • Gonadal atrophy • Hypertension • Deafness	

organic hemiplegia from hysterical hemiplegia. In unilateral pyramidal lesion (hemiplegia) when a patient in recumbent position flexes the thigh and lifts the paretic limb presses the bed with normal limb. This can be appreciated with the palm of the hand placed below the heel of the limb. This phenomenon is negative in hysterical hemiplegia.

Localisation of the Lesion

The site or level of the lesion can be deduced from the associated neurological findings.

1. Cortical or subcortical (corona radiata) lesion

The characteristic features are:
 i. Contralateral hemiplegia of uncrossed type. (Cranial nerve and hemiplegia are opposite to the side of lesion).
 ii. Supranuclear 7th nerve palsy.
 iii. Convulsions (Jacksonian) may occur.
 iv. Speech disturbance (aphasia) if dominant hemisphere is involved.
 v. Cortical type of sensory loss (asterognosis, loss of sense of position and two-point discrimination).
 vi. Anosognosia (disturbance of smell), visual field defect.

2. Internal capsular lesion (capsular hemiplegia)

- Commonest site.
- Contralateral hemiplegia of uncrossed type.
- UMN paralysis of 7th nerve.
- Contralateral hemianaesthesia.
- Dense hemiplegia—complete paralysis of face, upper and lower limbs
- No convulsion, speech, taste or visual disturbance.

Remember. Lacunar infarct (small vessel infarct) can produce pure motor or pure sensory hemiplegia.

3. Midbrain lesion

- Contralateral hemiplegia of crossed type. (Cranial nerve on the side of lesion with contralateral hemiplegia)
- The 3rd nerve nuclear paralysis with contralateral hemiplegia constitute *Weber's syndrome*.
- Contralateral hemianaesthesia and analgesia.

4. Pontine lesion

- Contralateral hemiplegia of crossed type
- Contralateral hemianaesthesia and analgesia

TABLE 5.39: Differential Diagnosis of Cerebrovascular Accidents with Hemiplegia

Feature	Cerebral thrombosis	Cerebral embolism	Cerebral haemorrhage
Onset	Sudden, may be slow (stroke-in-evolution)	Abrupt like bolt from the blue	Sudden, catastrophic
Premonitory symptoms	May be present in the form of TIA	Absent	May be present in the form of speech disturbance or attacks of weakness in a limb
Consciousness	Preserved or there may be slight confusion	Preserved, sometimes patient may be dazed	Usually semiconscious or unconscious
Headache	Absent but occurs if cerebral oedema develops	Absent	Severe, persistent
Neck stiffness	Absent	Absent	Present if bleed leaks into subarachnoid space
Neurological deficit	Slowly developing	Maximum at the onset, followed by initiation of recovery	Rapidly developing and progressive
Precipitating or predisposing conditions	Hypertension, diabetes, dyslipidaemia, hypothyroidism, hypercoaguable states (pregnancy, puerperium, oral contraceptives), dehydration or shock	Evidence of source of embolisation, i.e. heart disease (ischaemic, rheumatic), aneurysm (arterial ventricular), thrombosis (atherosclerosis, atrial)	Precipitated by stress, exertion, physical act, sudden rise in BP. Atheromatous arteries, aneurysm of arteries or AV malformations predispose to haemorrhage
Symptoms and signs of raised intracranial tension	Absent	Absent	May be present if bleed leaks into subarachnoid space
Recovery	Slow, may be partial or complete	Rapid, recovery is the rule	Slow, if patient recovers. Residual damage persists.

- Ipsilateral 6th or 7th cranial nerve paralysis (LMN type) with contralateral hemiplegia is called *Millard-Gubler syndrome*.
- Constriction of pupil (*Horner's syndrome*) on the same side of the lesion due to involvement of sympathetic fibres.
- Ataxic hemiplegia with or without dysarthria (due to a lacunar infarct).

5. Medulla oblongata lesion

I. *Features of medial medullary syndrome*
- Paralysis of half of tongue (XII nerve palsy) on the side involved
- Upper and lower limb UMN paralysis sparing the face on the opposite side
- Impaired tactile and proprioceptive sensations on the opposite side

II. *Features of lateral medullary syndrome (Wallenberg's syndrome)*

- Facial numbness (V) ⎫
- Ataxia, nystagmus (cerebellar) ⎬ Same side of lesion
- Horner's syndrome (sympathetic) ⎬
- IX and X nerves palsy ⎭

- Loss of posterior column sensation lateral ⎫
- Spinothalamic (pain, touch, temperature) sensory loss ⎬ Opposite to the side of lesion
- Hemiparesis (mild, unusual) ⎭

6. Spinal Cord ($C_1 - C_4$) lesion
- *Brown-Sequard syndrome* (read spinal cord lesion).

EPILEPSIES

Definition: They are a group of disorders of cerebral function characterised by chronic, recurrent paroxysmal nonsynchronous discharges of cerebral neurons

Seizure is defined as an episode of neuronal dysfunction, hence, epilepsies are seizural disorders with motor concomitants, e.g. limb jerking and incontinence.

Classification of Adult Epilepsy

I. **Primary partial/focal seizures**
 i. Simple partial seizure (consciousness preserved) with motor/sensory/visual/psychomotor signs.
 ii. Complex partial seizures (consciousness lost).

II. **Primary generalised seizures**
- Grand mal (tonic and clonic)
- Only tonic or clonic
- Petit mal
- Akinetic
- Myoclonic

Causes
1. Cerebrovascular accidents, TIA.
2. Space occupying lesion (neurocysticercosis, brain tumour).
3. CNS infections, e.g. encephalitis, meningitis, brain abscess.
4. Head injury/trauma.
5. Hypertensive encephalopathy.
6. Metabolic causes, e.g. uraemia, hepatic failure, hypoglycaemia, electrolyte disturbance, i.e. hyponatremia.
7. Alcohol withdrawl syndrome.
8. Illicit drug use.
9. Miscellaneous, e.g. neurosarcoidosis, neurotuberculosis, multiple sclerosis, Alzheimer's disease.
10. **Precipitating factors**, e.g. fatigue, insomnia, stress, pyrexia, drugs, infections, flashes of light/bright light, loud noise or music, alcohol ingestion or withdrawl, reading or writing, etc.

Jacksonian Epilepsy (Focal Epilepsy)

It is a simple partial seizure of focal onset arising from a small portion of precentral gyrus resulting in a fit involving one part of limb (e.g. thumb) and then spreads to the whole limb/one half of the body/whole body. It suggests usually an intracranial space occupying lesion. It may be followed by *Todd's paralysis* (transient paralysis of a limb or hemiplegia).

Characteristics of an epileptic fit. The characteristics of an epileptic fit and its differentiation from psychogenic fit are listed in Box 5.12.

POLYNEUROPATHIES

Definition. It is a group of disorders involving the peripheral nerves resulting in symmetric or asymmetric peripheral sensory loss. Polyneuropathy may be axonal (irreversible) or demyelinating (reversible). It may be pure sensory, pure motor or sensorimotor.

Causes
1. **Genetic**
 - Hereditary motor and sensory neuropathy (Charcot-Marie-Tooth disease).
2. **Toxins and drugs**
 - Alcohol
 - Heavy metals, e.g. gold salts, arsenic.

Nervous System

Box 5.12	Features Differentiating an Epileptic fit from a Hysterical fit
Grand mal fits	*Hysterical conversion fits*
• The fits occur in a coordinated fashion due to hypersynchronous discharge of neurons	• The fits may vary from simple falling to the ground to bizarre attacks
• Stereotyped movements of limbs occur	• There is wild bizarre movements of all the four limbs simultaneously
• Attacks can occur during any time of the day	• Attacks occur when patient is being observed or somebody is present
• Patient may injure himself or herself during an attack	• Patient does not hurt himself during an attack
• These are unprovoked fits. There is no purpose behind these fits. These are true seizures	• Attacks occur with some purpose, i.e. to draw the attention of nears and dears or to seek compensation or sympathy
• There may be an aura before a fit. Postictal phenomena are common	• These are pseudo-seizures. There is neither an aura nor any post-ictal phenomenon
• There may be biting of tongue during seizure. There is urine and faecal incontinence	• There is no biting of tongue during fit. There is no urine or faecal incontinence
• The seizures may be precipitated by some known factors	• There are no known precipitating factors
• Pattern of the fits is fixed	• Frequent change in the pattern of fits. There may either be an addition or deletion of some symptoms during the fit
• EEG may be abnormal	• EEG is normal

- Organic solvents.
- Drugs, e.g. amiodarone, vincristine, nitrofurantoin, hydralazine, metronidazole, phenytoin, dapsone, isoniazide.
- Toxins-diphtheria.

3. **Metabolic**
   - Diabetes mellitus, hypothyroidism.
   - Amyloidosis, paraproteinaemia.
   - Renal and hepatic failure.
   - Acute intermittent porphyria.

4. **Connective tissue diseases**
   - Polyarteritis nodosa (PAN), RA, SLE.

5. **Deficiency states**
   - Deficiency of vitamins, e.g. B_1, B_6, B_{12} (subacute combined degeneration) and folate.

6. **Infections**
   - Leprosy, typhoid, diphtheria and HIV.

7. **Malignancy and paraneoplastic syndrome**
   - Carcinoma of bronchus, lymphomas, multiple myeloma.

Clinical Features

Symptoms

The first manifestation is distal paraesthesia (tingling affecting the feet and then the hands) which progresses proximally up the limbs. This is followed by numbness. There may be history of slipping of shoes/slippers off the feet. There may be history of trophic changes.

Signs

i. There is loss of superficial sensations in a *glove and stocking distribution and calf tenderness* may be present on squeezing the calf muscles.
ii. There is distal weakness of hands and feet with diminished or absent ankle and palmar reflexes (e.g. *finger flexion reflex*). Plantar reflex may not be elicitable.
iii. High-steppage gait (*see* Fig. 5.64C). Patient while walking lifts the leg high from the ground due to bilateral foot drop.
iv. There may be burn marks or trophic changes.

Diagnosis is confirmed by nerve conduction velocity (slowing of nerve conduction).

Differential diagnosis rests between the causes of polyneuropathy.

POSTINFECTIVE POLYNEUROPATHY (GUILLAIN-BARRÉ SYNDROME)

Guillain-Barré syndrome is an acute demyelinating polyneuropathy mostly immunologically mediated. It develops 1–3 weeks following viral infection in 70% cases and more rarely following surgery or immunisation.

Clinical Features

The patient complains of weakness of distal limb muscles (Fig. 5.86) or distal numbness. This ascends over several days or weeks. The most striking findings on examination are diffuse weakness and widespread loss of reflexes (areflexic motor paralysis) with or without sensory disturbance. In mild cases, there is little disability but in some cases respiratory and bilateral facial muscles are affected making the patient totally paralysed.

Miller-Fisher syndrome—a variant of Guillain-Barré presents with ataxia, areflexia and external ophthalmoplegia followed by weakness of proximal muscles.

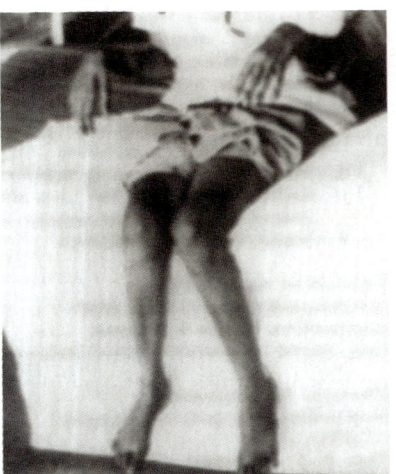

Fig. 5.86: Guillain-Barré syndrome. There is distal weakness with bilateral hand and foot drop.

Diagnosis is confirmed by CSF examination (albumino-cytological dissociation) and nerve conduction velocity (delayed velocity).

Differential Diagnosis
Acute porphyria and lead intoxication may cause neuropathy similar to Guillain-Barré syndrome.

MYASTHENIA GRAVIS

Definition: This is an acquired autoimmune neuromuscular junction disorder characterised by weakness and fatiguability of proximal limb muscles, ocular and bulbar muscles. It occurs in young females (2nd and 3rd decade), runs relapses and remitting course. It may be associated with other autoimmune disorders.

Symptoms
1. Muscle fatigue and weakness precipitated by exertion, exercise, infection, changes of climate pregnancy, hyper and hypothroidism
2. Intermittant ptosis or diplopia
3. Difficulty in swallowing, speaking or moving the limbs
4. Respiratory symptoms, e.g. cough, dyspnoea, respiratory failure. Asphyxia can occur.

Signs
1. Muscle fatigue and weakness which can be demonstrated by asking the patient to count up to 100. There is change in the speech which become inaudible
2. Intravenous edrophonium test (test reverses the symptoms).

Diagnosis. It is confirmed by serum acetylcholine receptors antibodies and EMG/nerve conduction velocities and edrophonium test.

Differential Diagnosis
1. It is to be differentiated from myasthenia myopathic syndrome (Box 5.13).
2. Oculopharyngeal myopathy.

MULTIPLE SCLEROSIS

Definition: Multiple sclerosis (MS) is a disorder of unknown aetiology in which there are multiple areas of demyelination (*plaques of demyelination*) within the brain and spinal cord. These plaques are disseminated in time and space, hence, also called *disseminated sclerosis*. An abnormal immune mechanism is presumed to be its cause.

It is rare in India and other countries of Asia and Africa, but is extremely common in west.

Clinical features: It occurs in young age and runs relapsing and remitting course. The symptoms and signs are:

 i. *Eye symptoms*, e.g. pain and visual disturbances.
 ii. *Brain stem sign and symptoms*, e.g.
   - Diplopia, vertigo, facial numbness, dysphagia, nystagmus.
   - Pyramidal signs in the limb (monoplegia) or limbs (spastic paraplegia/quadriplegia).
   - Cerebellar ataxia, e.g. ataxia of gait.

Box 5.13: Myasthenia vs Myasthenia Myopathic Syndrome

Myasthenia gravis	Myasthenic-myopathic syndrome
• An immunological disorder	• A non-metastatic manifestation of malignancy
• Common in females	• Common in males
• Anticholinesterase receptors antibodies present	• They are absent. Antibodies to Ca^{++} channels depress the release of ACh
• Tensilon test is positive	• It is negative
• Tendon reflexes are preserved	• They are lost or diminished
• Exercise induces muscle weakness	• Muscle strength improves with activity
• Spontaneous remission may occur	• No such remission
• Treatment is anticholinesterase drugs or immunosuppression	• Removal of the tumour, if found or by use of 3, 4 diaminopyridine

- Charcot's triad (dysarthria, nystagmus and intention tremors).
  iii. **Sensory symptoms**
    1. Paraesthesias (tingling and numbness).
    2. Loss of posterior column sensation (loss of position and joint sense). There may be positive Lhermitte's sign. (*Barbar chair sign*).
    3. Loss of pain, touch and temperature.
  iv. **Urinary symptoms**
    - Urgency, hesitancy, incomplete emptying or incontinence.
  v. **Other features**
    - Epilepsy, trigeminal neuralgia, hemifacial spasms, anxiety, depression, etc.

Diagnostic Criteria

1. Two or more separate episodes of worsening involving two or more different sites in the brain occuring at least one month apart with gradual progression over 6 months.
2. CNS involvement of more than two sites out of five, i.e. (i) pyramical tracts, (ii) cerebellum, (iii) optic nerve, (iv) medial longitudinal fasciculus and (v) posterior column.
3. MRI evidence plaques or evoked potential evidence for involvement of two sites.
4. Exclusion of other conditions by investigations.

Diagnosis is established by CSF changes (lymphocytosis and oligoclonal band of IgG), MRI brain and electrophysiological studies.

SYRINGOMYELIA

Syringomyelia (*syrinx*—cavity; *myelia*—spinal cord) is defined as a cavity in the cord not communicating with the central canal and is not lined by the epithelium. The cavity may be present in the lower cervical and upper thoracic lesion, or may extend into medullary region (*syringobulbia*).

Aetiology

- **Congenital defect** when it is associated with other developmental defects (Chiari malformations, platybasia, atresia of foramen of Magendie or cysts of posterior fossa (*Dandy-Walker syndrome*).
- **Acquired cavitary lesions** as a sequelae of trauma, meningitis or tumours. In majority of cases, no cause is detected in syringomyelia.

Clinical Features

- Insidious onset and slow irregular progression.
- Symptoms and signs of cervicothoracic cavity.

A. **At the level of cavity**
  i. There is LMN paralysis of upper limbs i.e. wasting of small muscles of hands, forearms with areflexia
  ii. Dissociated sensory loss over the upper limbs in a *"cafe fashion"*.
  iii. Trophic changes in hands, charcot joints.
  iv. Horner's syndrome

B. **Clinical features below the site of cavity**
  - Bilateral pyramidal signs (spastic paraplegia).

Diagnosis is confirmed by MRI of spinal cord.

Differential Diagnosis

1. Intramedullary spinal cord tumour.
2. Arachnoiditis.
3. Craniovertebral anomaly.
4. Spinal cord injury with cervical myelopathy.

MOTOR NEURON DISEASE (MND)

Definition: It is a degenerative motor disease involving anterior horn cells of spinal cord, motor cranial muclei of lower cranial nerves and pyramidal pathways. It is of 4 types:

1. Progressive spinal muscle dystrophy
2. Progressive lateral sclerosis
3. Amyotrophy lateral sclerosis
4. Pseudobulbar palsy

Characteristic Features

1. Rarely occurs before 40 years of age
2. Presence of both upper and lower motor neurons signs in at least two limbs or one limb and involvement bulbar cranial nerves. Fasciculations are characterstic and diagnostic
3. No sensory involvement in the limbs
4. No ocular muscle involvement
5. No cerebellar or extrapyramidal involvement
6. Sphincters are involved late
7. Disease is progressive with no remission.

> **Note:** Madras motor neuron disease has an early onset with asymmetric paralysis of limbs with sensorineural deafness.
> Fasciculations are marked. It is slowly progressive and benign condition.

Diagnosis is mainly clinical supported by raised serum muscle enzymes, EMG and nerve conduction *studies* and *muscle biopsy*. Genetic studies are also useful.

PARAPLEGIA

Definition: Complete paralysis or weakness of both the lower limbs is called *paraplegia* while partial weakness is labelled as *paraparesis*. It may be upper motor neuron type (spastic) or lower motor neuron type (flaccid).

Causes

Paraplegia may be *compressive* or *noncompressive* in nature.

Compression paraplegia may be due to extramedullary or intramedullary compression (Table 5.40).

TABLE 5.40. Compressive and Non-compressive Paraplegia with their Causes

Extramedullary compression	Intramedullary compression
Causes: Meningioma, neurofibroma, arachnoiditis Pott's disease, vertebral disease (neoplams, fracture, dislocation) prolapsed disc and epidural abscess	**Causes:** Syringomyelia, haematomyelia intramedullary tumour, spinal cord abscess
1. Root pain common	1. Rare
2. UMN signs are early and prominent	2. Late and less prominent
3. Segmental sensory loss or absent reflex at the site of compression	3. Extends to involve a few segments producing fasciculations and atrophy
4. Contralateral sensory loss with ipsilateral loss of proprioceptive sensations	4. Dissociated sensory loss
5. Sphincters involved late	5. Early involvement
6. Trophic changes absent	6. Present (common)
7. Vertebral tenderness may be present	7. Absent
8. Froin's syndrome common	8. Rare

The **clinical signs** of compression are:
I. LMN type of paralysis (areflexia, atrophy of the muscles) or segmental sensory loss at the level of the lesion.
II. UMN type of spastic paralysis with all signs below the level of compression.

Paraplegia-in-flexion: It means involvement of only pyramidal tract, hence, is mild disease.

Paraplegia-in-extension: It means complete compression of pyramidal as well as extrapyramidal tracts.

Causes of Non-compressive Paraplegia

1. Motor neuron disease.
2. Multiple sclerosis.
3. Acute transverse myelitis.
4. Subacute combined degeneration of the cord.
5. Lathyrism.
6. Syringomyelia.
7. Hereditary spastic paraplegia.
8. Tropical spastic paraplegia.
9. Radiation myelopathy.

Causes of LMN Paraplegia

1. Guillain-Barré syndrome.
2. Poliomyelitis or postpolio syndrome.
3. Radiculopathy.
4. Peripheral neuropathy.
5. Myasthenia gravis.
6. Myopathies.

Symptoms and Signs of LMN paraplegia

- Flaccid paralysis with areflexia below the level of the lesion.
- Muscle atrophy/fasciculations.
- Sensory loss may or may not be present.
- Trophic changes/contractures may or may not be present.

Unit VI

Gastrointestinal and Hepatobiliary Systems

- Symptoms and their Analysis
- History
- General Physical Examination
- Systemic Examination
- Diagnosis and Differential Diagnosis
- Brief Synopsis of GI and Hepatobiliary disorders

SYMPTOMS OF GASTROINTESTINAL SYSTEM

Read Box 6.1.

Box 6.1 Symptomatology of Gastrointestinal Tract

UPPER GI SYMPTOMS
- Pain abdomen
- Aerophagia
- Appetite
- Vomiting
- Hematemesis
- Heartburn and acid reflux (pyrosis)
- Dysphagia, odynophagia
- Hiccups
- Dyspepsia, flatulence
- Halitosis (bad breath)

LOWER GI SYMPTOMS
- Abdominal pain
- Diarrhoea
- Constipation
- Rectal bleeding
- Weight loss
- Malena
- Abdominal distension
- Tenesmus

PAIN ABDOMEN

Any ache or pain in or around the abdomen is referred as *abdominal pain*. It may be *specific* or *non-specific* such as burning, gnawing or vague fullness or discomfort.

Types of Pain

1. **Visceral pain:** It arise from the stretching of a hollow viscus due to its distension. The painful stimuli from the organ are transmitted through sympathetic nerve endings to thalamus.
2. **Parietal pain:** Parietal peritoneum has painful nerve endings which get stimulated when parietal peritoneum is involved (e.g. peritonitis). Such pain is usually *localized* or may be *diffuse* and associated with *muscular guarding* or *rigidity*.
3. **Referred pain:** It means that site of production of pain is different than where it is perceived over the abdomen. Anginal pain may be referred to epigastrium; pain of herpetic intercostal neuralgia may be referred to abdomen.
4. **Psychogenic pain:** It has no organic basis. Patient pinpoints the pain with tip of a finger. This indicates neurosis or depression.

Causes of Abdominal Pain
Also see Table 6.1 and Fig. 6.1.

Symptom Analysis

Ask about the following

Q. **What is the site of pain?** Pain may be epigastric quadrantic or back pain.
- The site and causes of pain are depicted in Fig. 6.1
- Back pain may occur due to kidney stone, pancreatitis, tabes mesenterica (tubercular lymphadenitis), diseases of the spine (secondaries), retroperitoneal deposits.

Q. What is its severity and nature?
- *Colicky pain* (severe pain due to which patient tosses in the bed or uses a hot water bottle) is characteristic of biliary, renal or intestinal spasms. It is intermittent.
- *Non-colicky severe pain* may be due to intestinal obstruction/perforation, haemorrhage or infection, inflammation or may be referred pain from myocardial infarction, pulmonary or pleural diseases.

Q. Is it continuous or intermittent?
- *Colicy pain* is intermittent while pain due to inflammation, infection or malignancy may be continuous.

Q. What is duration of pain?
- Pain of short duration is colicky pain.
- Pain of long duration indicates either inflammatory or neoplastic disorder.
- Paroxysmal pain with intervals of freedom indicates peritonitis.
- Constant pain indicates malignancy or low grade inflammatory process (peritonitis).

Q. Does it radiate to any site/direction?
- Renal colic pain radiates to testicle or labia.
- Gall bladder pain radiates to right scapula.
- Interscapular pain indicates pancreatitis/pancreatic cancer.
- Periumbilical pain could be due to appendicitis.

Q. Is pain related to meals?
- Pain of duodenal ulcer occurs three to four hours after food, i.e. empty stomach at midnight or early morning called *hunger pain*.

TABLE 6.1. Causes of Pain Abdomen

Structure involved	Causes
I. Abdominal wall	Myalgia, neuralgia, herpes zoster
II. Intra-abdominal	
• Visceral pain	*Colic* (intestinal, biliary, renal), *ulcer* (peptic, enteric, gastric), *infection* (amoebic or pyogenic liver abscess, cholecystitis, hepatitis, pancreatitis, ulcerative colitis) and *mesenteric artery insufficiency* (abdominal angina)
• Peritoneal pain	Peritonitis, malignant infiltration of peritoneum
• Referred pain	Myocardial infarction, pneumonia, diaphragmatic pleurisy, caries spine
• Functional	Munchausen syndrome

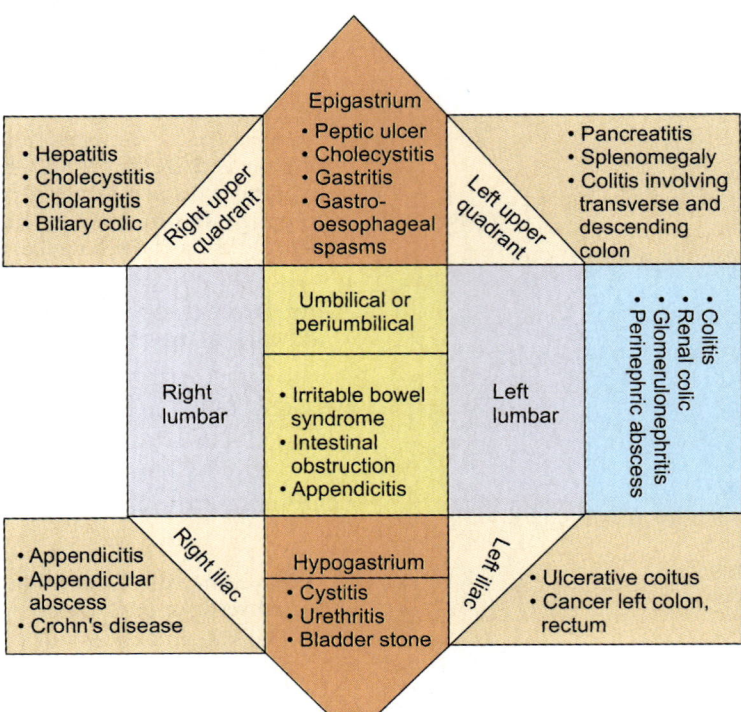

Fig. 6.1: Causes of pain.

- Attacks of biliary colic occur 3 to 5 hours after a heavy meal.

Q. Is it nocturnal? Does it disturb sleep?
- Pain of peptic ulcer is usually nocturnal and disturbs the sleep.

Q. Is there an aggravating or relieving factor?
- Physical effort exacerbates pain of renal or gall bladder colic.
- Musculoskeletal pain should be suspected if it is aggravated by exercise and relieved by rest.
- Fatty food aggravates gall bladder pain.
- Pain aggravation during lying down and relieved on sitting or bending indicates pancreatic disease (malignancy).
- Alcohol and smoking exacerbate pain of peptic ulcer.
- Pain aggravation during menses indicate premenstrual tension, pelvic inflammatory disease and endometriosis.
- Food and antacids relieve pain of peptic ulcer
- Epigastric pain worst during lying down and relieved by sitting up suggest hiatus hernia or pancreatitis.

Q. Is there an associated symptom?
- Vomiting is common in gall bladder colic, acute gastritis and pancreatitis.
- Dysuria and haematuria indicate renal disease.
- Alternating constipation and diarrhoea indicate intestinal tuberculosis, irritable bowel syndrome.

AEROPHAGIA (AIR SWALLOWING)

Excessive swallowing of air is called *aerophagia*. It may cause distension and abdominal discomfort. Some patients complain of belching and a moving ball of wind.

Normally, a small amount of air is swallowed during deglutition, gets expelled through mouth or rectum (passage of flatus). Whenever, a large amount of air is swallowed and its expulsion becomes difficult resulting in abdominal discomfort is called *aerophagia*. It is common in psychogenic states. The common **causes** are:
1. *Certain foods and drinks* such as cokes, beer, carbohydrate meal, chewing gum, milk and milk products can lead to it.
2. *Smoking*, alcohol and pan-chewing.
3. *Mouth breathing*.
4. *Gastrointestinal diseases*, e.g. gastritis, peptic ulcer, hiatus hernia, irritable bowel syndrome.
5. *Psychogenic*, e.g. anxious movements/states, depression and emotional disturbance.
6. *Postoperative swallowing* of air.

Clinical Significance

Aerophagia, itself is of no significance. It becomes important when it mask or simulate certain organic disorders such as cholecystitis, pancreatitis, angina, myocardial infarction, peptic ulcer, etc.

Secondly it causes discomfort, abdominal distension, early satiety, hiccups, passage of flatus and may give rise to gastric pneumatosis (feeling of suffocation), pseudoangina (cardiac neurosis) and splenic flexure syndrome (chest pain, palpitation, chocking) simulating ischaemic heart disease.

Symptom Analysis

Q. Ask about abdominal distension.

Q. Ask about moving ball of wind in the abdomen.

Q. Ask about aggravating or relieving factors.

Q. Ask about associated symptoms.

APPETITE

It is defined as *"desire to eat"*. Disorder of appetite includes increase or decrease in appetite or perversion of appetite.

Terms Related to Appetite

- *Anorexia* means loss of appetite or loss of desire to eat. It may be *psychogenic, physiological* or *pathological*.
- *Satiety* means lack of desire to eat.
- *Sitophobia* means "fear of eating". It is observed in peptic ulcer when patient does not eat due to fear of pain.
- *Polyphagia* means excessive appetite, is seen in metabolic disorders, commonly in diabetes mellitus and thyrotoxicosis. It can be psychogenic (hysterical or obsessional psychosis).
- *Perversion of appetite* means craving for unusual or abnormal food. Perverted appetite is seen in *worm infestations* in children, *during pregnancy*, etc.
- *Geophagia* or *pica* means craving for unusual substances, e.g. mud, plaster, hair, chalk, leaves, etc.

Causes of Decreased Appetite

1. *Physiological*, e.g. sedentary habits/physical inactivity or irregular eating.
2. *Metabolic and endocrine disorders*, e.g. Addison's disease, hypothyroidism, hypopituitarism.
3. *Liver and kidney diseases*, e.g. hepatitis, cirrhosis and chronic kidney disease.
4. *Congestive heart failure*.

5. *Malignancies* of stomach, colon, pancrease, leukaemias and lymphomas.
6. *Drug induced*, e.g. amphetamines, antiobesity drugs, digitalis and cytotoxics.
7. *Psychogenic*, e.g. anorexia nervosa.

Symptom Analysis

Ask about the following
- Is appetite decreased or increased?
- If reduced, is appetite poor or patient is afraid of taking food due to pain?
- Does the patient has history of pica? Is there any loss of weight?
- History of fever suggesting tuberculosis, etc.
- History of taking drug. Take full drug history.
- History of alcoholism and smoking.

Q. What is anorexia nervosa?
- It is a functional loss of appetite in which patient usually young girls eat less to reshape their body and lose weight. In **binge eating** or **purging**, the patient not only restricts so caloric consumption but tries to reduce weight by inducing vomiting or abuse the laxative or a diuretic.
- **Bulimia nervosa** is characterized by episodes of excessive eating due to central loss of appetite control. This binge eating is followed by periods of restricted eating, thus a viscious cycle is set up. Binge eating generates a feeling of guilt that can be relieved only by induction of vomiting or by self starvation.

NAUSEA AND VOMITING
- *Nausea* means an intense feeling to vomit.
- *Vomiting* or *emesis*: It is an act of expulsion of gastric contents.
- *Retching*. It is an urge to vomit with forceful expiratory contractions of the abdominal muscles with the glottis closed but there is no vomiting.
- *Regurgitation* implies expulsion of gastric contents back to mouth resulting in bitter acid taste in the mouth (*water brush*).

Causes of Vomiting
1. **Gastrointestinal**
   - Gastritis, peptic ulcer, gastric malignancy, duodenal ulcer, pyloric obstruction (gastric outlet obstruction), post-gastrectomy syndrome, gastroparesis.
   - Acute appendicitis, pancreatitis, gastroenteritis (food poisoning).

2. **Neurological**
   - Meningitis, encephalitis, migraine, raised intracranial pressure, subarachnoid haemorrhage, autonomic neuropathies.
   - Labyrinthitis, Meniere's disease, motion sickness

3. **Cardiovascular**
   - Congestive heart failure, acute MI.

4. **Hepatobiliary**
   - Hepatitis, portal hypertension, gallstones, cholecystitis.

5. **Endocrinal and metabolic**
   - Uraemia
   - Diabetic ketoacidosis, Addison's disease.

6. **Drugs and toxins**
   - Alcohol
   - Drugs, e.g. aspirin, digitalis, iron preparations, cytotoxics, narcotics such as morphine, sulphonamides, anaesthetics, theophylline, etc.

7. **Pregnancy**
8. **Psychogenic**
9. **Radiation therapy**

Symptom Analysis
Following questions are asked and analysed as follows.

Q. When does it occur? Does it occur in the morning?
- Early morning vomiting occurs in pregnancy, alcoholic gastritis, uraemia and raised intracranial pressure.

Q. Is it related to meals?
- Vomiting occurring during or immediate after eating is either psychogenic (*anorexia nervosa*) or peptic ulcer with pylorospasm.
- Vomiting occurring after 4–6 hours of eating indicates either pyloric obstruction, gastroparesis, cardia achalasia or Zollinger-Ellison's syndrome.

Q. What is duration of vomiting?
- A short history suggests toxic factor or food poisoning or some infective cause.
- A long duration indicates uraemia, malignancy or Addison's disease

Q. Is there any associated symptom?
- Associated symptoms of tinnitus, vertigo indicate vestibular disease.
- Associated fever with vomiting indicates infection or an inflammatory disorder.
- Epigastric pain with vomiting indicates peptic ulcer or pancreatic disease (pancreatitis, cancer pancreas). Colicky pain with vomiting

indicates either biliary or renal or intestinal colic (acute intestinal obstruction).
- Headache associated with vomiting indicates migraine.

Q. Does it contain residue of food taken the day before?
- Vomiting containing undigested food particles indicates pyloric obstruction, gastroparesis or cardiac achalasia.

Q. Does vomitus contain blood?
- Blood in vomitus (*hematemesis*) indicates peptic ulcer, gastric malignancy, drug induced, Mallory-Weiss syndrome (a tear at gastro-oesophageal junction after an alcoholic bout) or variceal bleed due to portal hypertension.

Q. Is there a history of drug intake?
- A large number of drugs already discussed can lead to vomiting.

Q. Ask about past history of:
- Peptic ulcer, gallstones, inflammatory bowel disease, irritable bowel syndrome.

HEMATEMESIS

Definition: Blood in the vomitus is called *hematemesis*. The blood may be in streaks or frank blood. It may be red or coffee ground colour. Bleeding in upper GI tract produces black coloured vomitus due to formation of acid hematin in stomach. The stools may remain black coloured for 3–4 days even after the bleeding has stopped.

> *Note:* Hematemesis is always associated with malena in upper GI bleed. Malena without vomiting or haematemesis indicates lesion below the pylorus.
> Blood in hematemesis and malena can be red-coloured in upper GI bleed if it is passed hurriedly without staying for sometimes in the stomach, i.e. its transition in stomach and intestine is short.

Causes
1. Acute gastric erosions commonly due to NSAIDs
2. Chronic duodenal ulcer, gastric ulcer or malignancy.
3. Variceal bleed due to rupture of oesophageal or gastric varices due to portal hypertension.
4. Oesophagitis, Mallory-Weiss syndrome (oesophageal tear)
5. Vascular anomalies (angiodysplasias) in upper GI tract
6. Acute pancreatitis (haemorrhagic)
7. Blood dyscrasias or coagulation defect.

Symptom Analysis
Proceed as follows:

Q. Ask about the age.
- Duodenal ulcer is common in young, portal hypertension in middle age and malignancy in old age.

Q. Ask about drug history or alcohol intake.
- Haematemesis is common after intake of NSAIDs or after a bout of alcohol.

Q. Is there a history of pain?
- Chronic periodic nocturnal pain indicates duodenal ulcer while acute pain indicates gastritis or pancreatitis or oesophagitis.

Q. Is the hematemesis recurrent?
- Previous episodes of hematemesis or malena suggest the possibility of portal hypertension or peptic ulcer

Q. Is there a history of jaundice?
- Jaundice and hematemesis indicate hepatic disease (portal hypertension).

Q. Ask about history of bleeding disorder.
- Bleeding disorder may be associated with hematemesis in addition to bleeding at other sites, i.e. epistaxis, ecchymosis, haematuria, etc.

Q. Ask about the amount of blood passed in vomitus.
- Small amount of blood passed indicates gastric oozing due to malignancy stomach; while large amount indicates peptic ulcer or variceal bleed.

> *N.B.* The hematemesis has to be differentiated from haemoptysis (read haemoptysis).

BLEEDING PER RECTUM/HEMATOCHEZIA

Bleeding through the rectum is a common symptom of lower GI bleed. It differs from malena being red in colour.

Causes
1. Anorectal conditions, e.g. pile (haemorrhoids) and fissure, rectal ulceration/prolapse
2. Inflammatory bowel disease (ulcerative colitis, Crohn's disease)
3. Drugs, intestinal polyposis, diverticular disease and angiodysplasias.
4. Uraemia and portal hypertension in elderly rectal carcinoma, ischaemic colitis and inflammatory bowel disease are common causes.
5. Blood dyscrasias

> **Warning:** Massive blood loss in upper GI bleed may manifest as bleeding per rectum due to rapid transit, hence, do not jump to the diagnosis of lower GI bleed straight way.

Symptom Analysis

Ask about the following

Q. **Age of the patient.**
- Piles, rectal prolapse, blood disorders, and angiodysplasia are common causes of rectal bleeding in young; while rectal carcinoma, ischaemic colitis, inflammatory bowel disease are common in old persons.

Q. **Does blood comes in streaks or spurts?**
- Bleeding in anorectal conditions usually comes in streaks while spurting of blood is common in angiodysplasias or during anti-coagulant therapy.

Q. **Is bleeding painful?**
- Painful bleeding indicates mostly anorectal conditions or inflammatory bowel disease.

Q. **Is blood mixed with loose stool?**
- Blood mixed with loose stool indicates dysentery or inflammatory bowel disease.

Q. **Is there history of drug intake?**
- The drug causing bleeding has already been discussed under hematemesis.

Q. **Is there any change in bowel habits?**
- Change in bowel habits with bleeding per rectum indicates right-sided colonic malignancy.

Q. **Is there bleeding from other sites?**
- Bleeding from many sites occur due to blood dyscrasias, leukaemias, anticoagulant therapy, liver or renal failure.

HEARTBURN AND ACID REFLUX

Definition: As the name suggests, a burning sensation behind the sternum (heart) or high up in the epigastrium is called *heartburn*, hence the causes originate in the oesophagus mostly due to reflux of acid or bile into the oesophagus called *gastro-oesophageal reflux disease (GERD)*.

Causes

Gastro-oesophageal reflux is the underlying mechanism in addition to oesophageal diseases for heartburn. The causes of gastro-oesophageal reflux are:
1. Intake of spicy food, alcohol, smoking, etc.
2. Heavy meal with full stomach. A full distended stomach is likely to produce regurgitation/heartburn.
3. Raised intra-abdominal pressure (pregnancy, ascites, GERD).

> **Note:** Normally short-lived bouts of regurgitation are physiological. Bouts of regurgitation staying for longer period produce oesophagitis called *reflex oesophagitis*.

4. *Organic causes*, e.g. oesophagitis (gastro-oesophageal reflux disease), peptic ulcer, pyloric spasms, hiatus hernia.
5. *Psychogenic*, e.g. neurosis, hypersensitive individuals.

Symptom Analysis

Ask about the following provoking factors

Q. **Ask about history of taking spicy food.**
Q. **Ask about dietary habits, history of alcohol, smoking, etc.**
Q. **Does patient sleep flat at night?**
- Sleeping flat exacerbates GERD

Q. **Are the bouts of heartburn short-lived or long-lived?**
- Short-lived heart burn after meals is of no consequence prolonged heartburn leads to oesophagitis.

Q. **Is there any associated history of hematemesis?**
- Hematemesis with heartburn indicates organic cause.

DIARRHOEA

Diarrhoea refers to more than 3 loss stools/day Quantitatively it is defined as stool content more than 200 g/day when dietary fibre content is low. The bulk of the stool increases with high dietary fibre intake.

Types

- **Acute diarrhoea** refers to loose motions of less than 2 weeks duration, rapid in onset, occurs otherwise in a healthy person, may lead to dehydration and hypotension. It is usually infective in origin.
- **Chronic diarrhoea** means loose motions of more than 2 weeks to a few months duration. Chronic diarrhoea of 3 months or more is referred as malabsorption syndrome. Chronic diarrhoea is insidious in onset, usually intermittent but can be constant resulting in nutritional deficiencies. It is usually a manifestation of systemic disorders.
- **Small bowel diarrhoea.** It refers to large loose watery stools without blood and mucus. It indi-

cates involvement of small intestines. It is either infective (bacterial, parasitic) drug-induced (ampicillin, digitalis), traveller's diarrhoea or consumption of shellfish.
- **Large bowel diarrhoea.** It refers to small viscid stools with blood and pus cells, indicates large bowel involvement. It results from inflammatory bowel disease, pseudomembranous colitis, pelvic inflammatory disease and faecal impaction (*spurious diarrhoea*).

Causes

Acute Diarrhoea

i. Infections
  - Viruses (rota, norwalk, adeno, HIV, corona), bacterial (*E.coli*, *V.cholerae*, Salmonella, Shigella, Campylobacter, Yersinia), parasitic (*Giardia lamblia*, *E. histolytica*).
ii. Food poisoning (*bacillus cereus*, Vibrio, Salmonella, *Shigella* spp).
iii. Drug-induced, e.g. amoxicillin, laxatives, digitalis, magnesium containing antacids prokinetics, antineoplastic, antibiotic induced pseudomembranous colitis, thyroxine.
iv. Traveller's diarrhoea.
v. Consumption of fish (e.g. shellfish).
vi. Miscellaneous, i.e. pelvic inflammatory disease, spurious diarrhoea (faecal impaction).

Chronic Diarrhoea

1. Dietary factors, e.g. high intake of fructose, sorbitol.
2. Intestinal infections, e.g. amoebiasis, tuberculosis.
3. Drug-induced as discussed above.
4. Malabsorption syndrome, lactose intolerance, functional bowel disorder (irritable bowel syndrome).
5. Inflammatory bowel diseases, e.g. ulcerative colitis, Crohn's colitis.
6. Metabolic diseases, e.g. diabetes, thyrotoxicosis, Addison's disease.
7. Neoplasms, e.g. carcinoid syndrome, WDHA syndrome, pancreatic cancer.
8. Faecal impaction (spurious) or faecal incontinence (diabetic autonomic neuropathy), anorectal surgery.
9. Large bowel secretory diarrhoea, e.g. bile salt induced, post-cholecystectomy, etc.

Symptom Analysis

Q. **Ask the age of the patient.**
  - Most common cause in young age is infections, in middle and old age is either colon carcinoma or laxative abuse.

Q. **Ascertain the sex.**
  - Colon carcinoma is more common in males.
  - Anxiety neurosis, thyrotoxicosis and use of laxatives are more common in females.

Q. **Does diarrhoea alternate with constipation?**
  - Alternate diarrhoea with constipation indicates intestinal tuberculosis, amoebic infection, irritable bowel syndrome, colon malignancy and laxative abuse.

Q. **Ask about relation to food.**
  - Diarrhoea occurring after certain food indicates food allergy.
  - Cramping pain with diarrhoea following ingestion of milk or milk products indicates lactase deficiency (lactose intolerance).

Q. **Ask about the duration.**
  - Causes of acute and chronic diarrhoea have been discussed.

Q. **Is there any tenesmus (gripping pain before defaecation)?**
  - Tenesmus indicates bacillary dysentery, tuberculosis, ulcerative colitis or diverticulosis.

Q. **Ask about the timing of diarrhoea.**
  - Nocturnal diarrhoea occurs in diabetic autonomic neuropathy and inflammatory bowel disease.
  - Diarrhoea occurring at any time of the day suggests small bowel disease.
  - Diarrhoea on rising in the morning suggests large bowel involvement.

Q. **Ask about nature of the faeces.**
  - *Large pale, pasty and frothy stools* indicate steatorrhoea.
  - *Bloody diarrhoea* indicates infections and infestations (amoebiasis, salmonellosis), inflammatory bowel disease, ischaemic colitis, malignancy colon, diverticulitis and radiation colitis.
  - Presence of *blood mixed with mucus* suggests amoebic or bacillary dysentery.
  - *Passage of large amount of mucus* without blood indicates mucus colitis/ulcerative colitis.

CONSTIPATION

Definition: It is defined as infrequent passage of hard stool. Because of the wide range of normal bowel habits, constipation is difficult to define precisely. Most patients have 3 bowel movements/weeks, hence, stool frequency is not a definite criteria. Similarly hard stool and intestinal transit time, not a criteria for diagnosis. Therefore, any patient who strains to defecate and does not pass at least one soft stool a day is said to constipated, hence, in addition to hard stool, straining and other abdominal symptoms such as abdominal distension, sense of incomplete evacuation and flatulence are corroborative to diagnosis.

Dyschezia: It means straining at stool due to constipation. It is associated with constipation.

Types

Constipation may result due to decreased bulk of stool (low fibre intake), retention of faeces due to disorders of colon and delay in the discharge of faecal matter due to anorectal conditions. Therefore, the main types of constipation are:

I. *Inadequate bulk of stool.* Inadequate bulk of the stool will not lead to sufficient peristalsis to propel the faeces.
II. *Colonic constipation.* Formation of faeces in colon may result in delay of excretion/propulsion of faecal matter in colon leading to constipation. This is most common cause of constipation in old age.
III. *Dyschezia.* It means defective evacuation of faeces. Here colonic movements are normal. This is accompanied by dissatisfaction with act of defaecation.

Causes

I. **Gastrointestinal (simple constipation)**
 - Low fibre/fluid intake
 - Old age (decreased expulsive power due to weakness of abdominal muscles or of pelvic floor).
 - Delay in rectal clearance due to voluntary suppression of defaecation as a result of travelling or improper lavatory facilities. This is common cause of simple constipation in females.
 - Motility disorders, e.g. irritable bowel syndrome, acute intestinal obstruction.
 - Colonic diseases, e.g. carcinoma, Hirschsprung's disease (congenital megacolon in children), diverticulosis, stricture, etc.
 - Painful anorectal conditions, e.g. piles, anal fissure, faecal impaction.

II. **Neurological**
 - Spinal cord diseases, e.g. compression, injury.
 - Parkinsonism.
 - CVA
 - Multiple sclerosis.

III. **Endocrinal/metabolic**
 - Diabetes, hypothyroidism, pregnancy, hypercalcaemia.

IV. **Drugs**
 - Opiates, anticholinergics, calcium antagonists, iron supplements, aluminium containing antacids.

Symptom Analysis

Q. Ask about the details of dietary intake.
 - Inadequate fibre intake in diet leads to it.

Q. Ask about the onset (acute/chronic).
 - *Acute onset* indicates either acute obstruction or acute inflammatory or infective disorder or malignancy colon in old age.
 - *Chronic constipation* may be due to neurological, metabolic and endocrinal causes. It leads to chronic abuse of laxative which further perpetuates constipation.

Q. History of drug intake.
 - List of drugs causing constipation has been given already.

Q. Does diarrhoea alternate with constipation?
 - Subacute intestinal obstruction (ileocaecal tuberculosis) and irritable bowel syndrome are common causes.

Q. Does pain accompany constipation?
 - Constipation with crampy abdominal pain with anorexia and fullness after meals may suggest a diagnosis of spastic colon.

Q. History of rectal bleeding and constipation.
 - Bleeding per rectum with constipation indicates anorectal condition, e.g. pile, anal-fissure.

ABDOMINAL DISTENSION/SWELLING

Definition: Increased girth of the abdomen is called *abdominal distension*.

Causes

Girth of the abdomen increases in four ways denoted by "**Fs**", i.e.
1. **Fluid**, e.g. collection of fluid due to ascites, ovarian cyst or distended bladder.
2. **Foetus:** Pregnant uterus.
3. **Faeces and flatus**, e.g. acute intestinal obstruction, paralytic ileus.
4. **Fat:** Truncal obesity and fatty hernia.

Symptom Analysis

Following questions should be asked

Q. Is there an increase in abdominal girth, i.e. tightness of clothes or belt?
 - Increase in abdominal girth confirms abdominal distension.

Q. Ask about history of passage of flatus.
- Non-passage of flatus suggests acute intestinal obstruction, paralytic ileus and adynamic ileus.

Q. Does the bowel move regularly?
- Increased bowel movements with constipation indicate intestinal obstruction while decreased bowel movments with constipation indicate paralytic ileus.

Q. Is there a history of pregnancy in a female?
- Pregnancy can lead to distension abdomen.

Q. Is the distension progressive?
- Ascites leads to progressive painless distension.

Q. Is there any history of tapping of fluid?
- Tapping of fluid confirms ascites as a cause of distension.

Q. Ask about past history of liver disease (jaundice), cardiac disease (dysponoea, palpitation) or renal disease (puffiness of face, oedema).
- Chronic liver disease, cardiac disease, renal disease can lead to abdominal distension due to ascites.

Q. Is the patient obese?
- Record weight and height. Calculate BMI to confirm obesity.

TENESMUS
Definition. It is a sensation of incomplete rectal emptying. Patient has frequent desire to pass stools.

Causes
- Ulcerative colitis/colitis.
- Irritable bowel syndrome.
- Prolapse rectum/carcinoma rectum.

Symptom Analysis

Q. Do you have frequent urge to pass stool?
- Patient has frequent desire and he/she is not satisfied after defaecation in irritable bowel syndrome.

Q. Is pain associated with defaecation?
- Pain is usually associated with defaecation in tenesmus due to colitis.

Q. Is there any prolapse rectum?
- Rectal prolapse can lead to tenesmus.

Q. Is blood associated with stool?
- Blood in stool with tenesmus indicates ulcerative colitis.

FLATULENCE
Definition: It refers to presence of excess of air (more than normal) in the abdomen, the expulsion of which either by belching or through rectum gives relief of symptoms.

Meteorism: It refers to abdominal distension or bloating due to presence of gas.

Clinical Presentations
Patient with flatulence presents in the following ways:
1. Belching
2. Intestinal distension or meteorism with gurgling (Borborygmi)
3. Passage of excessive flatus.

Causes

I. Gastric causes
- Aerophagy (excess swallowing of air), pyloric obstruction, gall bladder dyspepsia, hiatus hernia.

II. Intestinal causes
- *Excessive fermentation resulting in excessive production of gas*, i.e. excess carbohydrate or milk or milk product intake, chronic amoebiasis, malabsorption.
- *Defective absorption* of gas, e.g. congestive heart failure, cirrhosis of liver.
- *Defective elimination*, e.g. constipation.

Symptoms Analysis
Proceed as follows

Q. Ask about history of belching.
- Belching produces swallowing of air. Patient tries to expul the gas by belching and instead of expulsion, he/she swallows the air in return.

Q. Ask about pain or retrosternal discomfort.
- It suggests either gall bladder disease or hiatus hernia.

Q. Presence of abdominal discomfort, diarrohea.
- It suggests amoebic infection or lactose intolerance.
- History of ingestion of certain goods, e.g. beans, peas, nuts, cabbage, sprout, prunes, apples produce gaseous discomfort and may even lead to diarrhoea.

Q. Ask about history of food allergy.
- Food allergy and lactose intolerance can produce gas due to excessive fermentation.

Q. Ask also history of parasitic infestation.
- Parasitic infestation/amoebiasis and bacterial infection (malabsorption) produce flatulence.

HICCUP

Definition: An involuntary violent contraction of the diaphragm producing a characteristic sound is called *hiccup* or *singultus*.

Pathogenesis

It occurs through a reflex arc, where the afferent impulses from the various structures travel to respiratory centre via 9th and 10th cranial nerves and efferents stimuli travel down from the respiratory centre to the diaphragm through phenic nerves.

Causes
I. *Intra-abdominal*, e.g. diaphragmatic pleurisy, peritonitis, high spicy food, subphrenic abscess, distended stomach and liver abscess.
II. *Mediastinal causes*, e.g. mediastinitis, cardiomegaly, pericardial effusion, aortic aneurysm, mediastinal tumour, substernal goitre.
III. *Neurological* (stimulation of respiratory centre), e.g. meningitis, encephalitis, epilepsy, hydrocephalus, brain tumour.
IV. *Metabolic*, e.g. uraemia, diabetic ketoacidosis.
V. *Toxic*, e.g. high fevers, toxaemia and septicaemia.
VI. *Psychogenic*, e.g. neurosis, hysterical swallowing, too hot or too cold drink, etc.
VII. *Postoperative*: Dilatation of stomach, peritonitis.

Symptom Analysis

Hiccup following high spicy food, too hot or too cold drink is normal (physiological). For abnormal hiccup, ask about the GI disorders, neurological cardiovascular, metabolic and toxic causes as follows:

Q. **Ask about history of past surgery.**
- Persist and frequent hiccup could be due to neurosis, hysteria, GI surgery.

Q. **Is hiccup short-lived or persistent?**
- Short-lived hiccup occurs due to intake of spicy food, too hot or too cold drink and heavy meal.
- Persistent hiccup suggests GI disorder, CNS disorder, i.e. meningtis, encephalitis, uraemia, ketoacidosis, high fever due to toxaemia/septicaemia, etc.
- Chronic recurrent hiccup indicates neurosis or hysteria.
- Chronic frequent hic cough can occur in amoebic liver abscess, subdiaphragmatic abscess or any other pathology.

HALITOSIS

Definition: Halitosis means foul breath, is produced in the mouth by the action of gram-negative bacteria on proteinous materials such as degenerated epithelial cells, leukocytes, food particles and damaged tissue releasing volatile sulphur containing compound which lead to foul breath.

> An unpleasant breath on awakening is normal as self cleansing mechanisms of the mouth, i.e. saliva and movements of tongue and cheeks cease during the night.

Causes
I. **Oral and upper respiratory infections**
- Chronic nasopharyngeal catarrh, dental caries, oral sepsis and quinsy (peritonsillar abscess).

II. **Respiratory infections**
- Bronchiectasis, lung abscess, bronchopleural fistula.

III. **Gastrointestinal causes**
- Gastrocolic fistula, sialadenitis, Sjögren's syndrome.

IV. **Metabolic causes**
- Uraemia (urine-like smell of breath)
- Hepatic failure (fetor hepaticus, ammoniacal smell or smell of mice)
- Diabetic ketoacidosis (sweet odour or acetone odour)

V. **Drugs and poisons**
- Organophosphorous (garlic-like smell), aluminium phosphide (pungent smell) poisoning
- Anticholinergic, paraldehyde, disulfiram.

VI. **Fever and toxaemia**

VII. **Psychoneurosis**

Symptom Analysis

Q. **Ask about oral dental hygiene.**
- Poor orodental hygiene, sialadenitis, oral sepsis can lead to halitosis.

Q. **Ask about cough, sputum, etc.**
- Bronchiectasis, lung abscess, bronchopleural fistula can lead to fuel breath.
- Upper respiratory infections, i.e. sinusitis, dental caries quinsy can also lead to halitosis.

Q. **Ask about diabetes, chronic renal or hepatic disease.**
- Diabetic ketoacidosis, uraemia, hepatic failure lead to foul breath.

Q. Ask about drugs/poisoning.
- OP compound and aluminium phosphide poisoning lead to pungent breath.

FATIGUE/TIREDNESS

Definition: It is defined as progressive decline of stamina for physical work, is often described as lethargy, weakness, malaise, listlessness. It can be intermittent and variable in intensity.

Tiredness which is similar to fatigue can occur, for example, in anxiety neurosis, depression and emotional stress.

Exhaustion is a severe form of fatigue usually occurs due to psychological and physical causes such as prolonged emotional stress, asthenia, lack of sleep, bouts of physical effort, heat intolerance, trauma.

Chronic fatigue syndrome is now a recognised clinical entity arising due to a variety of causes, in which symptoms must last for 6 months.

Causes
- *Haematological*, e.g. anaemia, leukaemia, lymphoma.
- *Electrolyte disturbance*, e.g. hypokalaemia, hypercalcaemia.
- *Cardiovascular*, e.g. CHF, hypertension.
- *Neurological*, e.g. periodic paralysis, myopathies.
- *Endocrine*, i.e. hyper- or hypothyroidism, Addison's disease, Cushing syndrome.
- *Psychogenic*, e.g. anxiety, depression, emotional trauma.
- *Drugs*, e.g. diuretics, antihypertensive.

Symptom Analysis

Ask about the following

Q. Ask about the duration.
- Recent onset fatigue is mostly organic in origin.
- Long duration (>6 month) indicates chronic fatigue syndrome.

Q. Is fatigue continuous or intermittent?
- Intermittent fatigue is due to psychiatric illness.
- Persistent fatigue indicates organic cause.

Q. Ask about timing of fatigue.
- Fatigue in the evening after activity is organic in origin.
- Fatigue on awakening or in early hours of the day suggests chronic fatigue syndrome.

Q. What is its severity?
- Severe fatigue that affects physical and mental functioning indicate chronic fatigue syndrome.

Q. What are relieving or aggravating factors?
- Fatigue relieved by rest and sleep and occurring during effort is psychogenic. Motivation relieves psychogenic fatigue. Physical and mental stress aggravate symptoms of chronic fatigue syndrome.

Q. Ask for associated symptoms of anxiety and depression.
- Chronic fatigue syndrome as well as organic diseases associated with fatigue lead to depression.

Q. Is there history of any systemic disease?
- Read the causes of fatigue.

THIRST

Definition. Excessive craving for water or fluids is called *thirst*. A proper fluid balance is necessary for physiological requirement of our body, hence, thirst indicates a major fluid deficit within the body.

Pathogenesis

The sensation of thirst is attributed to:
I. Dryness of mouth with reduced secretion of saliva because of inadequate water balance.
II. Altered composition of blood.

Causes

I. Physiological
- Hot weather, physical exercises, food rich in salt.

II. Excessive loss of fluids
- *Through GI tract*, e.g. diarrhoea, vomiting.
- *Through skin*, e.g. perspiration, hyperhydrosis.
- *Through kidneys*, e.g. polyuria.
- *Through blood*, e.g. blood loss, i.e. hemorrhage.

III. Drugs, e.g. anticholinergics, antidepressants, diuretics.

IV. Local causes, e.g. mouth breathing, Sjögren's syndrome, parotitis, mumps.

V. Systemic diseases, e.g.
- *GI tract diseases*, e.g. pyloric obstruction, gastric cancer, gastric stasis.
- *Endocrinal*, e.g. diabetes mellitus, diabetes insipidus, hyperparathyroidism.
- *Renal*, e.g. renal failure

VI. Psychogenic

Symptom Analysis
- Ask about age, sex, occupation, habits
- Ask about history of drugs

- Ask about history of fluid/blood loss through mouth skin (perspiration), through urine (excessive urination).
- History of GI disorder/renal disease or diabetes mellitus or diabetes insipidus.

SYMPTOMS OF HEPATOBILIARY SYSTEM

1. **Constitutional or nonspecific symptoms**
   - Fatigue
   - Weakness
   - Nausea, vomiting
   - Anorexia or poor appetite
   - Malaise
2. **Specific symptoms** (i.e. they are liver-specific, suggest the cause such a hepatitis or cirrhosis and/or complications such as end-stage liver disease or encephalopathy)
   - Abdominal pain, hepatomegaly (mass abdomen)
   - Jaundice
   - Dark-coloured urine, high-coloured stools
   - Swelling or oedema feet
   - Fetor hepaticus
   - Flapping tremors
   - Encephalopathic features (disturbed consciousness, disturbed speech and sleep pattern, bizarre handwriting)
   - Bloating
   - Haematemesis and malena
   - Pruritus

HEPATIC (UPPER ABDOMINAL) PAIN

Right upper abdominal pain occurs in many liver diseases and is usually marked by tenderness in this area. The pain arises due to stretching or irritation of Glisson's capsule which surrounds the liver and is a pain sensitive structure. Hepatic pain in liver disease occurs in *liver abscess, severe veno-occlusive disease, Budd-Chiari syndrome* and *acute hepatitis*. Occasional colicky pain in right hypochondrium indicates biliary colic (stricture, stone, tumour). Pain radiating to shoulder is due to involvement of diaphragmatic pleura (pneumonia) or liver (liver abscess or malignancy liver) or due to subphrenic abscess.

Symptom Analysis

Q. Ask about site of pain, its severity and radiation.

Q. Ask about associated features, i.e. jaundice, urine discolouration, stool colour.

Q. Ask about history of dysentery, abdominal surgery or sepsis.

MASS ABDOMEN (ABDOMINAL LUMP)

Mass abdomen refers to intra-abdominal masses in relation to various viscera in the abdomen. Mass abdomen may produce fullness of abdomen or visible swelling, dragging sensation in abdomen, pain abdomen or may just be asymptomatic, i.e. patient is not aware of it. Malignant masses or tumours produce decreased/loss of appetite or weight loss. The possible sites of masses in the abdomen and specific to right hypochondrium are disscussed at the end of Unit in Box 6.6.

Mass due to liver disease occurs in hepatitis, malignancy liver, liver abscess, leukaemia, hemolytic anaemia, etc. (read the causes of hepatomegaly).

Symptom Analysis

Q. **Ask about mass, its site.**

Q. **Ask about dragging pain or diffuse pain.**

Q. **Ask about other masses in cervical, axillary and inguinal region.**

Q. **Ask about associated features, i.e. fever, cough, dyspnoea.**

Q. **Ask about diarrhoea, dysentery, discolouration of urine and stool.**

Q. **Ask about jaundice.**

JAUNDICE

Jaundice is yellowness of sclera, mucous membranes and skin, occurs due to raised serum bilirubin. Normal serum bilirubin is more than 0.3 to 1.5 mg%. Jaundice appears when serum bilirubin is more than 2.5 mg%. Serum bilirubin less than 2.5 mg but more than normal indicates *subclinical jaundice*. The clinical jaundice may be progressive or may appear intermittently.

Types and Causes

Jaundice is of three types; *hemolytic* (excessive destruction of RBCs), *hepatic* (involvement of liver) and *obstructive* (obstruction to biliary system within liver or outside the liver).

Depending on the type of bilirubin accumulation, it is further classified as *unconjugated* and *conjugated hyperbilirubinaemia* (conjugated hyperbilirubin exceeds 50% of total serum bilirubin). Conjugated hyperbilirubinaemia indicates intrahepatic or extrahepatic cholestasis while unconjugated hyperbilirubinaemia mainly occurs due to hemolysis, defective uptake or conjugation.

Causes

I. **Hemolytic Jaundice**
   - Defective shape of RBCs, e.g. spherocytosis, sickle cell anaemia.

- Defective haemoglobin, e.g. thalassaemia (hemoglobinopathies)
- Deficiency of enzyme, e.g. G6PD deficiency
- Drug-induced (warm and cold antibodies)
- Congenital, e.g. Gilbert's syndrome

II. Hepatic Jaundice
- Hepatitis, e.g. viral, drug-induced, auto-immune
- Neonatal jaundice.
- Congenital, e.g. Crigler-Najjar syndrome
- Biliary cirrhosis.

III. Obstructive Jaundice
- Intrahepatic cholestasis, e.g. viral hepatitis, drugs, cirrhosis, alcohol and pregnancy.
- Extrahepatic cholestasis, e.g. biliary duct obstruction due to stone, carcinoma pancreas, gallstones, biliary stricture, pancreatitis and secondaries liver.
- Cogenital (defective excretion), i.e. *Dubin-Johnson syndrome.*

Symptom Analysis
Ask the following questions
Q. Age and sex.
- Viral hepatitis is common in young while common bile duct stone common in middle and old age.
- Alcoholic cirrhosis, carcinoma liver and pancreas are common in males; while bile duct or gallstones, carcinoma gall bladder and biliary cirrhosis are common in females.

Q. Ask about occupation.
- Occupational handling of hepatotoxic chemicals, e.g. DDT, heavy metals and occupational exposure to viral heptitis in medical and paramedical staff can lead to jaundice. There is predisposition to Weil's disease (leptospirosis) in sewerage workers in rat infested regions.

Q. Contact with jaundiced patient or patient's blood.
- Contact with patient of jaundice, forceful kissing, sexual activity and contact with the infected blood of jaundice patient can lead viral hepatitis.

Q. Family history.
- Congenital or familial hyperbilirubinaemia runs in families.

Q. History of drug.
- Take detailed history of drug being taken or had been taken in the past.

Q. Ask about past history of recent surgery on biliary tract, alcohol intake and drugs.

> *Running Commentary about Jaundice*
> 1. Jaundice with fever, abdominal pain, anorexia. Distaste to food and smoking suggests viral or drug-induced hepatitis or liver abscess.
> 2. Jaundice in haemophilics, IV drug abuser and male homosexual indicates acute transfusion hepatitis B or C, chronic active hepatitis, if duration of jaundice is > 6 months.
> 3. Jaundice with dark-coloured urine and stool indicates haemolytic jaundice due to any cause.
> 4. Pruritus (itching) with jaundice, alcoholic white-coloured stool, xanthomatosis indicates cholestatic (obstructive) jaundice (intra- or extrahepatic cholestasis) or biliary cirrhosis.
> 5. Abdominal pain with fluctuating jaundice indicates either bile duct stone or stricture, pancreatitis.
> 6. Painless progressive jaundice indicates carcinoma of pancreas.
> 7. Jaundice, ascites with prominent abdominal veins and history of hematemesis suggest portal hypertension (cirrhotic, non-cirrhotic, Budd-Chiari syndrome).
> 8. Jaundice with pregnancy is either hepatic or cholestatic jaundice of pregnancy.
> 9. Recurrent jaundice is due to congenital hyperbilirubinaemia or recurrent benign cholestasis.

PRURITUS (ITCHING)
Definition. It is defined as desire to scratch. It is a dermatological symptom, can occur due to skin disorders but can occur due to certain systemic conditions commonly due to hepatic and renal diseases.

Causes
I. Localised pruritus
  a. *Pruritus ani* (anal itch), e.g. piles, fissure, fistula, thread worm infestation, fungal infection, psychogenic.
  b. *Pruritus valvae*, e.g. vaginitis (Candida, Trichomonas), leucorrhea (vaginal discharge), vaginal atrophy due to oestrogen deficiency, vitamin A deficiency, diabetes mellitus.
  c. Lichen simplex.

II. Generalised pruritus
  1. *Skin conditions*, e.g. scabies, dermatitis herpetiformis, eczema, psoriasis, pediculosis, senile, urticarias and carcinoid syndrome.
  2. *Systemic diseases*
     - Blood, e.g. polycythaemia

- Lymphatics, e.g lymphoma
- Endocrinal, e.g. diabetes, hyper- and hypo-thyroidism, hyper- and hypoparathyroidism.
- Renal, e.g. uraemia
- Liver diseases, e.g. cholestasis, biliary cirrhosis.
- Autoimmune diseases, e.g. SLE, Sjögren's syndrome, systemic sclerosis.

3. *Pregnancy associated*
4. *Drug-induced* (*drug allergy*)
5. *Parasitic infestation*, e.g. roundworm, trichinosis, onchocerciasis and schistosomiasis.
6. *Neurological*, e.g. herpes zoster, HIV associated
7. *Psychological*

Symptom Analysis

Q. **Ask about the history of systemic disorders described above.**

Q. **Ask about history of skin disease or skin eruption.**
- Skin diseases (read the causes) are common causes of pruritus.

Q. **Ask about history of drug intake.**
- Hepatotoxic drugs can lead to jaundice (read drug-induced hepatitis and jaundice).

Q. **Ask about history of jaundice.**
- Jaundice with pruritus suggests cholestasis.

Q. **History of worm infestation or worm expulsion.**
- Worm can occlude bile duct, hence can lead to obstructive jaundice.

> Pruritus in liver disease invariably indicates cholestasis (obstructive jaundice).

HAEMATEMESIS AND MALENA
It has already been discussed

DISCOLOURATION OF URINE
The normal urine is either clear or pale yellow in colour. The pale urine is due to normal excretion of urobilinogen (1:10) in urine. High-coloured urine can normally occur due to dehydration. Urine discolouration may be due to haemolysis, haematuria, haemoglobinuria, myoglobinuria, porphyria, can also be drug induced.

Causes
The causes of abnormal colouration of urine are:
1. **Haemolysis.** Haemolysis due to any cause produce dark colour urine either due to excretion of excessive urobilinogen or bilirubin in the urine. The bilirubinuria causing dark-coloured urine is characteristic of obstructive jaundice. Haemolysis can produce haemoglobinuria as discussed below.
2. **Haematuria.** Red colour urine is due to presence of RBCs in urine which can easily be seen on microscopic examination of urine. The causes of haematuria have been discussed in unit on genitourinary system.
3. **Haemoglobinuria.** Haemoglobin after haemolysis can be passed in the urine causing brownish discolouration of urine. The common **causes** of haemoglobinuria include *malaria (black water fever), paroxysmal nocturnal hemoglobinuria, Weil's disease. drug and congenital disorders of RBC or hemoglobin*. This can be detected by presence of haemoglobin not the RBCs in the urine.
4. **Myoglobinuria.** Myoglobin is the pigment presents in muscle, gets released into the circulation and excreted in urine in rhabdomyolysis (due to necrosis of skeletal muscle, i.e. crush injury, excessive exertion) and cardiac muscle, i.e. myocardial infarction. Myoglobin can be distinguished from haemoglobin by spectrophotometry of urine. Myoglobin also produces brownish discolouration of urine.
5. **Porphyria** (porphobilinogenuria). Porphobilinogen is the pigment released in porphyria. It does not produce immediate discolouration of urine but on standing for sometimes, it undergoes oxidation and produces bragandy-wine discolouration of urine.
6. **Drug-induced discolouration.** Excretion of rifampicin and phenolphthalein produces urine discolouration.

Symptom Analysis

Ask about the following

Q. **Fever.**
- Fever with discolouration indicates intravascular haemolysis due to infective cause (malaria, Weil's disease).

Q. **History of trauma.**
- Paroxysmal haemoglobinuria occurs during severe exertion (*marching disease*) or following crush injury.

Q. **History of acute MI.**
- Myoglobinuria can occur following acute MI.

Q. **Dark-coloured urine with discolouration of stool.**
- Dark-coloured urine with dark-coloured stool occurs due to haemolysis or diseases of the liver (hepatitis).

Gastrointestinal and Hepatobiliary Systems

Q. Ask about jaundice.
- Jaundice with dark-coloured urine indicates either hemolysis or hepatic or post-hepatic diseases.

Q. History of drug intake.
- Rifampicin and phenolphthalein produce dark urine.

Q. History of porphyria, i.e. intermittent colicky abdominal pain, diaphoresis, etc.

ABDOMINAL DISTENSION (ASCITES)

It has already been discussed.

HISTORY

Present History
- Write the complaints in chronological order.
- Detail each and every complaint/symptom with analysis as discussed above, i.e. age of the patient, onset of symptoms, duration, their progression, aggravating and relieving factors, associated symptoms and causative factors.

Past History
- History of such episodes in the past (haemolytic anaemia)
- History of alcoholism, smoking, spicy food, hepatotoxic drugs/toxin (bush tea).
- Transfusion, vaccination and injection
- Abdominal trauma/surgery
- History of diabetes, tuberculosis, hypertension.

Family History
- History of tuberculosis, polyposis, GI malignancy
- Family history of jaundice or liver disease (Wilson, hemochromatosis).

Personal and Occupational History
- Loss of appetite and weight for GI malignancy, tuberculosis
- Ask about addiction to alcohol and smoking
- Ask about lifestyle, i.e. sedentary habits
- History of travel to endemic area of hepatitis malaria, kala-azar.
- Sleep disturbance
- Colour of the urine and stool
- Occupation, e.g. labourer or sewer workers (leptospirosis) medical/paramedical staff (HIV, hepatitis)
- Vegetarian/non-vegetarian

Menstrual History
- Menses (normal/scanty/excessive).

EXAMINATION

General Physical Examination
- Built (normoasthenic/hypoasthenic)
- Nutrition (undernutrition/malnutrition)
- Look for anaemia (pallor)
- Look for alcoholic stigmatas, i.e. red tip of nose, ear lobules, sunken cheeks, shining eyeballs (cirrhotic facies), parotid glands, enlargement, pigmentation (biliary cirrhosis, hemochromatosis).

☞ **Examination of Mouth**
- Look at the face, lips, tongue (leukoplakia, Fig. 6.2), raw magenta-coloured tongue, Fig. 6.3), buccal mucosa, nails, creases of the palm for pallor (anaemia due to any cause, i.e. bleeding, nutritional, hookworm, etc.).

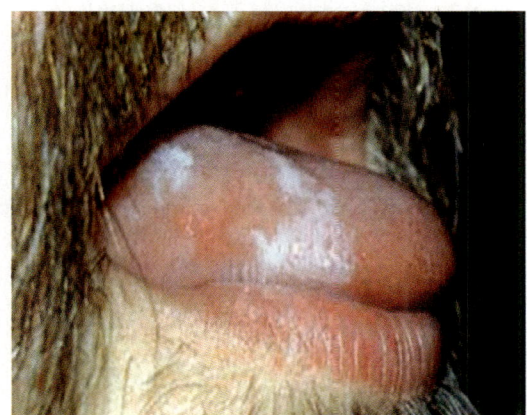

Fig. 6.2: Leukoplakia of tongue in a patient with AIDS.

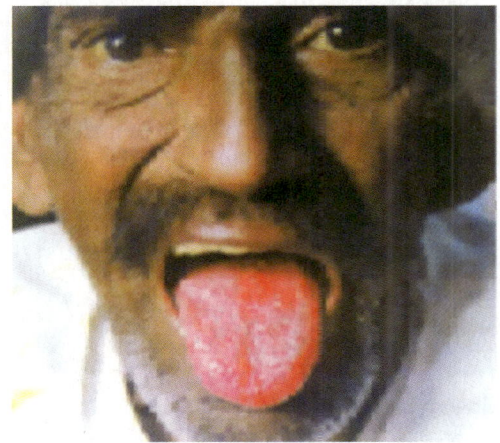

Fig. 6.3: Magenta-coloured tongue. Red, beefy, painful tongue is seen in Vit. B complex deficiency (megaloblastic anaemia).

- Look for signs of vitamins and mineral deficiency (Vit. C deficiency), angular stomatitis and cheilitis (for Vit. B complex deficiency), bald tongue (iron deficiency or nutritional anaemia (Fig. 6.4), magenta colour tongue (Vit. B_{12} deficiency), blue tongue indicates cyanosis (portal hypertension with AV shunting in lungs), aphthous ulceration (Fig. 6.5) (coeliac disease, malabsorption), Crohn's colitis, Behçet's syndrome, etc.), white (fur) mucous patches due to candidiasis (Fig. 6.6), red patches due to Vit. B complex deficiency (Fig. 6.7).

- Look for circumoral pigmentation (hereditary intestinal polyposis syndrome is called Peutz-Jeghers syndrome).

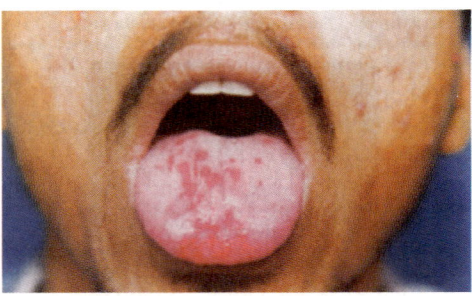

Fig. 6.7: Glossitis. Note the red patches over the tongue. The tongue was painful. There are cracks along the angles of the mouth (cheilosis) due to Vit. B complex deficiency.

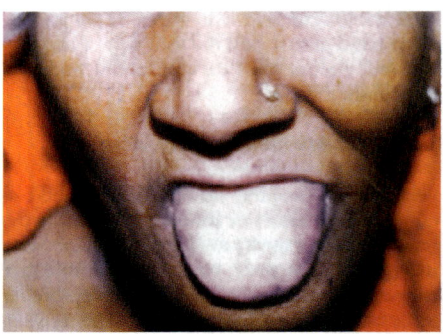

Fig. 6.4: Bald (atrophic) tongue. Pale, smooth, pigmented tongue with loss of papillae seen in the patient with iron deficiency anaemia (common in hookworm infestation).

☞ The Teeth

Ask the patient to show the teeth. If the patient has a denture, ask him/her to remove it and open the mouth widely. With the help of tongue depressor, retract first the lips and then the cheek so as to have a glimpse of all the teeth. Look for *erosion, gum hypertrophy*, *bleeding gum*.

- Gum hypertrophy occurs due to drugs (phenytoin, scurvy, leukaemias).
- Bleeding gums indicate bleeding diathesis, i.e. thrombocytopenia, anticoagulant therapy, leukaemia, lymphomas, scurvy, etc.
- Teeth erosion in children is common due to gastro-oesophageal reflux.

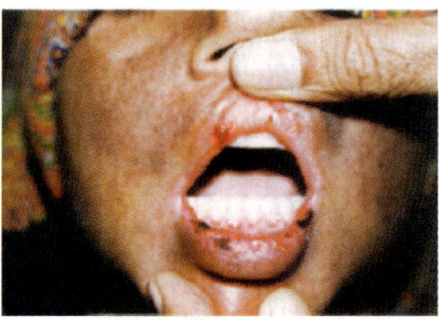

Fig. 6.5: Aphthous ulceration. Note the superficial ulcers on inner aspects of both lips with hyperaemia. The ulcers have whitish base.

☞ The Eyes

- Look for jaundice, xanthelasma.
- Examine the eyes for extra-intestinal manifestations of ulcerative colitis (i.e. iritis, episcleritis, conjunctivitis, keratitis, Sjögren's syndrome), and loss of hair on lateral third of eyebrows in obstructive jaundice.

☞ The Skin

- Look for scratch marks, pigmentation.
- Look for haemorrhagic diathesis, i.e. purpuric spots, ecchymotic patches/bruises on the skin and buccal mucosa due to Vit. C deficiency or due to chronic liver disease or pancreatitis.
- Look at the salivary glands for sialadenitis (acute and chronic) or parotitis (unilateral in mumps, bilateral in liver cell failure). Excessive salivation occurs in Wilson's disease.
- Look for subcutaneous nodules (cutaneous metastases due to gastric malignancy).

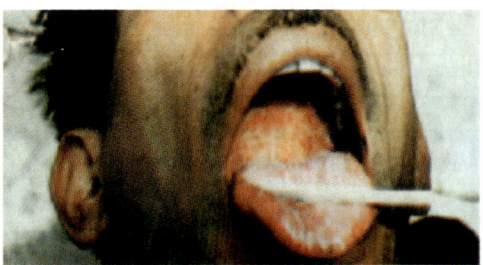

Fig. 6.6: Mouth thrush. White patches due to candidiasis.

☞ The Neck

Examine the neck for
1. *Lymphadenopathy.* Cervical lymph nodes enlargement could be due to tuberculosis, HIV and infections. Virchow's lymphadenopathy (deep cervical lymphadenopathy above the clavicle) on left supraclavicular region occurs in gastric cancer.
2. *Thyroid enlargement* (read endocrine system).
3. *Trachea* (read examination of respiratory system).

☞ The Extremities

Look at the hands and fingers.

- *Pale hands and nails* indicate anaemias, blue nails indicate cyanosis.
- *Koilonychia* (spoon shaped nails) occur due to iron deficiency anaemia as a result of hookworm disease, malabsorption and chronic diarrhoea.
- *Leukonychia* (white nails) are seen in cirrhosis of liver.
- *Clubbing of the fingers* is seen in ulcerative colitis, GI malignancy, chronic liver cell disease/insufficiency, hepatocellular carcinoma.
- *Dupuytren's contractures* occur in chronic liver insufficiency.
- *Pigmentation of hands* is seen in hemochromatosis.
- Look for the presence of *flapping tremors* (Fig. 6.8) for liver cell failure (hepatic encephalopathy) as follows:

Method

Ask the patient to outstretch his/her hands with widened fingers if patient is conscious. Note the flaps of the hands. In unconscious patient, hold the wrist with one hand and dorsiflex the patient's hand with your other hand and feel for the flap with palm of your hand.

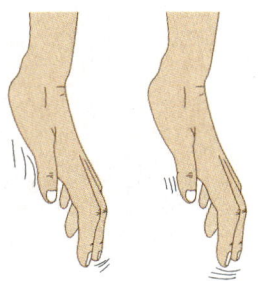

Fig. 6.8: Flapping tremors on extended hands (jerky forward movements every 2–3 sec).

☞ The Feet

Look for pitting oedema over the feet which may be isolated or a part and parcel of anasarca.

The oedema feet in GI tract and hepatobiliary diseases occur due to hypoproteinaemia, malnutrition, anaemia, cirrhosis of liver.

Examination of Abdomen for Gastrointestinal and Hepatobiliary Systems

The abdomen includes:
1. *Gastrointestinal system*
2. *Urinary system*—it is dealt separately as a Unit IV.
3. *Hepatobiliary system*

Applied Anatomy (an Anatomical Landmarks and Divisions)

For descriptive purposes, the abdomen is conveniently divided into 9 regions by intersection of imaginary planes; two horizontal and two sagittal. The upper horizontal plane is transpyloric, lies at the level of L1 vertebra, midway between the suprasternal notch and the symphysis pubis. The lower horizontal plane passes through the upper borders of the iliac crests. The sagittal planes are indicated on the surface by lines drawn vertically from the mid-inguinal points towards the midclavicular points on each side (Fig. 6.9).

The resultant regions are artificial but are used to localise the mass lesions. An alternative method is to divide the abdomen into 4 quadrants by imaginary lines crossing at the umbilicus, forming the right upper, right lower, left upper and left lower quadrants.

Normal Palpable Structures in the Abdomen

While examining the abdomen, one must know the palpable normal structures.

1. Sigmoid colon is palpable as firm tube in the left lower quadrant; while the caecum and part of the ascending colon forms a soft wider tube in the right lower quadrant. Portions of transverse and descending colon may also be palpable. None of these structures should be mistaken for tumour.
2. The liver is difficult to be felt through the abdominal wall but its lower margin or edge descends 1–3 cm during deep inspiration, hence, often becomes palpable in the right hypochondrium. Also in the right hypochondrium the lower pole of the right kidney also become palpable in thin individuals with relaxed abdomen.
3. Pulsations of abdominal aorta are frequently visible as well as palpable in the epigastrium.
4. A distended urinary bladder may be palpable above symphysis pubis.

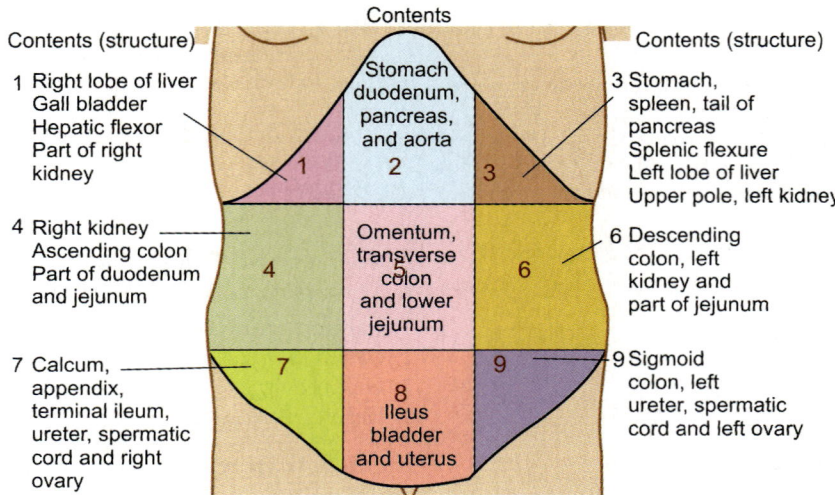

Fig. 6.9: Regions of the abdomen (diagram). 1. Right hypochondrium, 2. Epigastrium, 3. Left hypochondrium, 4. Right lumbar, 5. Umbilical, 6. Left lumbar, 7. Right iliac, 8. Hypogastrium, 9. Left iliac.

5. Other structures that become palpable in the lower abdomen include the uterus enlarged by pregnancy or fibroids, may rise above symphysis pubis, the sacral promontory and the anterior edge of the first sacral vertebra.
6. The *kidneys* are retroperitoneal structures and lie along the vertebrae, usually not palpable except lower pole of right kidney in thin abdomen. The costophrenic angle (the angle formed by the lower border, the 12th rib and the transverse process of the upper lumbar vertebrae) defines the region to be assessed for renal tenderness.

Sequence of Examination

1. Inspection
2. Palpation (conventional, hooking and dipping methods)
3. Percussion
4. Anscultation

☞ Inspection

Make the patient to lie supine in a comfortable position with arms by the side and head and neck supported on one or two pillows, so as to relax the abdomen.

The breathless patient should be examined in a standing or prop up position.

For proper inspection of the abdomen, the lighting must be adequate and the room should be warm.

A shivering patient makes the abdominal examination difficult.

Expose the abdomen properly by pulling up the clothes up to xiphisternum and sheet is folded down over the upper thighs so as to have proper look of the groin and the genitalia. Once the inspection of genitalia is over, the sheet may be pulled up to the level of symphysis pubis.

For inspection stand on the right side of the patient so as to have a close look on the abdomen.

☞ **Look for the following**

I. **Skin:** *Inspect the skin for scars*

- Shiny, smooth skin over abdomen indicates abdominal distension. Wrinkled skin suggests old distension.
- Common surgical scars produced by various incisions are depicted in Fig. 6.10. These weak scars can bulge with rise in abdominal pressure resulting in incisional hernias.

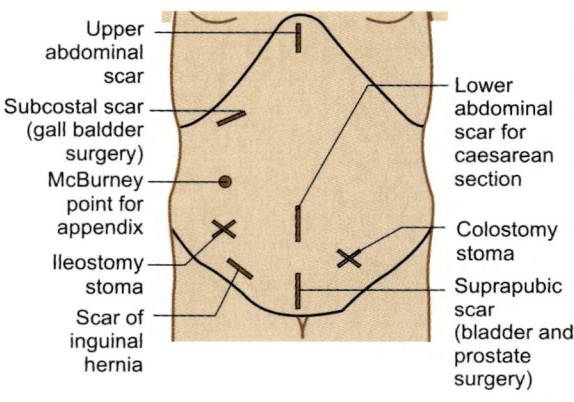

Fig. 6.10: Common surgical scars

Gastrointestinal and Hepatobiliary Systems

II. *Inspect the skin for striae*

- Silvery white striae appear on the abdomen either due to stretching of the skin in abdominal distension (e.g. ascites, pregnancy) or postpartum or due to wasting diseases or dieting.
- Pink white purple striae appear in Cushing's syndrome (see Fig. 9.17) or in patients receiving prolonged steroid therapy.

III. *Look for dilated prominent veins*

- Small thin veins over abdomen do not carry much significance.
- Dilated superficial veins on the abdomen could be due to either inferior vena cava obstruction or caput medusae due to portal hypertension (Fig. 6.11). To differentiate between the two, see the blood flow through these veins as follows:
  - Inferior vena cava obstruction, distended veins are present on the abdomen (flanks), back and lower chest wall. The flow of the blood is below upwards. Venous hum is not heard over dilated veins.
  - In portal hypertension (caput medusae), the dilated veins are present around the umbilicus and blood flow is away from the umbilicus (Fig. 6.11). Venous hum can be heard sometimes over dilated veins.

IV. *Look for rash/lesion or pigmentation*

Note any rash (drug induced, viral, vasculitis) or lesion (vesicular or maculopapular or papular) or pigmentation (linea nigra or erythema ab igne)

- *Linea nigra*—pigmentation in the midline below the umbilicus is a sign of pregnancy.
- *Erythema ab igne*—a brown mottled pigmentation produced by heat to the skin (hot water bottle or heating pad).

V. *Spider angiomata* (Fig. 6.11)

Look for spidery capillary dilatation or pin-head size macules over upper abdomen and thorax. The spider angiomatas blanch on pressure with head of a pin.

- Spider angiomatas appear in patients with cirrhosis of liver with decompensation, i.e. it is a sign of hepatic cellular failure. They may appear in vasculitis and chronic alcoholism.

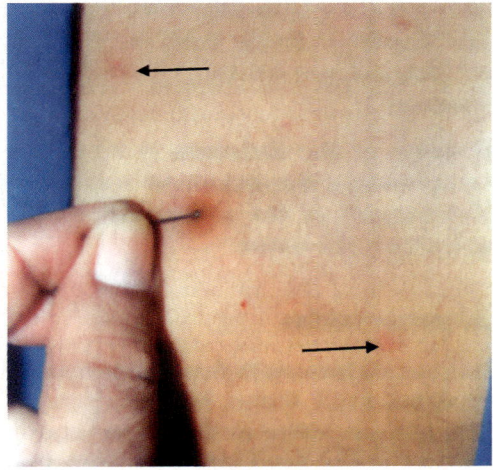

Fig. 6.12: Spider angiomata (→) that blanches on pressure.

Umbilicus: *Observe its location, contour, displacement, signs of inflammation or hernia.*

Normal umbilicus is retracted and inverted

- Umbilicus may be pulled up and down in lower and upper abdominal muscles paralysis respectively (*Beever's sign*).
- Any mass around the umbilicus may distort its position.
- Umbilicus may be transversely slit (smiling umbilicus) due to its stretching by distended flanks (ascites), everted in central abdominal distension (pregnancy, distended bladder) or displaced obliquely in ovarian cyst.
- Umbilicus is red in inflammation and sepsis (omphalitis)
- A cherry-red swelling of the umbilicus suggests inflamed Meckel's diverticulum.
- A bluish discolouration around the umbilicus (*Cullen's sign*) or bruising of the loins

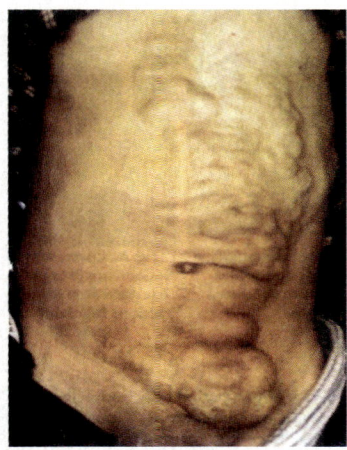

Fig. 6.11: Caput medusae. Note the dilated and tortuous abdominal veins around the umbilicus.

(*Grey Turner sign*) indicates hemorrhagic pancreatitis, ruptured ectopic pregnancy or leaking aortic aneurysm.

Shape of abdomen: *Note whether abdomen is of normal contour/shape, full, or distended. Is it sunken (scaphoid)? Do the flanks bulge? Is there any local bulge? Is the abdomen symmetrical or asymmetrical? Are there any visible masses or swellings?*

> The normal shape of the abdomen is boat-shaped or slightly scaphoid, i.e. abdominal wall sinks within bony rib margins and recede toward the centre. Flat abdomen (abdominal wall and the rib margins are at the same level) is common in normal young adults; obesity produces globular or round shape of abdomen.

- Generalised distended abdomen indicates one of the **5Fs**, i.e. *Fatty* abdomen (truncal obesity, flabby abdomen), *Fluid* (ascites), *Foetus* (pregnancy) and *Faeces* (constipation with impacted fecoliths) or *Flatus* (gaseous distension).
- Localised distension may be due to:
  i. Lower abdominal central bulge may be due to distended bladder, while peripheral bulge in this location could be due to ovarian and uterine mass/cyst.
  ii. Visible intra-abdominal mass in the right and left hypochondrium may indicate liver and spleen enlargement respectively. Kidneys may produce visible mass in the lumbar region(s).
  iii. Localised bulge in the upper abdomen with visible peristalsis indicates pyloric obstruction. Succussion splash test should be done to ascertain pyloric obstruction.
  iv. Sunken (extremely scaphoid) abdomen is common in thin emaciated persons (malnutrition), wasting diseases, malignancy, cachexia and dehydration.
  v. Divarication of recti (diastasis recti). It is wide separation of recti muscles in the midline which can be demonstrated by a linear midline bulge (Fig. 6.13) when patient is asked to rise from supine position without support (patient should raise head and shoulder).

Abdominal Respiratory Movements: *Note the abdominal movements for any abnormality*
- Normally the abdominal wall bulges during inspiration and falls during expiration. The movements are free and equal on both sides. In diaphragmatic paralysis, paradoxical abdominal movements (opposite to normal) are observed, i.e. the abdomen bulges during expiration and falls during inspiration.

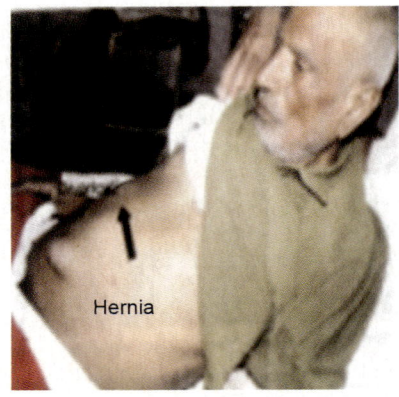

Fig. 6.13: Divarication of recti (↑) and umbilical hernia seen and felt when patient was asked to rise from supine position.

- In generalised peritonitis, the abdominal movements are diminished or absent.

Peristalsis: *Note the peristaltic (intestinal) movements*

Peristalsis is observed by watching the abdomen for sometimes. If, not visible, an attempt should be made to provoke it by tapping the abdomen with fingers.
1. Intestinal peristalsis may be seen normally through a thin abdominal wall (wasted abdomen).
2. Peristaltic waves may be seen spontaneously or after drinking some fluid from left to right (epigastrium to right hypochondrium) in upper abdomen above umbilicus in pyloric obstruction. Peristaltic waves in this region may be seen in colonic obstruction but they travel from right to left (reverse of pyloric obstruction).
3. Peristaltic waves in small gut obstruction are seen in the centre of the abdomen in worm-like fashion while in ileocaecal obstruction, distended coils of intestine appears as parallel ridges one above the other in step-ladder pattern.

Pulsations: *Note any visible pulsations in epigastrium or other abdominal areas.*

Normally, pulsations are not visible over the abdomen in normal built person. Pulsations of the abdominal aorta may become visible in thin anxious patients, anaemia, aortic regurgitation, thyrotoxicosis and lordosis of upper thorax.

Abnormal pulsations seen are:
- Expansile pulsations in epigastrium are seen in abdominal aortic aneurysm. These pulsations can be transmitted to any mass either adjacent or over the aorta. To differenitiate between a pulsatile tumour from true aortic pulsations, ask the patient to adopt a "knee-elbow' position. These pulsations will disappear if due to aorta.

- Right ventricular pulsation may be seen in epigastrium due to tricuspid regurgitation. These pulsations correspond with the apex beat. Even congested liver, sometimes, produces pulsations posteriorly in tricuspid regurgitation.

Hernias: *Look at the following sites for hernias* (Fig. 6.14)

If there is any swelling over the abdomen suspected to be hernia (ventral hernia), ask the patient to cough. Positive cough impulse (protuberance on coughing) suggests ventral hernia (Fig. 6.15).

Ventral hernia (e.g. epigastric hernia) is a small midline bulge through a defect in the linea alba, some where between the xiphisternum and the umbilicus. Ask the patient to raise both head and shoulders off the table or bed or couch, if hernia is present, a central bulge will appear.

☞ **Palpation**

Palpation of the abdomen is most informative method.

For palpation, patient is made to lie comfortable on a couch/bed with one pillow behind the head, legs are flexed and the feet resting on the bed. This position relaxes the abdomen. The patient is asked to breath quietly. Examiner either sits by the side of the patient on a stool/chair or bends down sufficiently when standing to bring himself/herself on a level with the patient so as to have tangential view. The palpating hand must be warm by rubbing the hands against each other in order to prevent the reflex contraction of abdominal muscles. Palpation must be gentle and firm. Do not poke the fingers into the abdomen, this will produce reflex spasm of the abdominal muscles. In nervous patients, the attention of patients can be diverted by engaging the patient in talking during palpation.

Knee-elbow or knee chest position is best for:
i. Palpation of small intra-abdominal lumps which are not palpable in supine position.
ii. Minimal ascites (Pudal's sign)
iii. Differentiating a pulsatile tumour from abdominal aortic aneurysm.

Methods of Palpation
1. Superficial (light) palpation
2. Deep palpation
3. Bimanual palpation
4. Palpation by dipping or ballottement.

1. Superficial palpation (Fig. 6.16)
- After making the patient to lie supine comfortably with arms alongside the body, explain the procedure to the patient to gain confidence and relaxation of the abdomen.
- Enquire about the site of any pain and examine that region last.

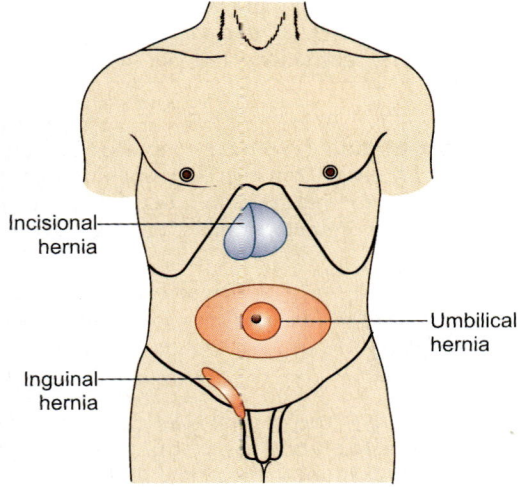

Fig. 6.14 : Sites of hernia.

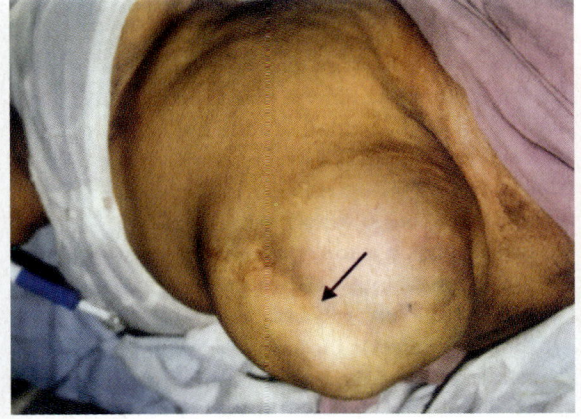

Fig. 6.15: Incisional ventral hernia. Note the incisional scar (←) and protuberance around the scar (e.g. ventral hernia).

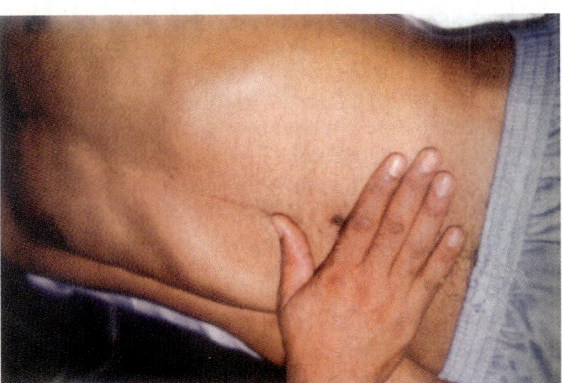

Fig. 6.16: Superficial (light) abdominal palpation.

- Ask the patient to report any pain elicited during palpation and observe the patient's face for any grimace/wince indicative of local pain/discomfort.
- Place the right hand (after rubbing against each other in cold weather) on the abdomen and thereafter maintain the continuous superficial contact with the patient's abdominal wall.
- **Test the muscle tone** by light dipping movements over symmetric areas. **Guarding** is local or generalised rigidity encountered as resistance due to increased muscle tone. Guarding is indicative of inflammation, enlargement or new growth involving the underlying organ.
- **To elicit rebound tenderness**, press your hand gently and firmly into the abdomen and then release the pressure suddenly. Observe for any grimacing/wincing of face due to pain. Sudden withdrawal causes pain due to movement of the inflamed organ. It is positive in acute appendicitis.

2. Deep palpation (Fig. 6.17)
- Palpate the abdomen more deeply and firmly with the flat of the hand. Poking of fingertips should be avoided as it is likely to induce muscular spasm or resistance.
- You can use both hands one over the other for deeper palpation if necessary.
- Examine each region in turn, starting away from any area of tenderness; start preferably from the left iliac fossa and proceed anticlockwise as follows:

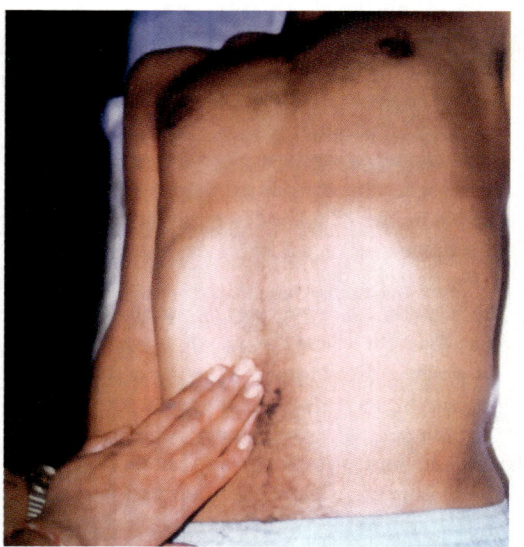

Fig. 6.17: Deep abdominal palpation by both hands one above the other.

- Feel for the left kidney (left lumbar region)
- Next feel for the spleen (left hypochondrium)
- Feel for the liver (right hypochondrium)
- Feel for the right kidney (right lumbar)
- Feel for the urinary bladder (hypogastrium)
- Feel for aortic pulsations and para-aortic glands (around umbilicus)
- Feel also the femoral vessels/pulses (groin).

Method

Start by placing the right hand flat on the abdominal wall in left iliac fossa. Palpate gently with firm pressure with the fingers held straight with slight flexion at the metacarpophalangeal joints.

Palpate each quadrant of the abdomen. Note the *feel of abdomen*, any *area of tenderness, guarding* or *rigidity*. If necessary, repeat the palpation using both hands; putting the left hand over the right to exert increased pressure (*reinforced palpation,* Fig. 6.17). It is the method of palpation in an obese or muscular patients.

> *Remember.* In patients who are unable to relax their abdominal muscles, the best way of examination is to ask them to breath deeply, bend their knees up and distract their attention by talking to them.

☞ *Elicit skin elasticity or turgor over abdomen by pinching a fold of skin and then releasing it. Note the skin wrinkling or slow recovery towards normal due to laxity of skin.*

Skin elasticity or turgor. The elasticity of the skin is a parameter to state of hydration; *loss of turgor* indicates dehydration, on the other hand, redundant skin folds indicate weight loss. Laxity of skin may be seen with advancing age, after child birth and ascitic tap.

☞ *Measure the girth of abdomen*

- Abdominal girth is measured with a measuring tape at the level of umbilicus. It is increased in conditions associated with distension of abdomen, i.e. 5Fs.

☞ *Elicit for tenderness of abdomen*

- Tenderness means pain on pressure (patient winces). Resistance accompanies tenderness (guarding), indicates inflammatory lesions of the underlying viscera and the surrounding peritoneum (Box 6.2).

Rebound tendernes is elicited by exerting firm pressure over a painful area with hand and then suddenly releasing it, provokes pain.

- *Rebound tenderness* may reveal deep-seated inflammation (parietal peritonitis) where local guarding may not be present.

Shifting tenderness (tenderness shifts due to change in position) is useful sign to differentiate mesenteric adenitis from appendicitis.

Box 6.2	Pain and Tenderness as a Clue to Diagnosis
Site	Condition
1. Epigastrium	Peptic ulcer
2. Right hypochondrium (intercostal tenderness)	Hepatitis, liver abscess, cholecystitis (gallstone)
3. Spine	Pott's disease
4. McBurney's point or right iliac fossa	Appendicitis
5. Lumbar region/lion	Renal colic

In mesenteric adenitis on shifting the patient to left lateral position for a few minutes, tenderness shifts to left side to its original position from the centre.

☞ *Palpate for feel of abdomen and guarding rigidity*
- Doughy feel of abdomen indicates tubercular peritonitis, may also occur in multiparus females.

Guarding. Guarding is the resistance offered by the patient during palpation. It is a protective or defense mechanism against pain in which abdominal muscles contract resulting in increased tone. It is commonly seen in anxious patients who are unable to relax their abdomen, can be overcome by talking and explaining them no undue pain will be caused by the examination.

Rigidity. Rigidity is a protective mechanism similar to guarding but cannot be voluntarily relaxed.

- *Generalised 'board-like' rigidity* invariably indicates peritonitis due to any cause. In peritonitis, abdomen does not move during respiration and bowel sounds are absent but rebound tenderness is present. *Diffuse rigidity* may be encountered in meningitis, tetanus, acute intestinal obstruction, lead colic, spinal injury, extensive intra-abdominal adhesions and uncooperative patient.

- *Localised rigidity* (limited to one side according to the organ affected) is due to pain of organ involved, i.e. right hypochondrial rigidity in amoebic liver abscess, cholecystitis, pancreatitis, etc. Iliac fossa rigidity occurs in appendicitis, salpingitis, torsion of right ovarian cyst, etc.

- Intestinal strangulation, ruptured ecotopic pregnancy and superior mesenteric artery thrombosis can lead to localised/generalised rigidity.

☞ *Elicit for oedema of the abdominal wall (Figs 6.18A and B)*

It is demonstrated by pinching a fold of oedematous skin between thumb and index finger of right hand and then on releasing it look for the pits or impression, i.e. thumb and index finger impression or stethoscope over the abdominal wall. The **causes** of oedema of abdominal wall are same as for pitting oedema of the feet. It is commonly associated with ascites also.

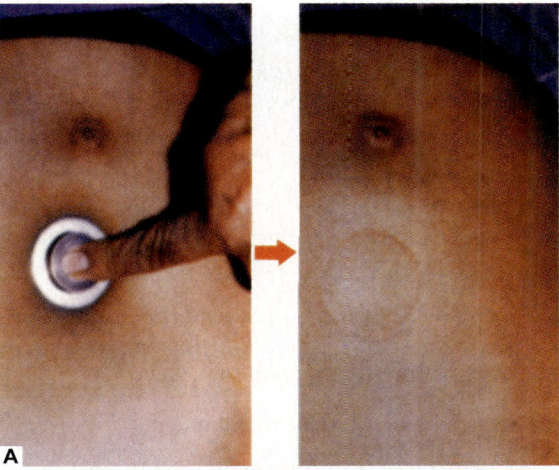

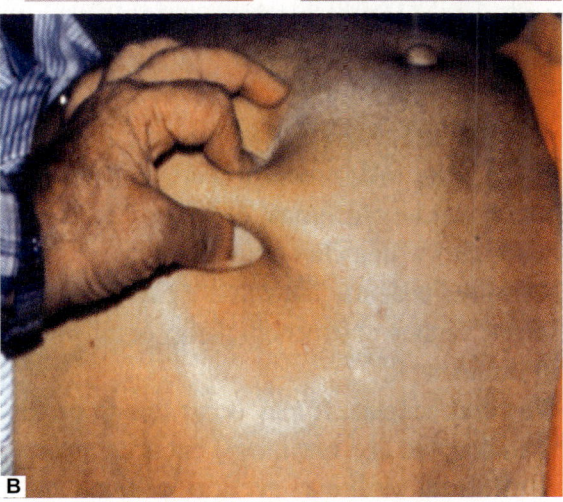

Figs 6.18A and B: Elicitation of abdominal wall oedema. (A) Pressure by diaphragm of stethoscope leaves behind a circular impression on the wall after withdrawal of stethoscope; (B) Pinching of the abdominal wall will leave behind the pits at the sites of pressure by the thumb and index finger.

Palpation of Various Visceras during Deep Inspiration

The liver, gall bladder, spleen and kidneys are palpated in turn during deep inspiration because they lie at some points with the contact of diaphragm.

Remember. Those organs which lie in contact with diaphragm move during respiration hence, are better palpable during inspiration as they descent down during the inspiration.

Palpation of Enlarged Organs

☞ The Liver

Conventional method is to place the right hand below and parallel to right subcostal margin. Palpate the edge of the liver with radial border of the index finger of right hand during deep inspiration which will be felt as something striking your hand (Fig. 6.19).

The *'hooking technique'* is useful to palpate liver in obese persons. Stand on the right side of the patient, place both hands, side by side on the right abdomen below the costal margin. Press in with your fingers and hook them up towards costal margin. Ask the patient to take deep breath. The liver edge becomes palpable with the fingerpads of both hands.

The liver is often palpable in normal persons without being enlarged (visceroptosis, thin abdomen). Hepatomegaly is described in centimeters below the right costal margin in midclavicular line.

Describe the liver enlargement as follows:
- *Enlarged* by so many centimetres.
- *Surface.* Rough (cirrhosis) or smooth (hepatitis, CHF, Budd-Chiari syndrome), nodular in malignancy (primary or secondary).
- *Consistency.* Soft (hepatitis, amoebic liver abscess, CHF), *firm* (cirrhosis) or *hard* (malignancy).
- *Tenderness* present or not.

  - Liver is tender in hepatitis, CHF, liver abcess and malignancy.

- *Bimanually palpable or not.* Enlarged liver is bimanually palpable, i.e. can be grasped between two hands, one in the front and other behind the liver mass. Kidney can also be palpated bimanually.
- *Ballotable or not.* Liver is not ballotable.
- *Movement with respiration.* Liver and spleen show free mobility during respiration while kidney shows restricted mobility.
- *Pulsatile or not* (Fig. 6.20). Liver becomes pulsatile due to hemangioma of liver or presence of tricuspid regurgitation (TR)

Separation of hands indicates pulsatile liver (Fig. 6.20)

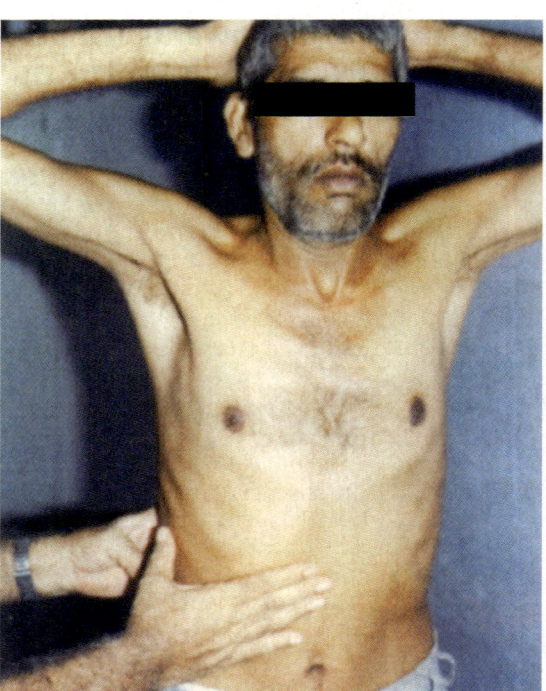

Fig. 6.20: Method to elicit pulsatile liver. Make the patient sit. Position the hands as if you are bimanually palpating the liver. Note the separation of hands during quiet breathing.

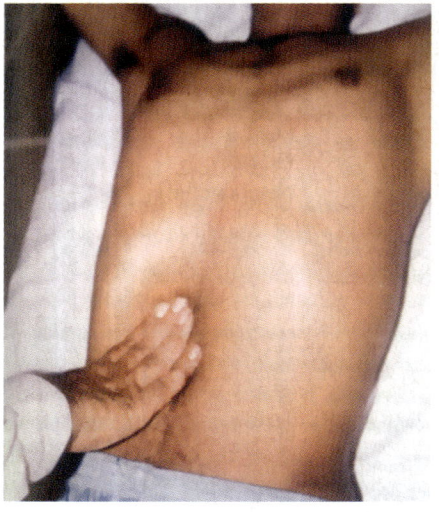

Fig. 6.19: Palpation of liver (conventional method).

- Fingers cannot be insinuated behind the costal margin in case of hepatomegaly.

The characteristics of liver mass are discussed in Box 6.6. (Read the differential diagnosis of mass in right hypochondrium.)

- *Assessing the tenderness of a nonpalpable liver.* Place your left hand flat on the lower right rib cage and then gently strike your hand with the ulnar surface of your right fist. Ask the patient to report pain or note the wincing. This is called *Murphy sign*. Murphy sign is positive in hepatitis, perihepatitis, amoebic liver abscess, cholecystitis.
- *Thumping sign* (Fig. 6.21). Strike your right fist over the lower right rib cage and note whether the patient winces/grimaces or feel pain. Tenderness by this manoeuvre indicates inflamed liver. It is positive in amoebic liver abscess, hepatitis, perihepatitis following liver biopsy. This is just like Murphy sign.

Differentiation between liver mass and right kidney mass (Table 6.2).

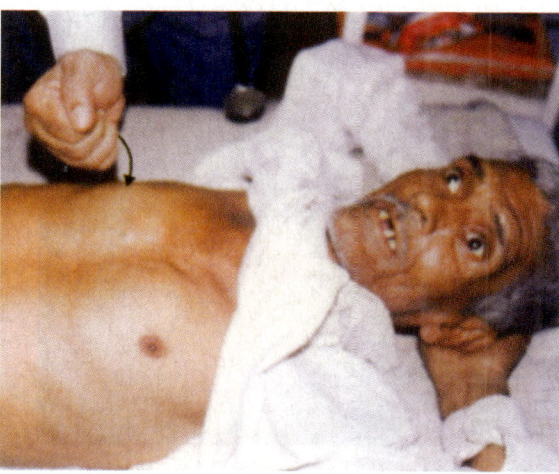

Fig. 6.21: Thumping sign for intercostal tenderness. Note the wincing following a gentle thump with fist of right hand.

TABLE 6.2: Differences Between Liver Mass and Right Kidney Mass

Liver mass	Kidney mass
• Present in right hypochondrium	• Present in right lumbar region, may extend upwards
• Mass freely moves with respiration	• Restricted mobility
• Mass has smooth surface with well defined lower border	• Smooth or irregular mass (lobulated due to multiple cysts)
• Dull on percussion. Dullness over the mass is continuous with liver dullness	• Resonant on percussion due to interposition of intestine.
• Bimanually palpable but not ballotable	• Both bimanually palpable and ballotable
• Fingers cannot be insinuated between the mass and costal marginal	• Fingers can be insinuated between the mass and costal margins
• Renal angle is empty	• Renal angle is full.

☞ Gall Bladder

The gall bladder is a pear-shaped organ lying under the right lobe of the liver.

Method

The gall bladder is palpated in the same way as the liver.

Place the examining fingers over the right hypochondrium and ask the patient to take a deep breath. Gall bladder if palpable is felt as a firm, smooth, globular swelling with distinct borders, just lateral to rectus abdominis muscle near the tip of 9th costal cartilage. Its upper border lies under the lower border of the liver or disappears underneath the costal margins, hence, its only fundus and a part of the body is palpable when it gets enlarged.

When both the liver and gall bladder are grossly enlarged, the latter may be felt not in the hypochondrium but in the right lumbar region or even as low down as the right iliac fossa.

> Once the gall bladder is palpable, note its shape, surface, consistency, tenderness and percussion note.

The characteristics of gall bladder mass/palpable gall bladder

1. The gall bladder mass is rounded or globular structure with well defined margins.
2. It moves freely with respiration similar to liver.
3. It is superficially placed, dull on percussion.
4. It is neither ballotable nor bimanually palpable.
5. The upper border of the mass cannot be reached.
6. The renal angle on the back is not full.

The differences between palpable gall bladder and palpable right kidney are given in Table 6.3.

TABLE 6.3: **Distinctive Features between Palpable Gall bladder and Palpable Right Kidney**

Feature	Gall bladder	Right kidney
1. Shape of mass	Globular, firm, smooth	Boat-shaped, firm, smooth
2. Movements with respiration	Free movement	Restricted movements
3. The upper border of the mass defined or not	Not defined, merges with the liver	Defined
4. Ballotability	Not ballottable	Ballottable
5. Bimanually palpable	No	Yes
6. Percussion note over the mass	Dull	Colonic resonance over the renal mass present
7. Renal angle	Empty	Full

☞ Elicit tenderness over gall bladder area (*Murphy's sign*). In acute cholecystitis, the gall bladder gets inflamed, swollen, painful and tender. Often, in acute cholecystitis tender gall bladder can be palpated as an indistinct mass. To elicit Murphy's sign, ask the patient to take deep breath and palpate for the gall bladder in the normal way. At the height of the inspiration, the breath is arrested with a gasp as the mass is felt. This sign is not found in chronic cholecystitis or uncomplicated gallstones. Hepatic tenderness with or without enlarged liver may also produce positive Murphy's sign, hence it is not *sine quanon* of cholecystitis.

Differential diagnosis of enlargement of the gall bladder/gall bladder mass

The gall bladder becomes enlarged and palpable in the following conditions:

1. *Carcinoma of the head of the pancreas* causing obstruction of the common bile duct. The gall bladder and biliary ducts become dilated painlessly and progressively leading to deep jaundice with palpable gall bladder (*Courvoisier's sign*). The gall bladder is firm as it is chronically distended.
2. *A stone in common bile duct (CBD)*. If a stone is present in CBD, then there is intermittent colic, intermittent jaundice and fever with chills and rigors. By *Courvoisier's law*, gall bladder is not palpable but becomes palpable in an impacted stone, stricture or fixed luminal obstruction. Here the gall bladder appears as smooth globular mass.
3. *Mucocoele of the gall bladder*. Occasionally, the inflammation in acute cholecystitis may be mild and subsides quickly; sometimes leaving a gall bladder distended by mucocoele. In this condition, there is pain with palpable gall bladder.
4. *Empyema of gall bladder*. It is a complication of acute cholecystitis, where the infection involves the whole wall of the gall bladder giving rise to localised peritonitis and acute pain. Occasionally, the gall bladder may become distended with pus (*an empyema*) and becomes tender.
5. *In carcinoma of the gall bladder*. The gall bladder will be felt as a stony hard, irregular swelling with jaundice. There is associated anorexia, weight loss. It is common in middle aged females denoted by *4Fs (female, forty, fair, fertile)*.
6. *Porcelain gall bladder*. The gall bladder wall may get calcified due to chronic inflammation. It may become palpable sometime.
7. *Emphysematous gall bladder*. Especially seen in diabetics and following hepatic artery embolisation. This is severe form of cholecystitis with gas forming organisms producing soft palpable gall bladder with gurgling sound. On plain X-ray abdomen, air within gall-bladder wall may be identified.
8. *Mirizzi's syndrome*. This consists of obstruction of common hepatic duct or common bile duct by a stone impacted in the cystic duct with surrounding inflammation (*Mirizzi's type-I*). In Mirizzi's type II, the stone erodes into the common bile duct creating a fistula (*calculous cholecystitis*).
9. *Chronic cholecystitis and cholelithiasis*. It is characterised by pain in the right hypochondrium radiating to inferior angle of the scapula, aggravated by a fatty meal and relieved by frequent belching or vomiting. The gall bladder may become palpable if full of stones and *Murphy's sign* may be positive.

☞ The Spleen

When the spleen enlarges, it expands anteriorly, downwards and medially, often replacing the tympany of the stomach and colon with the dullness of a solid organ in *Traube's region* (Fig. 6.22). It then becomes palpable below the costal margin.

Spleen can be palpated by the following methods:

☞ *Bimanual or conventional method* (Fig. 6.23A) The examiner's left hand is placed on the lower chest and patient is asked to roll slightly to right side, allowing the finger tips of the right hand to feel the tip of the spleen as it descends while the patient inspires quietly and deeply. Palpation is begun

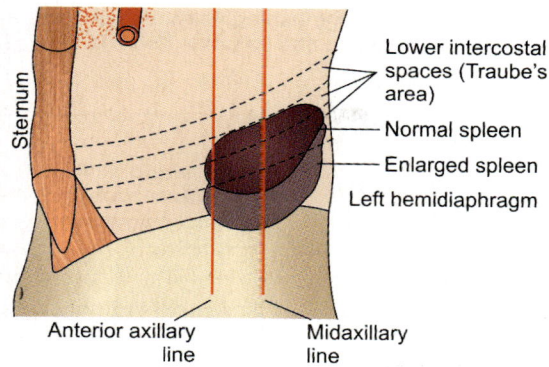

Fig. 6.22: Traube's area/region (diagram). It lies underneath the 9th to 11th intercostal spaces. Normally, this area is resonant, becomes dull on percussion in splenomegaly and left-sided pleural effusion.

with the right hand in the left lower quadrant with gradual upwards movement towards the left costal margin thereby identifying the lower edge of the enlarged spleen.

Once the splenic tip is felt, the finding is recorded by measuring the enlargement in centimetres below the left costal margin at some fixed point, i.e. *left midclavicular line*, the *xiphisternal junction or from midpoint of umbilicus*. Bimanual examination is done either in supine or right lateral position for massive splenomegaly (Fig. 6.23B).

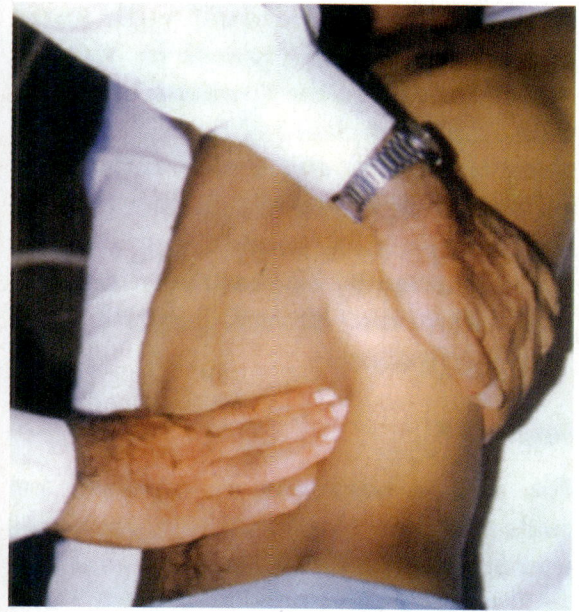

Fig. 6.23A: Bimanual method for mild splenomegaly. Tip of the spleen will strike the fingertips of palpating hand.

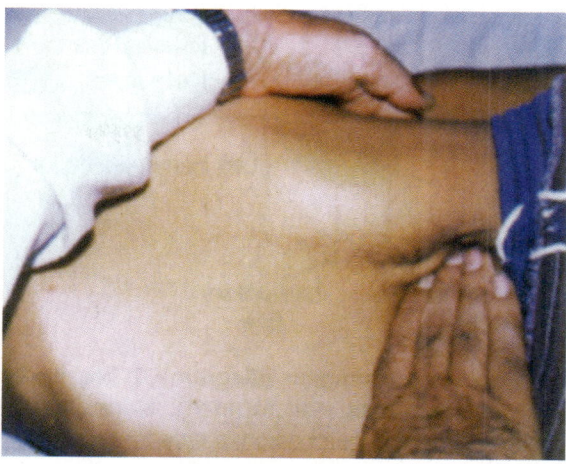

Fig. 6.23B: Palpation of spleen by bimanual method for massive splenomegaly. Start palpation from the right iliac fossa and proceed towards the umbilicus obliquely.

☞ *Hooking method* (Fig. 6.24): The patient is put in right lateral position and the examiner stands on the left side behind the patient, hook your both hands over the left costal margin. The tip of the spleen can be felt striking the pulp of fingertips when the patient takes deep breath.

☞ *Dipping method* (Fig. 6.25). This method is used to palpate the spleen in presence of ascites whereas the other methods are likely to displace the spleen.

- Stand on the right side of the patient. Palpate the spleen starting from the right iliac fossa moving towards the left hypochondrium. Dip your fingers into the abdomen with

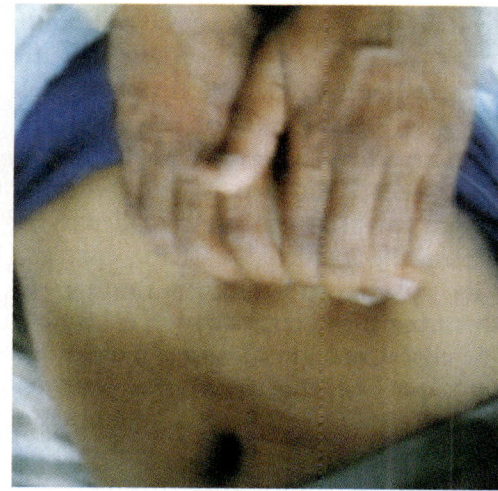

Fig. 6.24: Palpation of spleen by hooking method. This method is similar to palpation of the liver.

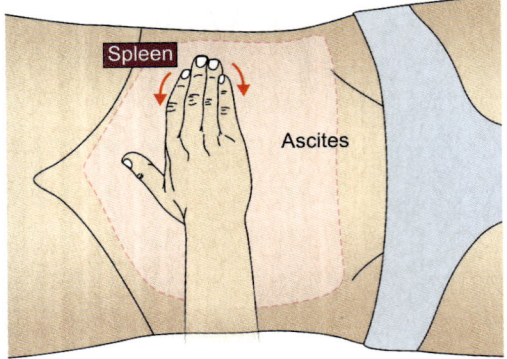

Fig. 6.25: Palpation of spleen in the presence of ascites (dipping method).

each palpation so as to displace the fluid to the side. If spleen is enlarged, it will strike back your hand, following each dip. By this method you can just judge the enlargement only while other characteristics are difficult to judge.

Note: Spleen is normally not palpable. It can become palpable only when it has enlarged two to three times its usual size.

Splenomegaly

Palpable spleen does not mean enlargement as it may be pushed down by the low descending diaphragm in emphysematous patients. Therefore, to define its extent of enlargement, its upper and lower borders have to be defined and span of the spleen (distance between upper and lower borders) may be measured. The spleen enlargement may be graded as *mild* (1–2 cm), *moderate* (3–7 cm) and *severe* (7 cm or more).

Causes (Read case discussion on splenomegaly in bed side medicine by Prof. SN Chugh). However, common **causes** include *infections* (hepatitis, malaria, kala azar, typhoid, endocarditis), *congestion* (pericardial effusion, CHF, portal vein or hepatic vein thrombosis), *haemolytic anaemias, collagen vascular disease* (SLE) and infiltrative disorders (*lymphomas and leukaemias*). (Read the differential diagnosis at the end of unit.)

The characteristics of splenomegaly and its differentiation from left kidney are described in Table 6.4.

When the spleen is palpable, describe its following features:
1. *Shape*: Normal spleen is pyriform or triangular in shape. In case of new growth, the shape may be distorted.

TABLE 6.4: Distinguishing Features between Palpable Spleen and Palpable Left Kidney

Spleen	*Kidney*
1. Mass is smooth and regular	Mass is irregular (boat shape)
2. It freely moves obliquely with respiration	It moves vertically and movements are restricted (e.g. slight movement possible)
3. Not ballotable	Ballotable
4. Fingers cannot be insinuated	Fingers can be insinuated between the mass and costal margins
5. A notch is felt on its surface if moderately or massively enlarged	No notch
6. Dull note on percussion over the mass	Resonant note over the mass due to interposition of intestine over the mass
7. The direction of the mass anterior, downwards and obliquely towards right	Anteroposterior mass
8. Spleen if massively enlarged crosses the midline	Never crosses (except with horseshoe kidney)
9. Renal angle empty	Full
10. Cannot be pushed back into the loin	Can be pushed back into the loin

Note: Both the masses are bimanual palpable.
Remember: Any large mass of the abdomen can be bimanual palpable.

2. *Size*: Enlargement of spleen is either described in terms of 'fingers breadths' or in centimetres below the costal margins. The degree of enlargement is graded *mild* (1–3 cm), *moderate* (4–6 cm), *massive* (≥7 cm).
3. *Site*: The mass arises from left hypochondrium, extends towards lumbar region. A grossly enlarged spleen may cross the midline obliquely to occupy the right lumbar or extend towards right iliac fossa.
4. *Consistency*: Spleen is *soft* in typhoid fever, SABE and septicaemia, *firm* in portal hypertension and myeloid leukaemia, lymphomas and *hard* in chronic malaria.
5. *Surface*: The surface of the spleen is smooth and has a notch on its medial border.
6. *Tenderness*: Spleen is non-tender but becomes tender when there is abscess formation or infarction of spleen (sickle cell anaemia).
7. *Depth*: The spleen is superficial structure, hence, when it enlarges, it just lies behind the costal

margin, hence fingers cannot be insinuated between the costal margins and spleen.
8. *Splenic rub*: A splenic rub due to perisplenitis or splenic infarct may be heard over the spleen.

☞ The Kidneys

Kidneys are usually not palpable but the lower pole of the right kidney may be palpable bimanually in thin patients as a smooth, rounded swelling which descends on inspiration. The kidneys being retroperitoneal in position enlarge anteroposteriorly in the lumbar region filling the costovertebral angle (renal angle).

Method: A bimanual method is used to palpate the kidneys.

Palpation from the same side (bimanual method)
A. Left Kidney
- Stand on the patient's left side. Place your right hand just below the costal margins with your fingertips just covering the costovertebral angle (renal angle). Place your left hand anteriorly in the left upper quadrant.
- Push the two hands together towards each other firmly. Feel for the lower pole as it moves down between the hands (i.e. try to capture the kidney between your hands) as the patient breathes in deeply. The lower pole of the kidney, when kidney is enlarged, is felt as a rounded solid swelling between two hands, i.e. bimanually palpable.
- *Test for ballotability*. Push the kidney from back to the front with one hand and feel its movement with the other. This movement is known as balloting.

Kidney is a ballottable structure.

- Assess the *size, surface* and *consistency* of a palpable kidney.

Normal kidney is ovoid structure with rounded margins, resilient to feel and move lightly with respiration. Kidney is resonant on percussion.

B. Right Kidney (Fig. 6.26)
The method of palpation is same. Now you have to stand on the right side and repeat the above process in the manner described above. Now use the left hand posteriorly and right hand anteriorly.

The differences between right kidney mass and liver mass have already been described.

Palpation from the Opposite Side
A kidney can be palpated from the opposite side by standing on the right side as follows:

- The left kidney can be palpated by placing the left hand posteriorly in the left loin and right hand anteriorly on the left upper quadrant. Feel the kidney's lower pole between two hands as described above.

Elicitation of tenderness of the kidney. The tenderness of the kidney is elicited posteriorly by gently tapping the renal angle using a fist or fingertips with the patient sitting forward.

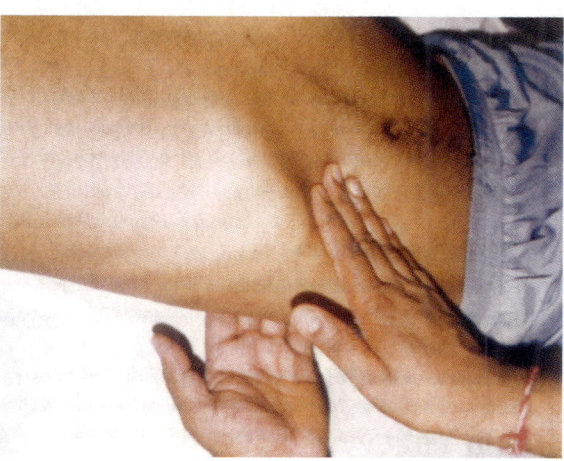

Fig. 6.26: Palpation of the right kidney by bimanual method from the same side.

Common Abnormalities
1. *Congenital horseshoe kidney*. The two kidneys are joined at their lower poles and may be palpable straddling the midline.
2. *Enlarged kidney(s)*. Owing to the varying degree of thickness of the abdomen, kidney enlargement is difficult for the inexperienced to assess unless there is gross enlargement. Irregularity of the surface or an abnormal consistency is more easily appreciated. The causes of enlargement are given in Box 6.3.
3. *Small kidneys*. The kidneys are smaller and naturally non-palpable in chronic renal disease (e.g. chronic renal failure) where the diagnosis is suggested on the history rather than from the clinical examination. Ultrasound confirms the diagnosis.
4. *Tenderness over the renal angle* is present in inflammatory disease of the kidneys or in musculoskeletal disorder.

The characteristics of the renal mass. The salient features of the renal mass and its differentiation from liver or gall bladder on right side and spleen on left side have already been described in Tables 6.2 to 6.4, respectively.

Box 6.3 Differential Diagnosis of Enlarged Kidney(s)

Unilateral
- Renal tumour
- Hydronephrosis, pyonephrosis
- Unilateral cystic disease (medullary cystic disease, medullary spongy kidney)
- Compensatory hypertrophy of one kidney due to renal agenesis or hypoplasia affecting the other kidney or following nephrectomy

Bilateral
- Polycystic kidneys
- Lower urinary tract obstruction with hydronephrosis, pyonephrosis
- Acute pyelonephritis in children
- Amyloidosis
- Diabetic nephropathy
- Acromegaly

Once kidney is enlarged, note the following features:

1. *Situation.* Kidney mass is situated in the lumbar region except floating kidney.
2. *Size.* The visible lump depends on the size of kidney as it is retroperitoneal organ. A very large kidney may produce a visible lump.
3. *Shape.* Kidneys are ovoid structures with rounded margins.
4. *Direction of the mass.* The kidneys enlarge anteroposteriorly.
5. *Consistency.* The normal kidney has a peculiar resilient feel. Cystic mass of kidney is *soft to firm* (hydronephrotic kidney, polycystic kidneys) while renal carcinoma is hard and nodular.
6. *Surface.* The surface is smooth and round in hydronephrosis, multiple grapes like clusters in polycystic kidneys due to multiple cysts.
7. *Tenderness.* Kidneys are non-tender but become tender in perinephric abscess. The tenderness is elicited over the renal angle (costovertebral angle).
8. *Renal angle.* The renal angle posteriorly is full in renal enlargement (normally it is empty).
9. *Movement with respiration.* Since the upper pole of the kidney lies on the lower part of diaphragm, hence, there is restricted motility during inspiration.
10. *Percussion note.* The renal mass exhibits a band of resonant due to interposition of colon over the mass.
11. *Fluctuation.* A large soft mass with fluctuation sign positive is either hydronephrotic or pyonephrotic kidney.
12. An arterial bruit may be heard on either side of umbilicus in case of renal mass.

☞ Urinary Bladder

The bladder normally cannot be examined unless it is full or distended above the symphysis pubis.

The Characteristics of Bladder Mass

- Distended bladder produces a globular swelling in the hypogastrium arising from the pelvis and extending to the umbilicus. Its lateral and upper borders can be made out but it is not possible to feel it lower border.
- The mass is smooth and tender.
- Pressure over the mass may produce sensation of urination.
- It is dull on percussion
- The mass disappears after micturition or catheterisation.

Differential Diagnosis

The mass has to be differentiated from masses of uterus, ovaries and fallopian tube (read differential diagnosis of mass in hypogastrium described in differential diagnosis of mass in different region at the end of unit).

Abnormality

- Bladder distension occurs from outlet obstruction due to urethral stricture, prostate enlargement, drugs and medications and also from neurological disorders such as stroke, multiple sclerosis as well as in spinal cord compression.
- Suprapubic tenderness indicates cystitis.

☞ Aortic and Other Pulsations

Aortic pulsations are not readily felt but can easily be made out with practice on deep palpation a little above and to the left of umbilicus. In older patients particularly women with marked lumbar lordosis and in thin individuals, the aortic pulsations are more easily palpable.

Method

- Palpation is done with finger tips to detect the pulsations and to assess the width of the aorta
- Press the extended fingers of both the hands, held side by side deeply into the upper abdomen on each side of aorta as illustrated in Fig. 6.27. Make out the left wall of the aorta by right hand and note its pulsations.
- Remove both hands and repeat the procedure slightly to the right of the midline in upper abdomen. Make out now the right wall of the aorta by left hand and note its pulsations.
- The width of the aorta, in this way, is assessed by measuring the distance between pulsations felt on either side of midline. Increased width more

Gastrointestinal and Hepatobiliary Systems

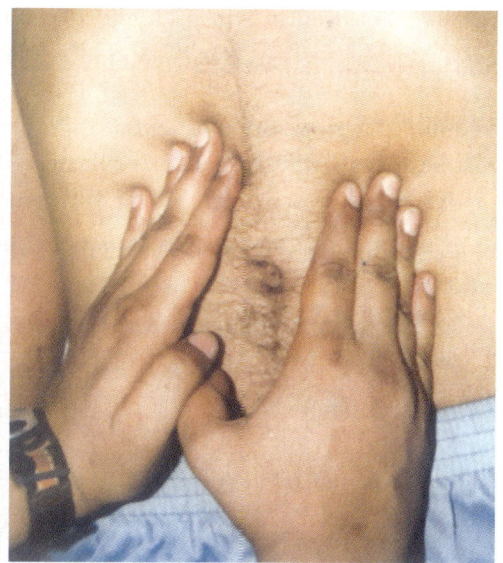

Fig. 6.27: Method for palpation of aortic pulsations (e.g. aortic aneurysm).

than normal suggests either a merely tortuous aorta or an aortic aneurysm (a pathological dilatation of the aorta), hence, an ultrasound is a mean to distinguish between the two.

Roughly, a normal aorta is 1–3 cm (average 2.5 cm) wide in adults; increase in width suggests an aneurysm.

Femoral vessels (palpation of femoral vessels is described under CVS examination).

☞ Percussion

The aim of abdominal percussion is to distinguish between *resonant* (gaseous distension) and *dull* (ascites, solid or cystic mass) *percussion note*. Normal percussion note is resonant over whole of the abdomen. Tympany (hyper-resonant note) of whole abdomen including, flanks indicate gaseous distension due to toxic states, paralytic ileus.

Fluid gravitates into flanks during lying down, hence, flanks are dull on percussion in ascites. Percussion is tympanitic in gaseous distension, e.g. ileus or intestinal obstruction and intussusception. Solid (tumour or gravid uterus) and cystic (ovarian cyst) masses in the abdomen are dull.

Percussion for Liver Dullness to Define its Span

Procedure

Percuss lightly for lower border of the liver over the upper abdomen and firmly for the upper border of the liver over the lower chest. Measure the vertical span of the liver dullness (Fig. 6.28) by mapping out the upper border of the liver dullness by percussing the chest starting from 4th intercostal space downwards in midclavicular line, and lower border by percussing the upper abdomen starting from the umbilicus towards right hypochondrium in midclavicular line. The distance between the upper border of dullness and lower border of dullness is the vertical span of liver dullness. Normal liver span is 10–14 cm.

The span of liver dullness is increased when the liver is enlarged.

The span of liver dullness is decreased when liver is small and shrunken (fulminant hepatitis) or when free air collects below the diaphragm (perforation of a hollow viscus) or interposition of the colon between the liver and diaphragm—*Chilaiditi's syndrome'*, serial observations may show a decreasing span of dullness with resolution of hepatitis, CHF.

Liver dullness may be displaced downwards by the low diaphragm in COPD (emphysaema).

The Stomach

The stomach is palpated for tenderness and presence of a mass.

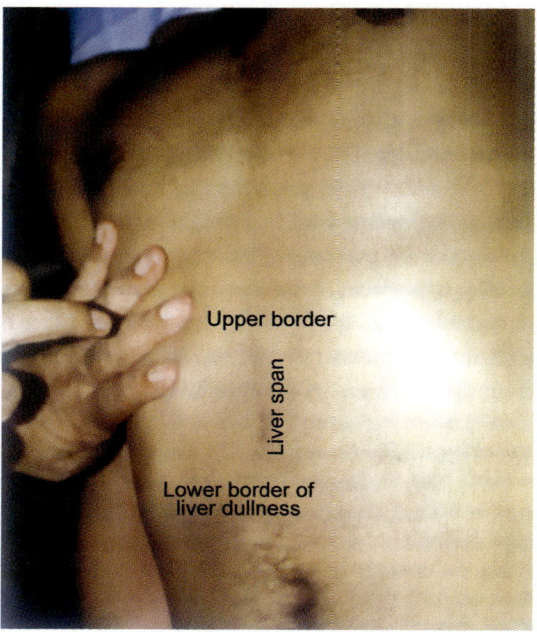

Fig. 6.28: Percussion for upper and lower borders of liver dullness and measurement of liver span. (Remember the best way to define liver span is ultrasound.)

1. *Tenderness*: Superficial tenderness is elicited by applying gentle pressure in epigastrium in peptic ulcer. Deep epigastric tenderness is elicited in case of pancreatic disease.
2. *Palpable lump or mass*: A stomach mass may be due to growth or an inflammatory mass due to thickening or induration of pylorus of stomach secondary to an ulcer.

   The growth of pylorus is frequently palpable through the anterior abdominal wall. The gastric tumour is felt as an ill-defined mass during deep inspiration.

The Pancreas

Because of deep position behind the stomach, the pancreas is felt by deep palpation by placing one hand over the other along the lateral margin of left rectal muscle in epigastrium and upper umbilical region in case there is a tumour or cyst (pseudopancreatic) involving the pancreas. The mass is ill-defined, slightly mobile on digital manipulation, does not move with respiration, frequently transmits the pulsation of abdominal aorta. Mass is resonant on percussion.

The Colon

- The pelvic colon is normally palpable in left iliac fossa and can be rolled as a sausage-filled structure. It is felt as a rigid tube filled with hard scybal masses (faecal pelvic colon is tender and spastic due to ulcerative colitis and diverticulitis).
- The transverse colon is normally palpable as tubular structure just above the umbilicus.
- A hepatic flexure mass (tumour of ascending colon) being frequently adherent to the under surface of the liver, tends to descend during deep inspiration. Assumption of erect posture render palpable lump of ascending colon lump to descend by a few inches.

- The ileocaecal mass is palpable in intestinal tuberculosis, amoeboma, appendicular lump or Crohn's colitis.

Differential Diagnosis of Protuberant Abdomen

Common **causes** of protuberant abdomen are:
- Ascites.
- A large ovarian cyst.
- Obstruction of the large bowel, distal small bowel or both.
- Enlargement of an intra-abdominal organ.

Percussion distinguishes between the above mentioned conditions (Fig. 6.29).

i. A protuberant abdomen with bulging flanks suggests ascites in which gas filled intestines float in the centre, therefore, percussion note is dull in flanks and resonant in the centre (Fig. 6.29A).
ii. The whole abdomen is tympanitic in intestinal obstruction (dilated gut above the obstruction) with increased peristalsis (Fig. 6.29C).
iii. A localised dullness on one side of lower half of the abdomen (Fig. 6.29B) in an ovarian cyst.

N.B. Abdominal girth measurement: A periodic measurement of abdominal girth is helpful in follow-up the progress of a case of ascites or of distension due to splenomegaly/hepatomegaly, etc. Abdominal girth is measured at the level of umbilicus.

Method

- Percussion is done from resonant to dull area. Start percussion in the centre and move to the periphery of the abdomen.
- Place the flat of the left hand with fingers spread on the abdomen.

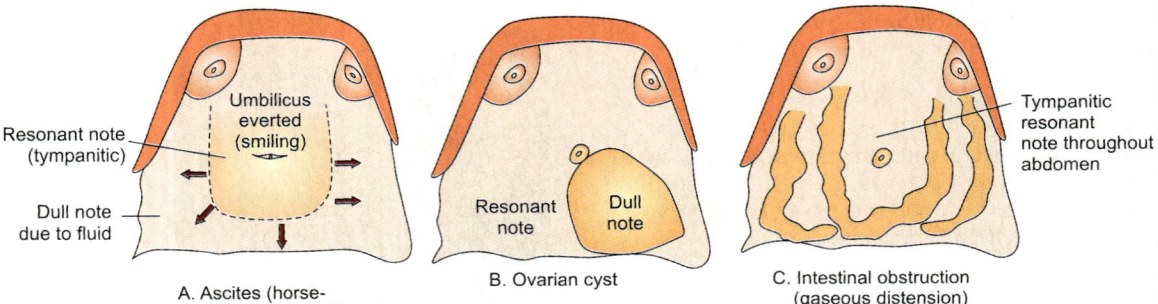

Figs 6.29A to C: Differentiating percussion note in a patient with distended abdomen. Percussion can distinguish the resonant structures from dull structures inside the abdomen. (A) Ascites (horseshoe) dullness; (B) Ovarian cyst (localised dullness over lower half of abdomen; (C) Resonant whole abdomen (tympanitic note) in intestinal obstruction.

☞ Elicit the Signs of Ascites

Two following important signs help to confirm the presence of moderate ascites.

1. *Shifting dullness* (Fig. 6.30). Make the patient to lie supine. Percuss from the centre (resonant area) at the level of umbilicus outwards towards one of the flanks (resonant area) at the level of umbilicus; say left flank keeping the fingers in the longitudinal axis, until dullness is detected. The dullness is detected over the flanks in ascites. Now keeping the hand here on the dull area on the abdomen, ask the patient to roll away from you on to the right side. Percuss again in this position, if the previously dull note has now become resonant then ascites is probably present (Fig. 6.30B). To confirm its presence, repeat the same manoeuvre on the right side of the abdomen.

> *Remember.* This sign is positive in moderate ascites but becomes absent when fluid is either too small or too large (no space to shift the fluid) or loculated.

2. *Fluid thrill* (Fig. 6.31). Ask the patient or an attendant to put the edge of one hand in the midline of the abdomen and press firmly as shown in Fig. 6.31. This pressure will stop the transmission

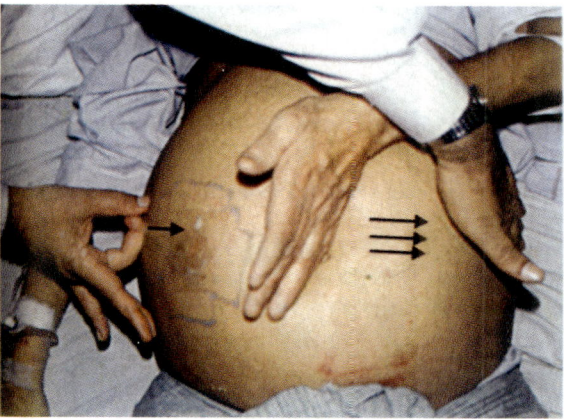

Fig. 6.31: Elicitation of fluid thrill.

of waves or thrill through the fat in the abdominal wall. Place your left hand flat in one of the flanks to detect the impulse while you tap or flick the opposite flank with your right hand (Fig. 6.31) for an impulse or thrill which will be transmitted to the receiving hand if fluid is present. Fluid thrill just suggests fluid under tension either in the peritoneal or a cyst (ovarian).

> Presence of fluid thrill indicates tense ascites. It may be absent in mild ascites and loculated ascites.

3. *Horseshoe-shaped dullness.* This can be demonstrated in ascites by mapping out dullness from the umbilicus outwards in different directions (Fig. 6.29A). Dull area accumulates in the dependent parts and the resonant intestines float up in centre.

4. *Ovarian cyst dullness.* Dullness is usually limited to one side of the umbilicus or midline but can cross the midline. Dullness is unequal on either side between umbilicus and superior iliac spine and umbilicus on either side is same in ascites but unequal in ovarian cyst. In a ascites the greatest circumference of the abdomen is at the umbilicus whereas in ovarian cyst, it is below the umbilicus.

5. *Pudal's sign* (dullness in knee-elbow position). The centre of the abdomen is percussed as the patient adopts a knee-elbow position. The fluid collects (gravitates) in the centre in this position, making it dull on percussion.

> Pudal's sign demonstrates minimal or mild detectable ascites (Fig. 6.32).

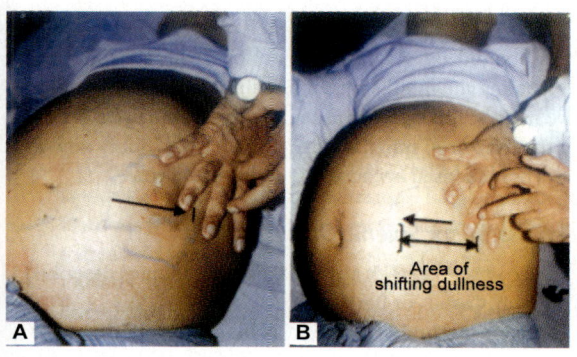

Figs 6.30A and B: Elicitation of shifting dullness. Start percussing from resonant area towards dull area till you reach a dull area (A indicated by →). Now while keeping the finger over dull area ask the patient to roll to the other side, now the area which was dull earlier becomes resonant due to shift of fluid, hence, shifting a dullness is present (B). To define the area of shifting dullness, now start percussion again from this newly found resonant area toward umbilicus to know where the dullness has shifted. Mark the line of demarcation at the start of dull area now (←). The distance between the previous resonant area in (B) and newly found dull area on change of position indicates the area of shifting dullness, i.e. the space over which fluid has shifted (indicated between arrows by an arrowhead lines ←→ Fig. 6.30B).

The various signs depending on the amount of fluid collection are summarised in Box 6.4.

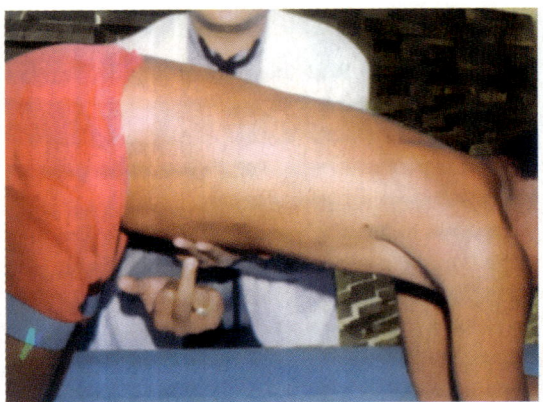

Fig. 6.32: Pudal's sign for mild ascites.

Box 6.4	Physical Signs to Different Grades of Ascites	
Grade	Approx. fluid	Physical sign
Minimal	300–500 ml	Pudal sign
Mild	500–1000 ml	Shifting dullness present, fluid thrill absent
Moderate	1000–2000 ml	Both fluid thrill and shifting dullness present
Massive	3 litres or more	Fluid thrill present, shifting dullness absent

☞ Ovarian Cyst

Ovarian cyst is one of the fluid fill masses lateralised to one of the lower half of the abdomen. It is dull on percussion and fluid thrill is present and shifting dullness absent (Box 6.5).

Box 6.5	Differentiation Between Ascites and Ovarian Cyst (Fig. 6.32)
Ascites	**Ovarian cyst**
1. Produces generalised distension of abdomen	• Localised distension on either side of lower abdomen
2. Flanks full	• An iliac fossa swelling (on one side)
3. Umbilicus is transversely slit (smiling umbilicus) or everted	• Vertically slit or everted umbilicus
4. Umbilicus to symphysis pubis distance is more than xyphisternum to umbilicus	• Umbilicus to pubis distance is less than unbilicus to xiphisternum
5. Swelling not well defined. One cannot reach above the swelling	• Swelling is rounded with well defined upper border. One can reach above the swelling
Ascites	**Ovarian cust**
6. Horseshoe shape dullness (flank dull, centre resonant)	• Dullness limited to one of the iliac fossae/ quadrants
7. Shifting dullness present (a characteristic)	• Shifting dullness absent

☞ Signs of Decompensated Cirrhosis of Liver

Flapping tremors (asteriaxis). Look for the presence of flapping tremors (Fig. 6.33) in a patient with cirrhosis of liver with ascites.

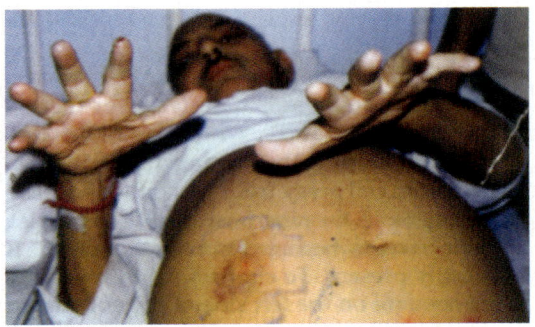

Fig. 6.33: Demonstration of flapping tremors in a conscious patient with decompensated cirrhosis of liver. This should be demonstrated in sitting position in conscious patients, if not able to sit then in lying down position

Ask the patient to outstretch his/her hands with widened fingers if patient is conscious. Note the flaps of the hands. In unconscious patient, hold the wrist with one hand and dorsiflex the patient's hand with your other hand and feel for the flap with palm of your hand.

☞ Hydatid Thrill/Sign

It is elicited by placing 3 fingers over the swelling and percussing the middle finger. After thrill will be felt by other two fingers. This sign was used to demonstrate a hydatid thrill in the liver or in other abdominal structures, but is nowadays not practised because of doubtful significance.

Percussion for Splenic Dullness when Spleen is not Palpable

As you know spleen becomes palpable when it enlarges two and half times than normal. If spleen is suspected to be enlarged but is not palpable then it is accomplished with any of the three techniques.
1. **Nixon method.** The patient is placed on the right side so that the spleen lies above the colon and stomach. Percussion begins at the lower level of

lung resonance in the posterior axillary line and proceeds diagonally along a perpendicular line towards mid and anterior axillary lines.

Normally, the upper border of splenic dullness is 6–8 cm above the lowest costal margin. Dullness >8 cm in an adult indicates splenomegaly.

2. **Castell's method.** With the patient supine, percussion in the lowest interspace in anterior axillary line (8th or 9th) produces a resonant note during deep inspiration if spleen is normal in size. A dull percussion note on full inspiration suggests splenomegaly.

3. **Percussion of Traube's semilunar space.** Read the borders of the Traube's space in Fig. 6.22. The patient lies supine with left arm abducted. During normal breathing, the space percussed from medial to lateral margins, yields a normal resonant sound; a dull percussion note suggests splenomegaly.

Note: All these techniques are less reliable in obese patients and in patients with full or distended stomach.

Percussion is of limited value in determining the size and position of the spleen as this can only be roughly assessed from the percussion note. However, dull left hypochondriac mass is invariably splenic in origin. In case the spleen is enlarged but not palpable, USG is helpful to diagnose the enlarged spleen.

Splenic area of dullness may be masked by expanding left lung in COPD (emphysema).

☞ **Auscultation**

The areas to be auscultated over the abdomen are represented in Fig. 6.34.

1. **Peristaltic sounds.** Place the stethoscope preferably in the centre just right to the umbilicus and keep it pressed there until bowel sounds are heard (Fig. 6.34).

Normal peristaltic bowel sounds are heard as intermittent low and medium pitched gurgles at a rate of 3–5/min with an occasional high-pitched noise.

Auscultate for at least 3 minutes for peristaltic sounds before you declare them as absent.
- *Increased and exaggerated bowel sounds (borborygmi)* are heard in mechanical small gut obstruction. If associated with bouts of colicky pain abdomen, then they are pathognomonic of it.

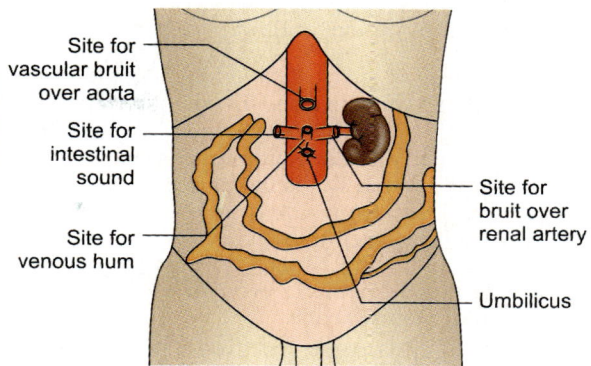

Fig. 6.34: Sites for auscultation for bruits over the abdomen.

- *High-pitched tingling sounds* may be heard after every 10–30 seconds in adynamic obstruction (paralytic ileus). This represents the fluid spilling over one distended gas or fluid filled loop to another. Later on the peristalsis ceases and bowel sounds become absent.
- *Silent abdomen* (absence of bowel sounds) occurs in:
  ◆ Generalised peritonitis
  ◆ Paralytic ileus.

2. Listen for *a vascular bruit over the aorta (Fig. 6.34) and over other vessels*. Place the stethoscope lightly on the abdominal wall in epigastrium above and to the left of the umbilicus and listen for aortic bruit. For *renal bruit*, place the stethoscope similarly just above and to the side of umbilicus (Fig. 6.34).
- Listen for *bruit in the corresponding iliac fossae*, and over the common femoral arteries in each groin.
- Listen for a *bruit in right hypochondrium* over the liver.

Arterial bruits (harsh systolic murmurs) in the abdomen may arise from the aorta, or any other narrowed or partially obstructed vessel (renal artery stenosis in renovascular hypertension). Rarely, a systolic bruit may be heard over the liver in hepatoma (due to increased vascularity) and hemangioma.

3. *Venous hum.* A humming sound may be heard between xiphisternum and the umbilicus in portal hypertension (*Cruveilhier-Baumgarten syndrome*).
4. *Auscultate for friction rub.* Auscultate over the splenic and hepatic area for any rub (friction sound).

A hub over hepatic area or splenic area is indicative of an infarct or perihepatitis or perisplenitis.

5. *Elicitation of succussion splash.* A splashing sound like shaking a half-filled bottle is termed *succussion splash*. To elicit a succussion splash in stomach, place one hand over the lower ribs or shoulder and shake the patient quickly and rhythmically from side to side and auscultate over the epigastrium.

The splash is particularly pronounced in case of atonic or dilated stomach.

It is heard in pyloric obstruction, acute intestinal obstruction (dilated loops of gut) and paralytic ileus.

Palpation of the femoral arteries have already been discussed (read CVS examination). Auscultation of femoral artery for any bruit has also been described.

☞ EXAMINATION OF INGUINAL REGION

A swelling over the groin is commonly either a *hernia* (inguinal/femoral) or a *lymph node mass*.

To differentiate between femoral and inguinal hernia, the index finger of the examiner is placed on the pubic tubercle (traced up along the tendon of adductor longus to inguinal canal) and the patient is asked to cough. If the impulse is medial and above the index finger, it is *inguinal hernia*. If the impulse tends to bulge straight through the posterior wall of the inguinal canal, it is *direct*, whereas if it travels obliquely along the inguinal canal, it is *indirect inguinal hernia*. The bulge below the finger indicate femoral hernia (Fig. 6.35).

Now palpate for inguinal lymph nodes (Fig. 6.36) for any enlargement along the femoral artery, beneath the inguinal ligament towards perineum. Repeat this examination on the other side also.

When the patient complains of a lump in the groin, he/she should be examined lying down and standing up. Note any scar or discharging sinus, if

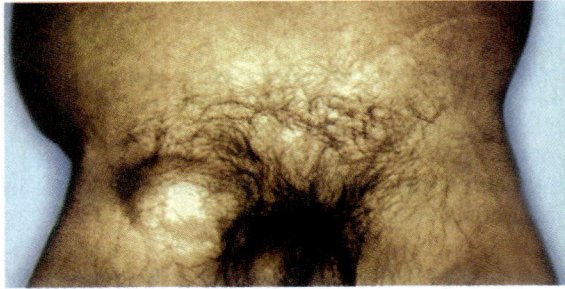

Fig. 6.35: Femoral hernia.

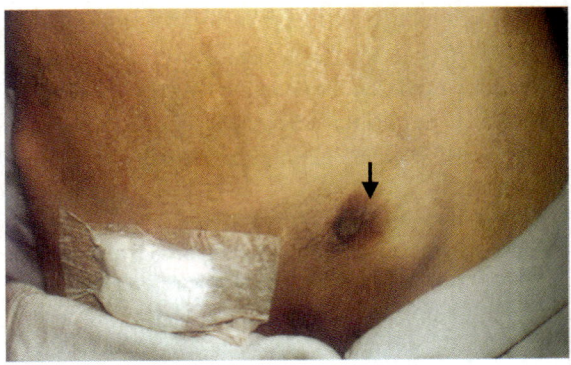

Fig. 6.36: Inguinal lymph nodes. The biopsy of the lymph node has been done on right side and the wound is dressed. The left inguinal region shows a mass with discharging sinus (↓).

nodes enlarged, then describe their characteristics, i.e. size, consistency, tenderness, matting, adherent to underlying or overlying structures, etc.

Remember. Lymph node enlarged up to 2 cm or more is significant clinically in inguinal region, less than that are usually insignificant, can be normal

THE BACK OF ABDOMEN

☞ Inspect the back of abdomen for any swelling, skin lesion or deformity of the spine or a tuft of hair (*spina bifida*). Palpate the spine and ribs for any deformity and tenderness.

A gibbus indicates Pott's disease of the spine.

EXAMINATION OF THE ANUS, RECTUM AND PROSTATE

Common Presenting Symptoms of Anorectal and Prostate Disorders

1. Change in bowel habits (occur in cancer).
2. Blood in the stool (polyps, cancer, piles, GI bleed).
3. Pain during defaecation, rectal bleeding and rectal prolapse.
4. Anal warts or fissures (*fissure in ano*).
5. Thinning of stream of the urine (prostate enlargement or uretheral obstruction).
6. Increased frequency and burning during micturition (urinary infection).

Examination

The examination includes inspection of the perianal area, anus and digital (per rectum) examination of anal canal and rectum.

Position: Make the patient to lie in left lateral position with knees drawn up and buttocks projecting over the side of bed/couch. A good source of light should be used for inspection. Put a disposable glove on the right hand and stand behind the patient's buttocks facing the patient's leg. Explain the procedure to the patient and assure him that you will be as gentle as possible.

☞ **Inspection**

After separating the buttocks, look at the anus and perianal area (Fig. 6.37) for any abnormality such as:
 i. *Inflammation of skin* or *dermatitis* or *rashes* or *excoriations*.

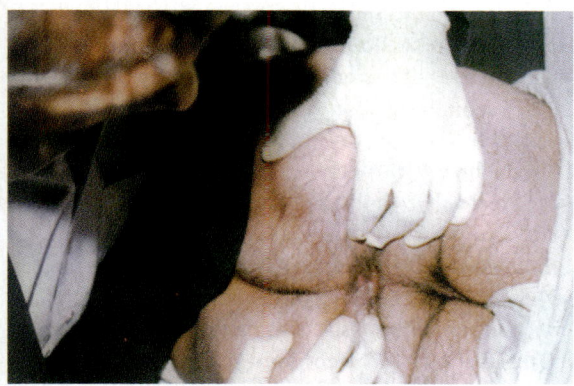

Fig. 6.37: Examination (inspection) of anus.

Pruritus and dermatitis around the anus is common in children due to worm infestation (thread worm).

 ii. *Anal skin tags* (occur in severe pruritus or prolapsed piles).
 iii. *Anal warts (condylomata accuminata)* which are sessile or pedunculated papillomata with red base and white surface and are numerous.
 iv. Note any *hole* or *dimple* near the anus with a tell-tale bead of pus or granulation (*fissure in ano*), commonly seen in Crohn's disease.
 v. A *sentinal pile* is a tag of skin which is pathognomonic of anal fissure. The fissure can easily be demonstrated by drawing apart the anus to reveal the linear tear in the lining of anal mucosa.

Anal fissures are common in proctitis and Crohn's disease.

 vi. *A perianal haematoma* (thrombosed external pile).
 vii. *Prolapsed piles* (prolapsed pile which is deep red or purple is surrounded by oedema of the anus and perianal skin).

Piles uncommonly occur due to portal hypertension, following constipation and local anorectal conditions.

 viii. *An abscess*. A tender fluctuant swelling which deforms the outline of the anus is perianal abscess, common in ulcerative colitis.
 ix. *Note the presence of any ulceration*.
 x. *Rectal prolapse*. If rectal prolapse is suspected, ask the patient to strain and note whether any pink rectal mucosa or bowel comes out through the anus.

Rectal prolapse can occuring following worm infestation.

 xi. *Perineal bulge*. Note whether the perineum bulges itself downwards.

Downward bulging of the perineum during straining or coughing indicates weakness of pelvic floor muscles usually due to denervation of these muscles. This sign is also seen in women after childbirth, in women with urinary—faecal incontinence or in patients with severe constipation.

☞ **Palpation (Digital Examination)**

Lubricate your gloved right index finger and place it flat on the anus. As the sphincter relaxes, gently insert the fingertip into the anal canal, in a direction pointing towards the umbilicus (Fig. 6.38). If severe

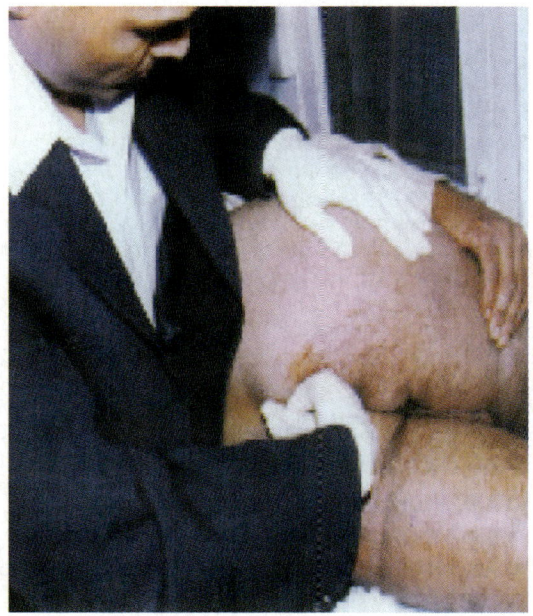

Fig. 6.38: Digital (per rectal) examination.

pain is elicited by this manoeuvre, then further examination must be stopped and now spread the anus with the fingers and examine it for any anal fissure which might explain this tenderness or pain.

If no pain or discomfort is elicited, then proceed further,

1. *Note the tone of the anal sphincter.* Normal tone of sphincter grips the finger.

Sphincter tightness occurs in anxiety, inflammation or scarring.
Sphincter is lax in neurological diseases.

2. Rotate the finger through 360° in the anal canal and *feel for any induration, thickening or irregularity of the wall of anorectum.*

Induration may be due to inflammation, scarring or malignancy.
The irregular border or nodularity of border indicates rectal cancer.

To bring the lesion (nodularity, irregularity or induration) within a reach of palpating finger, first take out the finger and ask the patient strain down and palpate again.

3. Try to visualize the anatomy of the rectum which can be assessed by sweeping movements of the finger at 2, 5, 8 cm inwards or until the finger cannot be pushed further anymore into the rectum. Repeat these movements as the finger is being withdrawn. In this way, one can *detect malignant ulcer, nodular or stenosing carcinomas, polyps and adenomas.*

4. Palpate also the hollow of sacrum and coccyx posteriorly and walls of the pelvis laterally for any abnormality.

5. In men, one should feel anteriorly the *rectovesical pouch, seminal vesicles* and the *prostate.*

Normally, rectovesical pouch and seminal vesicles are not palpable. Abnormally, pus may collect in this pouch producing swelling (pelvic abscess) or it may contain malignant deposits which may be felt as hard nodules. Infection of the seminal vesicle produces a tender tubular swelling on one side of midline above the prostate.

6. *Palpation of prostate gland.* It is felt as a rubbery firm swelling about the size of a large chestnut. Move the finger over each lateral lobe which is normally smooth, regular and has rubbery consistency. Between the two lateral lobes is a palpable median sulcus (a faint depression running vertically between lateral lobes). Assess the prostate for enlargement and any other abnormality.

Benign prostatic hypertrophy produces smooth enlargement of prostate. Its consistency and median sulcus are preserved.
In carcinoma, the gland becomes hard, nodular, the lateral lobes tend to become irregular and nodular and there is distortion or loss of median sulcus.

In women, the cervix is felt as a firm, rounded mass projecting back into the anterior wall of the rectum. Above the cervix, there is rectouterine pouch (pouch of Douglas) which is a common site of abnormality in females. Thus, rectal examination is an essential part of pelvic examination in females.

The body of the retroverted uterus, a fibroid mass, ovarian cyst, malignant nodule or a pelvic abscess, all can be palpated in the pouch of Douglas—a common site of abnormality.

7. Gently withdraw your finger and wipe out the patient's anus or give him/her tissue paper or a piece of gauge to do it. *Inspect your finger for mucus, blood or pus on the glove and test it for occult blood.*

In ulcerative colitis (proctitis), the withdrawn finger may show blood mixed with mucus, while only mucus will be seen in mucus colitis.

EXAMINATION OF ABDOMINAL LUMP/MASS

When a mass or a swelling is palpable in the abdomen, first of all make sure that it is not a normal structure. The normal palpable structures have already been described.

A mass felt over the abdomen may be *superficial* (in the abdominal wall such as haematoma, lipoma, cyst) or **deep** (arising from intra-abdominal organ). To differentiate between the two perform **Trendelenburg rising sign**. For Trendelenburg rising sign, ask the patient to lift his/her head while you press firmly against the forehead. Now feel the swelling and decide whether it disappears or becomes prominent or does not change.

If swelling becomes less prominent or disappears, it is intra-abdominal.
If it becomes more prominent, it is extra-abdominal.
If it remains the same, it must be within the layers of the abdominal wall.

Next consider whether it could be due to enlargement of liver, spleen, right or left kidney, gall bladder, urinary bladder, aorta or para-aortic lymph nodes. The mass in relation to these structures as well as other masses in the abdomen are discussed below.

Now palpate the mass carefully again and localise it to one of the anatomical regions and try to study the pathological nature of the mass. The points to be described about a mass include:

☞ **A. Inspection (look at):** Note the following:
- Site
- Size and shape
- Surface, edge
- Movements with respiration
- Skin overlying the mass

☞ **B. Palpation (to elicit and define):** Palpate for the following:
- Tenderness
- Rigidity
- Confirm the findings of inspection regarding size, shape, edge and surface.
- *Margins*, i.e. ill defined or well defined.
- Notch present or not.
- *Consistency*, i.e. soft, firm or hard. Hard swelling are usually malignant. Soft swellings are usually cystic. A solid undefined, tender mass suggests an inflammatory mass.
- *Abdominal (parietal) or intra-abdominal position*. To determine whether the mass lies in the abdominal wall or inside the abdomen, perform Trendelenburg rising sign.
- *Mobility or adherence*. Move the mass in all directions, i.e. from side to side and above downwards.

A mass arising from the small bowel, transverse colon, cysts in mesentery and large secondary deposits in the omentum move freely in all directions.

Fibroid uterus or pregnant uterus moves from side to side that differentiates it from bladder and ovarian mass.

A fixed mass indicates either an adherent inflammatory mass or infiltration of malignant tumour into the abdominal wall and surrounding structures or the mass is situated retroperitoneally (e.g. pancreas).

- *Boundaries or limits*. If the mass lies in the upper abdomen, feel the upper border and decide if it is possible to "get above it". Similarly, if the mass lies in the lower abdomen, decide whether one can "get below it".

If one cannot get above the mass (i.e. disappears under the costal margins), a hepatic, splenic, renal or gastric origin of the mass must be suspected.

If one cannot get below it (i.e. arising from the pelvis), a bladder, uterus, ovary or rectal origin should be suspected.

- *Movements on respiration*

Mass that lies in contact with diaphragm, i.e. mass of liver, spleen, kidneys, gall bladder and distal stomach descend on inspiration.

Swellings originating from aorta, lymph nodes and gut do not move with respiration.

- *Pulsations, if present*. Feel the pulsations and decide whether these are intrinsic (expansile mass) or extrinsic (transmitted aortic pulsations) to the mass. Put two fingertips at some distance over the mass and look what happens to them during systole. If fingers are separated while being lifted, it is expansile swelling, (e.g. aneurysm), and if just lifted not separated, it is transmitted pulsations. Secondly, disappearance of the pulsations in knee-elbow position (mass is off the aorta) suggests transmitted aortic pulsations.
- *Bimanual palpation and ballotability*.

Any mass that can be caught between two hands is bimanually palpable. Ballotability means mass if pushed from behind is felt anteriorly.

Renal mass is bimanually palpable and ballotable while a gall bladder mass may only be bimanually palpable.

- *Fluctuation*. Tap the mass from one side after fixing it between the fingers and thumbs, feel the impulse on the other side. Cystic mass and distended urinary bladder show fluctuation positive.

☞ **C. Percussion.** Light percussion should be employed.
- Decide whether mass is resonant or dull.

Masses originating from liver and spleen are dull on percussion while renal mass is usually resonant.

☞ **D. Auscultation.** Auscultate over the mass for rub (hepatic or splenic) or an arterial bruit (hepatic haemangiomas, renal artery stenosis).

DIFFERENTIAL DIAGNOSIS OF MASSES IN DIFFERENT AREAS OF ABDOMEN

The mass may be on the abdominal wall itself or inside the abdomen. This can be decided by head-raising sign or Trendelenburg sign (i.e. abdominal wall mass becomes prominent while intra-abdominal mass disappears on this manoeuvre).

A. Mass in or over the Abdominal Wall (e.g. cold abscess)

- A cystic swelling with no signs of inflammation (cold)
- Fluctuation sign is positive
- There may be irregularity in the affected rib or a gibbus or deformity of the spine (i.e. it usually arises from the caries of the spine or the rib).

B. Masses Inside the Abdomen

i. Mass in the right hypochondrium
- The differential conditions producing a mass in right hypochondrium are detailed in Box 6.6.

ii. Mass in epigastrium (Box 6.7).

iii. Mass in the left hypochondrium
- The splenic mass has been differentiated from the left kidney (Table 6.4).

iv. Mass in right and left lumbar regions (Box 6.8) shows differential diagnosis of renal mass. The distinction between kidney and spleen has already been discussed.

v. Periumbilical mass
- It could be either due to peritonitis or intestinal tuberculosis or intestinal obstruction, their characteristics have been highlighted in Table 6.6.

vi. Mass in right iliac fossa
- The masses in the right iliac fossa are related to either appendix, caecum, ileocaecal junction, ascending colon, iliopsoas sheath, uterus and its appendages.

1. Appendicular mass—characteristics
- History of severe pain around the umbilicus, settling down to the right lower quadrant.

Box 6.6 Differential Diagnosis of a Mass in Right Hypochondrium

1. Liver mass	2. Gall bladder mass	4. Subphrenic abscess	5. Gastric or duodenal mass (malignancy)	7. Hepatic flexor mass of colon
• It moves with respiration (descends during inspiration) but is not mobile from side to side • It has a sharp edge • Fingers cannot be insinuated between it and the costal margins • It is dull on percussion. Dullness of the mass is continuous with liver dullness above • Bimanual palpable but nonblottable mass • Liver span is increased (> 10 cm)	• Pear-shaped or globular swelling of the size of an egg • Cystic and smooth • Upper border is not reachable (hidden behind liver) • Moves with respiration • Can be moved from side to side but cannot be pushed down to the loin-like kidney **3. Kidney mass** • The difference between liver mass and right kidney mass have already been discussed	A diffuse tender swelling with fever and signs of toxaemia, e.g. sweating, tachycardia, rigors and chills and tachypnoea • Shallow respiration due to pain with frequent breath holding • Frequent hiccups • Pain in right hypochondrium referred to shoulders • Fluoroscopy shows raised and fixed diaphragm with gas under it	An irregular, firm lump that fully moves with respiration • Patient is anorectic, anaemic and emaciated with weight loss • If pyloric obstruction present peristalsis is visible from left to right • Succession splash is positive • Percussion note is tympanitic • Enlarged supraclavicular gland, if malignancy suspected **6. Omental mass** • A rolled up greater omentum due to tubercular peritonitis, produces a tender sausage-shaped lump in epigastrium • It hardly moves with respiration • A band of resonance between the mass and the lower border of liver. • Evidence of tuberculosis in the abdomen (lymph nodes) or elsewhere in the body	• Carcinoma of colon occurs in old age, produces alternate diarrhoea and constipation. The lump is firm and irregular, poorly moves with respiration. Stools are positive for occult blood • Barium enemas show a filling defect **Intussusception.** It occurs commonly in children, produces curved sausage-shaped lump in the line of colon with its convexity towards umbilicus. There is sudden intermittent pain and vomiting. Absolute constipation present without faecal odour. The lump may harden with screaming. Barium enema is diagnostic

- An irregular firm, tender mass initially fixed, may show slight mobility later on.
- Early voluntary guarding may be replaced by involuntary muscular rigidity.
- *Rebound tenderness* suggests peritoneal inflammation around the appendix.

- *A positive Rovsing's sign*. Pain in the right lower quadrant during left-sided pressure suggests appendicitis (*Rovsing's sign*). Similarly, the right lower quadrant pain on sudden withdrawal of hand (*referred rebound tenderness*) suggests appendicitis.

Box 6.7 Differential Diagnosis of Mass in the Epigastrium

Ventral hernia (abdominal wall mass)	Dilated stomach and duodenum (e.g. pyloric stenosis)	Pseudopancreatic cyst	Aortic aneurysm
• A small midline swelling in the abdominal wall due to defect in *linea alba*, lies between xiphoid process and the umbilicus	• A well defined intra-abdominal lump felt in the epigastrium in an infant (congenital stenosis) and adults (a complication of healed peptic ulcer)	• A well defined lump felt in the epigastrium following pancreatitis	• An expansile mass situated in the midline
• Dragging pain or discomfort after food resembling peptic ulcer	• Projectile vomiting and wasting	• It is a collection of fluid in the lesser sac of peritoneal cavity due to trauma or pancreatitis	
• Mass becomes prominent on Trendelenburg's rising sign	• Succussion splash may be positive	• The mass/swelling is smooth, rounded, cystic and fluctuation sign positive	• Pulsations will disappear on knee elbow position
	• Visible peristalsis from left to right		• An audible bruit over the mass
	• There may be past history of peptic ulcer in adults	• USG and barium meal study will show the mass posterior to the stomach (in the bed of stomach)	

Box 6.8 Differential Diagnosis of Lumbar Region Mass

Kidney mass. The characteristics of kidney lump have already been discussed in examination of abdomen.

Retroperitoneal tumour	Tumour of ascending colon	Perinephric abscess	Ovarian cyst	Riedel's lobe	Tabes mesenterica (lymph node mass)
• Tumour is situated in one of upper abdominal quadrants	• It is a hard nodular mass • Non-tender and mobile	• A bulging mass in the loin or flank • Mass is tender	• It occupies more anterior position • Exhibits greater range of mobility	• It moves freely with respiration like liver	• Young patient
• It is more centrally placed than renal mass	• Cannot be pushed behind the costal margin • Resonant on percussion	• Skin over the mass oedematous	• Fluid thrill present	• Its upper border merges with lower border of the liver	• Firm, nodular mass attached to the posterior wall of the abdomen
• Does not move with respiration	• Peristalsis may be visible sometimes	• Rigidity of abdomen over the mass	• Cannot be pushed back into the loin like a kidney lump.	• It is more superficial than kidney	• Oedema feet if there is pressure on inferior vena cava
• Dull on percussion • Renal angle full	• Anaemia, change in bowel habits are common accompaniments	• The thigh and the leg may be flexed on the affected side	• Renal angle is resonant and empty	• Its sharp lower edge can easily be palpated.	

- *A positive psoas sign.* This can be elicited in different ways:
  - Place your hand just above the patient's right knee and ask the patient to raise it against resistance. *Or*
  - Ask the patient to turn onto left side. Now extend the patient's right leg at the hip.

Increased pain on either manoeuvre constitutes a positive psoas sign indicating irritation of psoas muscle by an inflamed appendix.

- *A positive obturator sign.* Flex the patient's right thigh at the hip, with the knee bent, and rotate the leg internally at the hip. This manoeuvre *stretches the internal obturator muscle and produces pain.*
- Tympanitic note on percussion.

2. **Ileocaecal mass**
   i. *Hyperplastic ileocaecal tuberculosis*
      - An irregular, firm, tender mass that slips under your fingers.
      - More common in females than males
      - Intermittent subacute intestinal obstruction (i.e. vomiting, distension).
      - Caecum is pulled up (may be detected on USG)
      - Other manifestations of tuberculosis of lung or abdomen (lymph nodes).
      - Barium meal study shows pulled up caecum and a filling defect.

   Note: Barium meal study should not be done in presence of subacute intestinal obstruction)

   ii. *Carcinoma of caecum or ascending colon*
       The characteristics are:
       - Age above 45 years
       - An irregular firm lump
       - Change in bowel habits, e.g. alternate diarrhoea or constipation
       - Occult blood in the stool
       - Patient is anaemic and emaciated
       - Filling defect on barium enema
   iii. *Amoebic typhilitis*
       - History of amoebic dysentery (present or past)
       - An irregular, firm, tender lump
       - Stools are positive for *E. histolytica*
   iv. *Impaction by a bunch of round worms*
       - Irregular lump
       - History of intermittent abdominal colic, diarrhoea
       - History of passage of a large worm (patient may even bring the worm)

3. **Ileopsoas abscess**
   - It may be appendicular (read appendicular lump).
   - It may be infection of a haematoma in the traumatised iliopsoas muscle producing pain, tenderness, guarding, rigidity, etc.
   - It may be a cold abscess gravitating down deep to the inguinal ligament into the thigh, fluctuation on either side of the inguinal ligament is positive. There may be Pott's disease of the spine (e.g. gibbus or spinal deformity).

4. **Gall bladder mass**
   - A huge distended gall bladder may be palpable in this region as discussed (read examination of gall bladder).

5. **Undiscended kidneys**
   - Read characteristics of renal mass.

6. **Undescended testis**
   - When palpable, it is pathological (i.e. atrophic)
   - Hard, irregular lump
   - Absence of testis in the scrotum (scrotum is empty).

7. **Uterus or tubo-ovarian mass**
   - Usually a midline swelling extending into the right iliac fossa (uterine mass) or localised in one of the iliac fossae (tubo-ovarian).
   - One cannot get below the mass (mass arises from the pelvis).
   - Mass moves from side to side.
   - Menstrual disturbances are usual accompaniments.
   - Vaginal examination will confirm the diagnosis.

vii. Mass in the hypogastrium

1. **Distended urinary bladder** (read the characteristic of bladder mass as already discussed).
2. **Mass from uterus and its appendages**
   - A spherical midline mass arising from the pelvis; its lower limit cannot be reached.
   - Firmer than urinary bladder
   - Moves from side to side, not above downwards
   - Menstrual irregularity usually present.
   - Catheterisation will differentiate it from bladder mass. It does not disappear after catheterization.
3. **Tubo-ovarian** (salpingitis, ovarian cyst or tumour) mass
   - Mass arising from one side of the pelvis, may become central later on.

- Pain, fever and tenderness present in salpingitis due to surrounding pelvic peritonitis.
- Menstruation normal or scanty
- Ovarian cyst or tumour is dull on percussion but flanks remain resonant, i.e. a feature that distinguishes it from ascites.
- Vaginal examination confirms the diagnosis.

4. **Pelvic abscess (pelvic mass)**
   - It may follow acute appendicitis, salpingo-oophoritis and puerperal sepsis.
   - Constitutional symptoms, i.e. fever, pain abdomen, nausea present
   - Copious discharge of mucus per rectum due to irritation of rectum.
   - Increased frequency of micturition due to irritation of bladder.
   - Rectal examination shows bulging of anterior part of rectum.

viii. **Mass in the left iliac fossa**
   I. **Normally palpable masses**
      These masses are:
      - Thickened sigmoid or descending colon
      - Impacted faeces.
   II. **Abnormal masses**
      A. *Cold abscess of abdominal wall.* A parietal swelling, may present in any quadrant.
      B. *Carcinoma of sigmoid colon*
         - Increasing constipation
         - Loaded colon proximal to obstruction, signs of malignancy, i.e. anaemia, weakness, cachexia may be present.
         - Sigmoidoscopy/colonoscopy is diagnostic.
         - Barium enema shows a filling defect.
      C. *Diverticulosis/Diverticulitis*
         - *Diverticulosis of colon.* There is history of recurrent pain, flatulent distension of lower abdomen, diarrhoea or constipation. Barium enema is diagnostic, i.e. shows saw-tooth appearance of the colon.
         - *Diverticulitis*: There will be signs of inflammation, e.g. pain, fever, altered bowel habits, tender colon. Confirmation is done by CT scan after opacification of bowel.
      D. *Ileopsoas mass*—already discussed above
      E. *Undescended testis*—already discussed above
      F. *Unascended kidney*—already discussed above.

BRIEF SYNOPSIS OF COMMON GI TRACT HEPATOBILIARY DISORDERS

ACUTE EROSIVE (HAEMORRHAGIC) GASTRITIS

Definition: It refers to acute inflammation of the stomach with erosions and haemorrhages.

Causes
- Aspirin
- NSAIDs
- Alcohol abuse, streptococcal infections
- Other infections, e.g. viral and fungal
- Following stress (*Cushing's ulcer*) and burn (*Curling's ulcers*)
- It can occur postoperatively

Clinical Features
These patients present with acute pain in the abdomen associated with nausea and vomiting. Hematemesis is frequent with acute gastric erosions. The blood loss is small and does not require blood transfusions, may be detected as faecal blood loss. (tests for occult blood may be positive). This may lead to iron deficiency anaemia in severe cases. *Upper GI endoscopy* confirms the diagnosis.

PEPTIC ULCER

Peptic ulcer is ulceration of the gastric mucosa in, or adjacent to an acid bearing region due to acid and pepsin. The common sites are:
- First part of the duodenum (commonest).
- Stomach (gastric ulcer).
- Lower oesophagus (with oesophageal reflux).
- Jejunum (due to Zollinger-Ellison syndrome or after gastrojejunostomy.)
- Meckel's diverticulum (rare).

Causes
- Heredity.
- *H. pylori* infection.
- Excessive consumption of tea, coffee.
- Smoking and alcohol.
- Anxiety and stress.
- Steroids and non-steroids anti-inflammatory drugs (NSAIDs).
- Common in certain blood group.

Clinical Features
Duodenal ulcer occurs commonly in age group of 20–40 years, while gastric ulcer occurs a decade later. *Symptoms* of both duodenal and gastric ulcer are almost similar, hence discussed together.

1. **Recurrent abdominal pain** with the following characteristics:
   - Sharp, burning or gnawing pain of varying intensity, may be boring or aching.
   - Located to right of epigastrium or to restrosternal region. Posterior duodenal ulcer pain radiates to the back and may even erode pancreas (pancreatitis).
   - **Periodicity.** It is hunger pain, occurs 90 minutes to 3 hours after eating and frequently awakens the patient at night. A daily clock-like (fixed hours) recurrence of the pain is characterisic.
   - **Relation to food.** Pain is relieved by food or antacids.
   - **Known aggravating and relieving factors.** Tea, coffee, chillies, smoking, alcohol, mental stress aggravate the pain, while bland food, milk or antacids relieve it.
2. **Associated nausea and vomiting.** Nausea may accompany pain, occasional vomiting may occur in 40% patients but persistent vomiting occurring daily suggests gastric outlet obstruction.
3. **Uncommon presentations** such as recurrent acute bleeding or chronic severe anaemia.

Differential Diagnosis (read Table 6.5).

CARCINOMA OF OESOPHAGUS

The carcinoma of oesophagus is either adenocarcinoma or squamous cell carcinoma.

Sites
- Squamous carcinoma involves the middle of the oesophagus.
- Adenocarcinoma involves the lower third of oesophagus.

Predisposing Factors
- Common in men.
- Heavy drinkers/heavy smokers.
- Plummer-Vinson syndrome.
- Achalasia cardia.
- Coeliac disease.
- Hereditary tylosis (hyperkeratosis of palms and soles).
- Gastro-oesphageal reflux disease.

Clinical Features
It occurs commonly in old age (60–70 years). Most patients present with progressive painless dysphagia initially for solids and then to liquids also. In late stages weight loss and malnutrition occur. Impaction of food causes pain but more persistent pain indicates infiltration.

Sequelae/Complications
- Oesophageal obstruction.
- Hoarseness of voice.
- Regional lymphadenopathy.
- Metastases to distant organs.

Physical signs are usually absent. Cachexia, malnutrition, cervical lymphadenopathy are occasionally found. Upper GI endoscopy and biopsy confirms the diagnosis.

GASTRO-OESOPHAGEAL REFLUX DISEASE

Definition. It is defined as *"reflux of gastric contents"* into oesophagus resulting in inflammation of oesophagus (reflux oesophagitis) caused by H^+ ions, pepsin and bile salts.

Causes
- Old age and smoking
- Fat, chocolate, coffee, alcohol ingestion

TABLE 6.5: Differential Diagnosis of Peptic Ulcer

Acute gastric erosion	Peptic ulcer	Nonulcer dyspepsia
Acute onset of pain	Acute or chronic onset of pain	Subacute onset of pain
Epigastric pain may radiate to back	Epigastric pain non-radiating	Diffuse pain, non-radiating
Intermittent episodic, severe pain	Intermittent, periodic, excruciating colicky pain	Dull, boring pain
Aggravated by food	Relieved by food	No relation
No nocturnal frequency	Nocturnal frequency of pain	No nocturnal frequency
Alcohol, smoking, NSAIDs are common aggrevating/etiotogical factors	Smoking, alcohol, *H. pylori* and genetic predisposition are aetiological factors	Psychological stress is aggravating factor
Relieving factors. e.g. antacids	Food, antacids relieve pain	No relieving factor
Nausea, vomiting, hematemesis common	Nausea, vomiting, hematemesis are less common	No nausea, vomiting or hematemesis

- Hiatus hernia
- Gastric stasis (gastroparesis), e.g. anticholinergics, diabetes, systemic sclerosis
- Raised intra-abdominal pressure, e.g. pregnancy, ascites, etc.
- Obesity and sedentary habits.

Clinical Features

The disorder is common in middle age, frequently seen in obese females.

Heartburn is an early feature. It is deep seated retrosternal burning, brought on bending, lifting or straining due to rise in intra-abdominal pressure. It may be nocturnal or may occur after heavy meals during the day. Relief occurs with the use of antacids and food. It occurs commonly in recumbent position and relieved on sitting; this postural relationship is characteristic. In addition, other symptoms are: *Sour eructations or taste*, *acid erosion of teeth (incissors)* and *precipitation of an attack of asthma* in children, *hoarsenss of voice* and *pneumonia* due to aspiration of refluxed contents.

There may be *dysphagia, haematemesis* due to erosive oesophagitis in some patients. Retrosternal pain mimicing angina can occur due to oesophagitis.

The **diagnosis** is confirmed by continuous pH monitoring of stomach and upper GI endoscopy.

Complications

1. Stricture of oesophagus.
2. Ulceration of oesophagus.
3. Barrett's oesophagus.
4. Carcinoma of oesophagus.

GASTRIC MALIGNANCY

Most gastric cancers occur in the antrum (50%) and body of the stomach (20–30%) and are almost adenocarcinoma associated with *H. pylori* infection. These tumours may be polypoidal or ulcerating lesions.

Diffuse type adenocarcinoma with extensive submucosal infiltration resulting in schirrus cancer (*linitis plastica*) where stomach appears as rigid tube like on barium meal study is uncommon.

Aetiology

- Diet, alcohol, smoking
- *H. pylori* infection with chronic gastritis and gastric metaplasia
- Pernicious anaemia (autoimmune gastritis)
- Adenomatous gastric polyps
- Previous partial gastrectomy (>20 years)
- Menetrier's disease
- Family history of gastric cancer or polyposis

Clinical Features

- Asymptomatic, common in old age
- Two-thirds patients present with anaemia, anorexia and asthenia (AAA)
- Vomiting is frequent. Hematemesis, melana and dyspepsia are less common
- Dysphagia can occur but less common.

Physical signs. Vague-palpable abdominal mass, which is tender, firm and moves with respiration. It is present in upper abdomen (epigastrium or right hypochondrium). Peristalis may be visible. *Succession splash* may be positive. Lymphadenopathy i.e. supraclavicular (*Virchow's node*), or secondaries around umbilicus (*sister Joseph nodule*) or over ovaries (*Krukenberg's tumour*), can occur in advanced cases.

- *Acanthosis nigricans, thrombophlebitis, dermatomyositis* occur as nonmetastatic manifestations
- Secondaries occur in lungs (round opacities/cannon ball), peritoneum and bones.

Diagnosis is established by barium meal study, endoscopy and CT/MRI abdomen.

INTESTINAL TUBERCULOSIS

The intestinal tuberculosis is common in underdeveloped countries than in advanced countries. In recent years, however, there has been a global increase in the incidence of tuberculosis with upsurge in infection with HIV. It is generally a disease of adult population, most often of females with equal frequency in rural and urban population.

The human gut infection is due to *M. tuberculosis*. An isolated cases of infection by *M. bovis* have been reported. The ileocecal region is commonly affected. The colon and jejunum are also frequently involved. About two-thirds patients are 'primary' without evidence of any active or quiescent pulmonary disease.

Intestinal tuberculosis is either *ulcerative type* (multiple ulcers, scarring et) or *hypertrophic type* (ileocaecal mass)

Clinical Features

Patient with **ulcerative type** presents with chronic diarrhoea, oedema of face and feet, anaemia, muscles wasting and weight loss due to hypoproteinaemia.

The **hypertrophic variety or ulcero-hypertrophic variety** may produce acute or subacute intestinal obstruction characterised by colicky pain, abdominal distension and/or vomiting. There may or may not be passage of flatus. An *ileocaecal mass* is formed and becomes palpable in right iliac fossa.

Physical Signs

- The patient may be febrile and malnourished, anemic.

- An ileocaecal, tender mass may be palpable in the right iliac fossa.
- There may be distension of abdomen with visible peristalsis and *doughy* feel of the abdomen.

Diagnosis and Differential Diagnosis

The diagnosis of intestinal tuberculosis is difficult one; in some cases, presence of an associated active pulmonary tuberculosis may help. The differential diagnosis of ileocaecal lump has already been discussed under the head of appendicitis (appendicular lump). The distinguishing features between ulcerative intestinal tuberculosis and Crohn's disease are tabulated in Table 6.6.

TABLE 6.6: Differentiation between Intestinal Tuberculosis and Crohn's Disease

Feature	Tuberculosis	Crohn's disease
A. Gross		
Constitutional symptoms	• Fever with evening rise with night sweats, annorexia common.	• Fever, anorexia, vomiting may or may not be present • Localised pain with guardian
Feel of abdomen	• Pain abdomen is diffuse • Doughy abdominal feel	• Normal feel of abdomen
Frequency of stool	• Diarrhoea with no blood or mucus	• Diarrhoea with blood and mucus
Anal lesions (fissures, fistula)	Rare	Common
Length of strictures	Small (<3 cm)	Usually long
Internal fistulae	Very rare	Frequent
Perforation	Uncommon	Rare
Ulceration (location and direction)	Circumferential and transverse to long axis, large and confluent	Along the mesenteric attachment and longitudinal, small and discrete
B. Microscopic		
Presence of granulomas	Always present	Present in 75% of cases
Lymph node involvement	May be involved without intestinal involvement	Nodes not involved when intestine not involved
Caseation	Present	Absent
Fibrosis and hyalinisation	Common	Rare

INFLAMMATORY BOWEL DISEASE

Crohn's Disease and Ulcerative Colitis (Table 6.7)

These are non-specific inflammatory disorders of bowel having similar aetiopathogenesis, pathology, investigations, complications and treatment.

Aetiology

Exact aetiology is unknown. Factors responsible are:
1. Genetic predisposition/familial occurrence
2. Infective cause, e.g. some unknown bacterial/viral infection.
3. **Immunological basis.** Autoimmune aetiology is based on histopathological evidence (infiltration of lamina propria by lymphocytes) and response to steroid and immunosuppresive treatment.

Clinical Features

Read Table 6.7.

TABLE 6.7: Clinical Features of Inflammatory Bowel Disease

Crohn's disease	Ulcerattive colitis
Diarrhoea and pain abdomen in right lower quadrant with tenderness and guarding are presenting features	Diarrhoea with blood, mucus and pus. Pain abdomen and fever may be present. Tenderness in left side of abdomen or left iliac fossa
A mass may be palpable on abdominal and rectal examination. It is an inflammatory mass.	No mass palpable
Recurrent abdominal colics are common due to obstruction	No colicky pain. Toxic megacolon may produce diffuse pain associated with distension of abdomen and stoppage of loose motions
Moderate diarrhoea and fever. Stools are loose or well formed. Features of malabsorption of fat, carbohydrate, protein and vit. D and vit. B_{12} are common. These patients have anaemia, weight loss, growth retardation in children.	Patients have severe diarrhoea with tenesmus Anaemia, weight loss present. Malabsorptive features are less common but dehydration is common.
Relapses or remission common	Common

Contd.

Contd.	
Stricture/anal fissure common	Less common
Abscess and fistulae common	Less common
Carcinoma in situ less common	More common in long standing disease
Systemic involvement (hepatic, ocular, skin, ankylosing spondylitis, arthritis) less common	More common

Note: These distinctions in clinical features are arbitrary and should not be interpreted in absolute sense.

COLORECTAL CANCER

It is common cancer involving colon and rectum. It occurs commonly in the developed countries than underdeveloped countries. The condition occurs after the age of 50 years.

Aetology
- Genetic factors, e.g. *APC gene* and *K-ras* gene mutations facilitate the growth of adenoma into carcinoma.
- Dietary factors, e.g. reduced intake of fibres, fruits, vegetables, vitamins and selenium.
- *Lifestyle changes:* Obesity, sedentary habits, physical inactivity are associated with higher risk of cancer.
- *Familial occurrence.* A positive family history predisposed to it.

Clinical Features
- Abdominal colic, altered bowel habits, bleeding, intestinal obstruction and iron deficiency anaemia.

  Physical signs include an abdominal mass in one of the iliac fossa, lymph node enlargement, rectal mass, hepatomegaly and ascites.

Differential Diagnosis
Read the differential diagnosis of mass in right and left iliac fossa.
  Diagnosis. It is confirmed by sigmoidoscopy/colonoscopy and radioimaging.

ACUTE PANCREATITIS

Definition. It is defined as an acute inflammation of the pancreas presenting with acute abdominal pain and raised pancreatic enzymes in the blood, urine and peritoneal fluid.

Causes
1. **Common**
   - Gall stones, alcohol
   - Idiopathic
   - Iterogenic, e.g. ERCP, postsurgical
2. **Uncommon**
   - *Viral infection,* e.g. mumps, Coxsackie B
   - Pancreatic tumours
   - Drugs, e.g. azathioprine, oestrogens, corticosteroids, thiazides
   - Pancreas divisum
   - Metabolic, e.g. hypercalcaemia, hyperlipidaemia
   - Biliary microlithiasis
   - Sphincter of oddi dysfunction.
   - Miscellaneous, e.g. ischaemia, trauma to abdomen, scorpion bite, ascariasis, cardiac surgery

Clinical Features
The characteristic feature is acute upper abdominal (epigastric) pain which radiates to the back, is commonly associated with nausea and vomiting in majority of patients (65%). The pain may vary from mild discomfort to excruciating pain in severe cases.

Physical Signs
- Varying degree of shock, tachycardia, fever and signs of paralytic ileus (absent bowel sound, distended abdomen)
- There may be some degree of guarding and rigidity of abdomen, which is absent in mild cases.
- Discolouration of flanks (*Grey Turner's sign*) or periumbilical area (*Cullen's sign*) are features of severe pancreatitis with haemorrhage.
  Occasionally, in severe cases, there may be multisystem failure and or development of complications.

Local Complications
1. *Pancreatic,* e.g. pseudocyst, pancreatic abscess, ascites/pleural effusion.
2. *Gastrointestinal,* e.g. upper GI bleed, paralytic ileus, duodenal obstruction
3. *Hepatobiliary,* e.g. portal vein thrombosis, obstructive jaundice.

Systemic Complications
1. *Metabolic,* e.g. hypoglycaemia, hypocalcaemia and hypoalbuminaemia.
2. *Hematological,* e.g. DIC, variceal bleed.
3. *Renal,* e.g. acute renal failure (ARF).
4. *Cardiovascular,* e.g. shock.
5. *Respiratory,* e.g. ARDS.

Diagnosis. It is made on investigations, i.e.
1. Raised serum amylase and lipase.
2. Ultrasonography.
3. CT scan/MRI.
4. Blood biochemistry and blood gas analysis.

Differential Diagnosis: Read the differential diagnosis of acute abdomen (Table 6.8).

PANCREATIC CARCINOMA

The incidence of pancreatic carcinoma is steadily increasing in the West due to an increase in both smoking and alcohol consumption. Most patients are above the age of 60 years at diagnosis. Males are affected more than females.

Aetiological Factors

- Alcohol, smoking, high fat and protein diet are important aetiological factors. Coffee and tea consumption increase the risk.
- Calcinosis with chronic pancreatitis and diabetes are definite premalignant conditions.

Type and Sites of Involvement

Common neoplasm is adenocarcinoma. Common site is the head of pancreas and the body. The tumour spreads locally to involve lymph nodes.

Clinical Features

General features include *abdominal pain, steatorrhoea weight loss* and *obstructive jaundice*. The specific features are:

TABLE 6.8: Different Diagnosis of Acute Abdomen

Condition	History	Clinical examination
Perforated peptic ulcer with acute peritonitis	Vomiting at onset followed by acute severe abdominal pain, previous history of dyspeptic symptoms, ulcer disease, NSAIDs or corticosteroids therapy	Shallow breathing with diminished abdominal movements, generalised abdominal tenderness, guarding, board-like rigidity, distension of abdomen with absent bowel sounds
Acute pancreatitis	Anorexia, nausea, vomiting, epigastric pain radiating to back, previous alcohol abuse or cholelithiasis	Fever, epigastric or right hypochondriac pain, periumbilical bruising (*Cullen's sign*), loin bruising (*Grey Turner's sign*), epigastric tenderness or mass (*pseudocyst*), variable guarding or absent bowel sounds (*paralytic ileus*)
Ruptured aortic aneurysm	Sudden onset of tearing, severe back/loin/abdominal pain, circulatory collapse, history of peripheral vascular disease and/or hypertension	Shock and hypotension, pulsatile tender epigastric mass with an overlying bruit, asymmetrical femoral pulses, sometimes hypertension due to renal artery ischaemia
Acute mesenteric insufficiency	Anorexia, nausea, vomiting, bloody diarrhoea, constant abdominal pain in an old person (>60 yrs), previous history of cardiovascular disease	Atrial fibrillation, cardiac failure, asymmetrical peripheral pulses, absent bowel sounds, variable tenderness and guarding
Acute intestinal obstruction (strangulated hernia)	Central colicky abdominal pain, nausea, vomiting and constipation	Surgical scars, abdominal mass, hernia, distension, exaggerated visible peristalsis, increased bowel sounds (*borborygmi*)
Acute appendicitis	Nausea, vomiting, central abdominal pain settling into right iliac fossa	Fever, tenderness, guarding in right iliac fossa, a mass in right iliac fossa, pelvic peritonitis (rebound tenderness)
Ruptured ectopic pregnancy	Premenopausal, delayed/missed menstrual period, feeling of fainting, circulatory collapse, unilateral iliac fossa pain or shoulder tip pain, vaginal discharge: 'Late period' like prune juice	Suprapubic tenderness, periumbilical bruising (*Cullen's sign*), pain/tenderness on vaginal examination, swelling/fullness in the fornix on vaginal examination
Pelvic inflammatory disease (PID)	Sexually active female, previous history of STD/PID, recent gynecological procedure, pregnancy or use of intrauterine contraceptive device, irregular menses, dysuria, dyspareunia, lower or central abdominal pain, backache, pleuritic right upper quadrantic pain (*Fitz-Hugh-Curtis syndrome*)	Fever, vaginal discharge, pelvic peritonitis, right upper quadrant tenderness (perihepatitis), pain and/or tenderness on vaginal examination (cervical erosions), swelling/fullness in the fornix on vaginal examination

- Carcinoma of head of pancreas or the ampulla of Vater presents with painless progressive jaundice, pruritus and clay-coloured stools.
- Carcinoma of body and tail presents with abdominal pain, anorexia and weight loss. The pain is dull, boring in character, results from invasion of coeliac plexus. It often radiates to the back and is relieved by bending forwards.
- A few patients present with duodenal obstruction (vomiting, diarrhoea), diabetes mellitus (insulin resistance caused by islet amyloid polypeptide, a hormonal factor secreted by pancreatic β-cells), recurrent thrombophlebitis, acute pancreatitis.

Physical Signs
- Pallor, weight loss, jaundice.
- A palpable gall bladder mass. A palpable gall bladder in a jaundiced patient is usually due to biliary obstruction by a pancreatic tumour (**Courvoisier's sign**).
- Hepatomegaly may be due to biliary obstruction or metastases.
- Ascites may be present if peritoneum is involved.
- On rectal examination, nodules (*Brumer's shelf*) may be felt.
- Enlargement of the left supraclavicular node (*Virchow's node*).

Diagnosis: It is made by USG and CT scan and confirmed by fine needle aspiraton biopsy.

Differential Diagnosis: Read the differential diagnosis of obstructive jaundice.

ACUTE CHOLECYSTITIS
The acute inflammation of gall bladder is called *acute cholecystitis*.
- It can be due to obstruction of the gall bladder duct or neck by stone (calculous), mucus, parasite or tumour. It can be nonbostructive called *acalculous cholecystitis*.

Acalculous cholecystitis can occur in 5 to 10% cases; is associated with trauma or burns, postoperative and post-partum period and a variety of systemic disorders, e.g. diabetes, tuberculosis, cardiovascular.

Clinical Features
Acute cholecystitis often presents as an acute attack of biliary colic that progressively worsens. Recurrent attacks that resolve spontaneously are common. The cardinal feature is abdominal pain in right upper quadrant and the epigastrium, may radiate to the intercapular region, right scapula or shoulder. The pain may increase with jarring or on deep inspiration if there is associated peritoneal inflammation. Attacks of pain may be associated with nausea, vomiting and anorexia. Jaundice can occur in late stages due to involvement of bile ducts (common bile duct stone) and surrounding lymph nodes. A low-grade fever is characteristically present but shaking chills or rigors are uncommon.

Physical Sign
Right hypochondrial tenderness, rigidity and occasionally palpable gall bladder (25–50% cases). A light blow delivered to the right subcostal area may evoke pain (*Murphy's sign*). Localised rebound tenderness is common. Signs of peritonitis or paralytic ileus are lacking. **Diagnosis** is established by ultrasound.

CARCINOMA OF GALL BLADDER
(Read the textbook of surgery).

The commonest tumours are adenocarcinomas (>90% cases) followed by anaplastic carcinomas. These tumours occur in old age (>70 years of age) and commonly in females. The gallstones are predisposing factor.

The condition may be asymptomatic. Symptomatic cases present as recurrent *attacks of abdominal pain, persistent jaundice* and *weight loss*. The gall bladder is palpable as lobular firm or hard mass in the right hypochondrium. It may spread to other organs, i.e. liver, bones, lungs, etc. The **diagnosis** is confimed by ultrasound and CT scan.

HEPATOMEGALY
Definition. It is defined as acutal enlargement of liver with liver span more than 14 cm defined either on percussion or on USG. Palpable liver due to visceroptosis (drooping of liver) is not hepatomegaly (liver span is normal).

Causes
I. **Mild to moderate hepatomegaly.**
  1. *Infections*, e.g. typhoid fever, tuberculosis, infectious mononuclosis, subacute infective endocarditis.
  2. *Blood disorders*, e.g. anaemia, hemolytic anaemia, acute leukaemia.
  3. *Cardiac disorders*, e.g. CHF, pericardial effusion.
  4. *Hepatic diseases*: Budd-Chiari syndrome, post-necrotic cirrhosis, fatty liver.
  5. Miscellaneous, e.g. hemangioma, hepatic cyst.

II. **Massive hepatomegaly** (>8 cm below the costal margin)
  - Malignancy liver (primary, secondary)

- Amebic liver abscess
- Chronic malaria
- Kala-azar
- Hepatitis
- Lymphomas

III. **Tender hepatomegaly**
- Acute viral hepatitis
- Liver abscess (pyogenic or amoebic)
- Congestive hepatomegaly (CHF, pericardial effusion)
- Budd-Chiari syndrome
- Hepatoma
- Perihepatitis

IV. **Soft hepatomegaly**
- CHF
- Fatty liver/steohepatitis
- Hepatitis
- SABE

V. **Firm hepatomegaly**
- Cirrhosis
- Chronic malaria and kala azar.
- Hepatic amoebiasis
- Lymphoma

VI. **Hard hepatomegaly**
- Hepatocellular carcinoma (nodular liver)
- Metastasis in liver (hard nodular)
- Chronic myeloid leukaemia (non-nodular firm)
- Myelofibrosis (non-nodular, hard)

Causes of Left Lobe Enlargement of Liver

1. Amoebic liver abscess (left lobe)
2. Hepatoma
3. Metastases in liver

Diagnosis and Differential Conditions causing Hepatomegaly

Congestive Hepatomegaly

It is due to chronic venous congestion of liver, occurs as a result of:
i. *Congestive heart failure* due to any cause, e.g. constrictive pericarditis, pericardial effusion and hepatic vein, thrombosis (Budd-Chiari syndrome). **Symptoms** of dyspnoea, orthopnoea, paroxysmal nocturnal dyspnoea (PND) and cough with pitting oedema, crackles at both lung bases, heart murmurs, cardiomegaly and hepatomegaly indicate *congestive heart failure*.
ii. Nonvisible apex, pulsus paradoxus, low pulse pressure, widening of cardiac dullness and dullness of 2nd and 3rd left space, feeble heart sounds with other peripheral signs of congestive heart failure indicates hepatomegaly due to either *constrictive pericarditis* or *pericardial effusion*.
iii. In *hepatic vein thrombosis (Budd-Chiari syndrome)*, there is an intractable ascites, jaundice, prominent abdominal veins and collaterals formation due to development of portal hypertension. Hepatomegaly is a part of the syndrome.

In these *congestive* states, *liver* is moderately or massively enlarged, tender, has smooth surface and round well-defined edge.

Inflammatory Hepatomegaly

Inflammation of liver due to hepatitis or typhoid fever produces enlargement of liver.
i. In *hepatitis*, there is history of fever, distaste for food, nausea, vomiting followed by jaundice and pain in right hypochondrium.
ii. Typhoid fever is characterised by moderate to high grade fever, abdominal symptoms (nausea, vomiting, diarrhoea with or without blood), tenderness of abdomen, rose spots and slow pulse rate. At about 7 to 10th day of illness, spleen also becomes enlarged.

Liver in inflammatory disorders shows mild to moderate enlargement, is tender and has smooth surface.

Infiltrative Hepatomegaly

Liver becomes enlarged when it gets infiltrated with leukaemic cells or lymphoma cells or with fat and glycogen.
i. *Fatty infiltration* of liver occurs in *pregnancy*, *diabetes mellitus* and *alcoholism*. Fatty liver is mildly enlarged, non-tender and has smooth surface, can progress to steohepatitis.
ii. In leukaemia and lymphoma, there is evidence of anaemia, bleeding tendency (purpuric spots, ecchymosis, epistaxis, bruising, etc.), fever, lymph node enlargement and splenomegaly. Peripheral blood film examination will confirm the diagnosis.

In these disorders, liver is moderately enlarged, soft to firm in consistency, non-tender with smooth surface.

Hepatomegaly due to Parasitic Infection/Infestations

Malaria, kala-azar, hydatid disease and amoebic infection can produce hepatomegaly by various mechanisms.

i. *Malaria* produces massive enlargement of liver along with other characteristics, such as fever of several days duration with classical bouts on alternate day with shaking chills and rigors. Jaundice is also common due to hepatitis or haemolysis. There is splenomegaly. Hepatomegaly is non-tender. Peripheral blood film will confirm the diagnosis of this condition.

ii. Fever, hyperpigmentation of skin, especially face and hands, hepatosplenomegaly and anaemia support the diagnosis of *kala-azar* in endemic area. The *diagnosis* can easily be confirmed by demonstrating the parasite in stained smears of aspirate of bone marrow, lymph nodes, spleen or liver or by culture of these aspirates.

iii. *Hydatid disease of liver* produces cystic enlargement with positive hydatid sign on percussion with peripheral eosinophilia. USG is useful for confirming the diagnosis.

Haematological Disorders

All types of anaemia, especially *haemolytic* anaemia, lead to mild to moderate non-tender hepatomegaly. The presence of mild jaundice, dark coloured urine and stools with mild to moderate splenomegaly support the diagnosis of haemolytic anaemia. The diagnosis is further confirmed by tests for haemolysis and peripheral blood film examination. Malaria can also produce haemolysis, jaundice and hepatomegaly.

Tumours of Liver

The tumours (primary or secondary) can enlarge the liver. Liver in malignancy is massively enlarged, tender and has nodular surface and hard consistency. Friction rub may be audible in some cases. Jaundice, pruritus may or may not be present, depending on the presence or absence of cholestasis. USG of liver and biopsy of liver will confirm the diagnosis.

Hepatomegaly due to Postnecrotic Cirrhosis of Liver

Posthepatitic or postnecrotic cirrhosis can produce non-tender, mild to moderate hepatomegaly due to regenerating nodules with other stigmatas of cirrhosis and portal hypertension (muscle wasting, loss of axillary and pubic hair, gynaecomastia, palmar erythema, spider angiomata, ascites, caput medusae and splenomegaly). The diagnosis is confirmed by liver biopsy and by biochemical and radiological tests.

ASCITES

Definition. Fluid more than normal amount (50–150 ml of lymph) is called *ascites*. Ascitic fluid >300 ml is detected on ultrasound and > 500 ml is detected on clinical examination. Tense ascites means peritoneal cavity is full with fluid causing cardiorespiratory embarrassment.

Differential Diagnosis of Ascites

1. **Ascites due to nephrotic syndrome.**
   - Mild, moderate, severe transudative ascites
   - Associated puffiness of face, pedal oedema.
   - History of morning puffiness of face
   - History of renal disease.
   - Presence of massive proteinuria (>3.5 g/d)

2. **Ascites due to cirrhosis of liver.**
   - Moderate to severe transudative ascites
   - Past history of jaundice, haematemesis or malena.
   - Signs of portal hypertension, i.e. caput medusae, splenomegaly, fetor hepaticus, prominent abdominal vein.
   - Stigmatas of cirrhosis, i.e. sunken cheeks, shining eyeballs, parotid gland enlargement, gynaecomastia, testicular atrophy.

3. **Ascites of CHF/Pericardial effusion.**
   - Mild to moderate transudative ascites.
   - Presence of cardiac disease, i.e. valvular, pericardial, myocardial
   - Signs of CHF, i.e. raised JVP, cyanosis, tender hepatomegaly, pitting oedema feet

4. **Ascites due to hypoproteinemia**
   - Mild transudative ascites
   - Muscle flabbyness
   - Anaemia
   - Multiple nutritional deficiency signs
   - Evident cause of hypoproteinemia, i.e. malnutrition, chronic diarrhoea

5. **Tubercular ascites**
   - Slowly developing mild to moderate ascites (exudative)
   - Low grade fever, anorexia, night sweats
   - Past history of tuberculosis or associated pulmonary or extra-pulmonary tuberculosis.

6. **Malignant ascites**
   - Moderate/severe/tense exudative ascites.
   - Old age
   - Rapid filling ascites
   - Malignant cachexia present (emaciation, loss of appetite, anaemia)
   - There may be jaundice if liver is involved in malignancy.

7. **Ascites due to Budd-Chiari syndrome**
   - Large exudative ascites
   - Intermittent Jaundice
   - Hepatomegaly (tender, soft liver), splenomegaly
   - History of taking hepatotoxin. (Bush tea, drug, etc.)
   - Signs of portal hypertension may or may not be present.

8. **Pancreatic ascites**
   - Painless, mild to moderate exudative ascites
   - History of recurrent or chronic pancreatitis
   - Fluid amylase levels are high.

Difference between Transudative and Exudative Ascites

Transudative	Exudative
Clear fluid, serous or straw coloured	Thick, turbid or mucinous, hemorrhagic or straw coloured fluid
SAAG (Serum Ascitic fluid Albumin Gradient) is >1.1 g/dl	SAAG is <1.1 g/dl

Mostly non-inflammatory	Mostly inflammatory
Fluid protein content <3 g/dl or, ≤50% of serum proteins	Fluid protein content > 3 g or >50% of serum protein
Specific gravity low or normal	Specific gravity is high
Occasional cell (cell count <100 cells/mm^3) mostly mesothelial	Cell count 100–1000 cell mm^3 mostly mononuclear or neurophilis
Causes: Nephrotic syndrome, cirrhosis liver hypoproteinemia, CHF, pericardial effusion	Tubercular, malignant, pancreatic, Budd-Chiari syndrome

JAUNDICE

Bilirubin ≥ 1.5 mg/dl in blood is called *jaundice*.

Clinical Types of Jaundice

1. Haemolytic (excessive production of bilirubin)
2. Hepatocellular (decreased uptake and conjugation)
3. Obstructive (impaired excretion)

The differentiation and differential diagnosis of all three types is given in Table 6.9.

TABLE 6.9: Differential Diagnosis and Differentiation Amongst Three Types of Jaundice

Feature	Haemolytic	Hepatocellular	Obstructive
1. Congenital	Gilbert and Crigler-Najjar type I syndrome	Crigler-Najjar type 2	Dubin-Johnson syndrome
2. Causes	Hereditary, infections (malaria), drug induced in G6PD deficiency, immune hemolysis (warm and cold antibodies), paroxysmal nocturnal hemoglobinuria	Hepatitis (viral, drug induced, autoimmune), postoperative, alcoholic—hepatitis or steohepatitis, intrahepatic cholestasis, Budd-Chiari syndrome, Wilson's disease, malignancy liver	Primary biliary cirrhosis, secondary biliary cirrhosis, e.g. bile duct stone, strictures, cholangitis, worms (round worm), bile duct trauma, tumour of pancreas, bile duct and duodenum, pancreatitis, secondaries in liver or at porta-hepatis
3. Age and sex	Young	All ages	Adult and old age
4. Severity of jaundice	Mild	Moderate	Severe
5. Level of bilirubin (mg %)	5–10	10–20	> 20
6. Type of bilirubin	Unconjugated	Both (conjugated and unconjugated)	Mainly conjugated
7. Pruritus	Absent	May or may not be present	Present
8. Hepatomegaly	Present (non-tender)	Tender hepatomegaly	No hepatomegaly
9. Splenomegaly	Present	Absent	Absent
10. Xanthelasma	Absent	Absent	Present
11. Urine	Yellow (excess of urobilinogen)	Dark yellow	Dark brown (bilirubinuria)
12. Stool	Dark coloured	Normal to dark	Clay (white) colour

Diagnosis and Differential Diagnosis of Hepatitis

Diagnostic clue to acute hepatitis
- Acute onset of jaundice
- Fever, myalgia, distaste to food as prodromal symptoms
- Dark-coloured urine and stool.
- Pruritus may be present if there is intrahepatic cholestasis
- Tender hepatomegaly

Differential Diagnosis of Acute Hepatitis

Read Table 6.10.

PORTAL HYPERTENSION

Definition. It is defined as increased portal vein pressure more than normal (normal is 9–11 mm Hg). Nowadays, it is diagnosed by portal vein diameter >13 mm on ultrasonography.

Classification and Causes

They are discussed below.

Classification	Causes
1. **Presinusoidal** (obstruction lies outside liver between sinusoids and portal vein, also called *pre-hepatic portal hypertension.*)	• Congenital hepatic fibrosis • Drugs and toxins induced hepatitis • Schistosomasis, sorcoidosis • Portal vein thrombosis • Compression of portal vein by lymph nodes at porta hepatis
2. **Sinusoidal** (obstruction lies within liver). It is also called *hepatic portal hypertension*	• Cirrhosis of liver • Malignancy liver • Cystic liver disease
3. **Postsinusoidal** (obstruction lies beyond liver, i.e. at the level of hepatic veins or inferior vena cava). It is also called *post hepatic portal hypertensoin*	• Budd-Chiari syndrome • Veno occlusive disease • Constrictive pericarditis, long standing chronic CHF

Portal hypertension can be due to liver disease (*cirrhotic portal hypertension*) or without liver disease (*non-cirrhotic portal hypertension*). Read Table 6.11 for their differentiation.

TABLE 6.10: Differential Diagnosis of Hepatitis

Viral hepatitis	Autoimmune hepatitis	Alcoholic hepatitis	Carcinoma of liver	Drug-induced
• Fever is followed by jaundice. As soon as jaundice appears, fever disappears • Anorexia, nausea, headache, distaste pharyngitis, cough, fatigue, malaise • Dark-coloured urine and clay-coloured or normal coloured stool • History of exposure to a patient with jaundice or sex contact with a patient of jaundice, etc. • Hepatomegaly. (liver is moderately enlarged, soft, tender, smooth) • Splenomegaly in 20% cases only • Tests for viral hepatitis are positive	• Insidious onset • Common in females • Fever with jaundice, anorexia, fatigue, arthralgia, vitiligo, epistaxis. • Sometimes a "cushingoid" face with acne, hirsutism, pink cutaneous striae • Bruises may be seen • Hepatosplenomegaly, spider telangiectasis are characteristics • Other autoimmune disorders may be associated • Serological tests confirm the diagnosis	• History of alcoholism • Anorexia, weight loss • Stigmata of chronic liver disease (spider nevi, palmar erythema, gynecomastia, testicular, atrophy) • Dupuytren's contracture, parotid glands enlargement may be present • Jaundice with enlarged tender liver (steohepatitis) • May be associated with other manifestations of alcoholism, e.g. cardiomyopathy, peripheral neuropathy • USG may show fatty liver with altered echopattern	• Common in old age • Progressive jaundice with loss of appetite and weight • Anaemia, fever, lymphadenopathy in neck and marked cachexia may be present • Jaundice is deep yellow or greenish • Liver enlarged, tender, hard, nodular. Hepatic rub may be heard • Ascites may be present • Evidence of metastatic spread to lungs, bone, etc. • USG and liver biopsy will confirm the diagnosis	• History of underlying disease, i.e. tuberculosis, diabetes, thyrotoxicosis for which the drug is being taken for a long period • History of intake of hepatotoxic drugs, e.g. INH, rifampicin, oral contraceptives • Occasionally rash, fever, arthralgia present • Liver is enlarged and tender • Tests for viral hepatitis are negative

TABLE 6.11: Differentiation Between Cirrhotic and Non-cirrhotic Portal Hypertension

Cirrhotic	Non-cirrhotic
• Slow, insidious onset	• Acute or sudden onset
• Ascites present	• Ascites absent
• Recurrent hematemesis uncommon	• Recurrent hematemesis common and presenting feature
• Anaemia (mild to moderate)	• Severe anaemia
• Hepatic encephalopathy common	• It is uncommon
• Ascites and oedema usually present	• No oedema, ascites (rare)
• Liver biopsy shows cirrhosis	• No evidence of cirrhosis, only portal fibrosis is seen
• **Causes** include: Hepatitis due to any cause, cardiac cirrhosis, biliary cirrhosis, Wilson's disease, hemachromatosis, cryptogenic cirrhosis	• **Causes** include: Idiopathic portal fibrosis, Portal vein thrombosis, Schistosomiasis, congenital hepatic fibrosis, non-Hodgkin's lymphoma

Clinical Manifestations

Symptoms
- Weakness, fatigue, abdominal distension
- Hematemesis and malena
- Foul breath

Signs
1. Splenomegaly
2. Collateral vessels (*caput medusae*)
3. Variceal bleed (hematemesis and malena)
4. Fetor hepaticus
5. Ascites

The **diagnosis** of portal hypertension is suspected on history of hepatitis, hematemesis, malena and USG abdomen (portal vein diameter >13 mm) and portal manometry

Differential Diagnosis
1. *Splenomegaly*: Portal hypertension comes into differential diagnosis of splenomegaly (read splenomegaly).
II. *Ascites*: Read the differential diagnosis of ascites.

PRIMARY BILIARY CIRRHOSIS

It is an autoimmune disorders of intrahepatic biliary system leading to impaired billary excretion, destruction of hepatic parenchma and progressive fibrosis.

Clinical Manifestations
- It may be a symptomatic for many years.
- Commonly involves the middle-aged females
- Symptomatic cases present with slow onset of jaundice (Fig. 6.39), pruritus (scratch marks), hepatosplenomegaly.
- Progressive disease over the years produce malabsorption (steatorrhoea), easy bruising (vit. K deficiency), bone pain and osteomalacia (vit. D deficiency), osteoporosis (protein deficiency) and xanthelasma due to hyperlipidaemia.
- Diagnosis is confirmed by positive antimitochondrial M_2 antibody by ELISA (titre > 1:60).

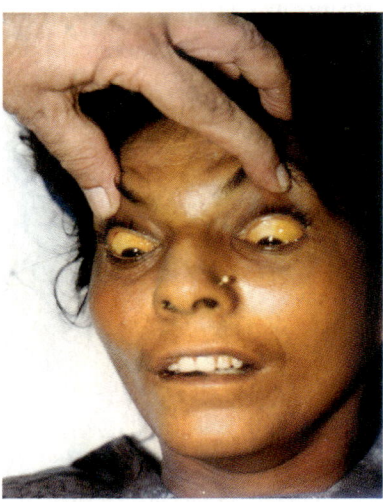

Fig. 6.39: Jaundice in a patient with primary biliary cirrhosis.

BUDD-CHIARI SYNDROME

It is an uncommon disorder resulting from occlusion of hepatic vein or inferior vena cava. The **causes** include: Primary polycythaemia, leukaemia, paroxysmal nocturnal hemoglobinuria, thrombophilia, hyperprothombinaemia, deficiency of antithrombin, protein S and protein C resistance (factor V Leiden mutation), pregnancy, use of contraceptives, antiphospholipid syndrome and malignancy liver. It may be acute (dehydration/shock) or chronic.

Clinical triad is jaundice, tender hepatomegaly and ascites with prominent abdominal vein.

Diagnosis is confirmed by CT scan/MRI.

HEPATIC INSUFFICIENCY/ENCEPHALOPATHY

Definition: It is defined as liver cell failure due to chronic liver disease (> 6 months) leading to mental features (hepatic encephalopathy).

Causes
1. Cirrhosis of the liver (viral, alcoholic, biliary cryptogenic)
2. Fulminant hepatitis
3. Wilson's disease, hemochromatosis
4. Budd-Chiari syndrome/veno-occlusive disease.

Clinical Staging of Hepatic Insufficiency

Stage	Mental features	Tremor	EEG change
I	Euphoria or depression confusion, disorientation	+/−	Normal EEG
II	Lethargy, moderate confusion	+	Abnormal EEG (High voltage triphasic slow waves)
III	Marked confusion, incoherent speech, drowsy but arousable	+	Abnormal EEG as described above
IV	Coma	−	Abnormal EEG (delta activity)

Clinical Manifestations

Precipitating Factors
Following are precipitaing factors in a patient with chronic liver disease or arrhosis.
- Hepatotoxic drugs (sedatives and hypnotics)
- Gastrointestinal bleeding (varices, peptic ulcer, congestive coagulopathy)
- High protein intake
- Diuretics
- Rapid removal of large amount of ascitic fluid
- Constipation
- Acute alcoholic bout
- Infection, surgery, septicaemia, uraemia
- Portosystemic shunts

Clinical Features
They arise due to endocrinal disturbance (hyperestrogenemia), bleeding disturbance (platelet and coagulation disturbance), hypoproteinemia, malnutrition, alcoholism, spironolactone therapy, etc. The features are:
1. *Mental features*, i.e. confusion, disorientation, behaviour changes, bizarre handwriting, sleep disturbance, constructional apraxia
2. Hepatomegaly (malignancy) or small shrunken liver (alcoholic cirrhosis)
3. Fever, jaundice
4. *Circulatory changes*, e.g. spider angiomata, palmar erythema, cyanosis, clubbing, bounding pulses, anaemia.
5. *Endocrinal features*
   - Loss of axillary and pubic hair
   - Loss of libido
   - Gynaecomastia, testicular atrophy (small, soft testes) impotence in males
   - Breast atrophy/irregular menses, amenorrhea in females
6. *Bleeding manifestations*, e.g.
   - Bruises, epistasis, purpura, menorrhagia
7. *Miscellaneous*
   - Diffuse pigmentation, flapping tremors (asterixis)
   - White nails (leuconychia)
   - Parotid enlargement (common in alcoholic cirrhosis)
   - Dupuytren's contracture (flexion deformities of fingers due to thickening and shortening).

SPLENOMEGALY
Enlargement of spleen is called *splenomegaly*.

Classification and Causes
1. **Mild Splenomegaly** (1–3 cm below costal margins). The conditions are:
   1. Typhoid fever, endocarditis, tuberculosis, infections mononucleosis.
   2. Felty's syndrome
   3. SLE.
   4. Acute leukaemia
   5. Anaemia
   6. Congestive heart failure
2. **Moderate splenomegaly** (between 3 and 7 cm below the costal margin). The conditions are:
   1. Haemolytic anaemia
   2. Cirrhotic portal hypertension.
   3. Lymphomas
   4. Sarcoidosis
   5. Constrictive pericarditis, pericardial effusion, CHF.
3. **Massive** (>8 cm below the costal margin, Fig. 6.40.)
   1. Chronic myeloid leukaemia (CML).
   2. Agnogenic myeloid metaplasia.
   3. Myelofibrosis.
   4. Chronic malaria, kala-azar.
   5. Hairy cell leukaemia.
   6. Gaucher's and Niemann-Pick disease.
   7. Hepatic vein obstruction (Budd-Chiari syndrome).
   8. Portal vein obstruction.

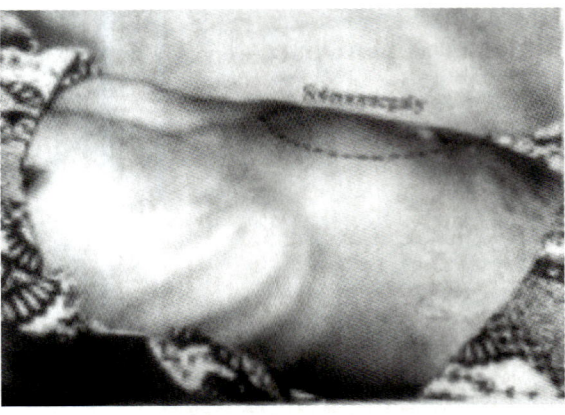

Fig. 6.40. Splenomegaly. Note the protuberance in left hypochondriac region in a patient with massive splenomegaly due to CML.

Differential Diagnosis of Splenomegaly

In evaluation of patients with splenomegaly, it is helpful to separate acute and chronic illness with splenomegaly.
1. An acute febrile illness associated with splenomegaly may be due to bacterial endocarditis, malaria, kala-azar, tuberculosis, histoplasmosis, typhoid fever. The chronic illnesses associated with splenomegaly include CML, CLL, lymphoma, myelofibrosis, anaemia, RA, SLE, cirrhotic portal hypertension, etc.
2. Fever, peripheral lymphadenopathy and splenomegaly with or without rash or arthralgia suggest infectious mononucleosis, sarcoidosis, Hodgkin's lymphoma, a collagen vascular disorder such as systemic lupus erythromatosis.
3. An acute illness with anaemia, splenomegaly suggests autoimmune haemolytic anaemia, acute leukaemia and myeloproliferative syndromes.
4. Splenomegaly may present with symptoms and signs of underlying or associated illness. Liver disease (cirrhosis) with portal hypertension is a common cause of splenomegaly.
5. In the presence of rheumatoid arthritis and leukopenia. Felty's syndrome should be considered.
6. The lymphadonopathy with splenomegaly suggests chronic lymphocytic leukaemia (CLL) or lymphoma.
7. Presence of symptoms and signs of right heart failure (cor pulmonale) or constrictive pericarditis suggest it to be the cause of splenomegaly.
8. Weight loss or other signs of chronic illness suggest leukaemia or other myeloproliferative disorders and haemoglobinopathies.

HYPERSPLENISM

It is defined as a clinical condition in which spleen removes excessive quanitities of erythrocytes, granulocytes and platelets from the circulation. Hypersplenism is a common feature in patient with cirrhosis of liver with portal hypertension and lymphoma.

Clinical Features

Clinical picture is not related to the size of spleen. Any grade of splenomegaly can be associated with hypersplenism. Hypersplenism, in strict sense, is hyperfunctioning spleen. The **clinical picture** will consists of (*i*) symptoms and signs of underlying disorder, for example, cirrhosis of the liver with portal hypertension, in addition to (*ii*) accelerated destruction of one or more formed elements of blood (bicytopenia or pancytopenia). Pancytopenia may manifest clinically with infections, easy bruisability or bleeding. The **diagnosis** is based on
1. Splenomegaly (moderate to massive)
2. Destruction of one or more cell line in peripheral blood (*bicytopenia or pancytopenia*)
3. Hypercellular bone marrow
4. Evidence of an accelerated cell turnover in the cell lines affected (*reticulocytosis, band forms of neutrophils and immature platelet forms*)
5. **Confirmation** is done by demonstration of sequestration of radioactive labelled RBCs in the spleen.

Clinical tip

The splenomegaly with pancytopenia and hypercellular marrow invariably indicate hypersplenism.

Unit VII

Examination of Breasts and Axillae

- Symptoms and their Analysis
- History
- Examination (Physical Signs and Systemic Signs)
- Diagnosis and Differential Diagnosis
- Brief Synopsis of Breast Diseases

COMMON SYMPTOMS RELATED TO BREAST

1. Breast lump or mass, asymmetry of breasts, breast pain or discomfort.
2. Skin dimpling.
3. Nipple discharge.
4. Nipple retraction.
5. Lymphoedema.
6. Galactorrhoea (milk ejection).
7. Men may present with gynaecomastia.

1. BREAST LUMP

The common **causes** of breast lump include; carcinoma of breast, fibrocystic change, fibroadenomas, cysts and breast abscesses. The commonest cause of breast lump varies with age (Table 7.1).

Symptom Analysis

Ask about the following

1. **Age.**
   - Advanced age is a risk factor. More than three-fourths breast cancer cases occur in women of 50 years or older; more than half in women older than 65. The chance of developing breast cancer is approximately 2–5% in young age (35–50 yrs).
   - Benign breast lumps (fibroadenoma, cyst) are common in young age.
2. **Ask about the family history.**
   - First degree relatives, namely a mother or sister with breast cancer establish a "positive family history". Inherited disease (genetic predisposition) in women with mutations in the breast cancer genes (BRCA1 and BRCA2) accounts only 5 to 10% of breast cancer. However, these genes confer a 50% risk in women under 50 yrs which increases further to 80% by age of 65 yrs.

TABLE 7.1: Palpable Masses in the Breast

Mass	Characteristics
Fibroadenoma occurs in young age	Usually fine, soft to firm in consistency, round, mobile and tender. It is well demarcated from surrounding tissue, *retraction sign* absent
Cysts	Common in young age. Usually single, soft, round, mobile, often tender, *retraction sign* absent
Fibrocystic changes	Occurs in middle age. Nodular, rope like, bilateral lumps in upper quadrant tender, rubery in consistency varies in size with menstrual cycle
Carcinoma breast	Occur in old age, irregular in outline, stellate, firm to hard, not clearly demarcated from surrounding tissue, may be fixed to skin and underlying tissue. *Retraction sign* may be present
Lactating adenomas	Same as above
Mastitis (abscess)	Common in middle age, mostly in lactating mothers. Tender breast lump, local temperature, raised, sign of inflammation present

3. **Ask about the menstural history and pregnancy.**

- Early menarche, delayed menopause, and first live birth after the age of 35 or no pregnancy, all raise the risk of breast cancer by two to three folds.

4. **Ask about associated conditions/diseases.**
   - Benign breast disease with biopsy findings of atypical hyperplasia or lobular carcinoma *in situ* carry significantly increased risk.

Q. **Is breast lump unilateral or bilateral?**
   - Fibrocystic disease of breasts is most common cause of bilateral than unilateral breast lump in the young women (35–50 years).
   - Unilateral lump include a cyst, breast cancer, breast abscess/mastitis.

Q. **Is breast lump painful/tender?**
   - Painful breast lump indicate fibrocystic disease, mastitis/breast abscess.

Q. **Is mother lactating or nonlactating?**
   - **Lactational breast abscess (es)** occur in women who are breast-feeding or lactating. They are usually peripheral in distribution.
   - **Nonlactational abscess(es)** occurs following mastitis and have a classical distribution at the edge of the nipple, causing nipple inversion. They are common among young women smokers. Occasionally, a nonlactating abscess may rupture spontaneously forming a fistula to the exterior.

Q. **Is there any nipple discharge?**
   - Blood stained nipple discharge suggests malignancy.

Q. **Is the breast lump(s) related to menstruation?**
   - Menstruation increases fibrocystic lumps in the breast as these are hormonal related.

2. SKIN DIMPLING

It may be just a benign simple skin dimpling due to retraction of the skin or indrawing of the skin due to infiltration of the dermis by malignant tumour. The differentiating features between the two are mobility of the skin. In *simple dimpling*, the skin remains mobile over the benign tumour but in *malignancy*, the tumour is fixed to the skin and is immobile. Similarly if the tumour is tethered to the chest wall (pectoral fascia), the tumour appears solid when pectoral muscle is contracted but it is possible to move it when the muscle is relaxed. In contrast, the tumours which infiltrate the chest wall become fixed whether the pectoral muscle is relaxed or contracted.

Q. **Is skin dimpling present?**
   - Skin dimpling indicates malignant breast tumour.

Q. **Is mass fixed to chest wall?**
   - Malignant tumour infiltrate the chest wall and become fixed while benign tumour remains mobile.

3. NIPPLE DISCHARGE

A small amount of clear fluid from the breast on massage is normal. Persistent discharge or blood-stained (macroscopic or microscopic), discharge is abnormal, should be investigated.

Blood stained discharge from breast (male or female) suggests malignancy, hence must be asked

4. NIPPLE INVERSION

The nipple retraction may be benign (shortening of the nipple ducts due to inflammation and fibrosis) in which the nipple retraction is symmetrical and slit-like. Nipple retraction due to malignant disease is asymmetrical and disfiguring pulling the nipple away from the central position (Fig. 7.1).

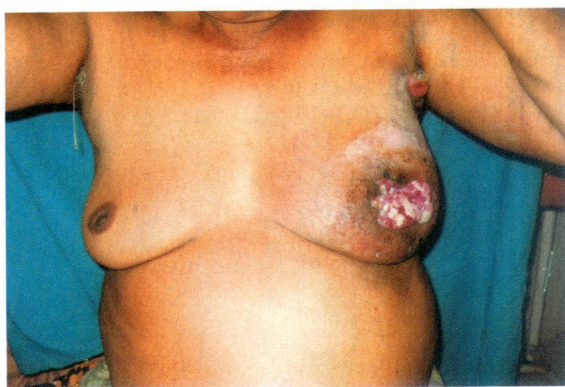

Fig. 7.1: Fulgrating growth causing disfigurement of breast (left) and displacement and retraction of the nipple.

5. LYMPHOEDEMA OF THE BREAST

It produced by obstruction of the intramammary lymphatics by the tumour. The skin is attached to the hair follicles but is swollen in between, giving the appearance of the skin of an orange (*Peau d'orange*, Fig. 7.2)

6. DISFIGUREMENT/ASYMMETRY

There may be fulgrating growth of the breast producing disfigurement (Fig. 7.1). Breast lump, mastitis, benign nodule produce asymmetry of breasts.

7. GALACTORRHOEA

A milky discharge from non-lactating mother is called *galactorrhoea* (Fig. 7.3). The causes of

Examination of Breasts and Axillae

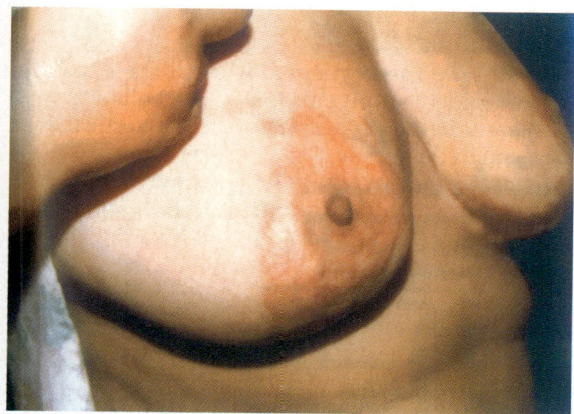

Fig. 7.2: Peau d' orange of the breast. The intramammary lymphatic obstruction by the tumour results in swollen (lymphoedema) breast and typical appearance like skin of an orange (Peau d' orange).

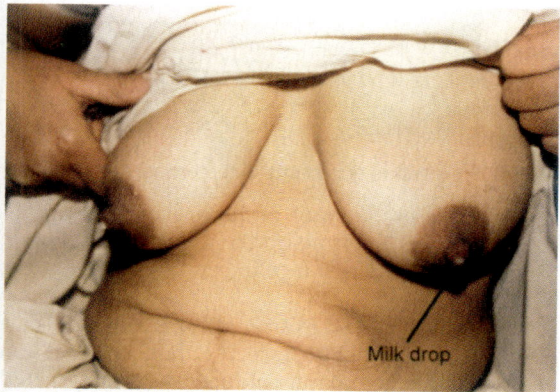

Fig. 7.3: Galactorrhoea in non-lactating women.

galactorrhoea are given below. It is commonly associated with hyperprolactinaemia.

Causes

- Prolactin secreting pituitary tumour.
- Hypothalamic-pituitary disease, i.e. tubercular meningitis.
- Drug-induced (phenothiazines, dopamine antagonists and dopamine depleting agents).
- Ectopic production of prolactin, e.g. hydatidiform moles, choriocarcinoma, lung cancer, hypernephroma.
- Primary hypothyroidism, acromegaly, Cushing's disease.
- Sucking reflex, herpes zoster intercostal neuralgia, breast trauma, stress, sleep, coitus, lactation may produce it called *physiological galactorrhoea*.
- Renal failure, cirrhosis of liver.
- Idiopathic.

Symptom Analysis

Q. Is mother lactating or non-lactating?
- Stress, puerperium, sleep, coitus, exercise, walking, running can produce galactorrhoea in lactating mother called *physiological galactorrhoea*.
- The non-lactating galactorrhoea is due to prolactinoma, hypothyroidism, prolactin secreting tumours, drugs, etc.

Q. Ask about symptoms and signs of hypothyroidism.
- Hypothyroidism can lead to galactorrhoea in married women.

Q. Ask about drug history (read the drugs causing galactorrhoea.

Q. Ask about history of wearing tight brassier.
- Running, jumping, exercise with tight brassier in lactating and non-lactating women can lead to galactorrhoea.

Q. History of associated symptoms.
- Associated amenorrhoea suggests galactorrhoea–amenorrhoea syndrome.
- Headache, visual disturbance, polyuria and polydispsia suggest pituitary tumour (craniopharyngioma).

GYNAECOMASTIA (Figs 7.4A and B)

Gynaecomastia refers to glandular enlargement of breast in the males, occurs in about 50% of pubertal boys probably due to elevated oestradiol levels. Growth of the breast in men, as in women, is mediated by oestrogen and results from disturbances of the normal ratio of the active androgen to oestrogen, hence breast enlargement results due to diminished testosterone production or action (old age, castration), enhanced oestrogen formation, or both.

Enlargement of the male breast can be a normal physiological phenomenon at puberty and in old age. It can be pathological. The causes are given in Table 7.2.

Symptom Analysis

Ask about the following

Q. Age of onset.
- Congenital or chromosomal disorders, hypogonadism, drugs produce gynaecomastia in younger age. Physiological gynaecomastia can occur in young and old (senile gynaecomastia).

Q. History of drugs.
- Drugs produce gynaecomastia are listed in Table 7.2.

TABLE 7.2: Common Causes of Gynaecomastia

1. **Physiological gynaecomastia**
   - Newborn, adolescents (Fig. 7.4A), ageing (senile)
2. **Pathological gynaecomastia**
   A. *Deficient testosterone production or action*
      - Trauma, castration, orchitis, leprosy.
      - Testicular feminisation
      - Congenital anorchia, Klinefelter's syndrome
   B. *Increased production of oestrogen*
      - Testicular tumours, carcinoma of lung or other tumours producing hCG
      - Adrenal disease
      - Cirrhosis of liver (Fig. 7.4B)
      - Thyrotoxicosis, malnutrition
   C. *Drug-induced*
      - Oestrogen used for treatment of prostate cancer
      - Androgen therapy
      - Diuretics, e.g. spironolactone and digitalis
      - Acid suppressants, e.g. cimetidine, omeprazole
      - Antidepressants, e.g. tricyclic.
      - Antimitotic drugs, e.g. busulfan, cisplatin
      - Antihypertensive, e.g. reserpine, methyldopa, calcium channel blockers, angiotensin-converting enzyme inhibitors
      - Antitubercular, e.g. isoniazid
   D. *Idiopathic*

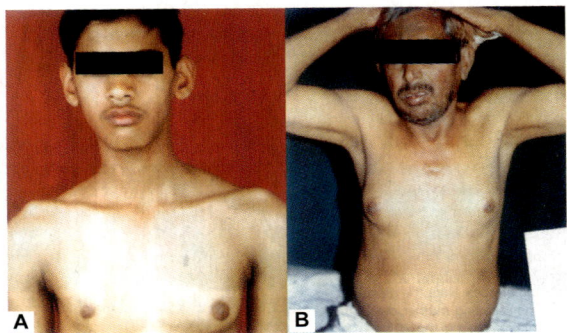

Figs 7.4A and B: *Gynaecomastia.* (A) In an adolescent male, more on the left than the right. It appears physiological, (to be investigated); (B) In a patient with cirrhotic portal hypertension. Note the ascites with everted umbilicus and bilateral gynaecomastia could be due to cirrhosis or spironolactone therapy or both.

Q. Ask about cirrhosis of liver, adreneal disease, thyrotoxicosis, CHF, testicular tumour.
   - These diseases can lead to gynaecomastia.

Q. History of mumps/orchitis.

Q. Ask about symptoms of hypogonadism.

Q. Is gynaecomastia painful?

☞ EXAMINATION OF BREASTS

To describe the clinical findings, the breast is often divided into the nipple, the areola and four quadrants based on the horizontal and vertical lines crossing at the nipple (Fig. 7.5). The nipple consists of erectile tissue covered with pigmented skin, which also covers the axilla. The opening of the lactiferous ducts may be seen near the apex of the nipple.

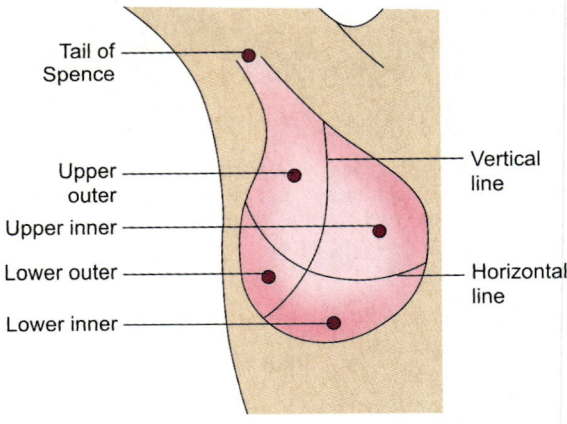

Fig. 7.5: Various quadrants of the breast (diagram).

Alternatively, instead of quadrants, finding can be localised as the time on the face of a clock (e.g. 6 o'clock) and the distance in centimeters from the nipple.

The clinical breast examination is an important part of women's health case; it enhances detection of breast cancers that may otherwise go undetected and also provides an opportunity to demonstrate techniques for self-examination to the patient.

Examination includes **inspection and palpation** of breasts in different positions with varying pressure and a circular motion used for palpation as described below.

Steps

1. Reassure the patient and adopt a gentle and courteous approach as women and girls are apprehensive about breasts examination.
2. Before you begin, explain to the patient that you are about to examine her breasts. Explain the purpose for the examination also.
3. **Position and exposure:** An adequate inspection requires full exposure of the chest. Ask the patient to sit upright on a well-illuminated chair/couch, undressed to the waist and with the hands resting on the thighs, so that the pectoral muscles are relaxed (Fig. 7.6A).
4. Sit facing the patient and *look for the size, symmetry, contour, local swelling and changes in the*

skin. Inspect the nipples also for size, shape, direction in which they point, any rash or ulceration or any discharge.

- Redness of a breast may be due to mastitis (local inflammation or inflammatory carcinoma).
- Thickening and puckering of the skin may suggest infiltrating carcinoma. Flattening of the normally convex breast, skin dimpling, *peau d'orange and blood-stained*, nipple discharge suggest breast(s) carcinoma.
- Asymmetry or direction in which nipple points suggests an underlying cancer (Fig. 7.7).
- Rash or ulceration of nipple occurs in Paget's disease of the nipple.
- A scar over the breast indicates the site of biopsy (Fig. 7.7).

5. Repeat the inspection with the patient's *hands pressed firmly on hips* (Fig. 7.6B) thereby contracting the pectoral muscles, then with arms raised above head (Fig. 7.6C) to stretch the pectoral muscles and the skin over the breasts, and finally leaning forward so that the breasts become pendulous (Fig. 7.6D). Such actions expose the whole breast and exacerbate skin dimpling.

6. Ask the patient to lie supine with the head supported on one pillow and with the hand on the side to be examined under the head (Fig. 7.8). Breast tissue gets flattened in this position.

7. With the hand held flat to the skin, palpate the rectangular area extending from the clavicle to the bra line, and from the midsternal line to the posterior axillary line and well into the axilla for the tail of the breast. Use the fingerpads of middle 3 fingers (2nd, 3rd, 4th) keeping them slightly flexed and applying gentle pressure over the breast against the chest wall. Use circular motion to palpate the breast.

8. To localise the lesion, consider the breast as a face of a clock and carefully examine each hour of the clock from outside towards the nipple, not forgetting the tissue directly under the nipple. Compare the texture of one breast with that of other.

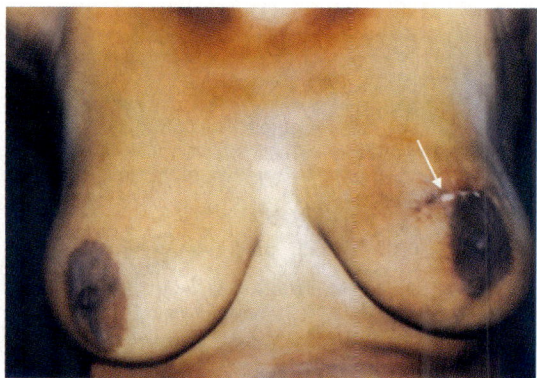

Fig. 7.7: Elevation of nipple in underlying carcinoma breast. The scar of biopsy is visible above the left nipple (↓). Left nipple is elevated and facing medially, while right nipple is directed laterally.

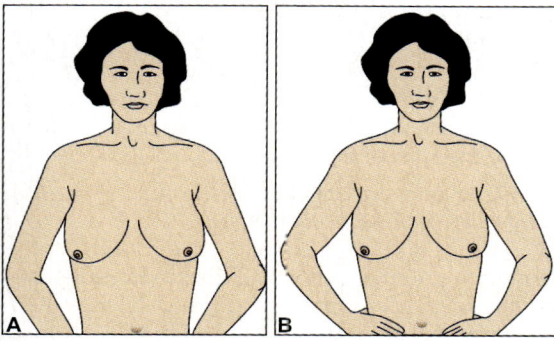

A Hand resting on thighs   B Hand pressed onto the hip

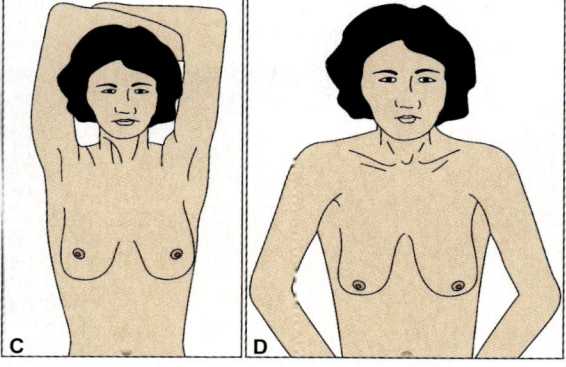

C Arms over the head   D Leaning forward with breast

Figs 7.6A to D: Examination of the breast in different positions.

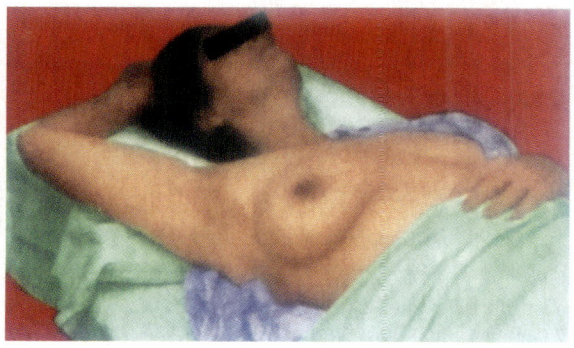

Fig. 7.8: Positioning for palpation of the right breast.

9. Define the following characteristics of a mass, if found:
   - *Location*—by quadrant or clock, with centimeters from the nipple.
   - *Size*—in centimeters.
   - *Shape*—round, or cystic, disc like, or irregular in outline.
   - *Consistency*—soft, firm, hard.
   - *Limits/extent*—well circumscribed or not.
   - *Tenderness*—present or absent.
   - *Mobility*—in relation to the skin, the pectoral fascia and the chest wall. Gently move the breast near the mass and watch for dimpling. Next try to move the mass itself by holding it between thumb and forefingers while the patient relaxes her arm and then while she presses her hands against her hip to contract the pectoral muscle.

Hard, irregular, poorly circumscribed nodule or nodules, fixed to the skin or underlying tissues strongly suggest malignancy (Fig. 7.9).

Note: Because breasts tend to swell and become more nodular before menses as a result of oestrogen stimulation, the best time for examination is 5 to 7 days after the onset of menses.

10. Examine the axillary tail between the thumb and finger as it extends towards the axilla.
11. Palpate each nipple gently between index finger and thumb and note its elasticity and try to express any discharge.
12. To examine the lateral portion of the breast, ask the patient to roll onto the opposite hip, placing her hand on her forehead but keeping the shoulders pressed against the bed or examining table. This flattens the lateral breast tissue. Now start the palpation from the axilla and move towards bra line. To examine the medial portion of the breast, ask the patient to lie with her shoulders flat against the bed or examining table, placing her hand behind her neck and lifting up her elbow until it is even with her shoulder. Palpate in a straight line down from the nipple to the bra line.
13. Complete the examination by palpating the regional lymph nodes, i.e. supraclavicular group.

☞ THE AXILLAE

Examine the axillae with the arm relaxed in order to expose the apex of the axilla.

☞ Inspect the skin of each axilla for any *rash* or *infection* or *unusual pigmentation*.

Deeply pigmented, velvety axillary skin suggests *acanthosis nigricans,* one form of which is associated with internal malignancy.

☞ Palpate the axillary region for any nodule or lymph node enlargement (Fig. 7.10) by asking

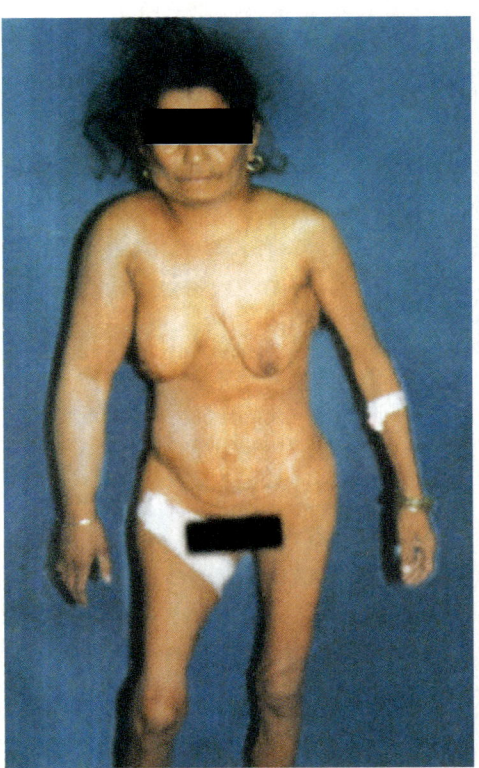

Fig. 7.9: Carcinoma of right breast producing an irregular hard poorly defined nodule in the breast. There is an associated lymphoedema of right upper and lower limbs due to metastases in the axillary and inguinal lymph nodes (biopsy has been taken).

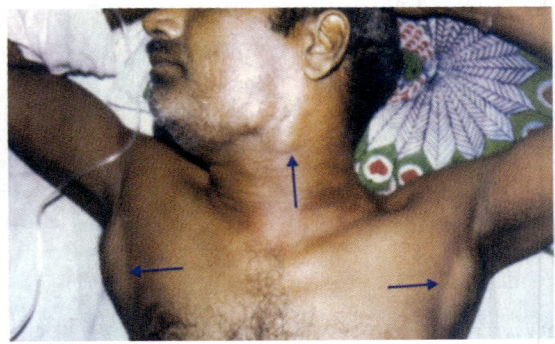

Fig. 7.10: Enlargement of axillary and neck lymph nodes (↑) in a male patient with carcinoma breast (not visible).

the patient to alternately contract and relax the pectoral muscles by pressing her hands on to the hip.

Nodules in the tail of the breast are sometimes mistaken for enlarged lymph nodes.

BRIEF SYNOPSIS OF BREAST DISEASES

CARCINOMA OF BREAST

This is one of the commonest malignancies in the women and its incidence increases with age. It is customary to regard any mass in the breast as potentially malignant until proven otherwise on histopathology. Cancer of the male breast is uncommon and there is strong genetic factor.

Characteristically carcinomas are solid masses with an irregular outline, often painless but firm or hard in consistency and cannot be delineated clearly from the surrounding tissue. The tumour may be localised within breast tissue or extend into the overlying structures such as skin or pectoral fascia, pectoral muscle or metastasise to regional lymph nodes through lymphatics or spread to distant organs through systemic circulation. When a tumour is fixed to the chest wall, it is immobile when the pectoral muscle is relaxed. When tethered to the pectoral fascia, but not muscle, it will be mobile when pectoral muscle is relaxed and adherent when the muscle is tensed.

The current TNM (tumour, nodes, metastases) classification of breast tumour is given in Table 7.3.

FIBROADENOMAS

These are tumours of main ductal lobules present as small, round, smooth mobile discrete rubbery lumps in young women (<35 years of age). The distinction between a juvenile fibroadenoma and phyllodes tumour (giant fibroadenoma) is made on distinct histopathological grounds and both are regarded as distinct pathological entities.

BREAST CYSTS

They are the commonest cause of lump in women between the ages of 35 and 50. Their clinical picture depends on the intracystic tension. They present as smooth lumps, which may be soft and fluctuant when intracystic tension (pressure) is low, become hard and painful when the cyst is under high tension or pressure. Cysts may occur in multiple clusters. Occasionally, a cyst may represent a malignant change.

Any cyst in which aspirate is blood-stained or there is residual mass following aspiration or which recurs after several aspirations should be excised and subjected to histopathology to exclude malignancy.

TABLE 7.3: TNM Classification of Breast Cancers

Tumour (T)

T_x	Cannot be assessed
T_0	No evidence of primary tumour
T_{is}	Carcinoma *in situ*, intraductal carcinoma, lobular carcinoma *in situ*, Paget's disease of the nipple
T_1	Tumour <2 cm in greatest dimension
	a. <0.5 cm
	b. >0.5 to 1 cm
	c. >1 cm to 2 cm
T_2	Tumour >2 cm to <5 cm in greatest dimension
T_3	Tumour >5 cm in greatest dimension
T_4	Direct extension into the chest wall or skin irrespective of the size
	a. Extension to chest wall
	b. Oedema including *peau d'orange* or ulceration of overlying skin
	c. 4a + 4b
	d. Inflammatory carcinoma

Nodes (N)

N_x	Regional lymph nodes cannot be assessed
N_0	No lymph node metastasis
N_1	Metastases with movable ipsilateral axillary nodes
N_2	Metastases to ipsilateral axillary nodes fixed to one another or to other structures
N_3	Metastases to ipsilateral internal mammary nodes

Metastases (M)

M_x	Presence of distant metastases cannot be assessed
M_0	No distant metastases
M_1	Distant metastases including supraclavicular nodes

Note: This classification is also applicable for classification of other primary malignancies.

Unit VIII

Haematological Disorders

- Symptoms of Pattern of Haematological Disorders
- History
- General Physical Examination
- Systemic Examination
- Brief Synopsis of Haematological Disorders

PATTERN OF HAEMATOLOGICAL DISORDERS

The haematological disorder presents with the following patterns:
1. Anaemia
2. Polycythaemia
3. Leucopenia, leucocytosis, leukaemia
4. Myelomatosis
5. Bleeding/haemorrhagic disorders
6. Thrombosis/thrombophilia

SYMPTOMS

The physical symptoms of each pattern are discussed below.

Anaemia

It is defined as haemoglobin level below the normal range of age and sex of the individual. A haemoglobin level of 12 g/dl is taken as anaemia in males and less than 11 g/dl in females.

Causes of Anaemia
1. Blood loss
   - Posthaemorrhagic
   - Chronic blood loss, e.g. piles, haematemesis, menorrhagia
   - Worm infestation, e.g. hookworm
2. Deficiency of haemopoietic factors
   - Iron deficiency (nutritional)
   - Folate and Vit. B_{12} deficiency (nutritional common)
   - Protein deficiency, e.g. diarrhoea, malabsorption

3. Hypoplasia or aplasia of marrow
   - Pure red cell aplasia
   - Aplastic or hypoplastic anaemia
4. Anaemia due to systemic disorders or chronic infections
   - Anaemia of chronic infection, e.g. tuberculosis
   - Anaemia of chronic renal disease, e.g. CRF
   - Anaemia of chronic hepatic disease, e.g. cirrhosis
   - Anaemia of disseminated malignancy
   - Anaemia of endocrinal disease, e.g. hypothyroidism
5. Anaemia of bone marrow infiltration (dyshaematopoietic anaemia)
   - Leukaemias, lymphomas, myelofibrosis or myelosclerosis
   - Multiple myeloma
   - Congenital sideroblastic anaemia
6. Anaemia due to haemolysis
   - Intracorpuscular defect (hereditary or acquired)
   - Extracorpuscular defect (acquired)

Morphological Classification of Anaemia

Based on the red cell size, haemoglobin content and red cell indices, anaemias are classified into:
1. **Microcytic hypochromic anaemia** (e.g. MCV, MCH, MCHC all are reduced). *Examples* include iron deficiency anaemia (Fig. 8.1A), sideroblastic anaemia, thalassemia.
2. **Macrocytic** (MCV is raised, MCH and MCHC are reduced relative to size of RBC). *Examples* include megaloblastic anaemia (folic acid and Vit. B_{12} deficiency.

3. **Normocytic normochromic** (e.g. MCV, MCH, MCHC are normal). Examples include anaemia of blood loss, haemolytic anaemia, aplastic anaemia, etc.
4. **Dimorphic.** When two populations of red cells (microcytes as well as macrocytes) are seen on peripheral blood examination, anaemia is said to be dimorphic due to combined deficiency of iron as well as folic acid/Vit. B_{12}.

The **symptoms and signs** of chronic severe anaemia are given in Box 8.1.

Box 8.1 Symptoms and Signs of Anaemia

Symptoms	Signs
1. General • Lassitude, fatigue	• Pallor of skin, mucous membrane, conjunctivae and creases of the palm
2. CVS • Chest pain (discomfort) • Exertional dyspnoea or dyspnoea at rest • Palpitation • Throbbing in head and ears • Precipitation of angina, intermittent claudication and vascular insufficiency	• Tachycardia and collapsing pulse • Raised JVP • Flow/haemic murmurs, e.g. midsystolic across the aortic and pulmonary valves • Cardiomegaly and congestive heart failure in chronic severe anaemia • Ankle oedema
3. CNS • Headache, dizziness, vertigo • Insomnia • Numbness and tingling of hands and feet	• Subacute combined degeneration (pyramidal and posterior column signs, i.e. ataxia) • Peripheral neuropathy
4. Genitourinary • Amenorrhea/menorrhagia, loss of libido	
5. GI tract • Abdominal pain • Anorexia, nausea, flatulence • Weight loss, diarrhoea • Dysphagia • Pica	• Mild hepatosplenomegaly

Symptom Analysis

Ask about the following

Q. Onset (acute or chronic).
- Acute onset of anaemia occurs following blood loss, haemolysis and leukaemias or lymphoma.
- Chronic anaemia occurs following poor nutrition, worm infestation, anaemia due to systemic diseases.

Q. Ask about the history of blood loss, i.e. through nose (epistaxis), through vomit (haematemesis), through urine (haematuria), through menses (menorrhagia) and after delivery (postpartum).
- Blood loss due to any cause can lead to anaemia

Q. Ask about history of loose motions, malabsorption and parasitic infestation.
- Malabsorption of nutrients and hookworm infestation can lead to anaemia

Q. Ask about the nutrition (diet) in details.
- Poor nutrition is a common cause of anaemia in India.

Q. Ask about history of drug intake.
- Drugs can lead to anaemia (read the causes of anaemia)

Q. Family history.
- Positive family history suggests possibility of haemolytic anaemia.

Q. History of repeated pregnancies and delivery.
- Repeated deliveries can result in anaemia.

Q. History of any renal, hepatic and musculoskeletal disorders.
- Chronic renal disease, chronic hepatic disease (cirrhosis of liver) and RA can lead to chronic anaemia.

Q. History of bleeding tendencies and bone pain.
- Hematological malignancies, i.e. leukaemia and multiple myeloma can lead to anaemia with bone pain.

Q. History of fever.
- Infections (malaria, typhoid, dengue, endocarditis) and SLE can lead to fever with anaemia)

Q. History of paraesthesia or weakness of limbs.
- Folic acid and Vit. B_{12} deficiency can lead to megaloblastic anaemia and neuropathy/subacute combined degeneration of spinal cord.

Q. Ask about specific symptoms of specific anaemia and look for their physical signs. Try to find out the cause(s) of anaemia.
- In a case of anaemia; one has to find out its cause. No single symptom and sign is diagnostic of a specific type of anaemia, but there may be specific findings related to the cause of anaemia, for example, a mass

in the abdomen such as in right iliac fossa may suggest caecal carcinoma. A patient having jaundice as well as anaemia is either due to cirrhotic portal hypertension with haematemesis or haemolytic anaemia. Anaemia with neurological signs such as peripheral neuropathy, dementia or subacute combined degeneration indicate vitamin B_{12} deficiency as its cause. Sickle cell anaemia may result in pain crises, and leg or digital ulceration.

- The specific symptoms and signs of various anaemias and their causes are briefed in Table 8.1.

Leucopenia and Neutropenia

The *leucopenia* refers to low leukocyte count (<4000/µl). *Neutropenia* means neutrophils count $<1.5 \times 10^9/L$. Virtual absence of granulocytes in peripheral blood is called *agranulocytosis*. The major consequence of neutropenia, leucopenia and agranulocytosis is infection, which in patients with blood disorders may be severe and lead to fatal septicaemia. Fever and pneumonia are common presentations.

Patients with neutropenia, leucopenia, agranulocytosis may develop opportunistic infections with unusual organisms such as fungi and viruses, i.e. *herpes zoster* and *herpes simplex* infections.

As a general rule; neutropenia or agranulocytosis is associated with bacterial infection while *lymphopenia* is associated with virus and other exotic infections, e.g. *Pneumocystis carinii* and *Toxoplasma*.

Causes of Neutropenia
1. Overwhelming infections, i.e. hepatitis, HIV, Gram-negative, septicaemia, chronic malaria, disseminated tuberculosis, Leishmania, etc.
2. Autoimmune diseases, i.e. Felty's syndrome, RA and SLE
3. Irradiation
4. Bone marrow suppression, i.e. pancytopenia
5. Drug induced
6. Idiopathic

Symptom Analysis
Ask about the following
Q. Onset of symptoms.
- Acute onset neutropenia is commonly drug induced (idiosyncratic) or induced by infections.

TABLE 8.1: Specific Symptoms and Signs of Various Anaemia and their Causes (Figs 8.1 and 8.2)

Specific symptoms and signs	Cause(s)
Iron deficiency anaemia	
• Glossitis with papillary atrophy (bald tongue) • Angular stomatitis (cheilosis)—fissuring at the angles with sore tongue • Dysphagia (Peterson-Kelly or Plummer-Vinson's syndrome) • Koilonychia or platynychia • Pica eating • Atrophic gastritis • Mild hepatosplenomegaly • Generalised pallor	• More prevalent in women and children • Common in agricultural workers • Strict vegetarian diet • Diarrhoea or malabsorption, gastrectomy • Chronic blood loss from *uterus* (menorrhagia, dysfunctional uterine bleeding), GI tract (e.g. NSAIDs, bleeding peptic ulcer, piles, varices, gastritis, colitis and hookworm disease), *renal* (e.g. haematuria), *nose* (epistaxis), *lungs* (haemoptysis) • Increased demands, e.g. growing children, pregnancy, lactation

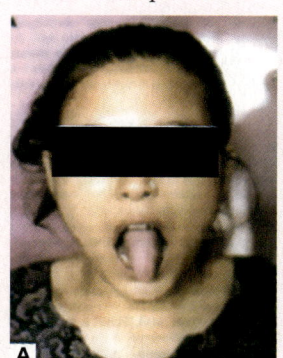
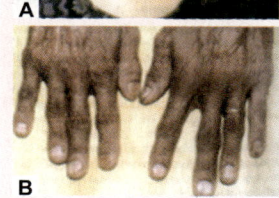

Figs 8.1A and B: A patient with iron deficiency anaemia and koilonychia.

II. Megaloblastic anaemias

• Mild jaundice • A lemon yellow tinge to skin, grey hair • Red-smooth (magenta coloured) sore tongue • Tinglings and paraesthesias • Weight loss • An abnormal gait • Mild hepatosplenomegaly • Skin pigmentation	• Inadequate dietary intake (vegetarian diet) • Malabsorption (diarrhoea) • Autoimmune gastritis resulting in loss of intrinsic factor • Previous surgery (gastrectomy)

Contd.

Contd.

Specific symptoms and signs	Cause(s)
• Mental features, e.g. poor memory, lack of concentration, depression, personality change and hallucinations	
• Optic atrophy and subacute combined degeneration	
• Neurological manifestation, e.g. spastic paraplegia due to folate deficiency	
III. Hemolytic anaemias	
• Mild jaundice	• Increased demand (pregnancy)
	• Poor intake (diet lacking in green vegetables)
• Dark-coloured urine and stool, e.g. smoky urine due to haemoglobinuria, or frank bloody or even black urine (black-water fever)	• Infection
	• Haemolytic anaemia due to any cause
	• Malabsorption
• Abnormal facies with frontal bossing (Fig. 18.3A)	• Congenital or hereditary defect
• Skin ulceration of legs or gangrenous toes or dactylitis (sickle cell anaemia)	• (spherocytosis, thalassaemia (Fig. 18.3), G6PD deficiency)
• Hepatosplenomegaly	• Drug induced (e.g. analgesics, anti-malarial, antibiotics)
• Pigmented gallstones (biliary colics)	• Autoimmune
	• Infections (malaria)
IV. Aplastic anaemia	
• Neutropenia results in infections, necrotic mouth ulcerations, throat ulcers	• Irradiation
	• Drugs
	• Chemicals
• Thrombocytopenia results in bleeding in skin, mucous membrane, epistaxis, haematuria or intracranial bleed	• Infection
	• Autoimmune disease
• Symptoms and signs of anaemia	

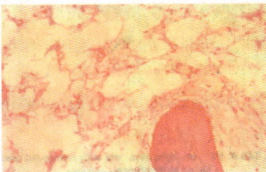

Fig. 8.2: Hypoplastic anaemia. Bone marrow examination reveals just fat and fibrosis with no cellular element.

Q. History of fever.
- Neutropenia with fever indicates underlying or superadded infection.
- Neutropenia can be associated with fever in patients with Felty's syndrome, SLE and RA.

Q. History of sore throat, mouth ulceration.
- Necrotic mouth ulcers and sore throat are common clinical presentation of neutropenia/agranulocytosis (Fig. 8.3) as these patients are predisposed to infections.

Q. History of drug intake.
- Antibiotics (chloramphenicol, sulpha group, cytotoxics, antidiabetic, antithyroid, analgesic, anti-rheumatoid arthritis drugs (DMARDs), insecticides, etc. can lead to it (read causes).

Q. Is there any bleeding manifestations
- Bleeding manifestation, infections, severe, anaemia, neutropaenia indicate bone marrow suppression.

Q. Is there any systemic illness
- SLE, RA, chronic disease can result in agranulocytosis.

Q. Is neutropaenia cyclic?
- Neutropenia can be cyclic, i.e. occur after 2–4 weeks. It is mild in nature.

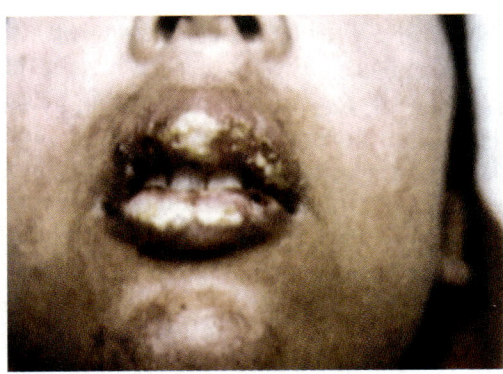

Fig. 8.3: A patient of agranulocytosis induced by drug; developed severe infection of the oral cavity with difficulty in swallowing and opening the mouth. Note redness, swelling and excoriation of lips and mucous membrane of oral cavity.

Leucocytosis and Leukaemoid Reaction

An increase in total leucocyte count more than 11,000/dl is called *leucocytosis*. This is usually due to an increase in a specific type of WBC, i.e. neutrophils, basophils, eosinophils, monocytes or lymphocytes. Sometime an increase in one type of leucocyte may not cause rise in total leucocyte count.

Neutrophilia or *neutrophilic leucocytosis* is a normal response to infection or injury and is often associated with symptoms of the disorder which have led to it. The *causes* of neutrophilic leucocytosis are:
1. Acute bacterial infection.

2. Drug and chemical intoxication.
3. Inflammatory diseases.
4. Metabolic diseases, e.g. diabetic ketoacidosis, uraemia, etc.
5. Acute haemorrhage.
6. Acute haemolysis.
7. Disseminated malignancies.
8. Myeloproliferative disorders (leukaemia, polycythaemia).
9. Following corticosteroid administration.

Symptoms and signs: The symptoms and signs depend on the cause, for example, a patient with neutrophilic leucocytosis with pneumonia will have fever, shaking chills, cough, sputum, haemoptysis, etc.; while a patient with infectious mononucleosis will have fever, malaise, sore throat, lymphadenopathy and lymphocytosis.

Eosinophilic leucocytosis (eosinophilia): It is seen in tropical eosinophilia, asthma, helminthic infections, Löeffler's syndrome, allergic disorders, eosinophilic leukaemia and hypereosinophilic syndrome.

Leukaemoid reaction: Leucocytosis with cell count of 10,000 to 25,000/μl occurs in response to infection and acute inflammation and results from release of mature WBCs. Leucocytosis with cell count of "30,000 to 50,000/μl and presence of immature cells in the PBF is called *leukaemoid reaction*, which is differentiated from leucocytosis. The differentiation between the two is given in Box 8.2. The difference between leukaemia and leukaemoid reaction is given in Box 8.3.

The leukaemoid reaction may be *myeloid* or *lymphoid*. The **causes** are:

I. Myeloid reaction
- Pneumonia, meningitis, diphtheria, pyogenic liver abscess, tumour with bone metastases
- Severe haemolysis or haemorrhage

II. Lymphoid reaction
- Disseminated tuberculosis, pertussis, infectious hepatitis, infectious mononucleosis.

Box 8.2 Leucocytosis vs Leukaemoid Reaction

Leucocytosis	Leukaemoid reaction
Cell count lies between 10,000 and 25,000/μl	Cell count is >25,000/μl
Mature cells are present in peripheral circulation	Immature cells are also present in addition to mature cells
Depending on the presence of mature cells, it can be neutrophilic, eosinophilic lymphocytic, basophilic, etc.	It is either myeloid or lymphoid due to presence of immature cells

Box 8.3 Differentiation between Leukaemoid Reaction and Leukaemia

Leukaemoid reaction	Leukaemia
• Count is between 30,000 and 50,000 cells/ml	• Count is >50,000 cells/ml
• Mostly mature cells. Immature cell may be present but are <25%	• Immature cells are present in all forms and account >30% of all cells
• Leucocyte alkaline phosphatase content is normal or increased.	• It is low

Leucoerythroblastic Anaemia
It is defined as anaemia with appearance of nucleated red cells and WBC precursors in peripheral blood.

Causes
Marrow infiltration with metastatic carcinoma, myelofibrosis, osteopetrosis, myeloma, lymphoma and occasionally severe haemolytic or megaloblastic anaemia are its causes.

Lymphocytosis and Leukaemias
(read bedside medicine by Prof SN Chugh)

Lymphocytosis refers to increase in lymphocyte count more than normal, occurs in infections, i.e. pertussis, infectious mononucleosis, infective hepatitis, tuberculosis, brucellosis, CLL and lymphoma.

Leukaemias, lymphoma and myeloma are malignant disorders of myeloproliferative and lymphoproliferative system. *Leukaemias* are a heterogenous group of diseases characterised by malignant proliferation or apoptosis of the blood cells resulting in infiltration into the blood, bone marrow and other tissues. If mature differentiated cells are involved, they will have a low growth rate and produce indolent neoplasms such as low grade lymphoma or chronic leukaemia. The differentiation between acute and chronic leukaemia is summarised in Table 8.2.

Symptoms and Signs of Leukaemias (Table 8.2)

Symptom Analysis

Ask about the following

Q. Age and sex of onset.
- Acute leukaemia occurs in younger age while chronic leukaemia occurs in middle (myeloid leukaemia) and old age (lymphatic leukaemia).

TABLE 8.2: Differentiation between Acute and Chronic Leukaemias

Acute leukaemia	Chronic leukaemia
Acute onset	Subacute or chronic onset
Involves young age	Middle or old age
Cell count varies in thousands from 50,000 onwards.	Cell count is very high, i.e. one lac onwards
Mostly immature blast cells (>25%), involves pleuropotential stem cells	Mostly mature differentiated cells (myelocytes, metamyelocytes and promyelocytes)
Rapid growth rate	Low growth rate
The *clinical features* include: Fever, bleeding, lymphadenopathy, splenomegaly and acute infections. Bone pain and tenderness, gum hypertrophy and DIC also occur.	The *clinical features* include: Massive splenomegaly, lymphadenopathy, tissue infiltration, symptoms and signs of anaemia. Bone tenderness may or may not be present
Poor response to treatment, hence, prognosis is a few months to 2 years	Response to treatment is good, prognosis is better than acute; varies from a few years to many years

- Acute leukaemias are common in males while chronic myeloid leukaemia is common in females.

Q. Is there any dragging pain?
- Dragging pain in the abdomen occurs in CML due to massive splenomegaly.

Q. History of bruising/bleeding.
- This is common in both acute and chronic leukaemias.

Q. Is there any history of breathlessness, fatigue, palpitation, weakness, etc.
- Breathlessness on exertion, fatigue, palpitations, weakness and signs of anaemia are usually present in leukaemia.

Q. Is there any history of fever, night sweats, tachycardia?
- Fever, night sweats, tachycardia indicate an infection which is common in leukaemias.

Q. Is there history of multiple swellings at other sites?
- Multiple swellings (lymphadenopathy) in neck, axillae and groin are common in chronic lymphatic leukaemia (CLL).

Myelomatosis

Definition: Multiple myeloma represents a malignant proliferation of plasma cells derived from a single clone, is characterised by the presence of a paraprotein (*an immunoglobulin*) in the serum which can be demonstrated by monoclonal dark-staining band on protein electrophoresis.

Clinical Features (Table 8.3)

It is common in old age. These patients usually present with anaemia, bone pain, tiredness, weakness, headache, blurring of vision and symptoms and signs of renal failure.

TABLE 8.3: Symptoms and Signs of Myelomatosis

Symptoms and signs	Underlying cause
• Bone pain	• Bone erosion
• Severe local pain	• Pathological fractures
• Thirst, lethargy, polyuria, weakness, depression, confusion	• Hypercalcaemia
• Tiredness, weakness	• Bone marrow failure
• Asymptomatic or symptomatic uraemia	• Renal damage
• When severe, produces blurred vision, headache, vertigo, stupor and coma	• Hyperviscosity
• Susceptibility to infection especially respiratory and urinary	• Immunodeficiency

Symptom Analysis

Ask about the following

Q. Age of the patient.
- Multiple myeloma occurs commonly in old age.

Q. History of bone pain and fractures.
- Bone pain and fractures (pathological) are common due to lytic bone lesions and weakened bones.

Q. History of lethargy, polyuria, polydipsia and weakness.
- Hypercalcaemia in multiple myeloma can lead to these symptoms.

Q. History of UTI and symptoms of uraemia.
- Renal involvements in multiple myeloma can lead UTI and uraemia.

Q. History of headache, vertigo and blurred vision.
- They are common in multiple myelma due to vascular occlusion by hyperviscosity of blood.

Q. History of repeated chest infections.
- Due to lowered immunity, repeated chest infections are common.

Polycythaemia (High Haemoglobin and PCV)

A haemoglobin level greater than upper limit of the normal (adult females 16.5 g/dl, adult males 18 g/dl) may be due to an increase in the number of red blood cells (*true polycythaemia*) or a reduction in the plasma volume due to dehydration, diuretic use or alcohol consumption (*relative or apparent polycythaemia*). True or primary polycythaemia (*polycythaemia rubra vera*) is defined as a myeloproliferative disorder involving the RBCs in the bone marrow. Polycythaemia may be secondary to *increased erythropoietin production* either as a consequence of chronic hypoxaemia (COPD, congenital heart disease), or because of *inappropriate erythropoietin secretion*, e.g. lung, renal tumours, etc.

Symptoms and Signs
1. Polycythaemia in the early stages may go unnoticed due to no symptoms. Relatives and friends may be the first to notice the red complexion or plethora of face due to polycythaemia.
2. The patient may complain of headache, tinnitus, a feeling of fullness in the head (hyperviscosity).
3. The patients are more at risk of developing heart attack, stroke and peripheral vascular disease due to thrombotic episodes.
4. In true polycythaemia, the patient, in addition to above features, have pruritus (itching) especially while taking a hot bath, gout and hepatosplenomegaly.

Smptom Analysis
Q. Does patient complain of headache, tinnitus, vertigo, fullness of head?
- These complaints may suggest polycythaemia.

Q. History of smoking.
- Smoking for prolonged period may result in COPD (hypoxaemia) and secondary polycythaemia.

Q. Does the patient has COPD or congenital heart disease?
- COPD and cyanotic congenital heart diseases produce secondary polycythaemia.

Q. Is there history of plethoric face and pruritus?
- Red face with pruritus indicates true polycythaemia.

Bleeding

Bleeding usually results from a breach of the vessel wall due to specific insult (e.g. trauma, peptic ulcer) or from haemostatic failure. The **haemostasis** is a complex process, involves interactions between vessel well, platelets and coagulation factors. Haemostatic failure may be *primary* (e.g. due to vessel wall abnormalities, qualitative or quantitative disorders of platelets) or *secondary* (a coagulation defect). Thus, bleeding may result from deficiency of one or more of the coagulation factors, thromboasthenia, thrombocytopenia or occasionally from excessive fibrinolysis which most often arises following therapeutic fibrinolytic therapy with streptokinase or with tissue plasminogen activator (tPA). Differences between primary (Fig. 8.4) and secondary (Fig. 8.5) hemostatic failure are given in Table 8.4.

Types of Bleeding
1. **Superficial,** i.e. purpura, bruises, petechiae, ecchymosis.
2. **Deep bleeding,** i.e. into joints (haemarthrosis) into the muscles (haematomas).

Symptom Analysis
Ask about the following

Q. **Age and sex.**
- Haemophilia is common in younger males while ITP is common in younger females.

Q. **Is bleeding spontaneous or occurs following minor trauma?**
- Spontaneous bruising or following minor trauma resembling devil's pinches in an old person (Fig. 8.6) indicate senile purpura; while in a younger patient indicates coagulation defect.
- Spontaneous bleeding following dental extraction or child birth also indicate hemostatic defect.

Q. **What is the site of bleeding?**
- Muscle or joint bleeding (haemarthrosis) indicates a coagulation defect.
- Purpura, epistaxis, prolonged bleeding from superficial cuts, GI bleed, menorrhagia suggest primary haemostatic failure due to a platelet defect, thrombocytopenia, von Willebrand's disease.
- Recurrent bleeding at a single site suggest a local structural abnormality (hereditary haemorrhagic telangiectasia, i.e. Osler-Weber-Rendu disease (Fig. 8.7).

Q. **What is the duration of history of bleeding?**
- A long history of bleeding episodes indicate a congenital disorder. Certain congenital conditions, such as haemophilia usually becomes obvious in early childhood but milder bleeding episodes may go undetected for long time even up to old age.

Q. **Is there any precipitating factor?**
- Trauma precipitate bleeding in haemostatic defect.

TABLE 8.4: Differentiating Features Between Primary and Secondary Haemostatic Defect

Defects of primary haemostasis (platelet defect, Fig. 8.4)	Defects of secondary haemostasis (Fig. 8.5)
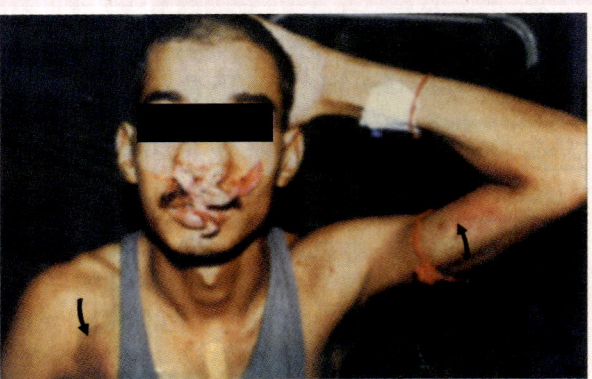	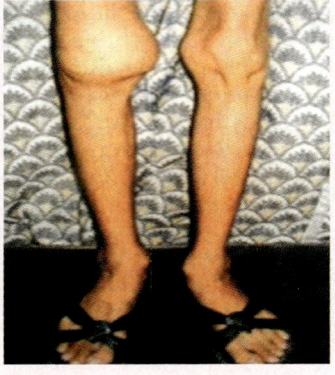
Fig. 8.4: Thrombocytopenic purpura. Epistaxis is present. Nasal packing is visible. There is an ecchymotic patch over the left forearm (↑) and another on right upper chest (↓).	**Fig. 8.5:** Haemarthrosis following trivial trauma in young haemophilic.
• Immediate bleeding following trauma	• Bleeding delayed for hours or days
• Superficial bleeding, e.g. skin, mucous membrane, nose, GI tract and genitourinary tract	• Deep bleeding into joints, muscles, retroperitoneal space, etc.
• More common in females	• 80–90% are males.
Physical signs	
• Purpura—collection of blood in the skin	• Haematomas into muscles
• Patechiae—pinpoint haemorrhages into dermis and ecchymosis—large subcutaneous collection of blood (Fig. 8.8)	• Haemarthrosis (joint swollen, tender due to bleed) as well as petechiae and ecchymosis
• Autosomal dominant	• Autosomal or X-linked recessive
• Immediate, local measures (local pressure) are effective in stopping the bleeding	• Requires sustained systemic therapy (coagulation factors)

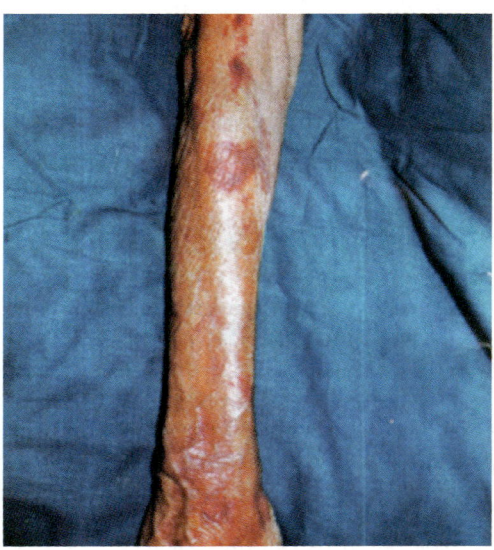

Fig. 8.6: Senile purpura. (Note the bruising resembling devil's pinches.)

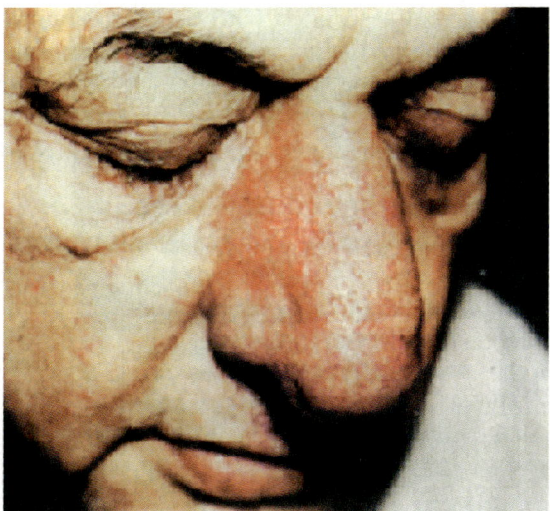

Fig. 8.7: Osler-Weber-Rendu disease. Note the multiple telangiectasis as red spots due to capillary dilatation. This is also called hereditary haemorrhagic telangiectasia.

Haematological Disorders

- Drugs can precipitate bleeding (read causes of purpura).

Q. Is bleeding occurring from multiple sites?
- Bleeding from two or more than two sites, i.e. nose, skin, urine, stool, mouth or genital tract suggest disseminated intravascular coagulation (Fig. 8.8).

Q. Enquire about all the operations and time of bleeding after surgery specifically dental extraction, tonsillectomy and circumcision as these are all stressful tests of haemostatic system.
- Bleeding that starts immediately after surgery indicates defective platelet plug formation; whereas that comes on after several hours indicates failure of platelet plug stabilisation by fibrin due to a coagulation defect.

Q. Is there any other family member suffering from blood disorder?
- A family history of bleeding may indicate both bleeding or coagulation disorder, hence, interview the relatives, if necessary.

Q. Does the patient suffer from a systemic disorder?
- Bleeding from multiple sites following trauma or surgery suggests a systemic disorder, i.e. hepatic, or renal failure, paraproteinaemia or a connective tissue disorder, snakebite (Fig. 8.8).

Q. Ask about full drug history, i.e. drugs taken in the past or being taken.

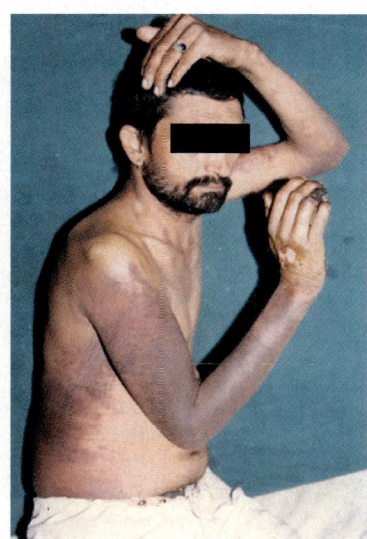

Fig. 8.8: Disseminated intravascular coagulation due to snakebite. Note the large ecchymotic patches over forearm and side of chest.

- Drugs can produce bleeding either by depressing bone marrow function with consequent thrombocytopenia or by interacting with coagulation factors (warfarin, NSAIDs inhibit platelet function).

Q. Ask about the occupation.
- Contact with dangerous chemicals may produce thrombocytopenia.

Physical Signs

Examination of bleeding site can differentiate platelet defect (primary haemostatic defect) from haemostatic defect (secondary haemostatic failure) as shown in Table 8.4.

Thrombosis/Thrombophilia

It is defined as an accelerated tendency for arterial and venous thrombosis with and without thromboembolic complications. The condition may be *inherited* (i.e. deficiency of protein C and protein S, factor V Leiden abnormality, anti-thrombin III deficiency and prothrombin mutation) or *acquired* due to antiphospholipid syndrome, 2–4 fold increase in coagulation factors, hyperhomocysteinemia and pregnancy.

N.B. Young patients with recurrent arterial and venous thrombosis must be screened for thrombophilia/antiphospholipid syndrome.

Arterial and venous thrombosis (deep vein thrombosis) may be presenting features of hypercoagulable or prethrombotic state. The thrombotic disorders are:

I. Inherited
A. *Defective inhibitors of coagulation factors/thrombophlilic conditions*
  - Antithrombin III deficiency, antiphospholipid antibodies.
  - Protein S and C deficiency, factor V Leiden deficiency.
B. *Impaired clot lysis*
  - Dysfibrinogenaemia, plasminogen deficiency and/or tPA deficiency.

II. Acquired
- SLE (lupus anticoagulant), malignancy, myeloproliferative disorders, thrombotic thrombocytopenic purpura, oestrogen treatment, hyperlipidaemia, diabetes, hyperviscosity, nephrotic syndrome, CHF.

III. Uncertain
- Homocystinuria.
- Paroxysmal nocturnal haemoglobinuria.
- Physiological states.

- Pregnancy, postpartum.
- Obesity, old age.
- Postoperative.
- Immobilisation.

> Thrombophilic conditions (proteins C and S deficiency, antithrombin III deficiency, antiphospholipid syndrome and factor V abnormalities have predilection for thrombosis (venous and arterial) and foetal loss.

Pancytopenia/Myelodysplastic Syndromes

Pancytopenia refers to the combination of *anaemia, leucopenia* and *thrombocytopenia*.

Pancytopenia with hypocellular or acellular marrow: It is due to reduced production of blood cells as a consequence of bone marrow suppression or infiltration. Common cause is aplastic anaemia.

Pancytopenia with hypercellular marrow: It is due to peripheral destruction or splenic sequestration of mature cells, seen in hypersplenism.

Myelodysplastic syndrome includes heterogenous group of diseases characterised by pancytopenia, hypercellular marrow with dysplastic changes in the RBC, WBC and platelets. Common diseases include mostly refractory anaemias, sideroblastic anaemias and some leukaemia.

Both *primary* (*idiopathic*) and *secondary* (*therapy induced*) myelodysplastic syndromes present with pancytopenia.

Lymphadenopathy (Read it in Unit I also)

Lymph node enlargement is called lymphadenopathy. It is usually symptomatic, but may be asymptomatic and an incidental finding. Infection or inflammation of lymph node is called *lymphadenitis*.

Symptoms of Lymph Nodes Enlargement

1. *Acute lymphadenopathy* may present with acute onset of fever, pains, sore throat, cough, indicates infection or inflammation as the cause.
2. *Superficial lymphadenopathy* presents with visible or palpable mass or masses in cervical, axillary or inguinal regions. This may present as a discharging sinus or sinuses in these regions.
3. *Nonsuperficial presentations* (thoracic or abdominal) of lymphadenopathy are:
   - May be detected on routine chest X-ray or during work up of superficial lymphadenopathy.
   - May present as a lump or lumps in the abdomen (mesenteric or para-aortic).
   - May present with pressure symptoms:
     – Cough and wheezing from airway obstruction.
     – Hoarseness and bovine cough from recurrent laryngeal nerve involvement.
     – Dysphagia from oesophageal compression.
     – Swelling of neck, face or arms due to compression of superior *vena cava* or subclavian vein
     – Paraplegia from spinal cord compression.

Symptom Analysis

Q. Is mass localised or generalised?
Localised lymphadenopathy is common with local acute and chronic infections (viral, bacterial) and metastases (secondaries).
Generalised lymphadenopathy indicate leukaemias, lymphomas, systemic infections, etc.

Q. Ask about age and sex.
- In children and young adults, the lymphadenopathy could be due to leukaemia, lymphoma and infections.

Q. Ask about occupation.
- Certain occupation or occupational diseases can lead to lymphadenopathy.

Q. History of extramarital relation.
- HIV is a common cause of lymphodenopathy. Syphilis and lymphogranuloma venereum—sexual transmitted diseases can lead to localised lymphadonopathy.

Q. History of associated symptoms.
- Associated fever indicates infection while fever, sweats, fatigue suggest tuberculosis.
- Anorexia, anaemia, fatigue, cachexia indicate internal malignancy, leukaemia, lymphoma.

Physical Examination for Evaluation
- Look for the site and size of lymph nodes, texture, presence or absence of tenderness, signs of inflammation over the node, skin lesions (petechiae, purpura) and splenomegaly.
- A thorough ear, nose and throat (ENT) check up.

Splenomegaly or Hepatosplenomegaly in Haematology

The spleen is a lymphoreticular organ, is capable of assisting the host in adapting to its hostile environment. It discharges following functions:
- Clearance of bacteria and particulates from the blood.
- The generation of immune response to certain invading pathogens.
- Reticuloendothelial activity (destruction of RBCs and other formed elements).

- Extramedullary erythropoiesis when the marrow is unable to meet the needs (e.g. myeloproliferative disorders). This is a recapitulation of the blood forming function the spleen performs during gestation. The spleen gets enlarged when its normal functions are exaggerated. **Causes** of enlargement of spleen have been discussed in the end under brief synopsis of blood disorders.

Symptoms Related do Splenomegaly or Hepatosplenomegaly

- Abdominal pain, left hypochondriac tenderness
- Lower chest pain or discomfort left lower chest
- Dragging pain due to large mass of spleen (massive splenomegaly)
- Symptoms and signs of anaemia or pancytopenia (hypersplenism)
- Symptoms and signs of hemolytic anaemia, i.e. jaundice, dark urine and dark stools.
- Symptoms and signs of underlying disease or cause of splenomegaly, i.e. anaemia, infection, SABE, leukaemias, lymphoma, ITP, Felty syndrome, myelodysplastic syndrome (read the causes of splenomegaly)
- Bilateral abdominal lumps producing pain due to hepatosplenomegaly.

Symptom Analysis

Ask about the following

Q. Abdominal discomfort and dragging sensation due to a mass itself.

Acute enlargement of spleen may produce pain due to stretching of its capsule.

Q. Ask about abdominal colicky pain/back pain.
- Back pain and abdominal bloating due to stomach compression.
- Severe abdominal colicky pain radiating to the left shoulder tip, associated with splenic rub due to splenic infarct (perisplenitis), commonly seen in myeloproliferative disorders and sickle cell anaemia.

Q. History of abdominal trauma.
- Rupture of the spleen, either from trauma or infiltrative disease that breaks the capsule, may result in intraperitoneal bleeding, shock and death. The rupture itself may be painless.

HISTORY

Present History

Ask about onset of symptoms, progression, blood loss, intestinal symptoms

- Iron deficiency anaemia is the most common type of anaemia worldwide. A thorough gastrointestinal history (anorexia, diarrhoea, worm infestation/haematemesis, malena, piles) must be recorded. History of ulcerating lesions in GI tract (peptic ulcer), gastric and colonic cancer, ulcerative colitis must be asked. Menorrhagia is a common cause of anaemia in females still menstruating, hence, a women must be asked about her periods. Ask about symptoms of leukaemias, lymphoma, bleeding and coagulation defect. Do the symptom analysis as discussed in the beginning of unit.

Past Medical History

Ask about
- Past history of diarrhoea, worm infection (roundworm, hookworm)
- History of walking bare-footed (hookworm) must be asked.
- Previous surgery (resection of the stomach or small bowel).
- Past history of any blood loss, e.g. piles, haematemesis, menorrhagia, epistaxis, PPH pregnacies, etc.
- Past history of drugs taken
- Any history of infection (e.g. tuberculosis, malaria) or hookworm infestation (chronic diarrhoea)
- Past history of chronic systemic illness, e.g. liver or kidney disease or rheumatoid arthritis, endocrinal problem.

Family History

Ask about anaemia in other family members. Ask about family history of haemophilia, Christmas disease, Glenzmann thromboasthenia and von Willebrand disease.

Haemolytic anaemias such as the haemoglobinopathies, thalassaemia, hereditary haemorrhagic telangiectasia and hereditary spherocytosis may be suspected from the family history. Pernicious anaemia may also be familial.

Drug History

Ask about the drugs being taken or have been taken as the drugs are known to cause blood loss (aspirin, NSAIDs), haemolysis (antimalarial in G6PD deficiency) or hypoplasia or aplasia of the bone marrow (chloramphenicol, arsenicals, anticancer, gold salt) and bleeding, i.e. antiplatelets and anticoagulants.

Dietary History

Full dietary history include whether person is vegetarian/nonvegetarian, intake of dietary articles rich in iron and folate (liver, meat, green vegetables, fruits), rich in B$_{12}$ (liver, meat and animal products) and Vit. C (rich source is citrus fruits).

A history must assess the intake of iron and folate which may become deficient in comparison to needs (e.g. in pregnancy, lactation, during periods of growth). Malnutrition due to diarrhoea and malabsorption may result in anaemia.

Menstrual History

Full menstrual history and amount of blood loss during each menstruation must be asked. History of repeated child birth may be recorded.

EXAMINATION OF A PATIENT WITH HAEMATOLOGICAL DISORDER

General Physical Examination

1. General Appearance

☞ *Look at the face for any abnormality*
- *Pale looking*—anaemia.
- *Plethoric face*—polycythaemia.
- *Mongoloid face,* frontal bossing, 'Hair on end' appearance—thalassaemia.
- *Emaciation*—anaemia, malnutrition, malignancy.
- *Puffy face*—hypoproteinaemia.

2. Conjunctivae

☞ *Look for pallor and jaundice*
- Pale conjunctivae suggest anaemia.
- Suffused conjunctivae are seen in polycythaemia or mediastinal compression.
- Jaundice indicates hemolytic anaemia or uncompensated cirrhosis as a cause of anaemia.

3. The Mouth

☞ *Look for glossitis and angular stomatitis.*

- Cracking of the skin at the corner of the mouth (angular cheilosis) glossitis (bald tongue) are due to iron deficiency anaemia.
- Necrotic mouth ulcers indicate neutropenia or aplastic anaemia or leukaemia.
- Red fiery tongue (magenta colour tongue) indicate vit. B$_{12}$ deficiency.

☞ *Look at the tongue and oral mucosa for any abnormality (Table 8.5).*

☞ *Inspect the lips for vesicles, ulceration, cyanosis, etc.*

TABLE 8.5: Oral Manifestations of Haematological Disorders

Oral lesion	Disease
• Gingival hypertrophy, gum bleeding, necrosis, petechiae and ulceration of oral mucosa	• All types of leukaemias especially acute monocytic type (Fig. 8.9)
• Multiple petechiae and ecchymosis	• Thrombocytopenias due to any cause
• Wide spread ulceration involving gums, buccal mucosa, tongue, pharynx, larynx, palate	• Agranulocytosis, leucopenia (neutropenia, Fig. 8.3)
• Atrophic papillae with red smooth sore tongue	• Iron deficiency combined with Vit. B complex deficiency
• Reddening of oral mucosa and tongue (magenta-coloured) with or without ulceration, swelling	• Vitamin B complex deficiency
• Petechiae in oral mucosa and swollen bleeding gums	• Scurvy
• Bald tongue (atrophy or loss of papillae)	• Pernicious anaemia, iron deficiency (Fig. 8.1) and pellagra
• Cyanosis of lips and tongue	• Methaemoglobinaemia
• White patches (mouth thrush)	• Oral candidiasis

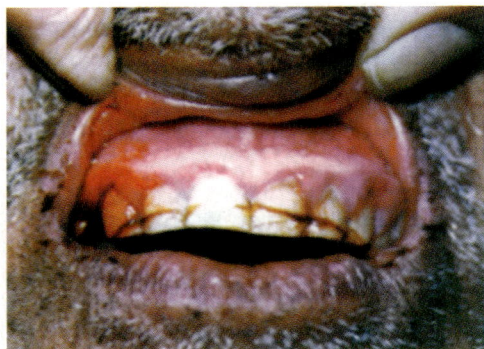

Fig. 8.9: Bleeding gums in a patient with acute leukaemia.

Cold sores (vesiculation of the lips) is seen in herpes simplex infection which is associated with certain blood disorders.

4. Legs/Feet

☞ *Look for oedema and necrotic ulcers (sickle cell anaemia)*

- Oedema may be present in anaemia due to any cause
- Necrotic ulcers are seen in sickles cell anaemia, vasculitis.

5. The Skin

☞ *Look for evidence of infection/ulceration/swelling*
- The skin surface may be infected, ulcerated or infiltrated by tumour (leukaemia, lymphoma).

☞ *Look at the skin and subcutaneous tissue for bleeding.*
The bleeding points are classified as follows:
  i. *Purpura, i.e. [(purpuric spot are 2–5 mm in diameter) (Fig. 8.10)] and petechial haemorrhages (haemorrhagic spots <1 mm)* are tiny pinpoint haemorrhages into the skin which do not blanch on compression with a glass slide.
  ii. *Ecchymotic patches* (Fig. 8.8) are larger haemorrhages than petechiae. They are ≥5 mm in diameter.
  iii. *Bruises* are larger areas of haemorrhages resulting as a result of confluent deposition of blood, often multicoloured in appearance as the bruise resolves.

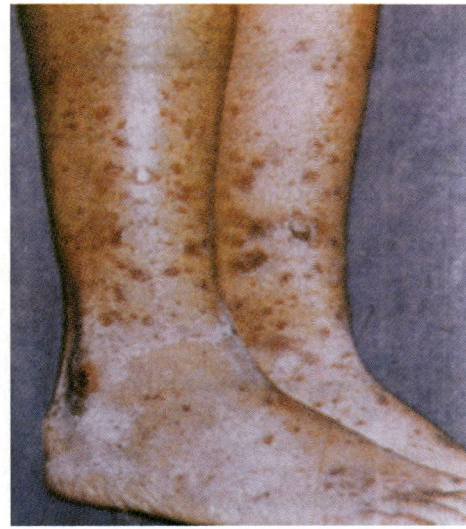

Fig. 8.10: Large purpuric spots in Henoch-Schönlein purpura.

Purpuric spots, petechial haemorrhages, ecchymotic patches and bruises indicate a bleeding disorder due to platelet dysfunction.
Bruises if large, extensive with an obvious firm haematoma beneath them, may indicate a coagulation defect.

  iv. *Telangiectasias* (Fig. 8.7) are small dilated blood vessels which may be visible on the skin surface particularly the lips. They blanch on pressure.
  v. *Vasculitis*: Skin lesions in vasculitis may be in the form of a rash (papulovesicular) or palpable purpura, ulcers or subcutaneous nodules. Henoch-Schönlein purpura (Fig. 8.10) is also a form of vasculitis.

Telangiectasia and vasculitis are not blood disorders, indicate vessel wall abnormalities but are important because sometimes they may be a source of severe haemorrhage.

☞ *Note the colour of the skin, pigmentation and depigmentation, pruritus.*

- Bright red skin (Phomme rouge) may be seen in dermatitis, sometimes associated with lymphoma.
- Dusky pigmentation (deposition of iron and melanin) is seen in hemochromatosis and hemosiderosis (haematoma).
- Patchy depigmentation (vitiligo) is a feature of pernicious anaemia but often has no clinical significance.
- Pruritus occurs in lymphoma, polycythaemia and mycosis fungoides.

☞ *Look for infiltrating skin lesions.*
- Infiltration into the skin occurs in leukaemia and lymphoma.

5. Ocular Fundi

☞ *Look at the ocular fundi for haemorrhages*
Fundal haemorrhages are often visible in:
- Thrombocytopenia, leukaemia
- Hyperviscosity syndrome due to macroglobulinaemia and promyelocytic leukaemia. Papilloedema may also be present.

6. The Muscle and Joints

☞ *Examine the muscles and joints for swelling and tenderness.*

Bleeding into the muscles (intramuscular haematoma) or in between muscles and into the joints (haemarthrosis, Fig. 8.5) indicate a coagulation disorder. The muscles and joints involved are swollen, hot and tender.

7. The Lymph Nodes Examination

Inspection and Palpation

☞ *The lymph nodes in a patient suspected of a lymphoreticular disorder must be examined as a whole not in* isolation. Note the following points on the lymph node examination

i. Size and the group involved (location).
ii. Consistency (soft, firm, hard, rubbery).
iii. Are they discrete or matted or confluent?
iv. Are they mobile or fixed to the underlying or overlying structure?
v. Are they tender or nontender?

Under normal conditions in adults, the inguinal lymph nodes may be palpable up to, 0.5 to 2.0 cm in size, hence, large lymph nodes >2 cm in diameter are considered as abnormal. Smaller lymph nodes elsewhere may be palpable due to past infection. Therefore, new lymph nodes enlargement more than 1 cm in size anywhere except in inguinal region is considered as abnormal and needs further evaluation.

Method of palpation of different groups of lymph nodes

1. *Preauricular* (Fig. 8.11): Using the pads of the 2nd and 3rd fingers, palpate the preauricular nodes with a gentle rotatory motion in front of the ear.
2. *Posterior auricular and occipital lymph nodes.* Palpate them in similar manner as described above by standing in front or behind the patient. Palpate them behind the ear.
3. *Cervical lymph nodes:* Examine the cervical lymph nodes with the patient sitting. Palpate the anterior cervical chain, located anterior and superficial to the sternomastoid. Standing in front of or behind the patient palpate the submental (in the midline below the mandible), submandibular glands (Fig. 8.12) and supraclavicular (Fig. 8.13) and scalene node behind the middle of clavicle (Fig. 8.14). (Read Clinical Methods in Medicines by Dr. S.N. Chugh for their examination.)
4. *Axillary lymph nodes:* Sit or stand in front of the patient, supporting the arm on the side under examination. Palpate the left axilla with right hand and *vice versa* (Fig. 8.15). Insert the finger tips into the vault of the axilla and then roll them downwards while palpating the medial, anterior and posterior axillary wall in turn.
5. *Epitrochlear lymph node:* Support the patient's left wrist with the right hand and grasp the partially flexed elbow with the left hand and use the thumb to feel for the epitrochlear lymph node.
6. *Inguinal lymph nodes:* Let the patient lie down for examination of inguinal and popliteal lymph nodes.

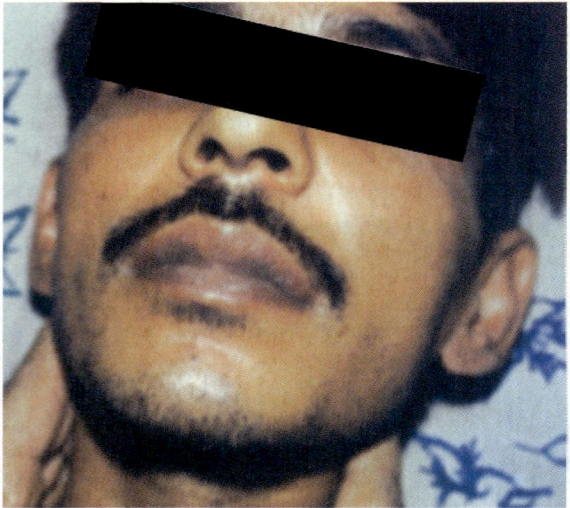

Fig. 8.12: Palpation of submandibular lymph nodes.

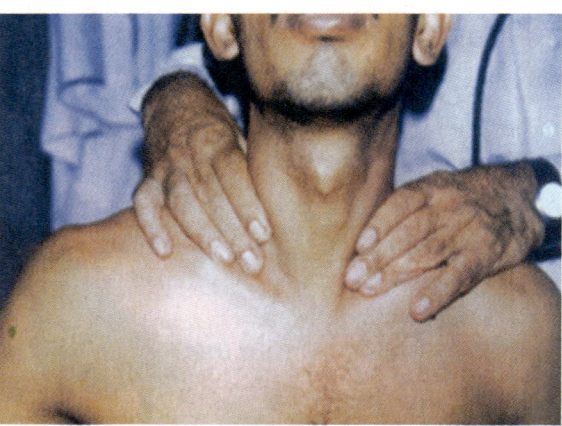

Fig. 8.13: Palpation of supraclavicular lymph nodes.

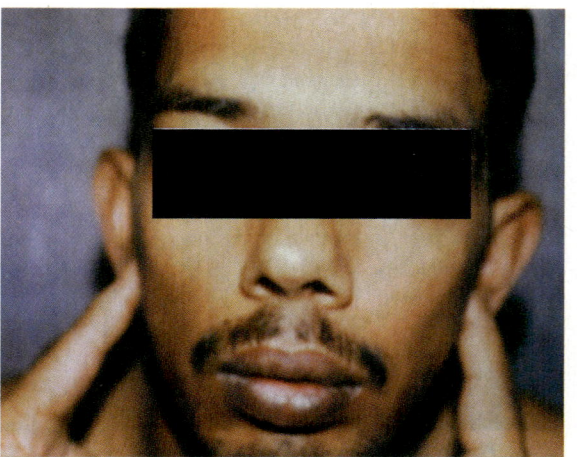

Fig. 8.11: Preauricular node.

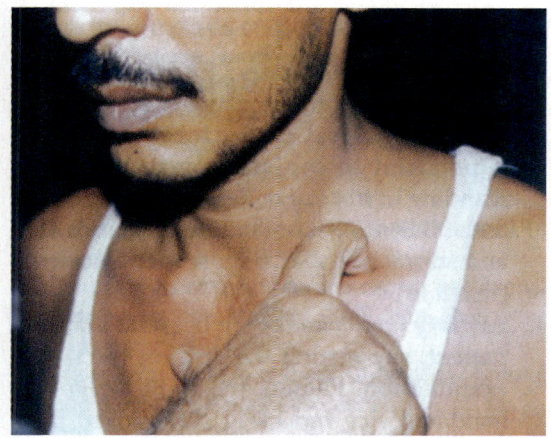

Fig. 8.14: Palpation of scalene lymph node.

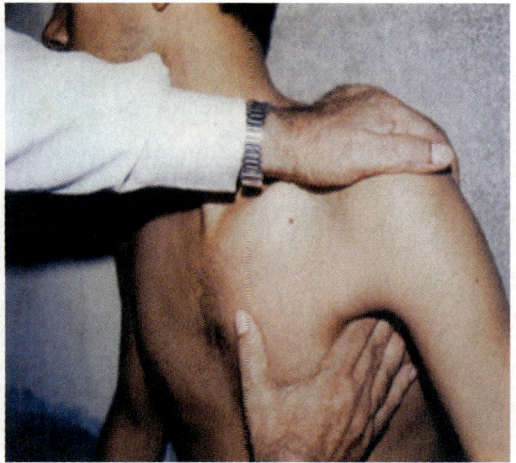

Fig. 8.15: Palpation of axillary lymph nodes.

Palpate inguinal nodes over the horizontal chain, which lies just below the inguinal ligament, and then over the vertical chain along the saphenous vein.

7. *Popliteal lymph nodes* (Fig. 8.16): Use both hands to examine the popliteal fossa with the knee flexed to less than 45°. Occasionally, a lymph node may be mistaken for a band of muscle or an artery. To differentiate between them, roll the mass or node in two directions; up and down; and side to side. The lymph node moves in both the directions; while muscle or an artery moves from side to side only.

☞ *If enlarged or tender lymph nodes found, proceed for:*
  i. Re-examination of the region they drain.
  ii. Careful assessment of lymph nodes elsewhere so that you can distinguish between regional and generalised lymphadenopathy.

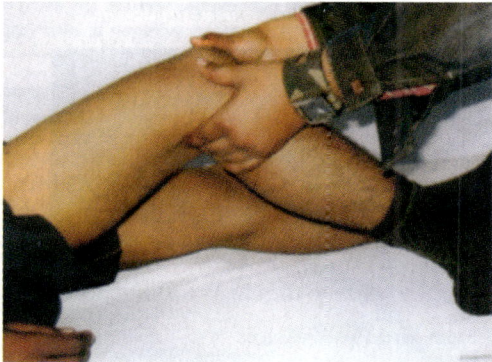

Fig. 8.16: Palpation of popliteal lymph node.

  iii. Look for the presence or absence of enlargement of the liver and spleen to determine whether the cause of lymphadenopathy is infection or haematological malignancy.
  iv. Look for any haematological manifestations, e.g. bruising, purpura or petechiae.
  v. Perform fluctuation test and transillumination test if mass is cystic.
  vi. Auscultate over the mass for bruit.

- Perform fluctuation test by compressing the swelling or mass suddenly with one finger, using another finger to determine if a bulge is produced. Positive fluctuation means a bulge is created, indicates cystic degeneration of lymph node.
- Confirm the presence of fluctuation in two planes.
- Auscultate the mass for vascular bruits and other sounds to differentiate between lymph node mass and any other vascular mass.
- Elicit transillumination in the dark. Press the lighted end of the torch into one side of the swelling (mass). A cystic mass will light up if the fluid is translucent provided that the covering tissues are not too thick. A solid lymph node mass is negative to transillumination.

EXAMINATION OF LYMPH NODE MASS(ES) TO DEFINE ITS CHARACTERISTICS

The examination involves not only the detection of lymphadenopathy but also an assessment of its significance and the various features described below:

- Inspect the mass carefully, noting change in colour or texture of the overlying skin.
- Elicit any tenderness by gentle palpation. Note any change in skin temperature by palpation with dorsum of the fingers.

- Define the size, shape of the mass.
- Keep the hand on the mass to determine whether it is pulsatile.
- Assess the consistency, surface, texture and margins of the mass.
- Try to pick up a fold of the skin between fingers and thumb over the swelling to determine fixation to the skin.
- To determine fixation to the deeper underlying structures, try to move the mass in different planes relative to the surrounding structures.

1. Onset and Progression

The sudden onset of lymphadenopathy with rapid progression indicates malignancy involving the lymph node. Lymphadenopathy in hematological malignancies are painless.

> The lymph nodes in lymphatic leukaemia are diffusely enlarged, firm, discrete and painless, involves the cervical, axillary and inguinal regions.
>
> The lymph nodes in Hodgkin's disease are painless, discrete and rubbery in consistency while they are firm in non-Hodgkin's lymphoma. Systemic symptoms, extranodal involvement (bone, brain or skin), compression symptoms, e.g. gut obstruction, ascites, superior *vena cava* obstruction and spinal cord compression are common in non-Hodgkin's lymphoma.

2. Consistency

The consistency of the lymph nodes may provide the following informations.

- In Hodgkin's disease, the lymph nodes are "rubbery" soft.
- In tuberculosis, the lymph nodes are firm and may be matted. There may be discharging sinus or involvement of skin (*scrofuloderma*, Fig. 8.17).
- In metastatic carcinoma, they feel hard or "craggy". Calcified nodes feel stony hard.

3. Tenderness

Tenderness of the nodes is a feature of acute infection. Therefore, if the lymph nodes are acutely tender, look for the evidence of infection in the region they drain, for example, the possibilities for tender cervical lymphadenopathy include; dental sepsis, tonsillitis and mastoiditis. In acute leukaemia, the lymph nodes are tender. Nodes in lymphoma and metastatic cancer are non-tender.

4. Fixation

The lymph nodes which are fixed to the underlying or overlying structures are usually malignant.

5. Site of Involvement

- *Supraclavicular nodes* enlargement occurs in tuberculosis, sarcoidosis, toxoplasmosis, metastatic cancer (Virchow's gland-enlarged left supraclavicular).
- *Axillary lymphadenopathy* is common due to injuries, infection in the upper extremities.
- *Inguinal lymphadenopathy* is due to infection, inflammation of lower limbs.
    - *Mediastinal (hilar) lymphadenopathy* is due to:
        - Metastatic carcinoma
        - Fungal infection
    - *Intra-abdominal or retroperitoneal lymphadenopathy is due to:*
        - Lymphomas
        - Tuberculosis (tabes mesenterica)
        - Metastatic

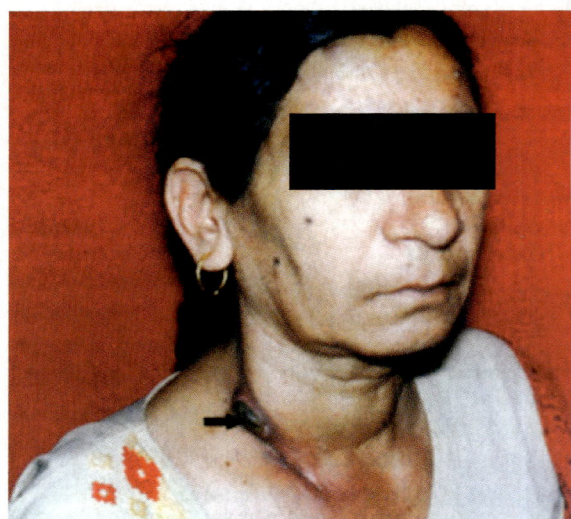

Fig. 8.17: Tubercular lymph node enlargement with extension into the skin (scrofuloderma→).

SPLEEN AS A HEMATOLOGICAL ORGAN

Examination and Evaluation

Normally, the spleen is not palpable. A palpable spleen is the major physical sign that warrants investigations because spleen becomes palpable when it has already enlarged two to three times than normal. The spleen is examined under four heads.

1. **Inspection:** Inspection may reveal a fullness in the left hypochondrium that descends on inspiration, a finding associated with massive splenomegaly.
2. **Palpation:** The spleen can be palpated by bimanual, ballottement method and palpation

from above (Middleton manoeuvre). Splenomegaly is just palpable if its tip descends during deep inspiration in right lateral position.
  - Bimanual method of palpation is as good as other methods. This method has already been described in examination of the abdomen (*see* Unit VI).
3. **Percussion:** For splenic dullness (read examination of abdomen).
4. **Auscultation:** A splenic rub may be heard in the splenic area in splenic infarct leading to perisplenitis in sickle cell anaemia.

Other Methods of Splenic Detection

On ultrasonography, radionuclide scan, the spleen has a maximum cephalocaudal diameter of 13 cm, the increased diameter indicates splenomegaly.

Note: Evaluation of splenomegaly and its importance causes diagnosis and differential diagnosis has been discussed in unit on examination of gastrointestinal and hepatobiliary system.

SYSTEMIC EXAMINATION

CARDIOVASCULAR SYSTEM EXAMINATION

☞ Examine for hyperdynamic circulation and hemic murmurs in anaemia. Cardiomegaly and CHF can occur in chronic severe anaemia. Arterial and venous thrombi may occur in polycythaemia and thrombophilia.

ABDOMINAL EXAMINATION

☞ Abdomen should be examined for:
  i. Liver enlargement
  ii. Spleen enlargement
  iii. Para-aortic lymph node. They are difficult to palpate unless patient has thin abdomen or lymph nodes are sufficiently large.

N.B. The thoracic lymph node cannot be palpated at all. Their enlargement is suspected when there are symptoms and signs of mediastinal compression. They are detected on X-ray or CT scan of chest.

☞ NERVOUS SYSTEM EXAMINATION

☞ Look for altered consciousness due to bleeding, infection in brain and meninges, polycythaemia, hyperviscosity, etc.
  - Examine for neuropathy (leukaemia, lymphoma, myeloma, Vit. B_{12} deficiency) and myopathy (paralysis).
  - Examine for subacute combined depenelation of spinal cord if megaloblastic anaemia is suspected.

RESPIRATORY SYSTEM EXAMINATION

☞ Examine for mediastinal compression (thoracic lymphadenopathy); for cough, rib and sternal involvement producing chest pain in lymphoma, myeloma, nerve root compression, zoster infection, acute chest syndrome in sickle cell anaemia and sternal tenderness in leukaemias.

Sexual Examination

☞ *Look for priapism*

THE ANUS

☞ The anus should examined because it is lined by mucosa which is vulnerable to infection, ulceration and bleeding similar to oral mucosa in patients with leucopenia, pancytopenia or agranulocytosis.

BRIEF SYNOPSIS OF COMMON BLOOD DISORDERS

IDIOPATHIC THROMBOCYTOPENIC PURPURA

It is an autoimmune disorder of platelets, where autoantibodies lead to an accelerated destruction of platelets with normal or increased megakaryocytes in the bone marrow.

Causes of Purpura
I. **Thrombocytopenic purpura**
  - Idiopathic thrombocytopenic purpura (ITP)
  - Thrombotic thrombocytopenic purpura (TTP)
  - Disseminated intravascular coagulation (DIC)
  - Infections, e.g. viral, septicaemia
  - Drug induced (e.g. quinine, quinidine, sulpha group, rifampicin, cytotoxics)
  - Leukaemias, aplastic anaemia, myelofibrosis, lymphomas, etc.
  - Hypersplenism

II. **Non-thrombocytopenic purpura**
  - Hereditary haemorrhagic telangiectasia
  - Allergic/immune complex (Henoch-Schönlein purpura)
  - Vasculitic purpura, drug-induced vasculitis
  - Senile purpura, steroid-induced purpura
  - Hemolytic uraemic syndrome

Diagnostic features of ITP in adults are
1. Chronic history of bleeding with relapses and remissions.
2. Mostly females (20 to 40 years) involved.
3. Purpura, epistaxis, bleeding into mucous membrane, ecchymoses and menorrhagia are major manifestaions.
4. BT is prolonged.
5. Platelet count is reduced.
6. Platelet antibodies present.
7. Bone marrow shows increased megakaryocytes indicating its response to peripheral destruction of platelets.

Differential Diagnosis of Purpura
It lies between three common conditions associated with purpura:
1. ITP
2. Anaphylactoid purpura (Henoch-Schönlein)
3. Thrombotic thrombocytopenic purpura.

DISSEMINATED INTRAVASCULAR COAGULATION (DIC)
It is a thrombohaemorrhagic disorder in which both platelets and coagulation factors are consumed leading to thrombocytopenia, prolongation of clotting time and partial thromboplastin time. Fibrinogen levels are low. Fibroinogen is degraded to its fibrinogen degradation products (FDPs) which form a diagnostic feature of DIC.

Causes of DIC
1. Infections, e.g. Gram-negative septicaemia, meningococcal septicaemia, malaria and viral infection.
2. Snakebite
3. Abruptio placentae, dead foetus, amniotic fluid embolism, pre-eclampsia.
4. Trauma, surgery, malignancies.
5. Aortic aneurysm
6. Hemolytic uraemic syndrome
7. Severe burns
8. Acute glomerulonephritis

Diagnosis
It is made from the history of bleeding from multiple sites (more than 2 sites) corroborated by following investigations:
- Platelet cout is low.
- Blood film shows schistocytes and fragmented red cells.
- Prothrombin time—prolonged.
- Thrombin time—prolonged.
- Partial thromboplastin time—prolonged.
- Plasma fibrinogen levels—low.
- Fibrinogen degradation products (FDP)—raised.
- D-dimer levels are increased.

POLYCYTHAEMIA
An increase in RBC count, red cell mass with rise in haemoglobin and PCV is called *polycythaemia*. Polycythaemia is suspected when the haemoglobin level is > 16 g/dl and PCV > 55% in males and haemoglobin level > 15.5 g/dl and PCV > 50% in females.

It may be relative (normal cell mass) or true polycythaemia (increased red cell mass). It may be *primary* (polycythaemia vera) due to malignant transformation of RBCs or *secondary* due to hypoxia of pulmonary disease, heavy smoking, high altitude and congenital cyanotic heart disease or tumours producing erythropoietin.

Clinical Features
- The disorder commonly occurs in middle age (around 40 years), more common in males than females.
- Raised haemoglobin produces red face (plethora) and conjunctivae.
- The cerebral symptoms include headache, dizziness, vertigo, black-outs, lack of concentration.
- Both thrombotic or haemorrhagic events occur. Bleeding may occur from nose (epistaxis) or from peptic ulcer disease. Bruising is also common. Peptic ulcer is 4–5 times more common, splenomegaly may occur in 75% cases. Hyperuricaemia, urate stone formation and uric acid nephropathy are also common.

The **diagnosis** is confirmed by raised haemoglobin, RBC count and PCV. The blood count of all the three elements, i.e. WBC, RBC and platelets are high. Blood viscosity is increased. Bone marrow is hypercellular with increased erythropoiesis, granulopoiesis and thrombopoiesis.

VON WILLEBRAND'S DISEASE
von Willebrand's disease is a coagulation disorder occuring due to defect in von Willebrand factor (vWF). It is autosomal dominant disorder. It is characterised by platelet dysfunction as well as low level of factor VIII.

Clinical Features
Superficial bleeding, i.e. bruising, epistaxis, menorrhagia, GI bleed due to platelet dysfunction.

Spontaneous bleeding: Following dental extraction, trauma, surgery, etc.

It is a mixed bleeding and coagulation disorder.

The **diagnosis** is suspected when bleeding occurs both into the skin and joints. It is confirmed by normal to low platelet count defective platelet aggregation, low level of plasma vWF factor and reduced factor VIII activity.

Differential Diagnosis
It has to be differentiated from other bleeding and coagulation disorders (haemophilia).

HAEMOPHILIA A
It is an inherited disorder of factor VIII deficiency and is second commonest disorder of coagulation system after von Willebrand's disease. The disorder being inherited as X-linked recessive trait manifests clinically in males, while females act as carriers.

All daughters of haemophilics are obligate carriers and sisters have a 50% chance of being a carrier. If a carrier has a son, he has 50% chance of having haemophilia and a daughter will have 50% chance of being carrier.

The reduction of factor VIII/vWF ratio as compared to normal indicates carrier. Now antenatal diagnosis of haemophilia A and identification of a carrier has been made possible due to advances in molecular genetic techniques. Haemophilic gene can be traced within families using gene probes.

Clinical Features
The clinical features according to its severity are given in Table 8.6.

Diagnosis: It is made from clincial features and positive family history. The diagnosis is confirmed by deficiency of factor VIII and prolongation of PT and aPTT levels.

Differential Diagnosis
It has to be differentiated from von Willebrand's disease.

TABLE 8.6: Severity and Clinical Manifestations of Haemophilia

Grade	Factor VIII or IX level	Clinical features
Severe	<2%	Spontaneous bleeding into joints (haemarthroses, Fig. 8.5) and muscles (haematomas)
Moderate	2–10%	Haematomas following minor trauma or surgery (cuts or wounds)
Mild	10–50%	Bleeding after major surgery or injury

LYMPHADENOPATHY
(Read Unit VI also for lymphadenopathy)

Significant lymphadenopathy which needs further investigations means enlargement of lymph node > 1 cm in size anywhere in the body except inguinal region where > 2 cm in size is considered as significant.

Lymph node constitute a part of lymphoreticular system, hence, get involved during infection, neoplasm, connective tissue diseases and lipid storage diseases (Table 8.7).

TABLE 8.7: Common Causes of Lymphadenopathy
1. **Infective**
   i. *Bacterial*
      - Streptococcal, brucellosis, tuberculosis, syphilis, leprosy, glanders, plague, diphtheria
   ii. *Viral*
      - Epstein-Barr, HIV, infectious mononucleosis
   iii. *Protozoal*
      - Toxoplasmosis, filariasis, leishmaniasis, trypanosomiasis
   iv. *Fungal*
      - Histoplasmosis, coccidioidomycosis
2. **Neoplastic**
   i. *Primary*
      - Leukaemias (acute and chronic lymphatic leukaemia), lymphomas (Hodgkin and non-Hodgkin)
   ii. *Secondary*
      - Lung, breast, thyroid, stomach metasteses
3. **Connective tissue disorders**
   - Rheumatoid arthritis
   - SLE
4. **Others**
   - Lipid storage diseases (Gaucher's, Niemann-Pick), sarcoidosis, amyloidosis, histiocytosis X.
5. **Drug-induced**
   - Phenytoin (pseudolymphoma), gold, hydralazine, allopurinol.

Differential Diagnosis
The differential diagnosis of lymphadnopathy depending on the characteristics of lymph nodes has been discussed during the examination of the lymph nodes. However, three common malignant conditions causing lymphadenopathy are compared in Table 8.8.

ACUTE LYMPHADENITIS
The characteristics are:
- Enlarged, tender and fixed lymph nodes.
- Overlying skin may be red, hot and indurated.
- Primary infective focus may be found.

TABLE 8.8: Differential Diagnosis of Malignant Lymphadenopathy

Features	Lymphoblastic leukaemia	Non-Hodgkin's lymphoma	Hodgkin's lymphoma
1. Cellular derivation	80% B, 20% T cells	90% B; 10% T	Unresolved
2. Age	Children	Young age	Middle age around 30–40 years
3. Site of the disease			
• Localised	Uncommon	Uncommon	Common
• Nodal spread	Common, non-contiguous lymph nodes involved	Discontiguous nodes involved	Contiguous nodes involved
• Nodal characteristics	Discrete, painful, soft	Painless, discrete lymph nodes, soft to firm	Rubbery consistency
– Common groups involved	Cervical and axillary groups	Involvement of Waldeyer's ring, epitrochlear node	Cervical group is involved early, but later all groups may be involved
– Mediastinal (pressure symptoms common, e.g. superior vena cava, bronchus, spinal cord compression)	Common	Common	Common
– Abdominal	Uncommon	Common	Uncommon
4. Extranodal involvement	Common	Common	Uncommon
5. Bone marrow involvement	Always	Common	Uncommon
6. B. symptoms (e.g. fever, weight loss)	Common	Uncommon	Common
7. Chromosomal defects	Common (translocations, deletion)	Common (translocations, deletion)	Common (aneuploidy)
8. Curability	40–60%	30–40%	75–85%

CHRONIC LYMPHADENITIS

Two common groups of infections are compared in Table 8.9.

CHRONIC LYMPHOCYTIC LEUKAEMIA (CLL)

Chronic lymphocytic leukaemia (CLL) is a haematological neoplasm, characterised by the accumulation of mature appearing lymphocytes in the peripheral blood associated with infiltration into bone marrow. It is a disorder of old age, peak incidence is at 60–65 years. Males are affected more than females. This is the commonest type of leukaemia. It is B cell type (95% common) and T cell type (uncommon 5%).

Clinical Features

The onset is insidious. 25% cases are asymptomatic and detected on routine blood film examination. The development of anaemia is slower than in CML. The **symptoms and signs** of CLL usually relate to lymphocytic tissue infiltration include peripheral *lymphadenopathy*, *splenomegaly* and *anaemia*. The stages are as follows:

1. Clinical stage A
   • No anaemia or thrombocytopenia and less than three areas of lymphoid enlargement.

TABLE 8.9: Chronic Infective Lymphadenitis (Septic vs Tubercular)

Septic	Tubercular
• Lymph nodes are discrete, firm, slightly tender and non-matted	• Lymph nodes may or may not be tender, firm and often matted, may be adherent to skin
• Symptoms of sepsis may be present, e.g. high temperature, tachycardia, tachypnoea, sweats	• Fever, weight loss, night sweats and respiratory symptoms present
• Abscess formation common, hence, fluctuation in the centre is common.	• Occasionally caseation may lead to cold abscess formation (fluctuation sign positive)
• Rupture is uncommon	• The lymph nodes may extend to involve skin and may burst forming tuberculous ulcer or sinus

2. **Clinical stage B**
   - No anaemia or thrombocytopenia with three or more areas of lymphoid enlargement.
3. **Clinical stage C**
   - Presence of anaemia and thrombocytopenia regardless of number of areas of lymphoid enlargement.

Diagnosis
The insidious onset of anaemia, weakness, lassitude with lymphadenopathy, splenomegaly in older persons (> 60 yrs) suggest the diagnosis of CLL. It is confirmed by PBF and bone marrow examination.

Differential Diagnosis
Read the differential diagnosis of lymphadenopathy.

CHRONIC MYELOID LEUKAEMIA (CML)
It is a myeloproliferative disorder characterised by excessive proliferation of myeloid series of cells in the marrow resulting in appearance of large number of immature cells (> 30%) in the peripheral blood film (PBF). It may be Philadelphia chromosome positive (Ph' positive: 90–95%) or negative (Ph' negative: 5 to 10%)

Clinical Features
1. *Symptoms of anaemia*, e.g. pallor, dyspnoea, weakness, tachycardia.
2. *General symptoms*, e.g. lassitude, weight loss, anorexia, night sweats.
3. *Symptoms and signs of infection*, i.e. fever, sweating.
4. *Bleeding tendency*, i.e. easy bruising, epistaxis, ecchymoses, menorrhagia, haematomas, etc.
5. *Bone pain* and *sternal tenderness*.
6. *Dragging abdominal pain* and massive *splenomegaly*.

Diagnosis is based on anaemia with massive splenomegaly, bleeding tendency, etc. It is confirmed by high WBC count (in lacs) with more than 30% immature cells with hypercellular bone marrow. It has to be differentiated from leukemoid reaction where most of the cell are mature with leucocytosis (Box 8.3).

Differential Diagnosis
Read the causes and differential diagnosis of massive (> 8 cm) splenomegaly in Unit VI on gastrointestinal and hepatobiliary system.

HAIRY CELL LEUKAEMIA
- It is lymphoid neoplams of B cell type of lymphocytes, also called *leukaemic reticuloendotheliosis*.
- It occurs in middle and old age in both sexes.
- It is characterised by bicytopenia or pancytopenia, splenomegaly and abnormal lymphocytes with hairy projections on their surface in PBF and bone marrow smear.
- **Symptoms** include weakness, fatigue, fever infections and bleeding tendency (bruising, ecchymosis)
- Hepatomegaly is also common.
- A characterisic diagnosic test is to demonstrate characterisitic hairy cells on histochemical staining with tartrate resistant acid phosphate (TRAP).

MYELODYSPLASTIC SYNDROME
It comprises a group of disorders characterised by pancytopenia and hypercellular marrow with dysplastic changes in all three cell lines (RBC, WBC, platelets).

Classification
The FAB (French-American-British) group classified this disorder into five subtypes:
1. Refractory anaemia.
2. Refractory anaemia with ring sideroblasts.
3. Chronic myelomonocytic leukaemia.
4. Refractory anaemia with excess of blast cells.
5. Refractory anaemia with excess of blasts in transformation.

Clinical Features
- Occurs in older persons (>60 yrs)
- *Symptoms and signs of anaemia*, i.e. pallor, fatigue, dyspnoea and murmurs. The anaemia is refractory.
- Infections are common due to neutropaenia
- Bruises, ecchymosis, gum bleeding occur due to thrombocyopenia
- Splenomegaly.

Diagnosis and Differential Diagnosis
Diagnosis is made by cytopenias (bicytopenia or pancytopenia) with hypercellular bone marrow and dysplastic changes in the WBC (hypogranular neutrophils with hyper or hyposegmentation)
It has to be differentiated from
1. *Aplastic anaemia*. The bone marrow in this condition is hypocellular with no dysplastic changes.
2. *Refractory anaemia* with blast cells/ring sideroblasts
3. *Leukaemias* (high WBC count with immature cells)

ACUTE LEUKAEMIAS

Acute myeloid leukaemia is common in adults while acute lymphoid leukaemia is common in children (<15 yrs). They are characterised by acute onset of symptoms, i.e. fever, bleeding tendencies, infection, etc. The diagnosis is based on more than 30% immature cells and 10% blast cells in PBF. Prognosis remains poor. The contrasting features of acute leukamias are presented in Table 8.10.

Depending on the high WBC count, one has differentiate acute leukaemia from chronic leukaemia; leukaemoid reaction and myelodysplastic syndrome (Table 8.11).

MYELOID METAPLASIA AND MYELOFIBROSIS

Myeloid metaplasia means extramedullary erythropoiesis due to loss of marrow activity. It may be idiopathic called *agnogenic myeloid metaplasia*. It could also be *secondary* to myelofibrosis.

Myelofibroris is defined as loss of marrow elements due to fibrosis which may be *primary* or *secondary* to toxic action of chemical and irradiation.

Symptoms
- Onset is insidious. Disease is progressive.
- Pallor, weight loss, lassitude, night sweats.
- Symptom of infections, i.e. fever.
- Dragging abdominal pain due to hepatosplenomegaly.

Signs
- Anaemia/pancytopenia.
- Splenomegaly (massive).
- Moderate hepatomegaly.
- No bone tenderness.

Diagnosis and Differential Diagnosis

It is based on clinical picture of massive splenomegaly with hepatomegaly and anaemia. Diagnosis is confirmed by cytopenias and dry bone marrow tap.

Differential Diagnosis

It depends on the causes of massive splenomegaly with anaemia (read splenomegaly Unit VI).

LABORATORY DIAGNOSIS OF HEMATOLOGICAL DISORDERS

LABORATORY DIFFERENTIAL DIAGNOSIS OF BLEEDING AND COAGULATION DISORDERS (TABLE 8.12)

I. The bleeding disorders are
   1. Thrombocytopenia
   2. Thromboasthenia
   3. Capillary wall as normalities

II. The coagulation disorders are:
   1. Haemophilia and Erishmas disease
   2. Anticoagulant therapy
   3. Liver and kidney diseases

TABLE 8.10: Contrasting Features of Two Types of Acute Leukaemias (AML and ALL)

Feature	AML	ALL
Age	Adult 15-40 years	Children < 15 years
Incidence	It comprises 20% of childhood leukaemia	Comprises 80% of childhood leukaemia
Physical findings	Hepatosplenomegaly (+) Lymphadenopathy (+) Gum hypertophy (+) Bone tenderness (+)	Hepatosplenomegaly (++) Lymphadenoapathy (++) Gum hypertophy (++) Bone tenderness (++)
Laboratory findings, i.e. blood and bone marrow examination	Low to high WBC count with predominant myeloblasts and promyelocytes. Thrombocytopenia is moderate	Low to high WBC count with predominant lymphoblasts. Thrombocytopenia is moderate
Cytochemical stains	Myeloperoxidase positive Sudan black positive	PAS positive
Specific therapy for remission induction	Cytosine-arabinoside, daunorubicin, etoposide and 6-thioguanine	Vincristine, prednisolone, L-asparaginase, daunorubicin
To therapy	Remission rate is low, (60–80%), duration of remission short 12–18 months	Remission rate is high (90%), duration of remission prolonged Children without CNS prophylaxis: 33 months and with CNS prophylaxis: 60 months; Adults: 12–18 months

Signs used: (+) means present; (++) means a marked feature.

TABLE 8.11: Differential Diagnosis of Leukaemia, Leukaemoid Reaction and Myelodysplastic Syndrome

Parameter	Acute leukaemia	Chronic myeloid leukaemia	Chronic lymphatic leukaemia	Leukaemoid reaction	Myelodysplastic syndrome
Total WBC count	Mild increase (20–30,000/cumm)	Very high (1,00,000/cumm) or above	About 50,000/cumm	20-25000/cumm	Normal, low or high
Blasts cells	>20%	only a few (<5%)	None	Very few	Scanty
Myelocytes	Present in small numbers except in promyelocytic leukaemia	Present in large numbers (30–40%)	Nil	Predominantly present in myeloid reaction	May be seen
Lymphocytes	Variable	Very few	All cells are adult lymphocytes	Predominant cell in lymphatic leukemoid reaction	Normal
Platelets	Reduced	Normal or increased	Normal or decreased	Normal or increased	Decreased
Nature of disease	Primary neoplasm	Primary neoplasm	Primary neoplasm	Secondary to other non-neoplastic conditions	Premalignant condition
LAP (leucocyte alkaline phosphatase)	Variable	low	Not applicable	Increased	Variable but low
Chromosomal change	Several changes	Philadelphia (Ph') chromosome diagnostic	Diagnostic changes present	Nil	Present and diagnostic
Dysplastic changes	None	None	None	None	Present in all the lines

Note: For classification of leukaemia and their immunological markers, read Textbook of Medicine for MBBS by Dr. S.N. Chugh.

III. *Combined bleeding and coagulation disorders*
  1. von Willibrand's disease
  2. Disseminated intravascular coagulation DIC.

APLASTIC ANAEMIA

1. Haemoglobin is low
2. Blood count
   - Neutropaenia
   - Thrombocytopenia
   - Anaemia
3. Blood film
   - Normocytic normochromic anaemia with reduction in platelets and leucocytes.
   - Low reticulocyte count (<1%).
4. Bone marrow (aspiration or trephine)
   - Dry tap. No marrow is aspirated (Fig. 8.2). In such cases trephine biopsy should be attempted.
   - Hypoplasia of marrow in the form of hypocellularity and increased fibrosis.
   - Cytogenic studies of the bone marrow for confirmation.

HAEMOLYTIC ANAEMIA

1. **Tests of increased red cell breakdown**
   - Normocytic normochromic or dimorphic anaemia.
   - Unconjugated serum bilirubin is raised.
   - Urine urobilinogen is raised but no bilirubinuria occurs.
   - Serum haptoglobin is reduced or absent.
   - Plasma LDH is raised.
   - Evidence of intravascular haemolysis, i.e. haemoglobinaemia, haemoglobinuria, methaemoglobinaemia, haemosiderinuria present.

2. **Tests of increased red cell production**
   - Reticulocyte count – Raised
   - Blood film – Macrocytosis, polychromasia and presence of normoblasts

TABLE 8.12: Tests For Assessment of a Case with Bleeding

Investigation	Result	Normal range	Bleeding disorder
Profile for bleeding disorders			
Platelet count	↓	1,50,000–400,000 per cubic	• Thrombocytopenia (congenital or acquired)
Bleeding time (BT). It is done by noting the time taken for spontaneous asset of bleeding from a cut in the capillary bed, i.e. finger tip	↑	2–7 min (Ivy method)	• Thrombocytopenia • Thrombopathy (aspirin, von Willebrand's disease)
Profile for coagulation disorders			
Prothrombin time (PT) or INR	↑	12–14 seconds (The patient's PT is compared with a control)	• Deficiency of factors II, V, VII, X
It screens the extrinsic (tissue of coagulation. It is the time taken for extrinsic thromboplastin to form a clot in recalculated placelet poor plasma at 37°C	↑		• Liver disease • Anticoagulant therapy • Disseminated intravascular coagulation (DIG)
Activated partial thromboplastin time (aPTTK). It screens the intrinsic pathway. It measures the time taken for the formation of thrombin and fibrin clot by intrinsic pathway	↑	30–40 seconds	• Deficiency of factors II, V, VIII, IX, X, XI, XII • Haemophilia A and B • vonWillebrand's disease • DIC
Thrombin time (TT) [These are employed when both PTT and PT are prolonged]	↑	About 12 seconds	• Hypofibrinogenaemia, afibrinagenaemia PTTK • Dysfibrinogenaemia
Fibrinogen	↓	1,5–4.0 g/l	• Hypofibrinogenaemia
FDP	↑	< 2.5 mg/l	• DIC

Note: Correction tests are used to differentiate prolonged times in PT, PTTK and TT due to coagulation factor deficiencies and inhibitors of coagulation. Prolonged PT, PTTK or TT due to coagulation factor deficiencies are corrected by addition of normal plasma to the patient's plasma, while no correction occurs in case of an inhibitor(s) of coagulation being present

↑ — means increased; ↓ — means decreased; INR—international normalised ratio. It ranges 1.5 to 3 and used to monitor the anticogulent therapy

| Clotting time (CT). This is done by noting the time taken for spontanous clotting of blood at | ↑ | 5–10 minutes | • Cogulation disorder or anticoagulation therapy |

- Bone marrow - Erythroid hyperplasia with raised iron store
- X-ray bones - Expansion of marrow space in the bones such as skull

3. Tests of damage to red cells
- Blood film—Microspherocytes, fragmented red cells.
- Osmotic fragility—Increased.
- Electrophoresis for abnormal haemoglobin.
- Estimation of haemoglobin A_2.
- Estimation of haemoglobin F (by alkali denaturation test).
- Test for sickling (a drop of blood incubated with 1% sodium bisulphite and examined under microscope).
- Screening test for G6PD deficiency.

4. Tests for shortened red cell survival
- Chromium-labelled method—red cell lifespan shortened.

5. Immunological studies
- Coombs' test (direct and indirect to detect antibodies. Direct test detects antibodies on the surface of RBCs while indirect test detects antibodies in serum.)
- **Heinz bodies.** These are inclusion bodies which develop in RBCs in the presence of hemolysis, hence, give clue to the diagnosis.

IRON DEFICIENCY ANAEMIA
- Haemoglobin and RBC count are low.
- MCV is <76 ft, MCH < 27pg and MCHC < 32% respectively. All are reduced.

Haematological Disorders

- Reticulocyte count is low for degree of anaemia (hypoproliferative anaemia).
- Platelet count and WBC count normal.
- PBF shows microcytic hypochromic picture with anisocytosis, poikilocytosis, elliptocytosis, etc.
- Bone marrow is hypercelular and iron stores (Prussian Blue Staining) are reduced.
- Serum iron is low (<80 mcg/dl), Serum Ferratin level low (<15 mg/ml) in males and <12 mg/ml in females. Transferrin saturation is low <2.5%
- Serum transferrin receptor (STFR) estimation is increased in iron deficiency and this distinguishes it from anaemia of chronic disease.

The various types of microcytic anaemia, i.e. iron deficiency, anaemia of chronic disease, Thalassaemia and Sideroblastic anaemia are differentiated on the basis of iron studies as follows:

Feature	Iron deficiency	Anaemia of chronic disease	Thalassaemia trait	Sideroblastic anaemia
MCV	Reduced	Normal or near normal	Very low	Low in inherited type but raised in acquired type
Serum iron	Low	Low	Normal	Raised
Iron binding	Raised	Reduced	Normal	Normal
Serum ferritin	Low	Normal or raised	Normal	Raised
Iron in marrow	Absent	Present	Present	Present
Iron in erythroblasts	Absent	Absent or reduced	Present	Ring forms

MEGALOBLASTIC ANAEMIA

1. Haemogloblin is reduced.
2. Mean cell volume (MCV) is usually raised (>120 ft.).
3. Red cell count is low for degree of anaemia.
4. Reticulocyte count is low for degree of anaemia.
5. WBC count is low to normal or reduced.
6. Platelet count is low or normal.
7. Peripheral blood film shows macrocytosis, poikilocytosis, red cell fragments, hypersegmentation of neutrophils
8. Bone marrow reveals hypercellular marrow with megaloblastosis, giant metamyelocytes and platelets, non-ring sideroblasts seen. Increased bone marrow iron is present

9. Plasma LDH level is markedly elevated
10. Serum iron is also elevated
11. Serum ferritin is also elevated
12. Bilirubin is raised with unconjugated hyperbilirubinaemia.

> **N.B.** Specific tests for cause of specific deficiency, i.e. Vit. B_{12} or folic acid may be carried out in addition to described above.

ACUTE LEUKAEMIAS

1. Haemoglobin is low.
2. Platelet count is low.
3. WBC count is markedly high (50,000–1,00,000 etc.)
4. Reticulocyte count is high
5. Blood film shows large number of blast cells (>10%)
6. Bone marrow examination shows hypercellularity with leukaemic blast cells (>30% of cells). The presence of auer rods in the cytoplasm of blast cells indicate myeloblastic leukaemia. Erythropoietic and megakarycytic cells are reduced.
7. Cytochemical stains differentiate different types of cells, i.e. myeloperoxidase and sudan black stains give positive reaction with myeloid series of cells (Table 8.11).
8. *Immunophenotyping*: The recent development of monoclonal antibodies as well as advances in flow cytometry have made immunophenotyping easy. It is useful to define definite lineage (B cell vs T cells), helps to differentiate acute leukaemia from other nonhaematological disorders.
9. *Chromosomal abnormalities*: Three major technique of molecular analysis such as *Southern blot analysis* (commonly used), the *PCR* and *fluorescent in situ hybridisation* demonstrate chromosomal abnormalities in acute leukaemia (read Text Book of Medicine by Dr. S.N. Chugh).
10. LDH, uric acid and alkaline phosphatase levels are elevated in acute leukaemia indicating rapid turn over of the cells.
11. *Coagulation profile*: DIC may be seen in acute promyelocytic leukaemia (M3).
12. CSF examination is mandatory in all patients of ALL to evaluate CNS involvement at presentation and during follow up.
13. X-ray chest for any mediastinal mass which may be seen in T-cell ALL.
14. Renal functions, e.g. urea and creatinine.

> **N.B.** Some patients present with pancytopenia and have a few blast cells in peripheral blood (subleukaemic leukaemia) or no blast cell (aleukaemic leukaemia). Both these conditions now-a-days are included under myelodysplastic syndromes.

CHRONIC LEUKAEMIA

1. Haemoglobin is low. There is normocytic normochromic anaemia.
2. WBC count is high usually more than a lac, but varies greatly from 50,000/µl to many lacs.
3. Platelet count is high initially but becomes low later on. It is low during acute blastic crisis in chronic leukaemia.
4. *Peripheral blood film examination.* In CML there is full range of granulocyte precursors (promyelocytes, myelocytes and metamyelocytes >30% and myeloblasts < 10%). There is increase in eosinophil and basophil counts. Blast cells >30% indicate blastic crisis. In CLL, there is lymphocytosis with atypical lymphocytes.
5. **Bone marrow:** It is done for cytogenetic studies (*Philadelphia chromosome*). The Ph'chromosome is present in 90% cases of CML. DNA analysis is done to demonstrate the presence of *Chimeric Abelson—BCR gene* in CML.
   Cytogenic studies not only help in the diagnosis of chronic leukaemia/lymphoma but help to monitor the response to therapy, detect relapse and distinguish relapse from a new therapy-related leukaemia or lymphoma during follow up.
6. **Other investigations**
   - Neutrophil alkaline phosphatase is low in CML
   - Plasma vitamin B_{12} levels are high in CML
   - LDH levels are elevated in CML

Unit IX

Endocrinal Disorders

- Symptoms and their Analysis
- History
- General Physical Examination
- Local and Systemic Examination
- Brief Synopsis of Endocrine Disorders

SYMPTOMS OF ENDOCRINE SYSTEM (TABLE 9.1)

Ask about the following symptoms for:

TABLE 9.1: Symptoms and their Analysis

Symptoms	Most likely endocrine disorder(s)
I. General	
Lethargy and depression	Hypothyroidism, diabetes mellitus, hyperparathyroidism, hypogonadism, adrenal insufficiency, Cushing's syndrome
Weight gain and oedema	Hypothyroidism, Cushing's syndrome, adiposogenital syndrome, obesity
Weight loss	Hyperthyroidism, adrenal insufficiency, diabetes mellitus (type 1), hypopituitarism, anorexia nervosa
Increased sweating (hyperhidrosis)	Hyperthyroidism, hypoglycemia, phaeochromocytoma
Pigmentation (e.g. axillary fold, soles, palmar creases, mucous membranes)	Addison's disease, Cushing's syndrome, hypothyroidism
Coarsening of features	Acromegaly, hypothyroidism
II. Cardiovascular	
Palpitations and dyspnoea	Hyperthyroidism, phaeochromocytoma, Conn's syndrome
Oedema	Hypothyroidism, Cushing's syndrome, Conn's syndrome, obesity
III. Respiratory	
Hoarseness of voice	Myxoedema, retrosternal goitre, thyroid surgery
Cough and stridor	Pressure over trachea by enlarged thyroid/parathyroid glands
IV. Gastrointestinal	
Increased appetite	Diabetes, hyperthyroidism, phaeochromocytoma
Anorexia	Addison's disease, anorexia nervosa, hypothyroidism
Polyuria and polydipsia	Diabetes mellitus, diabetes insipidus, hyperparathyroidism, Conn's syndrome, hyperthyroidism, phaeochromocytoma
Vomiting	Diabetic ketoacidosis, Addison's disease, pituitary tumour with raised intracranial pressure (ICP), hyperparathyroidism
Pain abdomen	Diabetic ketoacidosis, hyperparathyroidism
Diarrhoea	Thyrotoxicosis, Addison's disease, diabetic autonomic neuropathy, hyperparathyroidism
Constipation	Hypothyroidism
V. Neurological	
Visual dysfunction	Pituitary tumour, Graves' disease (e.g. *exophthalmic ophthalmoplegia*)
Headache	Acromegaly, pituitary tumour, phaeochromocytoma
Muscle weakness (usually proximal)	Hyperthyroidism, Cushing's syndrome, hypokalaemia (e.g. Conn's syndrome and iatrogenic steroid therapy), hyperparathyroidism, hypogonadism, acromegaly, Vit. D deficiency and osteomalacia

Contd. *Contd.*

Physical Signs, Symptoms, Diagnosis and Differential Diagnosis

Symptoms	Most likely endocrine disorder(s)
Paraesthesiae and tetany	Hypoparathyroidism
Coma	Diabetic coma, non-ketotic hyperosmolar coma, Addisonian crisis, hypoglycaemic coma

VI. Reproductive system

Amenorrhoea/ oligomenorrhoea	Menopause, polycystic ovarian syndrome, hyperprolactinaemia, hyperthyroidism, premature ovarian failure, Cushing's syndrome
Galactorrhoea	Hyperprolactinaemia, hypothyroidism, drug-induced, idiopathic, hydatidiform
Impotence	Hyperprolactinaemia, hypogonadism, diabetes mellitus
Precocious puberty	Congenital adrenal hyperplasia, hyperthyroidism
Virilisation	Congenital adrenal hyperplasia, ovarian/adrenal tumour
Hirsutism	Idiopathic, polycystic ovarian syndrome congenital adrenal hyperplasia, Cushing's syndrome, androgen secreting ovarian and adrenal tumours, gonadal dysgenesis, androgen therapy

VII. Urinary system

Polyuria	Read polyuria and polydipsia in gastrointestinal symptoms
Nocturia	Diabetes insipidus
Recurrent ureteric colic	Hyperparathyroidism

VIII. Endocrinal gland

Thyroid nodule	Solitary thyroid nodule, dominant nodule in multinodular goitre
Generalised thyroid enlargement	Simple goitre (nodular or diffuse), Graves' disease, Hashimoto's thyroiditis
Heat intolerance	Hyperthyroidism, menopause (hot flushes) oestrogen secreting tumours, Liver disease, drug-induced, Klinefelter's syndrome, true hermaphroditism
Gynaecomastia	
Delayed puberty	Hypothalamopituitary dysfunction, gonadal failure (tumour, radiation, chemotherapy) orchitis, undescended testes, Klinefelter's syndrome, Turner's syndrome, malnutrition, chronic systemic illness
Pain over thyroid	Haemorrhage into nodule, de Quervain's thyroiditis rarely Hashimoto's thyroiditis
Prominence of eyes	Graves' disease
Hair loss	Hypopituitarism, hypothyroidism, hypogonadism

HISTORY

Present History

Maximum informations can be gathered on the history in a patient with endocrinal disease. The patients of endocrine disorders present with multiplicity of symptoms pertaining to various systems, hence, symptomatic enquires are essential for differential diagnosis of the symptoms. Similarly endocrinopathy may involve one gland or multiple glands simultaneously, subsequently needs a high degree of suspicion on the history. This is because treatment of one condition may cause worsening of other and because familial endocrinal syndromes do occur, hence, it is mandatory to take detailed history for systemic effects of the disease. In the present history, ask for:

- Write chronological order of the symptoms and do their analysis (Table 9.1)
- Onset of symptoms, their progression and course.
- Full drug history including oral contraceptive pills and replacement hormonal therapy.

About the age and sex
- Endocrine diseases are more common, and often more obvious, in women than men such as hyperprolactinoma, hypothyroidism (Hashimoto's thyroiditis), puberty, goitre, etc.

Past History

- Details of previous pregnancies or abortions (number of pregnancies, postpartum haemorrhage—PPH)
- Previous surgery (e.g. thyroidectomy or orchidopexy)
- Radiation to neck, gonads, thyroid
- Drug treatment, e.g. chemotherapy, oral contraceptives
- In children—ask for developmental milestones and growth.
- History of severe bleeding and shock for pituitary apoplexy and hypopituitarism.
- Exanthematus fever, i.e. measles, mumps, rubella.

Family History

Ask about the family history of
- Autoimmune disease
- Endocrine disease
- Essential hypertension
- Diabetes mellitus
- Hyperparathyroidism
- Multiple endocrine neoplasia (MEN) syndrome

Endocrinal Disorders

Social History
- Details of alcohol intake
- Details of occupation, e.g. access to drugs, chemicals
- Diet, e.g. salt, iodine (overdose of iodine may lead to *jodbasedow's phenomenon*), liquorice
- Menstrual history particularly in young women.

GENERAL PHYSICAL EXAMINATION (GPE)

The physical signs in endocrine diseases arise either locally such as thyroid enlargement and or by its local effects, or due to systemic effects of the hormones. The physical signs to be examined in endocrine system are depicted in Table 9.2.

TABLE 9.2: Physical Signs of Endocrinal Diseases

I. General
- Appearance/look/external features
- Stature (short or tall)
- Enuchoidism (measure upper and lower body segments and calculate their ratio)
- Weight (increased or reduced)
- Temperature (high or low)
- Pulse rate (high/low)
- Respiration (rate/rhythm)

II. Local signs
- Blood pressure (lying down and standing), local signs
- Neck swelling
- Thyroid enlargement, e.g. note size, shape, temperature, nodularity, tenderness and bruit

III. Signs due to systemic effects

(i) *Cardiovascular*
- Look for postural drop of BP
- Signs of autonomic dysfunction
- Arrhythmias (irregularly irregular pulse due to atrial fibrillation or VPCs)
- Signs of congestive heart failure

(ii) *Eyes*
Look for:
- Xanthelasma
- Corneal calcification-band keratopathy
- Proptosis/exophthalmos (unilateral/bilateral)
- Ophthalmoplegia (external/internal/complete)
- Lid retraction
- Lid lag sign
- Failure of furrows on looking up
- Visual acquity/field defect
- Fundus examination for retinopathy or optic atrophy

Contd.

Contd.

(iii) *Neurological*
- Generalised muscle wasting
- Proximal myopathy
- Peripheral neuropathy
- Carpal tunnel syndrome
- Gait abnormalities/ataxia
- Tendon reflexes (exaggerated/delayed/absent)
- Induction of tetany in a patient with hypocalcaemia

(iv) *Reproduction and sex*
- Failure of appearance of secondary sexual characters
- Gynaecomastia
- Delayed puberty
- Galactorrhoea
- Precocious puberty
- Enlargement of clitoris

(v) *Skin*
- Hirsutism, loss of hair
- Thin and sparse hair
- Skin thickening/thinning (localised, generalised)
- Dry/wet skin
- Pigmentation (localised, generalised, mucous membrane)
- Striae (pink/white)
- Palmar erythema
- Necrobiosis lipoidica diabeticorum

(vi) *Extremities*
- Long or short limbs
- Long/short hands and fingers
- Spade-like hands
- Finger clubbing
- Short 4th and 5th metacarpals
- Subcutaneous nodules (xanthomatosis), gangrene of fingers or toe(s)
- Ulceration or pressure sores
- Loss of finger(s) or toes
- Oedema of feet (pitting or non-pitting)

☞ Observe the general appearance. Assess the state of hydration. Measure the height, weight and calculate the BMI (kg/m^2).

- Frightening look/staring look with wide palpebral fissure and bulging eyeballs suggest *Graves' disease*.
- Expressionless round, pale face with periorbital oedema and dry thick skin with coarse features suggest *myxoedema*.
- Ape-like appearance (prognathism-prominent lower jaw, coarse features, large nobe, ear-lips and widely paced teeth) occurs in *acromegaly*.
- Rounded, moon-like appearance of face is seen in *Cushing's* syndrome.

- Signs of dehydration can develop in patients with type I DM, thyrotoxic crisis and phaeochromocytoma, hyperparathyroidism.

Stature and Obesity

Normal BMI in men is 20–25 and in women is 18–24. The BMI >30 kg/m² is labelled as obesity. Obesity in endocrinal disorder is associated with Cushing's syndrome, hypothyroidism, adiposogenital syndrome, etc.
The causes of weight loss and weight gain have been described in Table 20.1.
- *Tall stature* (increased height) is seen in endocrinal diseases, e.g. gigantism, Kallmann's syndrome (hypogonadotrophic hypogonadism), Laurence-Moon-Biedl syndrome, Klinefelter's syndrome, and connective tissue diseases (e.g. Marfan's syndrome).
- *Short stature (dwarfism)* may be seen in *heredofamilial disorders* (Down's syndrome, Turner's syndrome), *metabolic disorders* (rickets, osteomalacia, PEM, chronic renal failure), *endocrinal disorders* (hypothyroidism, Frohlick's syndrome, hypopituitarism) and *GI disorders* (e.g. coeliac disease, Crohn's disease, steatorrhoea, cystic fibrosis).

☞ *If person is tall, measure body proportions. In case of obesity, note the redistribution of fat.*

- *Enuchoidism* is confirmed by measurement of body proportions (e.g. lower body proportion or leg length measured from the ground to symphysis pubis) exceeds the upper body proportion or sitting height (symphysis pubis to top of head). It can also be confirmed by measuring the arm span (distance between middle fingers of extended arms of both upper limbs) that exceeds total height (ground to top of the head). Enuchoidism is a feature of hypogonadism Marfan's syndrome and Klinefelter's syndrome (Fig. 9.8.).
- *Truncal obesity* is seen in patients with Cushing's syndrome, adiposogenital syndrome and obese type 2 diabetes mellitus.

THE FACE

☞ *Examine the face for colour, oedema, pigmentation, etc.*
  The characteristic **facies** in endocrine disease are:
  i. **Acromegalic face** (large nose, lips, ears, prognathism (protuding jaw, widely separated teeth, large tongue and prominent forehead and cheek bones)
  ii. **Hypothyroid face** (pale, puffy face, dull expression, emotionless, thick, dry skin and loss of hair over lateral third of eyebrows)
  iii. **Face in Addison's disease** (sunken cheek and eyeballs, dry, pigmented skin and mucous membrane and signs of nutrition and vitamins deficiency)
  iv. **Moon-face** (round face, flushed or plethoric skin with acne and hirsutism)
  v. **Hyperthyroid face** (frightened or anxious look, prominent eyes, i.e. exophthalmos, shiny and moist skin)
  vi. **Eunuchoid face** (shallow, pale skin) with wrinkles or furrows and absence of facial hair.

THE TONGUE

☞ *Examine the tongue (large or small), teeth and buccal mucosa*

- *Macroglossia* means large protruding tongue beyond teeth or alveolar ridge producing indentation of teeth at its margins. It can be *primary* (true hypertrophy) due to acromegaly and tumour of the tongue or *secondary* (infiltration by anomalous elements) due to hypothyroidism, amyloidosis, angiodema, etc.
- Tongue is small (*microglossia*) and dentition is delayed in hypopituitarism. The permanent teeth get separated in acromegaly due to enlargement of jaw.
- *Delayed dentition* may be due to cretinism, juvenile hypothyroidism.
- *Wide spacing of teeth* is a sign of acromegaly, hyperparathyroidism.
- *Serrated teeth* (transverse groove on the teeth) suggest hypoparathyroidism.
- *Projecting teeth with malalignment* could be due to acromegaly.
- Buccal mucosa is hyperpigmented in *Addison's disease*.
- *Mouth thrush (candidiasis)* can occur due to steroid replacement therapy in adenocortical insufficiency.

Vital Signs

☞ *Look for the vital signs, e.g. pulse, BP, temperature and respiration.*

- *Tachycardia* is seen in hyperthyroidism, phaeochromocytoma and Conn's syndrome
- *Bradycardia* is seen in hypothyroidism
- *Hypertension* is seen in hyperthyroidism, hypothyroidism, phaeochromocytoma, Conn's syndrome
- *Hypotension* is seen in Addison's disease

- Rise in temperature is seen in hyperthyroidism while low body temperature occurs in hypothyroidism
- Respiration may be increased in thyrotoxicosis, slow in hypothyroidism.

Examination of the Skin and Hair

☞ Examine the skin for hair (thin, sparse, hirsutism or loss) moistness (dry or wet), thickness (rough and thick or fine and thin), pigmentation (localised, generalised), striae (pink, white) and for any erythema (redness of palms) and nodules.

- *Androgenetic alopecia* or *frontal baldness* (miniaturisation of hair follicle) is seen in males and females due to androgen excess.
- *Diffuse hair loss* is seen in both hyperthyroidism and hypothyroidism.
- *Thin, shiny hair* is seen in hyperthyroidism; while *sparse hair* is seen in hypothyroidism.
- *Hirsutism* in females associated with acne and seborrhoea, is seen in polycystic ovarian syndrome, ovarian tumour, congenital adrenal hyperplasia, etc. (read the symptoms of endocrine disease in the beginning).
- *Thick (toad-like), rough and dry skin* is seen in hypothyroidism; while skin is fine and moist in hyperthyroidism and phaeochromocytoma. Localised thickening particularly on the anterior aspect of the leg (*pretibial myxoedema*) is one of the features of Graves' disease (*dermopathy*).
- *Marked thinning of skin* (*skin atrophy*) with ulceration in the anterior tibial region may be due to *necrobiosis lipoidica diabeticorum* seen in diabetes mellitus.
- *Generalised pallor* occurs in panhypopituitarism. In hyperthyroidism, the skin is wet, hot not flushed while in hypothyroidism, it is dry, pale-yellow and there is loss of hair on the lateral third of eyebrows.
- *Diffuse skin pigmentation* (palmar creases, exposed parts of the body) with buccal and circumoral pigmentation is seen in Addison's disease. Excessive pigmentation occurs in Cushing's syndrome.
- *Patches of depigmentation* or *vitiligo* may also be seen in Addison's disease and autoimmune hyperthyroidism or prolonged steroid therapy.
- *Pink or violaceous striae* are seen in Cushing's syndrome (refer to Fig. 9.17).
- *Multiple small subcutaneous nodules/xanthomas* are seen in hypothyroidism or hyperlipidaemia in patients with diabetes mellitus or familial hyperlipidaemia. There may be associated xanthelasmas.

☞ In a patient with diabetes, look for the following skin lesions common in diabetics

1. **Skin infections,** e.g. boils, carbuncle, cellulitis, abscesses, mucocutaneous candidiasis, gangrene.
2. **Diabetic dermopathy**—hyperpigmented atrophic skin due to microangiopathy.
3. **Diabetic stiff hands** (e.g. cheiroarthropathy) There is stiffness of small joints with tight waxy skin over the dorsum of fingers.
4. **Scleroderma** like thickening of skin starting from neck and trunk, may become generalised.
5. **Diabetic bullae or burn marks**—blistering and bullae formation on the skin of hands and feet without trauma and burn marks may be associated with polyneuropathy.
6. **Granuloma annulare**—the condition is similar to necrobiosis lipoidica. In this, fleshy coloured annular, crescentic skin lesions are seen on the skin of extensor surface of fingers, hands, wrist, toes and ankles.
7. **Eruptive xanthomas.** These are yellow-coloured papules on the knee, elbow, back and buttocks due to associated hyperlipidaemia in diabetes.
8. **Diabetic foot** (*see* Fig. 1.27): Foot ulceration at pressure points, digital necrosis, gangrene and infection are its components. It is due to neuropathy combined with vasculopathy and ultimately bone may be involved leading to osteomyelitis.
9. **Lipodystrophy or lipoatrophy** (Fig. 9.1). There is atrophy or dystrophy of skin at the site of insulin injections.
10. **Acanthosis nigricans** (Fig. 9.2A). There will be hypopigmented plaques in fluxes of skin.

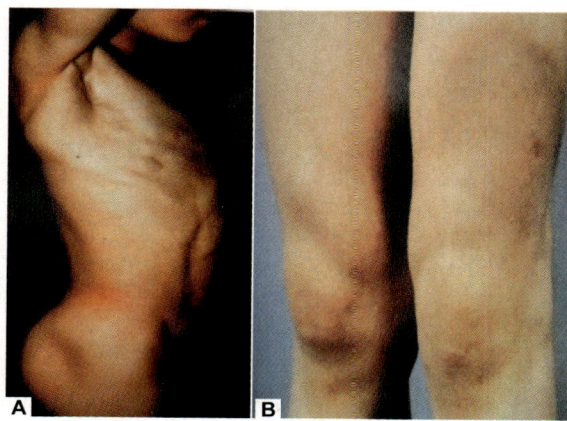

Figs 9.1A and B: Insulin induced sequela. (A) Lipoatrophy of abdominal wall; (B) Lipodystrophy of thighs.

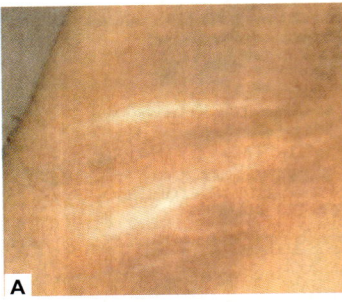

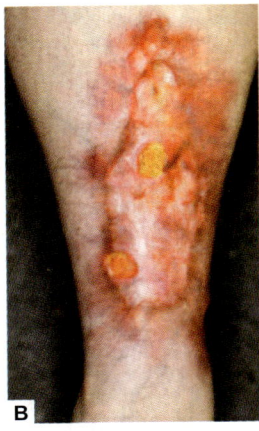

Figs 9.2A and B: (A) Acanthosis nigricans in diabetes: Velvety, hypopigmented plaques in major flexures of skin. (B) Necrobiosis lipoidica diabeticorum. Note the erythematous plaques with atrophy of skin.

11. **Necrobiosis lipoidica diabeticorum** (Fig. 9.2B). There are erythematous plaques with browny waxy discolouration followed by atrophy and scarring of the skin in front of shin (pretibial region).

Examination of the Eyes

☞ Look at the eyebrows, eyelids, eyelashes, eyeball, cornea, conjunctivae for any abnormality.

- *Lid retraction* leading to exposure of cornea is seen in Graves' disease.
- *Unilateral or bilateral exophthalmos (proptosis)* is common in Graves' disease (Fig. 9.3).
- NOSPECS represents eye signs in Graves' disease, i.e. N = no sign, O = only upper lid retraction with or without proptosis, S = soft tissue involvement, P = proptosis, E = extraocular involvement, C = corneal ulceration, S = slight loss.
- *Oedema of lids or periorbital oedema* with thickening of skin and loss or sparsity of hair is seen in hypothyroidism.
- *Recurrent styes, chalasion or blepharitis, conjunctivitis* are common due to infection in diabetics.
- *Xanthelasmas* over the eyelids are seen in diabetes, hypothyroidism and hyperlipidaemia.
- *Paralytic squint* occurs due to cranial nerve involvement in diabetes and external ophthalmoplegia in Graves' disease.
- *Exposure keratitis, corneal ulceration* may be seen in Graves' disease.
- *Corneal calcification* and *band keratopathy* is seen in hypercalcaemia due to hyperparathyroidism.

☞ Test for visual acquity, visual field and ocular movements

Examine the ocular fundus for optic atrophy or retinopathy.

- *Visual acuity* is reduced in exophthalmic goitre (Graves' disease), hypothalamic-pituitary space occupying lesions and diabetes.
- *Visual field* defects are seen in pituitary tumours.
- *Visual loss* is seen in diabetes and rapidly enlarging pituitary tumours.
- *Optic atrophy* is seen in compression due to pituitary tumour.
- *Retinopathy* is seen in hypertension associated with endocrine diseases and due to diabetes (read diabetic retinopathy).
- Look for various eyes signs (read synopsis of thyrotoxicosis later in this chapter) in case of thyrotoxicosis.

Examination of Neck

☞ Look for pulsations in the neck, look for redistribution of fat and webbing of the neck. Examine the thyroid gland.

Pulsations of carotid vessels and of other neck vessels are visible in thyrotoxicosis.
Buffalo hump at nape of neck occurs in Cushing syndrome.
Webbing of neck with skin fold on either side of the lower parts occurs in Turner's syndrome.

Examination of the Extremities

☞ Look at the hands, fingers, nails, feet and toes for any abnormality in shape and size or any other abnormalities.

- *Trident hands* (the fingers are pointed and are of equal lengths) are seen in achondroplasia.

- *Spade-like hands* and large feet with frequent change in shoes are seen in acromegaly.
- *Polydactyly* (presence of supernumerary digits) is seen in Turner's and Laurence-Moon-Biedl syndrome.
- *Finger clubbing* occasionally seen in thyrotoxicosis.
- Generalised *pitting oedema over feet* indicates Cushing's syndrome, Conn's syndrome, thyrotoxic heart disease; while *non-pitting oedema* indicates hypothyroidism.
- *Pedal spasms* occur due to hypoparathyroidism.
- *Ulteration and gangrene* of fingers and toes, loss of fingers, toes occur in diabetes.
- *Palmar erythema* may be seen in thyrotoxicosis.
- *Brittle nails* are characteristically seen in thyrotoxicosis and hypoparathyroidism.

Examination of Thyroid Gland

Thyroid gland is examined by *inspection, palpation* and *auscultation*.

Inspection of Thyroid

☞ Look at the thyroid region for the enlargement of thyroid (Fig. 9.3A). If thyroid is enlarged, look at the right and left lobes for their shape, size and presence of nodule(s). Next see the isthmus for any nodule. Note the movement of the swelling on deglutition.

- Prominence of thyroid beyond sternomastoid muscles and obliteration of suprasternal notch indicate thyroid enlargement (thyromegaly).

If thyroid swelling is mild, then Pizzalo's method of inspection is used which makes the thyroid swelling more prominent (Fig. 9.3B).

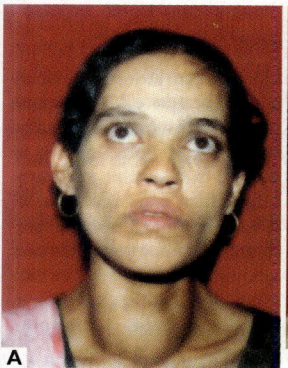 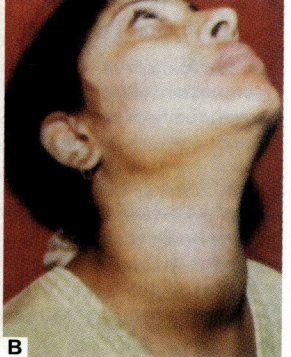

Figs 9.3A and B: Inspection of thyroid. (A) Note the huge enlargement of thyroid with the obliteration of supraclavicular fossa. There is exophthalmos with visible sclera both above and below the cornea; (B) Pizzalo's method of demonstration of mild enlargement of thyroid.

In case of thyroid swelling, look for the distension of neck veins and veins over the upper thorax.

- Neck veins and veins over the upper thorax are distended and visible in retrosternal goitre.

☞ If thyroid enlargement is suspected to be extending into the mediastinum and veins are prominent, try to establish the retrosternal extension of the goitre by asking the patient to raise both arms over the head and keep it therefore a while (Pamberton's sign).

Congestion of the face and increased dilatation of the veins over the neck and chest during this manoeuvre indicates retrosternal goitre. This is due to obstruction of veins at thoracic inlet by the goitre.

Palpation and Auscultation of Thyroid

☞ Palpate the thyroid for enlargement (goitre) and for movement during swallowing. Note the type of enlargement (nodules/diffuse).

- Patient is seated comfortably and minimum neck flexion is done.
- Examiner stands behind the patient and encircles the patient's neck with fingertips of both the hands at the level of cricoid cartilage to identify the isthmus of thyroid.
- Examiner moves the right thumb laterally to identify the right lobe as he compresses it against trachea.
- Same procedure is adopted on the left side to identify the left lobe.
- Palpate the lower margin particularly when the patient swallow on order to determine whether mass is extending down into the mediastinum.

The causes of diffuse thyromegaly are:
- *Goitre*, e.g. simple or puberty, diffuse toxic (Graves' disease) and nontoxic goitre.
- *Thyroiditis*, e.g. viral, postpartum and autoimmune (Hashimoto's thyrciditis)

The causes of nodular thyromegaly
- Nodular (single or multiple nodules): *Malignancy of thyroid, cyst*.

A single *focal nodule* suggests either a cyst or adenoma or thyroid carcinoma.

The swelling moves with deglutition.

☞ In case of localised nontoxic thyroid swelling in the neck in a young person, ask the patient to protrude the tongue to differentiate thyroid nodule from thyroglossal cyst.

- *Thyroglossal cyst* also produce midline swelling in the neck in thyroid region. Thyroid swelling and the thyroglossal cyst both move upwards on deglutition, but thyroglossal cyst also moves upwards with protrusion of the tongue while thyroid swelling does not a differentiating feature.

☞ If thyroid is enlarged, note its severity, tenderness, temperature, mobility, consistency and pulsations. Look for its pressure effects, e.g. dysphagia (pressure on oesophagus), dysphasia or stridor (pressure on trachea) or hoarseness of voice (recurrent laryngeal nerve involvement) or Horner's syndrome (sympathetic trunk involvement). Auscultate over thyroid for bruit, while the patient holds his/her breath.

- *Thyroid enlargement* is **mild** in simple goitre, **moderate** in thyroiditis, a single thyroid nodule and in benign tumour and some cases of carcinoma, **large** in Graves' disease (Fig. 9.4B) and multinodular goitre (Fig. 9.4A).

Goitre is **soft** in Graves' disease, **firm** in Hashimoto's thyroiditis and **hard** in thyroid malignancy and Riedel's thyroiditis.
- *Thyroid tenderness* is seen in thyroiditis.
- *Thyroid temperature* is raised in Graves' disease, multinodular goitre.
- A localised *systolic or continuous bruit* may be heard" in hyperthyroidism.

Pressure on the trachea can be confirmed by *Kocher's test*, i.e. pushing the trachea from one side will compress the lateral lobe and subsequently the trachea leading to stridor.

- **Mobility.** It is tested by moving the gland from side to side with the neck flexed and turned to ipsilateral side to relax the sternomastoid muscle.

Most of the goitres are mobile. The thyroid gets fixed to the deeper structures in malignancy and thyroiditis.

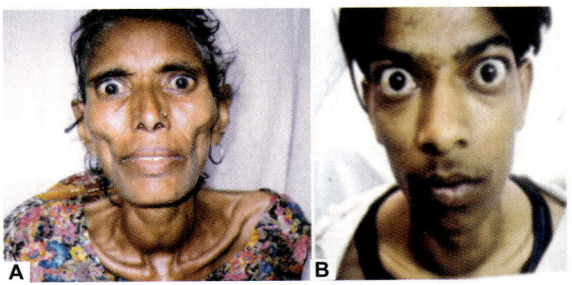

Figs 9.4A and B: Toxic goitre. (A) Multinodular; (B) Graves' disease.

- It is difficult to measure the thyroid gland in isolation, however, measurements of neck at the most prominent part of the swelling is employed to assess the increase or decrease in the size of the thyroid swelling during treatment.

☞ Note the toxic manifestations. These are discussed under thyrotoxicosis. Fine tremors can be seen on extending hands in front of the body.

☞ Ascertain whether there are features of hypothyroidism (read hypothyroidism). Elicit deep tendon jerks for myxoedema.

In myxoedema, the deep tendon jerks show delayed relaxation after a normal contraction.

☞ To complete the examination of neck, palpate the cervical lymph nodes.

Palpable and enlarged cervical lymph nodes with goitre indicate malignancy of thyroid.

☞ Measurement of thyroid swelling.

Examination of Parathyroid Glands

Normally all the four parathyroid glands are embedded into the under surface of thyroid, hence, are not palpable unless they are enlarged too much. Therefore, in a patient with hyperparathyroidism, one should carefully palpate the parathyroid in the neck if parathyroid tumour is suspected as the cause. Most of the times, parathyroid enlargement or tumour is visualised radiologically by CT scan or radioactive scan.

On the other hand, hypoparathyroidism is manifested by tetany characterised by spontaneous twitchings or contractions of muscles in part or full. It occurs due to hypocalcaemia; hypokalemia, alkalosis and hypomagnesaemia.

Tetany can be latent which can be provoked by certain tests/manoeuvres discussed below:

☞ **Elicitation of Tetany (Fig. 9.5)**

1. *Trousseau's sign:* Apply a sphygmomanometer cuff above the elbow, inflate it above the systolic BP and maintain it for 3 minutes. Latent tetany will manifest with *accoucher's hand* (Fig. 9.5) in which wrist is flexed, the fingers and thumb get adducted and extended due to carpal spasms induced by hypocalcaemia.
2. *Chvostek's sign:* Tapping with hammer in front of tragus of the ear evokes facial spasms (twitchings) with each tap. About 5% normal persons may also give positive response.
3. *Schultz's sign:* Tapping at the centre of the tongue with finger produces local depression due to contraction of tongue muscles.

Endocrinal Disorders

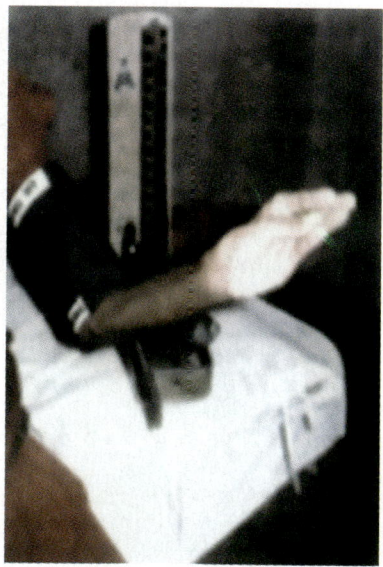

Fig. 9.5: Latent tetany: Trousseau's sign. Inflation of a sphygmomanometer cuff for a few minutes induced typical carpal spasm with flexion of wrist and thumb with hypertension of remaining fingers (*main d'accoucheur hand or obstetric hand*).

EXAMINATION OF THE BREAST AS A PART OF ENDOCRINE SYSTEM

Examination of breast and axilla has been described as separate unit VII.

Examine the breast for endocrinological point of view as follows.

A. Examination of Male Breasts

☞ *Examine the male breasts for gynaecomastia*

Gynaecomastia means enlargement of male breast similar to female. This can be detected by palpation with palm of the hand or palpation of breast tissue with fingers for any nodule.

The presence of subareolar nodule >0.5 cm in diameter suggests gynaecomastia which may be **physiological** or **pathological**.
Pathological gynaecomastia must be suspected when the glandular tissue or nodule is >4.0 cm in diameter and is gradually progressive.

Gynaecomastia must be distinguished from subareolar fat deposition by texture and shape of the breast. Comparison of the breast with nearby subcutaneous tissue provides a definite diagnosis.

☞ Note whether gynaecomastia is unilateral (Fig. 9.6) or bilateral.

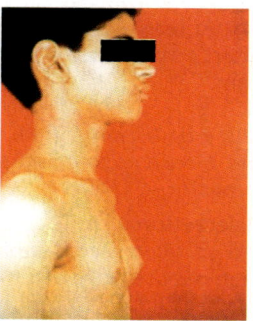

Fig. 9.6: Unilateral (left breast) gynaecomastia in an adolescent.

- The causes of gynaecomastia have already been given at the beginning in Table 9.1.
- Read the gynaecomastia in cirrhosis of liver (Unit VI).

True gynaecomastia is hard and tender.
Mammoplasia is soft gynaecomastia, occurs following oestrogen therapy.

☞ *Note whether breast enlargement is associated with generalised adiposity. Note the consistency and tenderness.*

Adiposogenital syndromes are characterised by breast enlargement, obesity and hypogonadism.

☞ *Examine the enuchoid features, i.e. body proportions, secondary sexual characters and gonads*

- Gynaecomastia, enuchoidism, small testes (hypogonadism) are characteristics of Klinefelter's syndrome.

B. Examination of Female Breasts

☞ *Examine the female breast for atrophy (Fig. 9.7)*

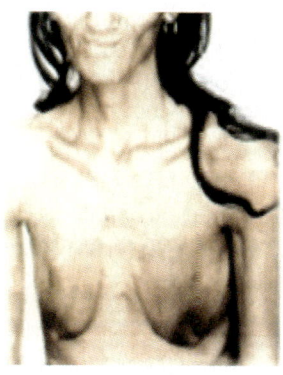

Fig. 9.7: Sheehan's syndrome. Note the atrophy of the breasts with failure of lactation.

Breast atrophy in females is seen in Addison's disease, Sheehan's syndrome (Fig. 9.7) and panhypopituitarism.

☞ *Also ask about any discharge from the nipples and when it occurs. Does it occur on squeezing the nipple or is spontaneous?*

Inappropriate secretion of milk in a non-lactating female is called *galactorrhoea* (see Fig. 7.3) may be *physiological*, i.e. occurs only after squeezing the nipple or *pathological* (i.e. occurs spontaneously and can be seen as wetting of bra or night clothes without local stimulation.

☞ *Try to demonstrate galactorrhoea by compressing the areola with your index finger placed in radial position around the nipple.*

Milky discharge in non-lactating female should be investigated. It could be due to hormones or drugs.

☞ *Is it unilateral or bilateral?*

Galactorrhoea invariably is bilateral occurs either due to hyperprolactinaemia (prolactin secreting tumour, hypothyroidism, drugs, idiopathic) or due to increased sensitivity to prolactin.

EXAMINATION OF ADRENAL GLANDS

Adrenals are situated just in relation to upper poles of kidneys. Adrenal glands are not palpable normally but become palpable as renal masses if they assume large size. Adrenal tumours are common in childhood (neuroblastomas) or in adults (phaeochromocytoma, adrenal adenoma/carcinorna).

Bilateral adrenal hyperplasia, a common cause of Cushing's syndrome, produces mild enlargement of adrenals which are not palpable. Special radiological procedures, i.e. ultrasonography, CT scanning, MRI and isotope scanning are done to detect them. Their functional status is determined by estimating hormonal levels in peripheral venous blood or blood obtained by selective venous adrenal catheterisation.

EXAMINATION OF GENITALIA

The genital examination has already been discussed under the examination of genitourinary system examination in Unit IV. Here, the examination of testes and ovaries being a part of endocrine system, will be discussed.

☞ *Inspection of testes and secondary sexual characters*
- Look at the amount and distribution of body hair including beard growth, axillary hair and pubic hair. Note the presence of male pattern baldness. Note the presence of gynaecomastia and galactorrhoea as already described.

- The failure of development of secondary sexual character indicates prepubertal hypogonadism (Fig. 9.8). While loss of libido and impotence suggest post-pubertal hypogonadism.
- Appearance of primary and secondary sexual characters in a male or female before 7 years of age is called *isosexual precocious puberty*.

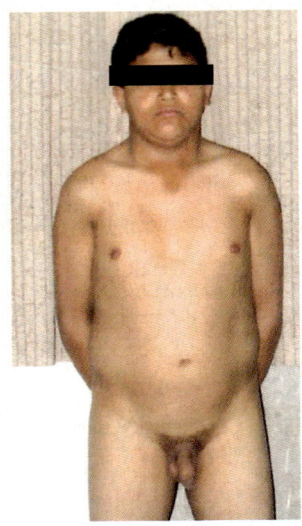

Fig. 9.8: Prepubertal hypergonadotrophic hypogonadism (Klinefelter's syndrome—46 XXY). Note the small penis with very small testes which are firm on palpation. Note the bilateral gynaecomastia and enuchoidism.

☞ *Note the presence or absence of testes in the scrotum.*

- Absence of testes in the scrotum is called **anorchia** while hidden testes with empty scrotum is called **cryptorchidism**.

☞ *Assess the testicular volume by palpation as well as measure its volume by Prader orchidometer.*

Prepubertal testicular volume is <4 ml. Increased volume implies pubertal gonadotrophin stimulation.

The approximate ranges of testicular size are as follows:

Age	Testicular volume (ml)	Testicular length in cm	Testicular width in cm
Prepubertal	3–4	<3	<2
Postpubertal	4–15	3–4	2–3
Adult	20–30	4.5–5.5	2.8–3.3

☞ Note the consistency of the testes

> The testes are small and firm in Klinefelter's syndrome and prepubertal hypogonadism (Fig. 9.8).
> The testes are soft and small in acquired hypogonadism or postpubertal hypogonadism.

☞ Inspect the external genital parts in female. Note the signs of virilisation.

> Enlargement of clitoris is a feature of androgen excess. The signs of virilisation are deepening of the voice, temporal balding, clitoromegaly and increased muscle mass.

SYSTEMIC EXAMINATION

The main systems involved in endocrinological disorders are cardiovascular and nervous system. The examination of both these systems have been dealt as separate chapters. The same steps of examination are applied here. However, the findings in system in relation to endocrine glands are discussed below:

- In case of carcinoma thyroid, always look for the metastatic manifestations in the lungs, liver and bone both clinically and on investigations.
- In case of anaplastic carcinoma of thyroid, even non-metastatic manifestations may occur. These should be looked and patient should be investigated for the following features and hormones.

Manifestation	Hormone/peptide secreted
1. Syndrome of inappropriate secretion of ADH	ADH-like peptide/substance
2. Hypercalcaemia	Parathormone-like peptide
3. Hypoglycaemia	Insulin-like peptide
4. Hyperthyroidism	TSH-like substance
5. Cushing's syndrome	ACTH

Rarely bronchial carcinoid produces growth hormone or GHRH. Carcinoma lungs and kidney may produce chorionic gonadotrophins.

Cardiovascular System

Pulse: Both tachycardia (hyperthyroidism, phaeochromocytoma, Conn's syndrome) and bradycardia (hypothyroidism) may be recorded. Bounding pulses and dancing carotid indicate hyperthyroidism. Arrhythmias (AF) are common in thyroid disorders, e.g. thyrotoxicosis.

BP: High BP suggests Conn's syndrome, Cushing's syndrome, phaeochromocytoma, hyperthyroidism, hypothyroidism while **low BP or hypotension** is recorded in Addison's disease, postural hypotension due to diabetic autonomic neuropathy or hypoglycaemia, Addison's disease. **Apex beat** may be **hyperdynamic** (thyrotoxicosis, phaeochromocytoma) or **hypodynamic** (hypothyroidism). **Cardiomegaly** can occur due to thyrotoxic heart disease and diabetic cardiomyopathy.

Auscultation of the heart may reveal benign flow murmur (thyrotoxicosis), arrhythmias, etc.

NERVOUS SYSTEM

Higher function. Cognitive function may be sometimes impaired in diabetes and due to repeated episodes of hypoglycaemia.

Cranial nerves. Cranial nerves (3, 4, 6th) may be involved in diabetes. Cerebrovascular accidents are also common in diabetes.

Motor System

- *Proximal myopathy* with positive *Gower's sign* is seen in Cushing's syndrome, thyrotoxicosis and diabetic amyotrophy.
- *Periodic muscle paralysis* is seen in Conn's syndrome.
- *Peripheral neuropathies* (sensorimotor) with loss of tendon jerks are seen in diabetes.
- *Hyper-reflexia* is seen in thyrotoxicosis and phaeochromocytoma while delayed relaxation of jerks is seen in myxoedema.

Sensory System

- *Carpal tunnel syndrome* or entrapment neuropathy is seen in hypothyroidism, pregnancy, etc.
- *Peripheral neuropathy* (loss of all types of sensation) occurs in diabetes.
- *Autonomic neuropathy* with postural hypotension, decreased libido, etc. occurs in diabetes.

Gait Abnormalities

- Ataxia or gait abnormalities are common due to peripheral neuropathy, myopathy and osteomalacia.

BRIEF SYNOPSIS OF ENDOCRINAL DISORDERS

GOITRE

The enlargement of thyroid gland is called *goitre*. It may be *physiological* (puberty) or *pathological*. It may be *diffuse* (Graves' disease, Hashimoto's thyroiditis, iodine deficiency, congenital or dyshormonogenesis) or *nodular* (single nodular or multinodular toxic or non-toxic goitre).

The **causes** of goitre are:
1. *Physiological*
    - Puberty (Fig. 9.9A)
    - Pregnancy
2. *Autoimmune*
    - Graves' disease (Fig. 9.4B)
    - Hashimoto's disease (Fig. 9.9B)
3. *Thyroiditis*
    - Acute (de Quervain's thyroiditis)
    - Chronic fibrotic (Riedel's thyroiditis)
4. *Iodine deficiency goitre*
5. *Dyshormonogenesis*
6. *Goitrogens* (e.g. sulphonylureas)
7. *Multinodular goitre* (Fig. 9.9C)
8. *Diffuse goitre* (unknown cause)
    - Colloid
    - Simple
9. *Cysts and tumours*
    - Adenoma
    - Carcinoma
    - Lymphoma
10. *Miscellaneous*
    - Sarcoidosis
    - Tuberculosis

Grading of Goitre (WHO)
Grade 0: Neither palpable nor visible goitre
Grade 1: Palpable goitre
 A: Goitre detectable only on palpation.
 B: Goitre palpable and visible with neck extended
Grade 2: Goitre visible with neck in normal position
Grade 3: Large goitre visible from a distance

Differential Diagnosis of Goitre
Differential diagnosis is discussed depending on the characteristics of the goitre as follows:
1. *Shape*. The regular, smooth, symmetric enlargement of thyroid occurs in Graves' disease and thyroiditis; while irregular enlargement is seen in solitary nodule or multinodular goitre.
2. *Size*. Large goitres are usually autoimmune, multinodular or malignant in origin whereas small goitres are seen during puberty, pregnancy, thyroiditis and dyshormonogenesis.
3. *Mobility*. Most goitres move upwards with swallowing except vary large goitre occupying the all available space in the neck. However, absence of mobility indicates invasive thyroid carcinoma leading to fixation of thyroid gland.
4. *Consistency*. The goitre is **soft** in Graves' disease, **firm** in Hashimoto's thyroiditis, and **hard** in malignancy.
5. *Surface*. The **surface is smooth** in Graves' disease, thyroiditis (Hashimoto's or viral) and iodine deficiency or puberty goitre. It is **nodular** in multinodular goitre or malignancy of thyroid.
6. *Tenderness*. Diffuse tenderness indicates infection or inflammation of thyroid (thyroiditis) while localised tenderness may occur following bleeding into a cyst.
7. *Bruit and a thrill*. **A palpable thrill** or an **audible vascular bruit** may be associated with Graves' disease, indicates increased blood flow through the thyroid gland (murmur), must be distinguished from a murmur arising in the carotid artery or transmitted from the aorta and from a venous hum originating in the internal jugular vein.

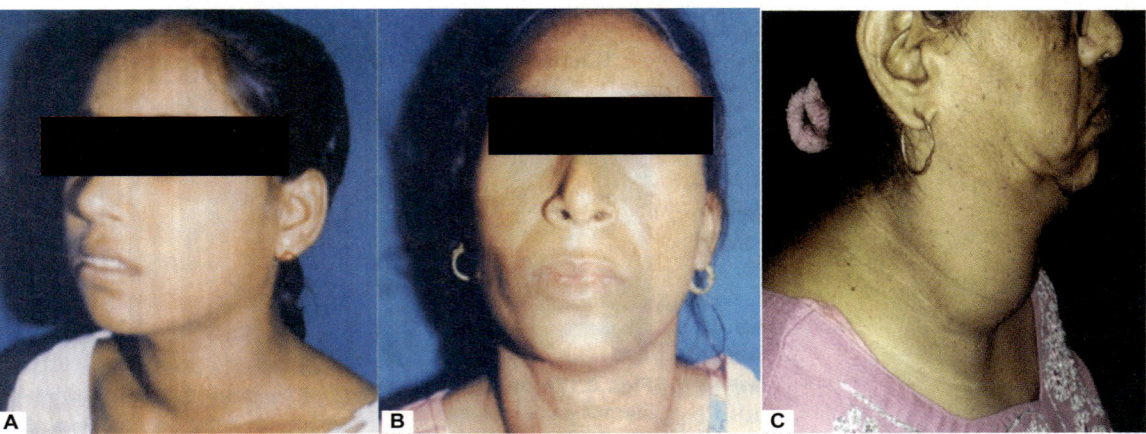

Figs 9.9A to C: (A) Puberty goitre (physiological); The thyroid is mildly enlarged in a 14-year-old girl; (B) Hashimoto's thyroiditis. The thyroid is diffusely enlarged; (C) Multinodular goitre. Note the multiple thyroid nodules enlargement of the thyroid.

8. *Other features*. The goitre may or may not be associated with systemic features (hyper- or hypothyroidism).

THYROTOXICOSIS

Definition: Thyrotoxicosis implies a state of hyperthyroidism in which the thyroid hormone is toxic to the tissues producing clinical features; while hyperthyroidism simply implies excessive thyroid function. However, both are not synonymous, yet are used interchangeably.

Graves' disease: It is an autoimmune disorder characterised by *hyperthyroidism, diffuse goitre, ophthalmopathy, dermopathy (pretibial myxoedema)* and *thyroid acropatchy (clubbing fingers)*. A thyroid scan and anti-thyroid antibodies (TPO, TRAb) are diagnostic.

Causes of Thyrotoxicosis

- Graves' disease.
- Multinodular goitre.
- Autonomously functioning solitary thyroid nodule.
- Thyroiditis, e.g. subacute (de Quervain's) and postpartum.
- Drug-induced (e.g. amiodarone, radioactive contrast media or iodine prophylaxis programme).
- Factitious (self-induced).
- Struma ovarii.
- Pituitary or ectopic TSH.
- Thyroid carcinoma.

Clinical Manifestations (Table 9.3)

Eye Signs and their Methods of Demonstration

☞ One should look for the various eye signs (Table 9.4)

1. **Lid Lag and Lid Retraction:** Lid retraction means the upper eyelid is pulled higher up than the lower leading to exposure of the upper cornea (Fig. 9.3). It is due to overactivity of smooth muscles inserted into levator palpebral superioris. In exophthalmos, the lower eyelid is also retracted exposing the lower sclerae (Fig. 9.3).

    Lid lag (*von Graefe's sign*) means the upper lid lag behind the movements of the eyeball when patient looks downward following an examiner's finger moving downwards from above (Fig. 9.11).

Both lid retraction (Fig. 9.13, Daivympie's sign) and lid lag are not synonymous with exophthalmos. They are part of exophthalmos.

TABLE 9.3: Clinical Features of Hyperthyroidism

1. **Goitre** (diffuse or nodular)
   - Diffuse goitre indicates Graves' disease while nodularity indicates toxic nodular (single or multiple) goitre
2. **Gastrointestinal**
   - Weight loss inspite of good appetite
   - Vomiting, diarrhoea or steatorrhoea
3. **Cardiovascular**
   - High resting pulse rate or sinus tachycardia
   - Good volume pulse with wide pulse pressure (more than 60 mm of Hg)
   - Exertional dyspnoea
   - Arrhythmias (artrial fibrillation is commonest). To and fro murmur may be present.
   - Precipitation of angina in patients of ischaemic heart disease
4. **Neuromuscular**
   - Nervousness, irritability
   - Restlessness, psychosis
   - Tremors of hands
   - Muscular weakness, mostly proximal
   - Exaggerated tendon reflexes
5. **Dermatological**
   - Perspiration (increased sweating or hyperhidrosis, wet red palms)
   - Clubbing of fingers (rare)
   - Loss of hairs
   - Pre-tibial myxoedema
6. **Reproductive**
   - Menstrual irregularity (amenorrhoea is commonest)
   - Abortions, infertility
   - Loss of libido or impotence
7. **Ophthalmological**
   - Lid lag or lid retraction
   - Staring look, wide palpebral fissures
   - Exophthalmos, excessive watering of eyes
   - Diplopia (double vision) or ophthalmoplegia
8. **Miscellaneous**
   - Heat intolerance (an important symptom)
   - Excessive thirst (polydipsia)
   - Outburst of anger
   - Fatiguability and apathy

2. **Exophthalmos (proptosis):** It means protusion of the eyeballs within the orbit due to push from behind due to increase in retrobulbar fat or oedema or cellular infiltration. This results in the prominence of the eyeball, staring look, retraction of the eyelids, and clear visibility of

TABLE 9.4: Various Eye Signs in Thyrotoxicosis

Joffroy's sign: Slightly flex the neck with face looking downward. Now ask the patient to make wrinkles over forehead by looking up. Absence of wrinkling indicates the sign is positive (Fig. 9.10).

Moebius sign: This means inability or failure to converge the eyeball (Fig. 9.12) when a finger is brought in front of the eyes.

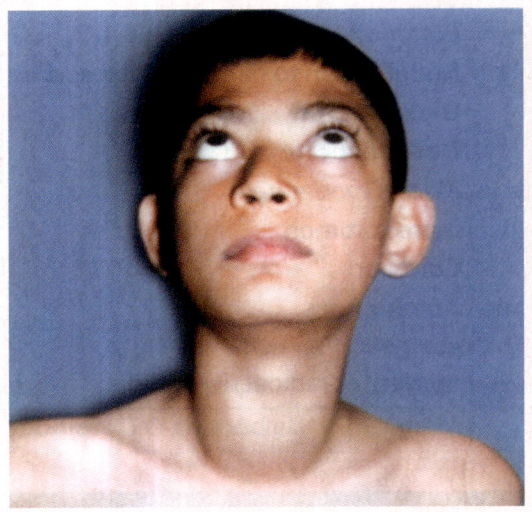

Fig. 9.10: Loss of furrows on looking up—Joffroy's sign positive.

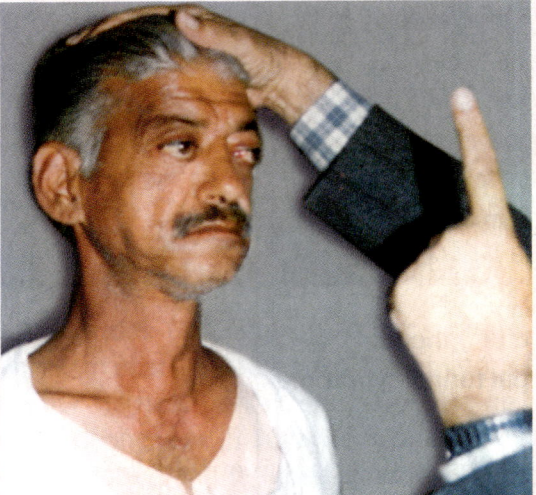

Fig. 9.12: Failure of accommodation (internal opthalmoplegia) in a patient of exophthalmos (Moebius sign positive).

von Graefe's sign (lid lag, Fig. 9.11). Ask the patient first look straight. Bring your index finger in front of one eye. Now instruct the patient to follow the movements of the finger which is moved slowly from above downwards. The upper eyelid lags behind the eyeball which is easily appreciated.

Daivympie's sign (lid retraction): This means the visibility of lower sclera due to retraction of the lower eyelid (Fig. 9.13). Ask the patient to look straight, the visibility of lower sclera indicates positive sign.

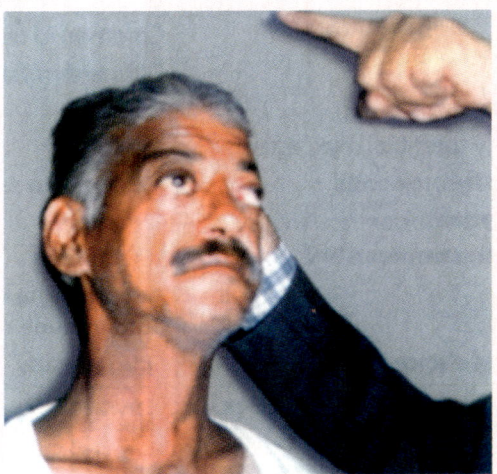

Fig. 9.11: Failure of elevation of upper eyelids on looking upwards due to inactivity of levator palpebral superioris. The upper lid does not move or lags behind due to levator palpebral muscle paralysis.

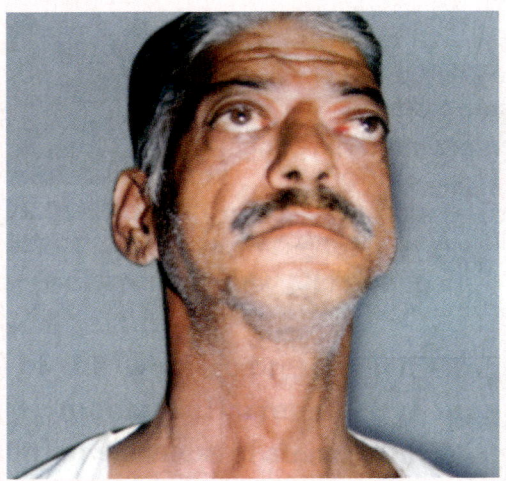

Fig. 9.13: Lower palpebral conjunctiva is clearly visible in a patient of thyrotoxicosis with bilateral ptosis (external ophthalmoplegia). In a patient with ophthalmoplegia with ptosis, the visibility of the lower sclera indicates lid retraction.

the upper and lower sclerae. Note the following signs:
- **Ophthalmoplegia:** This means weakness of extraocular muscles due to oedema or cellular infiltration leading to ptosis as a result of involvement of levator palpabral superioris, inward eyeball movement (lateral rectus palsy) or outward deviation of the eyeball (medial rectus palsy). These muscles palsy result in diplopia and prevents the patient looking upwards and inwards.
- Internal ophthalmoplegia (Moebius sign) due to failure of accommodation (Fig. 9.12).
- *Inability to wrinkle* (Joffroy's sign (Fig. 9.10). There is inability to wrinkle the forehead.
- **Chemosis:** It means oedema of the conjunctivae which become oedematous, thickened and wrinkled. It is due to venous and lymphatic obstruction of conjunctivae by proptosis.

As a mnemonic, the NO SPECS scheme is used to class the eye signs as follows:
0 = No sign or symptom
1 = Only sign (lid lag or retraction), no symptoms
2 = Soft tissue involvement (pretibial myxoedema)
3 = Proptosis (>22 mm)
4 = Extraocular muscle involvement (diplopia)
5 = Corneal involvement
6 = Sight loss

☞ One should look for pretibial skin thickening

Pretibial myxoedema (Fig. 9.14): It is a sign of Graves' disease. The name justifies the site of skin changes, i.e. over the anterior and lateral aspects of the lower leg. The typical skin change is non-inflamed, indurated, pink or purple colour plaque giving an 'orange-skin' appearance. Nodular involvement can uncommonly occur.

Diagnosis of Thyrotoxicosis

It is made by clinical features, and confirmation is done by increased RAIU, high T_3 and T_4 with low TSH (Graves' disease) or high TSH (pituitary disease) and presence of antithyroid antibodies in Graves' disease or autoimmune thyroiditis with thyrotoxicosis.

Differential Diagnosis of Thyrotoxicosis

The two common conditions causing thyrotoxicosis are compared in Table 9.5.

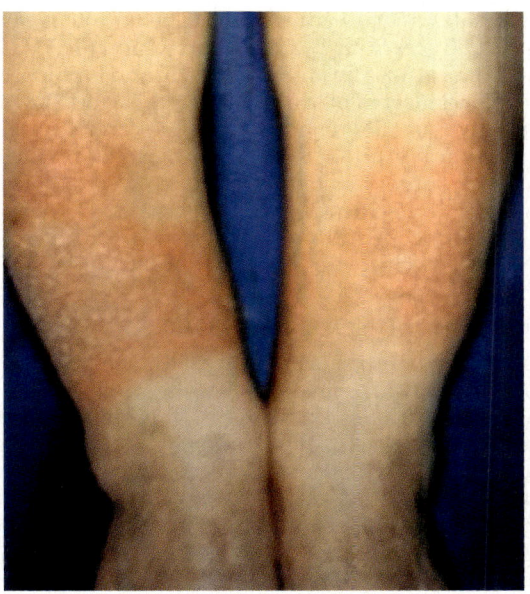

Fig. 9.14: Pretibial myxoedema.

TABLE 9.5: Differential Diagnosis of Thyrotoxicosis

Feature	Graves' disease	Toxic multi-nodular goitre
Age	Young age	Old age
Sex	Common in females	Common in females
Goitre	Diffuse, firm, smooth. Bruit is heard commonly	Nodular, firm to hard, irregular surface. No bruit
Eye signs	Common	Uncommon
Dermopathy (pretibial myxoedema)	May occur	Does not occur
Severity of thyrotoxicosis	Moderate to severe	Mild to moderate
Atrial fibrillation	Common	More common
Compression symptoms	Uncommon	Common
Cause	Autoimmune, may be associated with other autoimmune diseases	Autonomous
Treatment of choice	Drug therapy	Surgery or radioactive iodine

SOLITARY TOXIC NODULE

It is less common cause of thyrotoxicosis than multinodular goitre (MNG). It occurs commonly in females over 40 years of age. The nodule is toxic and produces both T_3 and T_4 and inhibits TSH. The adenoma is usually large 2.5–3.0 cm and is palpable. The **diagnosis** is made by elevated T_3 and T_4 with low levels of TSH. The radioisotope scan will reveal a hot nodule in one of the lobes of thyroid. **Treatment** is either surgery or radioactive ablation with large dose of ^{131}I (15–25 mCi). Permanent hypothyroidism does not occur following surgery or radioactive therapy.

TOXIC MULTINODULAR GOITRE

It is more common in females over the age of 60 years. Thyroid hormone levels are elevated. The goitre is large and nodules are seen or felt on palpation of thyroid (Fig. 9.4A). These patients of MNG present with cardiovascular complications (atrial fibrillation or CHF) more frequently than other systemic manifestations. **Treatment** is radioactive ablation by high dose of ^{131}I (15–30 mCi). If symptoms of compression are present (dysphonia or dysphagia, hoarse voice), then partial thyroidectomy is preferred to relieve the symptoms. Hypothyroidism is less common. Antithyroid drugs cannot be used for long time due to frequent relapse after drug withdrawal.

HYPOTHYROIDISM

Definition: Hypothyroidism is a clinical condition characterised by low levels of circulating thyroid hormones. It is called *primary* when the cause of it lies in the thyroid gland itself. It becomes *secondary* when hypothyroidism occurs due to disease of anterior pituitary or hypothalamus.

Goitrous hypothyroidism means enlargement of thyroid gland associated with hypothyroidism.

Subclinical hypothyroidism means biochemical evidence of hypothyroidism (normal T_3 and T_4 but raised TSH) without any symptoms of hypothyroidism (*asymptomatic hypothyroidism*).

Causes of Adult Hypothyroidism

1. *Idiopathic or spontaneous or atrophic*
2. *Goitrous*
   a. Hashimoto's thyroiditis.
   b. Deficiency of iodine.
   c. Drug-induced (para-aminosalicylic acid, phenylbutazone, lithium and iodides).
   d. Dyshormonogenesis (heritable biosynthetic defect).
3. *Postablative*
   a. Following surgery.
   b. Following ^{131}I.
4. *Transient* due to thyroiditis (self-limiting).
5. *Maternally transmitted* (iodides, antithyroid drugs).

Transient hypothyroidism refers to a state of reversible thyroid function, often observed in following situations:
   i. During the first 6 months after subtotal thyroidectomy or radioactive ^{131}I treatment for Graves' disease.
   ii. Post-thyrotoxic phase of subacute thyroiditis.
   iii. Post-partum thyroiditis.
   iv. In some neonates, transplacental passage of TSH receptor-binding antibodies (TRABs) from the mother with Graves' disease or autoimmune thyroid disease may cause transient hypothyroidism.

Transient hypothyroidism may persist for many years as sub-clinical hypothyroidism. Treatment with replacement therapy with small dose of thyroxine is indicated.

Congenital hypothyroidism is asymptomatic state detected during routine screening of TSH levels in blood spot samples obtained 5–7 days after birth. It results either from thyroid agenesis, ectopic hypoplastic glands or from dyshormonogenesis. Early detection and early treatment with replacement thyroxine therapy is mandatory to prevent irreversible brain damage.

Clinical Features (Fig. 9.15)

1. **General features**
   - Tiredness, weight gain, cold intolerance, hoarseness of voice and lethargy are common.
   - Somnolence and goitre are less common.
2. **Cardiovascular**
   - Slow pulse rate or bradycardia, hypertension and xanthelasma are common.
   - Pericardial effusion, precipitation of angina and cardiac failure less common.
3. **Neuromuscular**
   - Aches and pains, delayed relaxation of ankel jerks, muscle stiffness are common.
   - Carpal tunnel syndrome, deafness, psychosis, depression, myotonia are less common.
4. **Haematological**
   - Anaemia may be present
5. **Dermatological**
   - Dry thick skin (toad skin, Fig. 9.15B), sparse hair, non-pitting oedema are common.
   - Vitiligo and alopecia are rare.

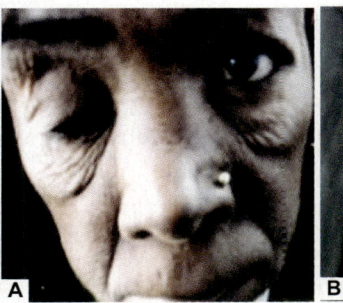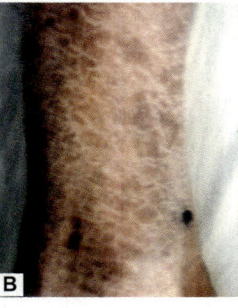

Figs 9.15A and B: Myxoedema. (A) Periorbital oedema; (B) Toad-like skin: Note the skierry, thick, rough skin with fine demarcations. There is diffuse hair loss.

6. **Reproductive**
   - Menorrhagia, infertility (common), galactorrhoea and impotence (less common).
7. **Gastrointestinal**
   - Constipation (common) and adyamic ileus (less common).

Differential Diagnosis of Goitrous Hypothyroidism

The difference between simple diffuse goitre and Hashimoto's thyroiditis is given in Table 9.6

TABLE 9.6: Differentiation Between Two Common Causes of Diffuse Goitre

Simple diffuse goitre	Goitre due to Hashimoto thyroiditis
No symptom except swelling	Pain, fever and difficulty in swallowing
Common in young girls (15–25 years) or during pregnancy.	Common in young or middle-aged females (30–50 years)
Mild, tends to be noticed by friends and relative	Large goitre
Soft, non-tender	Firm, tender
Endemic or sporadic	Sporadic
Asymptomatic or there is a tight sensation in neck	Pain radiating to jaw or neck, increased during swallowing, coughing and neck movement
Suboptimal dietary iodine intake and minor degrees of dyshormonogenesis are its causes	Autoimmune disease
Normal thyroid status	25% cases are hypothyroid at presentation, others become later on
Negative antithyroid antibodies	Positive (95% cases)

HASHIMOTO'S THYROIDITIS

It is a common cause of goitre with hypothyroidism. It is an autoimmune disorder. It has slow insidious onset. It affects mostly females in the age group of 30–50 years. The thyroid is diffusely enlarge, occupies major portion of neck, soft or rubbery in consistency and tender on palpation (Fig. 9.9B). Enlargement of thyroid is due to infiltration of thyroid with lymphocytes and there is follicular cell hyperplasia. There is fibrosis at the end and thyroid enlargement starts regressing. It may be associated with other autoimmune disorders.

About one-fourth of patients are hypothyroid at the time of presentation and have symptoms and signs of hypothyroidism. In the remainder, the euthyroid status is maintained by normal T_4 and normal or raised TSH levels, majority of these patients also develop hypothyroidism later on. Antithyroid antibodies and thyroid peroxidase antibodies are present in high titres and are diagnostic.

GIGANTISM AND ACROMEGALY

Gigantism is a disorder due to excess of GH before fusion of epiphyses resulting in tall stature with stout muscular built; while GH excess after fusion of epiphyses results in normal stature with enlargement of acral parts (hands and feet), a condition called **acromegaly** (Fig. 9.16). If GH excess occurs during puberty before fusion of epiphyses and continues after that will lead to a clinical picture of **gigantoacromegaly**. The most common cause is a pituitary tumour or prolactinoma. The effect of excess of GH is visible on all tissues, bones, hands and feet (Fig. 9.16). In addition, compression effects of the pituitary tumour may be noticeable if present. The symptoms and signs of GH excess are given in Table 9.7.

CUSHING SYNDROME (Table 9.8 and Fig. 9.17)

Cushing's syndrome is a clinical condition characterised by increased levels of free circulating

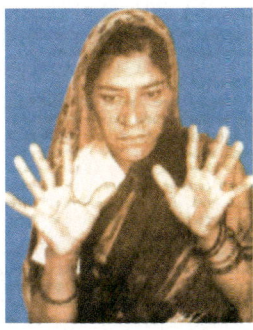

Fig. 9.16: Acromegaly (excess of GH after the epiphyses have fused). Note the stout stock built with spade-like hands and short stubby fingers.

TABLE 9.7: Clinical Manifestations of GH Excess (Gigantism/Acromegaly)

System	Symptoms	Signs
General	Fatigue, perspiration, heat intolerance and weight gain	Stout built, overweight and coarse facial features.
Skin and soft tissues	• Large hands and feet leading to increased in size of shoes and gloves • Oily skin • Hypertrichosis	• Moist, warm, stout hand with doughy hand shake, increased heel pad (>23 mm) • Skin tags • Acanthosis nigricans
Head	Headache, large head with increase in size of hat	• Frontal bossing, parotid enlargement
Eyes	Decreased vision	• Visual field defects
Ears and paranasal sinuses	Large ears and sinusitis	• Large ears and paranasal sinuses
Oral cavity and mouth	Large tongue, voice change, malocclusion of teeth; large thick lips • Prognathism	• Enlarged furrowed tongue with teeth indentation on it • Widely spaced teeth
CVS	Congestive heart failure	• Hypertension, cardiomegaly
Genitourinary system	Decreased libido, impotence, oligomenorrhoea	• Infertility
Neurological system	Paraesthesias, hypersomnolence, weakness	• Carpal tunnel syndrome, proximal myopathy
Skeletal system	Joint pains (shoulder, knees)	• Osteoarthritis

glucocorticoids and their effects on the various systems of the body. It occurs most often following the therapeutic administration of synthetic steroids or rarely a pituitary tumour or adrenal hyperplasia. It may be *primary* (e.g. adrenal disease) or *secondary* (hypothalamic-pituitary disease). Cushingoid features (pseudo-Cushing's syndrome) may be due to obesity or alcohol consumption.

Causes of Cushing's Syndrome

1. **Adrenal hyperplasia secondary to hypothalamic-pituitary involvement**
   - Pituitary-hypothalamic disorder
   - ACTH secreting tumour
   - Non-endocrine ACTH/CRH secreting tumours (para-neoplastic syndromes)
2. **Adrenal nodular hyperplasia**
3. **Neoplasm of the adrenals, e.g.** adenoma, carcinoma
4. **Iatrogenic,** e.g. prolonged use of corticosteroids, prolonged use of ACTH.

Clinical Manifestations (read Table 9.8)

The **clincial diagnosis** suggested by the clinical features is confirmed by raised plasma cortisol levels, loss of circadian rhythms of cortisol secretion and non-suppression of cortisol secretion by dexamethasone suppression test. ACTH levels differentiates between primary (↑ACTH) and secondary (↓ACTH) disease.

ADDISON'S DISEASE

It is defined as adrenocortical hormones insufficiency. It may be *primary* (adrenal disease) or *secondary* (pituitary or hypothalamic disease).

Causes

Common (in middle aged females)
- Autoimmune
- Sporadic
- MEN type I, II syndromes
- Tuberculosis
- Bilateral adrenalectomy

Rare
- Metastatic tumours
- Amyloidosis
- *Waterhouse-Friderichsen's syndrome* (adrenal haemorrhage in meningococcal infection)
- Haemochromatosis
- Adrenal infarction

Clinical features (Table 9.9 and Fig. 9.18)

PANHYPOPITUITARISM

Panhypopituitarism means deficiency of more than 2 pituitary hormones. It may be due to pituitary (*primary*) or hypothalamic involvement (secondary).

TABLE 9.8: The Clinical Features of Cushing's Syndrome

Symptoms	Figure	Signs
• Weight gain (94%) • Obesity, weight gain • Hirsutism (excessive facial hair) • Fatigue, muscle weakness and backache (85%) • Psychological changes and depression • Blackening of skin • Increased chances of fever, cough and other symptoms of infection • Menstrual irregularity, i.e. amenorrhoea (70%) • Polyuria, polydipsia (25%)	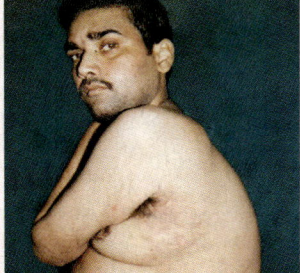 **Fig. 9.17:** Cushing's syndrome. Note the presence of moon-facies, truncal obesity and pink striae.	• Hirsutism (80%) • Oedema (60%) • Hypertension (80%) • Truncal or centripetal obesity (97%) • Camel hump • Moon-facies (Fig. 9.17) • Acne • Scanty menses • Cutaneous striae (65–70%), pinkish (Fig. 9.17) • Easy bruisability (55–60%) • Back pain, fracture and osteoporosis • Emotional lability and personality changes (60%) • Pigmentation • Hypokalaemic alkalosis • Predisposition to infection • Clitoromegaly (15%)

Note: The incidence of some symptoms and signs is indicated within bracket.

TABLE 9.9: Clinical Manifestations of Addison's Disease

Symptoms and signs

I. **Glucocorticoids insufficiency (↓ cortisol)**
 • Weight loss • Malaise
 • Nausea and anorexia
 • Vomiting

II. **Mineralocorticoids insufficiency (↓ aldosterone)**
 • Postural hypotension
 • Salt loss
 • Syncope

III. **Low of androgens levels**
 • Loss of axillary and pubic hair in females
 • Sparse body hair

IV. **Increased ACTH secretion**
 • Hyperpigmentation of sun-exposed areas, elbow, knees, creases of palm, knuckles, mucous membrane of mouth, scars, etc.

V. **General**
 • Fatigue
 • Asthenia or generalised weakness
 • Sunken eyeballs, cheeks, thin legs and oedema

Fig. 9.18: A patient of Addison's disease. Note sunken cheeks, eyeballs, dry pigmented skin and mucous membrane. Patient had long duration of diarrhoea and developed pedal oedema. Such a patient is likely to develop acute crisis during sepsis or surgery.

Diagnosis is clinical and confirmation is done by low levels of cortisol, aldosterone, androgens and high ACTH

Causes

1. **Hypothalamic causes**
   (a) *Congenital*
   • Gonadotrophin releasing hormone (GnRH) deficiency, i.e. Kallmann's syndrome
   • Isolated GH deficiency.
   (b) *Acquired*
   • Tumours such as craniopharyngioma
   • Radiation
   • Head injury
   • Tuberculosis or sarcoidosis
   • Histiocytosis X
2. **Pituitary causes**
   • Tumours
   • Surgery
   • Radiotherapy
   • Head injury
   • Postpartum necrosis (Sheehan's syndrome)
   • Autoimmune
   • Haemorrhage.

Clinical Features

Manifestations occur due to deficiency of pituitary hormones (Table 9.10). **Diagnosis** is confirmed by hormones assay.

CONGENITAL ADRENAL HYPERPLASIA

It is an inborn error of metabolism caused by defects in the biosynthesis of cortisol resulting in decreased secretion of glucocorticoids with compensatory oversecretion of ACTH by the pituitary which in turn leads to overproduction of intermediary compounds which are androgenic and cause virilisation. It is inherited as autosomal recessive trait, therefore, there is a 1:4 chance that the sibling of an affected parent will also have the disease.

The most common cause is C-21 hydroxylase deficiency. In about one-third of cases, the defect is severe (salt-losing variety) resulting in hypotension and hyponatremia. In non salt-losing variety, the secretion of aldosterone does not suffer, but features of cortisol deficiency and androgen excess are present.

Clinical Features

1. Hypotension, hypoglycaemia, salt loss (hyponatremia)
2. Signs of virilisation, i.e. clitoromegaly, ambigous genitals in girls, precocious pseudopuberty, hirsutism, amenorrhoea, infertility, pigmentation.

PHAEOCHROMOCYTOMA (CATECHOLAMINE EXCESS)

Phaeochromocytomas are uncommon, benign tumours of chromaffin tissues commonly arising from adrenal medulla (90%) which secrete epinephrine and norepinephrine. These tumours are associated with other endocrine tumours in MEN type I and type II syndrome.

Clinical Features

- Episodic or non-episodic hypertension with postural drop.
- Attacks of tachycardia, palpitation, sweating, pallor due to catecholamine excess.
- Headache, chest discomfort
- Anxiety, apprehension
- Abdominal pain, vomiting, constipation
- Glucose intolerance
- Weight loss and weakness.

Diagnosis and Differential Diagnosis

Diagnosis is made on clinical features and confirmed by high levels of plasma and urinary catecholamines (epinephrine, norepinephrines). It comes in differential diagnosis of all types of hypertension.

HYPERPARATHYROIDISM

A clinical condition characterised by excessive secretion of parathyroid hormone is called *hyperparathyroidism*. It may be *primary hyperparathyroidism* (autonomous parathyroid adenoma), *secondary hyperparathyroidism* (due to prolonged hypocalcaemia) and *tertiary hyperparathyroidism*. (Transformation of adenoma from prolonged secondary hyperparathyroidism.)

TABLE 9.10: Clinical Manifestations of Hypopituitarism

Deficiency of hormone	Manifestations
GH deficiency (Fig. 9.19)	• Short stature or growth failure in children • Fine wrinkling around the eyes and mouth, muscle mass decreased.
Gonodotrophin deficiency	• *In males:* Decreased libido, decreased beard and body hair and preservation of scalp hairline • *In females:* Amenorrhoea and infertility, loss of axillary and pubic hair
TSH deficiency	• Hypothyroidism features, e.g. fatigue, cold intolerance, thick puffy skin, no goitre
ACTH deficiency	Fatigue, decreased appetite, weight loss, decreased skin and nipple pigmentation, hypotension. No hyperpigmentation, hyperkalaemia or potassium loss—these are features of primary Addison's disease
Prolactin	• Failure of lactation in postpartum female
ADH deficiency	• Diabetes insipidus with polyuria and polydipsia

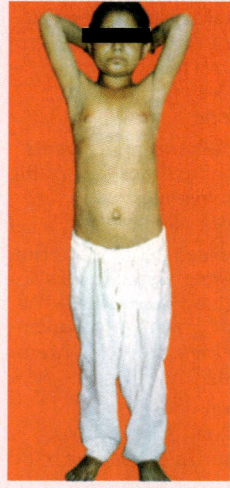

Fig. 9.19: An adolescent girl (16 years) with panhypopituitarism. Note the stunted growth, failure of secondary sexual characters, No menarche, thick skin, cold intolerance, weight loss.

Primary Hyperparathyroidism

This is the commonest parathyroid disorder seen in clinical practice (multiple renal calculi or recurrent renal stones). Most of the cases are asymptomatic or mildly symptomatic, hence, go undetected in early stage of the disease. It is more common in females than males (3:1). Majority of patients are above 50 years of age.

Clinical Features

I. **General**, e.g. weight loss, tiredness, lassitude
II. **G.I. tract**, e.g. nausea, vomiting, anorexia, constipation, peptic ulceration
III. **CNS**, e.g. drowsiness, lack of concentration, depression, myopathy (proximal)
IV. **Renal**, e.g. polyuria, polydipsia, stone formation and nephrocalcinosis
V. **Bone**, e.g. bone pain, tenderness, fractures, deformities, osteitis fibrosa cystica
VI. **Cartilage**, e.g. chondrocalcinosis
VII. **CVS**, e.g. hypertension
VIII. **Skin**, e.g. pruritus
IX. **The eyes**, e.g. corneal calcification
X. **Soft tissue**, e.g. ectopic calcification

Diagnosis is based on clinical features, family history, confirmation is done by hypercalcaemia with low PTH level.

Differential Diagnosis of Hypercalcaemia vis à vis Hyperparathyroidism

In addition to hyperparathyroidism, there are large number of conditions that are associated with hypercalcaemia with high or low PTH levels, i.e.
1. Hypercalcaemia with raised PTH levels
   - Hyperparathyroidism.
   - Chronic renal failure (tertiary hyperparathyroidism).
2. Conditions associated with hypercalcaemia and low or undetectable PTH levels
   a. Multiple myeloma
   b. Sarcoidosis
   c. Hyperparathyroidism
   d. Thiazide diuretics
   e. Milk-alkali syndrome
   f. Familial

HYPOPARATHYROIDISM

It is a disorder of parathyroid glands characterised by low levels of calcium either due to deficient production of *parathormone* (PTH) or its unresponsiveness. It may be *true* (↓PTH level) or *pseudohypoparathyroidism/PTH resistance* (normal or high PTH).

Causes
1. Postablative or postoperative
2. Idiopathic (autoimmune)
3. Infantile hypoparathyroidism (DiGeorge's syndrome)
4. Pseudohypoparathyroidism mostly congenital
5. Pseudopseudohypoparathyroidism

Clinical Features
- Tetany
- Cataract
- Psychosis
- Basal ganglia calcification
- Epilepsy
- Papilloedema
- Candidiasis of nails, skin and mucous membrane, if associated with candidiasis endocrinopathy.

Diagnosis and Differential Diagnosis

Diagnosis is made by clinical features of tetany and confirmation is done by low PTH level. For differential diagnosis, read Table 9.11.

TABLE 9.11: Distinguishing Features of Idiopathic Hypoparathyroidism and Pseudohypoparathyroidism

Idiopathic hypoparathyroidism	*Pseudohypoparathyroidism*
• Acquired	• Congenital
• Autoimmunity plays role in some cases	• Non-responsiveness to PTH either due to receptor or post-receptor defect
• PTH levels are low	• PTH levels are elevated
• Besides tetany, other features are epilepsy, psychosis, cataract, calcification of basal ganglia and papilloedema	• Besides tetany, other features include mental retardation and skeletal abnormalities, i.e. short stature and short 4th and 5th metacarpals and metatarsals

TETANY

This is a clinical condition characterised by low levels of ionised calcium leading to increased neuromuscular excitability. In this condition, total levels of calcium may even remain normal.

Causes
It may be due to hypocalcaemia, hypomagnesaemia and alkalosis.

Hypocalcaemia (Fig. 9.5) is due to;
1. Malabsorption
2. Osteomalacia

3. Hypoparathyroidism
4. Chronic renal failure
5. Acute pancreatitis
6. Anticonvulsants, e.g. dilantin

Hypomagnesaemia, alkalosis and hypokalaemia result from:
1. Repeated vomiting.
2. Excessive intake of alkalies.
3. Hysterical hyperventilation leading to alkalosis.
4. Primary hyperaldosteronism.
5. Acute anion load (citrate, lactate, HCO_3, etc.).

Clincial Features

Children: A characterisitic *triad of carpopedal spasm, stridor* and *convulsions* is common. The hands in carpopedal spasm adopt a peculiar posture in which there is flexion at metacarpophalangeal joints and there is opposition of thumb (*main d'accoucheur hand, see Fig. 1.18*). Pedal spasms are less frequent. The stridor (loud sound) is caused by closure of glottis.

Adults: Tingling sensations in the peripheral parts of limbs or around the mouth. Less often, painful carpopedal spasms may occur. Stridor and convulsions are rare.

Latent tetany: The absence of symptoms and signs of tetany in a patient with hypocalcaemia is called *latent tetany*. The signs of tetany can be induced by provocative tests.

Trousseau's sign: Raising the blood pressure above systolic level by inflation of sphygomomanometer cuff produces characteristic carpal spasm within 3–5 minutes (Fig. 9.5).

Chvostek's sign: A tap at facial nerve at angle of jaw produces twitchings of facial muscles.

HYPOGONADISM

Hypogonadism means hypofunctioning of the gonads which manifest either by deficiency in gametogenesis and/or decreased secretion of gonadal hormones. **Symptoms** of hypogonadism depend primarily on the age of the patient at the time of development. Hypogonadism is seldom recognised before the age of the puberty unless it is associated with growth retardation or other anatomic or endocrine abnormalities. The causes of hypogonadism are listed in Table 9.12.

The features of hypogonadism in males and females are given in Table 9.13. The *primary* hypogonadism means involvement of gonads while *secondary* is due to hypothalamic pituitary disease.

DIABETES MELLITUS (Fig. 9.19)

It is a metabolic disorder characterised by hyperglycaemia, glycosuria due to either lack of insulin

TABLE 9.12: Causes of Hypogonadism

1. **Primary gonadal disease**

In males: Cryptorchidism, torsion of testis, castration (removal, chemotherapy, irradiation), orchitis, systemic diseases (CRF, hepatic failure, sickle cell anaemia), alcohol and drugs

In females: polycystic ovarian syndrome, oophrectomy, castration (irradiation/chemotherapy), systemic diseases (CRF, liver failure), drugs, alcoholism

2. **Secondary (hypothalamic-pituitary disease hypogonadism)**
   - Hypopituitarism, hyperprolactinaemia
   - Kallmann's syndrome (hypogonadotrophic hypogonadism)

Diagnosis is established on history and physical examination corroborated by low gonadal hormones (testosterone/oestrogen) and high or low gonadotrophins (LH and FSH) depending on the cause.

TABLE 9.13: Clinical Features of Hypogonadism

In male	In female
I. Prepubertal hypogonadism	
• Scanty pubic and axillary hair	• Scanty pubic and axillary hair
• Enuchoidism	• Enuchoidism
• Reduced muscle mass and strength	• Reduced muscle mass
• Gynaecomastia	• Small atrophic breasts
• Persistent high-pitched voice	• Change in voice
• Small testes, phallus and prostate (Fig. 9.8)	• Small atrophic uterus and tubes
II. Postpubertal hypogonadism	
• Loss of libido	• Loss of libido
• Impotence	• Infertility
• Progressive decline in muscle mass	• Dry vagina and dyspareunia
• Oligospermia or azospermia	• Primary amenorrhoea

(type I) or insulin resistance (type 2). Diabetes mellitus (DM) may be *primary* (type 1 and type 2) or *secondary* due to pancreatic disease, endocrinopathies, drugs or genetic disorders. Type 1 diabetes is HLA-linked autoimmune insulinitis with destruction of Langerhans' cells in the pancreas while type 2 is related to insulin resistance due to several factors. The diagnostic criteria are given in Box 9.1.

Clinical Presentations of Diabetes Mellitus

1. **Type 1 diabetics** present with a *tetrad* of symptoms of hyperglycaemia, e.g. *polyuria, polydipsia, polyphagia* and weight loss. In some cases, the disease is heralded by the appearance

of ketoacidosis during an intercurrent illness or following surgery. The diagnostic criteria are given in Box 9.1.

Box 9.1 Diagnostic Criteria (ADA and WHO) for DM

Condition	Venous plasma glucose in mg% (mmol/L)	
	Fasting	Post-prandial (2 hr GTT)*
Normal	<110 (6.1)	<140 (7.3)
DM	>126 (7.0)	>200 (11.1)
Impaired fasting glycaemia (IFG)	>110 and <126	<140
Impaired glucose tolerance (IGT)	<126	>140 and <200

* 2 hr GTT means following 75 g of oral glucose.

Box 9.2 Clinical Presentations of Type 2 DM

Organ/system involved	Features
• Eye	Recurrent styes, chalazion, anterior uveitis (hypopyon), refractory errors with frequent change of glasses, cataract, keratitis, conjunctivitis and retinopathy, ocular nerve palsy.
• Urinary tract	• Urinary tract infection, acute pyelitis, or pyelonephritis, acute papillary necrosis, sterile pyuria, stone formation, nephrotic syndrome (diabetic nephropathy)
• GI tract	• Chronic diarrhoea, malabsorption, gastroparesis, adynamic ileus, GI infections
• Genital tract	In females: pruritus vulvae, vaginal discharge, menstrual irregularities, recurrent abortions, infertility
In males: loss of libido, impotence, urethritis
• Cardiovascular	Ischaemic heart disease (silent angina or acute coronary syndrome), hypertension, peripheral vascular disease (cold extremities, digital gangrene, diabetic foot).
• Nervous system	TIA, recurrent strokes, peripheral neuropathies, autonomic neuropathy, mononeuritis multiplex, diabetic amyotrophy, cranial nerve palsy
• Skin	Multiple boils, carbuncle, abscesses, cellulitis, pressure sores
• Respiratory	Pneumonias, lungs abscess, tuberculosis
• Immunity	Diabetes is an immunocompromised state, predisposes to infection at each and every site/system

2. **Type 2 diabetics are mostly** overweight and obese, present to different specialists and superspecialists with features of complications pertaining to various organs/system (Box 9.2).

DIABETIC NEUROPATHY (Box 9.3)

Patients with diabetes present with *sensorimotor symmetrical peripheral neuropathy* (glove-stocking type), *asymmetric motor neuropathy* (amyotrophy), *mononeuritis* (single long nerve involvement) or *mononeuritis multiplex* (more than one long nerve involvement), *cranial nerve palsies* (III, IV, VI, VII) and *autonomic neuropathy* (postural hypotension, gastroparesis, noctural diarrhoea, gustatory sweating, etc.).

Box 9.3 Classification, Clinical Features of Neuropathy

Classification	Symptoms and signs
I. Somatic	
(i) Symmetric sensorimotor (distal glove–stocking type)	• Tingling or burning sensation in the extremities (hands and feet), nocturnal pain in limbs, numbness and coldness of extremities
• Glove and stocking type of anaesthesia
• Loss of ankle jerks and muscle wasting
• Disorganisation of joints (Charcot joints)
• Abnormal gait (wide based, thumping gait)
• Nerve conduction velocity delayed
(ii) Asymmetric, motor, proximal (diabetic amyotrophy due to femoral nerve involvement)	• Lower motor neuron paralysis with wasting of thigh muscles
• Hyper- or hypoaesthesia presents on anterior aspect of thighs
• Thigh muscles (proximal) are commonly involved
• Difficulty in rising from sitting position or climbing stairs
• Knee jerks are lost on affected side or both sides.
• Lumbosacral area is the site of involvement
Mononeuropathy	
• Mononeuritis (cranial or spinal)	• 3rd and 6th cranial nerves involvement common producing diplopia and loss of eye movements. Median or ulnar nerve (long nerve palsy)

Contd.

Classification	Symptoms and signs
• Mononeuritis multiplex	• Carpal tunnel syndrome with distal ulnar and median nerve involvement (*wrist drop*)
II. Autonomic (visceral)	
a. Cardiovascular	• Vertigo, giddiness and blurring of vision due to postural hypotension, resting tachycardia and fixed heart rate
b. Gastrointestinal	• Nausea, vomiting, abdominal distension, nocturnal diarrhoea, constipation due to colonic atony, gastroparesis, dysphagia due to oesophageal atony
c. Genitourinary	• Loss of libido, impotence, urinary incontinence, difficulty in micturition (atony of bladder)
d. Sudomotor and vasomotor	• Abnormal or gustatory sweating, anhidrosis, fissuring of feet, cold extremities, dependent oedema
e. Eye (pupils)	• Constriction of pupils, absent or delayed light reflex

DIABETIC NEPHROPATHY

The involvement of kidney in diabetes irrespective of its type is called *diabetic* nephropathy. It occurs as a microvascular complications in long-standing patients of diabetes. Diabetic nephropathy is the leading cause of end stage renal disease (ESRD) and diabetes-related mortality and morbidity. A triad of *neuropathy*, *nephropathy* and *retinopathy* is common in diabetes.

Pathogenesis. Like other microvascular complications, it is also related to chronic hyperglycaemia, effects of soluble factors (i.e. growth factors, angiotensin II, endothelin and AGEs), haemodynamic alteration in microcirculation (glomerular hyperfiltration and hyperperfusion) and ultimately structural changes in the glomeruli (increased extracellular matrix, thickening of basement membrane, mesangial expansion and fibrosis). Other factors such as hypertension and smoking accelerate it.

Clinical Features

The symptoms and signs depend on the clinical staging (Box 9.4). It remains asymptomatic up to stage of microalbuminuria, asymptomatic urinary abnormalities develop as the disease advances followed by features of nephrotic syndrome, renal insufficiency and renal failure as disease further progresses.

Box 9.4 Clinical Staging of Diabetic Nephropathy

I. Hyperfiltration (GFR↑)
II. Microalbuminuria (GFR >90 ml/min)
III. overproteinuria (non-nephrotic range) with GFR 60–90 ml/min
IV. Nephrotic syndrome (GFR 30–60 ml/min)
V. Renal insufficiency (GFR 15–30 ml/min)
VI. End stage renal disease (GFR <15 ml /min)

Clinical Work up of a Case with Endocrine System (Fig. 9.20)

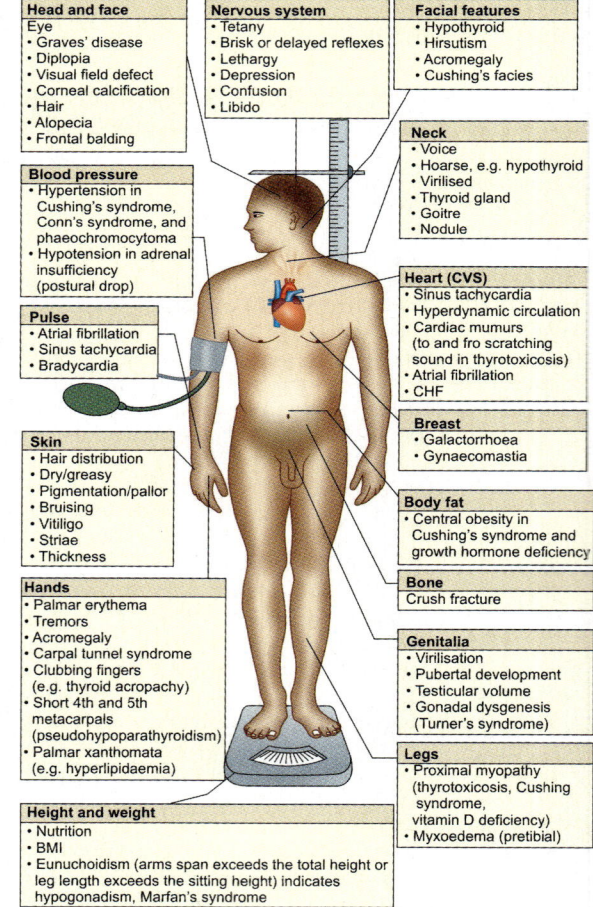

Head and face
Eye
• Graves' disease
• Diplopia
• Visual field defect
• Corneal calcification
Hair
• Alopecia
• Frontal balding

Nervous system
• Tetany
• Brisk or delayed reflexes
• Lethargy
• Depression
• Confusion
• Libido

Facial features
• Hypothyroid
• Hirsutism
• Acromegaly
• Cushing's facies

Neck
• Voice
• Hoarse, e.g. hypothyroid
• Virilised
• Thyroid gland
• Goitre
• Nodule

Blood pressure
• Hypertension in Cushing's syndrome, Conn's syndrome, and phaeochromocytoma
• Hypotension in adrenal insufficiency (postural drop)

Pulse
• Atrial fibrillation
• Sinus tachycardia
• Bradycardia

Heart (CVS)
• Sinus tachycardia
• Hyperdynamic circulation
• Cardiac murmurs (to and fro scratching sound in thyrotoxicosis)
• Atrial fibrillation
• CHF

Breast
• Galactorrhoea
• Gynaecomastia

Skin
• Hair distribution
• Dry/greasy
• Pigmentation/pallor
• Bruising
• Vitiligo
• Striae
• Thickness

Body fat
• Central obesity in Cushing's syndrome and growth hormone deficiency

Bone
Crush fracture

Hands
• Palmar erythema
• Tremors
• Acromegaly
• Carpal tunnel syndrome
• Clubbing fingers (e.g. thyroid acropachy)
• Short 4th and 5th metacarpals (pseudohypoparathyroidism)
• Palmar xanthomata (e.g. hyperlipidaemia)

Genitalia
• Virilisation
• Pubertal development
• Testicular volume
• Gonadal dysgenesis (Turner's syndrome)

Legs
• Proximal myopathy (thyrotoxicosis, Cushing syndrome, vitamin D deficiency)
• Myxoedema (pretibial)

Height and weight
• Nutrition
• BMI
• Eunuchoidism (arms span exceeds the total height or leg length exceeds the sitting height) indicates hypogonadism, Marfan's syndrome

General observations
• Most examination in endocrinology is by observation
• Acute observation can often yield 'spot' diagnosis of endocrine syndrome
• The emphasis of examination varies depending on which gland or hormone is thought to be involved

Fig. 9.20: Examination of endocrine system.

Unit X

Examination of Musculoskeletal and Locomotor System

- Symptoms and their Analysis
- History
- General Physical Examination
- Systemic Examination
- Brief Synopsis of Different Comas

RHEUMATOLOGY

MAJOR SYMPTOMS OF RHEUMATIC DISORDERS

Rheumatic symptoms are common, may reflect primary rheumatological disorders or an underlying systemic disorder; for example, bleeding into a large joint (haemarthrosis) may be the presenting symptom of a coagulation disorder—haemophilia. The various symptoms of joint disease are:

1. **Pain** (joint pain/bone pain)
   - *Usage pain*—worst on use, relieved by rest (mechanical strain, damage).
   - *Rest pain*—worst after rest, improved by movement (inflammation).
   - *Night 'bone' pain*—mostly at night, poorly related to movement occurs in septic and gouty arthritis
2. **Stiffness** (subjective feeling or inability to move freely).
   - Stiffness that can be *"worn off"* suggests inflammation
3. **Swelling** (symmetrical/asymmetrical)
   - Symmetric, i.e. fluid (fluctuant swelling), soft tissue (inflammatory) or asymmetric, i.e. bone swelling (joint deformity)
4. **Weakness/wasting**
   - *Primary* myopathy
   - *Secondary* to joint disease, e.g. overuse, disuse.
5. **Deformity**
   - *Joint* (RA, OA), *bone* (Paget's disease, rickets, tumour, fracture)
6. **Nonspecific symptoms**
   - Reduced appetite, weight loss
   - Fatigue, mood disturbance
   - Night sweats, chills
   - Feeling ill, low esteem, irritable

The first aim of clinical assessment of the musculoskeletal system is to determine whether symptoms are derived from *bone, joint, muscle* or other *soft tissue structures*. The pain due to soft tissue rheumatism is described in Table 10.1

TABLE 10.1: Symptoms and Signs of Soft Tissue Rheumatism

1. **Pain due to tendon involvement** (e.g. tenosynovitis, tendinitis, tendon rupture, etc.)
   Characteristics
   - Localised pain/tenderness at attachment (enthesitis) or in tendon substance
   - Swelling, pain and crepitus along the line of sheath in tendosynovitis.
   - Pain on resisted action
   - Complete loss of active movements with preservation of passive movements in tendon rupture.
   - Sometimes pain on stretching (e.g. Achilles)
   - Formation of contracture
2. **Ligament and joint capsule pain**
   Characteristics
   - Localised pain/tenderness at attachment or in ligament substance or joint capsule in incomplete tear of joint capsule or ligament (sprain)
   - Pain on stretch and movements is limited by muscle spasm.
   - Instability and swelling, if major tear or ruptured ligament. Passive movements are painful.

Contd.

Contd.

3. **Pain due to bursa involvement**
   Characteristics
   - Localised tenderness
   - Swelling
   - Pain on stretching the adjacent structures
4. **Muscular pain**
   Characteristics
   - Localised or diffuse pain and tenderness
   - Pain on resisted action
   - Pain on stretching (e.g. hamstring)

Causes and Characteristics of Soft Tissue/Bone/Vascular/Neuralgic Pain

Periarticular pain: It relates the pain to activity, wringing clothes can bring on the pain of a tennis elbow. The pain of planter fascitis occurs during walking in the morning or getting up from sitting position and first few steps are most painful. Pain around the shoulder with stiffness indicates periarthritis.

Joint pain: *Acute joint* pain occurs in rheumatic fever, traumatic arthritis, reactive arthritis, acute gout and acute onset of chronic arthritis. *Chronic joint pain* occurs in OA, RA, ankylosing spondylitis, etc. Osteomalacia and osteoporosis produce chronic aching pain over the spines and weight-bearing bones aggravated by physical activity.

Muscle pain. Muslce pain is felt over big muscles (calves, trunk, shoulder and back) with aches and associated with tenderness. It occurs when the muscle is in action. Unaccustomed overuse is the commonest cause. Pain is self-limiting. Electrolyte disturbance produces pain due to muscle cramps. Wandering muscle pain and tenderness associated with irritability and insomnia is common manifestation of fibromyalgia. Myalgia is common manifestation of infection, i.e. leptospirosis and ARBO-virus infections, i.e. chikungunya is cause of joint and muscle pain.

Bone pain. The bone pain is deep-seated and localised. The spontaneous bone pain may suggest Paget's disease of the bone (with bony enlargement e.g. skull or tibia), or metastatic deposits, infection in younger patients or immunocompromised hosts. In case of pain due to fracture, there is always a history of trauma/injury.

Bone pain around shoulder, back and thighs associated with proximal muscle weakness (*waddling gait*) in multiparous women indicate osteomalacia. *Backbone pain* on assuming erect posture and movement indicate vertebral involvement due to tuberculosis, multiple myeloma and secondaries bone. *Sciatic pain* starts from the back, radiates to thigh and legs, increases with coughing and sneezing, occurs due to prolapse intervertebral disc. Pain in lumbosacral region which spreads to other parts with stiffness of back indicate ankylosing spondylitis.

Neuralgic pain. Entrapment neuropathy leads to pain in the distribution of nerve roots. Nerve compression causes pain and sensory loss, i.e. compression of lateral cutaneous nerve by deep fascia in the thigh leads to pain over the lateral aspect of the thigh (*meralgia paresthetica*). In *peripheral neuritis*, pain and paraesthesia occur in distal parts of the extremities (**gloves and stocking fashion**). *Intermittent neurogenic claudication* of lower extremities produce pain and numbness in calves as the patient walks. This is due to ischaemia of lower segments of spinal nerve root and spinal cord.

Vascular pain: It occurs due to ischaemia of the nerve roots or cord (intermittent neurogenic claudication) during walking and relieved by rest and reappears on activity. Resting pain occurs due to vascular occlusion of small arteries of the distal extremities, is charactered by cold extremities with absence of peripheral pulsations (Read peripheral vascular system) resulting in vascular gangrene.

Pain of soft tissue rheumatism: Symptoms of soft tissue rheumatism include pain, dull ache, tenderness or swelling. In elderly, these symptoms often appear spontaneously, but in younger persons, there is history of trauma or overuse especially as a result of occupation, for example, tenosynovitis of long flexor tendons of hand in labourers, or achilles tendinitis in athletes. The severity of pain is judged by the presence of night pain and sleep disturbance. Persistent pain is also frequently associated with anxiety, depression, hence, one should be careful while interpreting the joint pain. The musculoskeletal pain is often referred to other sites (somatic referral).

The features of **mechanical** (degenerative or meniscal tear) and **inflammatory joint** disease are compared in Box 10.1.

Symptom Analysis

Joint Pain

Ask about the following

Q. Onset of pain (acute/gradual or chronic).

- Acute joint pain occurs is septic arthritis, rheumatic arthritis (rheumatic fever), gouty arthritis (podagra)
- Gradual onset of pain or chronic pain occurs in RA and OA

Examination of Musculoskeletal and Locomotor System

Box 10.1 Features of Two Common Types of Joint Disease

Mechanical (OA)	Inflammatory (RA)
• Pain on activity that improves on rest	• *Rest pain* that improves on activity
• *Inactivity stiffness* of joint disappears on activity	• Early morning stiffness persists for more than 30 minutes
• No signs of inflammation	• Signs of inflammation, i.e. pain, redness, warmth, swelling and tenderness present
• *Joints involved* include large joints of hip, knee, ankle, shoulder and spines	• Any joint may be involved but commonly the smaller joints of big toe (gout), small joints of hand and feet (RA), interphalangeal joint in reactive or psoriatic arthritis
• Loose bodies in the joint may be present	• No loose body
• No periarticular involvement	• Periarticular inflammation, e.g. erythema, soft tissue swelling and dactylitis present
• No triggering factor except old age	• Triggering factors include dysentery or new sexual contact, intercurrent illness, sore throat and surgery
Example: OA (osteoarthritis)	Example: RA (rheumatoid arthritis)

Q. Does pain occur at rest or on usage?

- Rest pain improved on movements indicates inflammatory joint disease.
- Usage pain (worst on use) relieved by rest indicates mechanical strain, degenerative arthritis

Q. Is pain migratory/fleeting type or constant?

- Migratory/fleeting pain indicates rheumatic arthritis
- Constant pain indicate inflammatory or degenerative joint disease.

Q. Does pain occur at night?

- Severe pain disturbing sleep occurs in septic and gouty arthritis.

Q. Does pain gets referred to other sites?

- Cervical pain gets referred to head or shoulder
- Lumbar pain gets referred to buttocks/thighs
- Shoulder pain is referred to upper arm
- Elbow pain is referred to forearm
- Hip pain is referred to thigh/knee or both.

Q. Does pain increase on coughing, sneezing, straining at stool?

- Cervical and lumbar pain may increase on coughing, sneezing and straining at stool.

Stiffness

It means inability to move, may be due to inflammatory and non-inflammatory arthritis.

I. **Inflammatory arthritis** (RA, SLE arthritits)
   Stiffness is due to inflammation of joint structure.
   - Early morning stiffness persists for more than 30 minutes in SLE
   - Morning stiffness persisting for more than 1 hour is characteristic of RA.
   - Stiffness is precipitated by prolonged rest and lasts for several hours.
   - Stiffness improves with activity and anti-inflammatory drugs.
   - Stiffness is associated with pain, swelling and warmth (signs of inflammation)

II. **Non-inflammatory arthritis** (i.e. OA)
   - Stiffness is due to pain or deformity.
   - Stiffness is usually intermittent
   - Stiffness may increase with activity
   - Stiffness lasts for a short-while (<1 hour)
   - Stiffness is not associated with signs of inflammation.

Symptom Analysis

Ask about the following

Q. Does stiffness occur in the morning?

- Early morning stiffness occurs in inflammatory arthritis and rheumatoid arthritis (RA)

Q. Is it precipitated by prolonged rest or acitivty?

- Stiffness precipitated by prolonged rest and improved with activity "Worn-off stiffness" suggests inflammatory arthritis.
- Stiffness that increases on activity suggest non-inflammatory arthritis.

Physical Signs, Symptoms, Diagnosis and Differential Diagnosis

Q. Is there any deformity associated?

- Stiffness associated with pain or deformity suggests non-inflammatory arthritis.

Deformities (Table 10.2)

Deformities occur both in *inflammatory arthritis* (hand and legs deformity in rheumatoid arthritis, Jaccoud arthritis in rheumatic fever) and *degenerative arthritis* (deformity of skull and spine in Paget's disease, hands and feet in acromegaly, large joints in haemophilia, thoracic kyphosis and lumbar lordosis in ankylosing spondylitis).

Symptom Analysis

Ask about the following

Q. Is deformity/deformities present?

- Deformity(ies) indicate inflammatory or degenerative arthritis, bone disease and fractures.

Q. Which part of the body is involved in deformity?

- Deformity of skull occurs in Paget's disease.
- Hand and foot deformities occur in RA.

TABLE 10.2: Analysis of Hand Deformities

Deformities	Significance
A. Joints	
Trident hand (short hand with divergent fingers)	Achondroplasia
Spindle shaped fingers (swelling of PIP joints)	Rheumatoid arthritis, scleroderma
Swan-neck (hyper-extended PIP joints and flexed DIP joints, see Fig. 10.10), and *Boutonniere'* or *button-hole* deformity (flexed PIP and hyperextended DIP joints, see Fig. 10.10)	Rheumatoid arthritis (Fig. 10.6)
Volar subluxation with ulnar deviation of hand, Z-deformity of thumb (Fig. 10.10)	Rheumatoid arthritis
Swelling of distal interphalangeal joints (DIP)	Osteoarthritis, psoriatic arthropathy (Fig. 10.2)
Claw hand (hyperextension of metacarpo-phalangeal joints and flexion of PIP and DIP)	Paralysis of interosseous and lumbricals
Prayer's Hand (Fig. 10.10)	Diabetic chiroarthropathy
Jaccoud's arthritis	Very rarely seen in rheumatic arthritis
Main D'accoucheur or obstetric hand	Tetany (see Fig. 1.17)
B. Subcutaneous tissue	
Dupuytren's contracture (thickening and shortening of palmar fascia resulting in flexion deformities of the 4th and 5th fingers)	Repeated trauma, alcoholic cirrhosis, phenytoin therapy, diabetes mellitus and working with vibrating tools
C. Tendons	
de Quervain's tenosynovitis (swelling over the tendon sheath) and trigger finger or thumb flexor tendon	Excessive use of the tendon
D. Muscles	
Flattening of palm, prominent knuckles and hollow interosseous spaces	Wasting of small muscles of the hand
Carpal tunnel syndrome	Rheumatoid arthritis, disuse atrophy, diabetes, amyloidosis, autoimmune hypothyroidism, acromegaly, pregnancy
Wrist drop	Radial nerve palsy peripheral neuropathies, lead neuropathy
E. Bones	
Tapering and conical fingertips with or without trophic changes (subperiosteal reabsorption)	Hyperparathyroidism, leprosy
Bone deformity due to pathological fractures or bowed legs	Paget's disease of the bone, surgical conditions, trauma
F. Nerves	
Trophic changes, e.g. ulcerations, burns	Peripheral neuropathies

- Jaccoud arthritis (deformity) involving hands occurs in rheumatic arthritis.
- Heberden's nodes over fingers occur in OA.
- Deformities of the spine can cause loss of height and curvature.

Q. Is there any weakness/wasting of muscles or impairment of movements?

- Joint and bone disorders can result in myopathy and impairment of movements due to overuse/disuse, deformities, tendon damage, etc.

Joint Swelling

Swelling of the joint may be due to
1. Inflammation of joint with resultant oedema and swelling (inflammatory arthritis).
2. Swelling may be due to synovitis or excessive accumulation of fluids in RA.
3. Swelling can be due to bony outgrowths or hypertrophy in degenerative arthritis, for example, OA.

Symptom Analysis
Ask about the following

Q. Is joint swelling present?

- Joint swelling indicates infective or inflammatory arthritis, rheumatoid and degenerative arthritis (bony swelling).

Q. How many joints are involved?
- Read terminology and patterns of joints involvement in Box 10.2.

Q. Is arthritis symmetrical or asymmetrical?
- Symmetrical arthritis is RA
- Asymmetrical arthritis are gout, rheumatic and seronegative arthritis and OA (osteoarthritis).

Q. Which joints are predominantly involved?

- Small joints involvement indicate RA, gout and SLE
- Large joint are involved in OA, septic arthritis, seronegative arthritis
- Axial joints are involved in OA and ankylosing spondylitis (AS)

Q. Is arthritis associated with fever?

- Fever in arthritis indicate septic arthritis, gout, reactive arthritis and RA (rheumatoid arthritis)

Crackling sensation of the Joint(s)
Symptom Analysis
Q. Is there any crackling or gritty sensation in the joint?

- Crackling sensation in the joint(s) suggests degenerative joint disease, i.e. OA (commonly felt as crepitus in osteoarthritis of the knees on palpation of the joint).

Locking of Joint
Symptom Analysis
Q. Is there any locking of joint during walking?

- Locking/jamming of joint may involve knee during walking due to interference with the movements of articular surfaces in degenerative arthritis or osteoarthirits.

Associated symptoms (i.e. extra-articular manifestation)
Symptom Analysis

Q. Ask about the following associated symptoms.
  i. *Fever and sweating*: Common in *septic* and *rheumatic fever*
  ii. *Skin lash*: Occurs in *SLE*, *psoriatic arthritis rheumatic fever*, *Reiter's disease*
  iii. *Dyspnoea and chest pain*: can occur in *ankylosing spondylitis, RA, SLE,*
  iv. *Eye symptoms,* i.e
   - Conjunctivitis occurs in *Reiter's disease*
   - Dry eye/eye grittiness occurs in *Sjögren's syndrome*
   - Blue sclera occurs in *osteogenesis imperfecta*
  v. *GI symptoms*
   - Transient diarrhoea indicates *enteropathic arthritis*
   - Recurrent mouth ulcer indicate *Behçet's syndrome*
  vi. *Urethritis*
   - It occurs in *Reiter's disease*
  vii. *Recurrent abortions*
   - It indicates *APLA (antiphospholipid) syndrome*
  viii. *Neuropathy*
   - Entrapment neuropathy occurs in *RA*
  ix. *ENT symptoms* **(nasal/sinus/middle ear disease)**
   - They indicate *Wegener's granulomatosis*

Pattern of Joint Involvement

Some diseases have specific prediction for specific joints (Box 10.2).

Box 10.2 Some Common Patterns of Joint Involvement of Rheumatic Diseases

I. Inflammatory disorders (synovitis)

Patterns of joints involved	Diseases
i. Polyarticular (many joints involved)	
• MCP, PIP, and MTP joints (small joints)	RA, SLE, psoriasis
• DIP joints (small joints)	Psoriasis
ii. Girdle joints (large joints)	Polymyalgia rheumatica, RA
iii. Oligoarticular (two, three or four joints affected)	
• Asymmetrical large joints or dactylitis (sausage digit)	Reactive arthritis, Reiter's syndrome, psoriasis or AS
iv. Monoarticular (single joint involved)	
• Acute	Gout, pseudogout, infection, psoriasis
• Chronic	Psoriasis, RA, AS, chronic infection (tuberculosis)
v. Axial, sacroiliac, girdle joints	AS

II. Degenerative disorders (bony swelling ± synovitis)

i. Polyarticular	
• DIP, or PIP joints and/or first-CMC joint	nodal OA
ii. Monoarticular	
• Chronic	OA
iii. Axial joints	Spondylosis (cervical or lumbar)

Abbreviations
MCP = Metacarpophalangeal joint
DIP = Distal interphalangeal joint
CMC = Carpometacarpal joint
RA = Rheumatoid arthritis
OA = Osteoarthritis
PIP = Proximal inter-phalangeal joint
MTP = Metatarsophalangeal joint
SLE = Systemic lupus erythematosus
AS = Ankylosing spondylitis
Small joints: Joints of hands and feet
Large joints: Any other joints except hands and feet

HISTORY

History of Present Illness

Main features in the history of a patient with rheumatological problem to be recorded are;

1. *Age and gender of the patient.* Juvenile idiopathic arthritis is restricted to children, haemophilia to boys; reactive arthritis most common in young men, gout in middle aged men while pseudogout in older women and osteoarthritis occurs in old age.
2. *Race:* Some arthropathies (e.g. sickle cell disease) occur in particular races.
3. *Occupation.* It is important in soft-tissue rheumatism or osteoarthritis.
4. *Joint symptoms.* A combination of *pain, swelling* and *stiffness* causing loss of function is a frequent presenting symptom of joint disease, however, pain and swelling can also result from the overuse of normal joint. Usually one component predominates, i.e. swelling in inflammation and pain in mechanical joint problems, hence ask specific questions to analyse whether symptoms are mechanical (e.g. degenerative joint disease) or inflammatory (rheumatoid arthritis or gout).

Write the symptoms in chronological order and analyse them regarding mode of onset, progression, aggravating and relieving factors and other associated symptoms.

Past Medical History

- A history of trauma or of some other disease like tuberculosis, psoriasis, sore throat (rheumatic fever) and enteritis (inflammatory bowel disease) may be sought.
- History of new sexual contact (for reactive arthritis), intercurrent illness or surgery (for crystal synovitis) must be asked in the past history.

Family History

- Some conditions run in families, e.g. rheumatoid arthritis, osteoarthritis, Behçet's disease ankylosing spondylitis and gout.
- Patients with psoriatic arthritis do not necessarily have psoriatic skin lesions but may give a family history of psoriasis. Psoriatic genes may be expressed in either skin, joints or both in any order and at any time.
- There is a common genetic basis to some common arthritis. HLA-B27 is found frequently in ankylosing spondylitis and reactive arthritis than other spondyloarthropathies (psoriatic arthropathy, enteropathic arthritis due to inflammatory bowel disease).
- Family history may be positive in patients with hypermobile joints (e.g. Marfan's syndrome. Ehlers-Danlos syndrome, benign familial hypermobility).

Social or Occupational History

The occupation of the patient may have a bearing on the arthritis. Soft tissue rheumatism may be related to physical stress and such forms are known as *overuse syndrome* or *repetitive stress syndrome*. The booming computer industry requiring prolonged sitting and bad human postures have unleashed

Examination of Musculoskeletal and Locomotor System

a variety of stress related neck-shoulder-limb and spine disorders, for example osteoarthritis of neck common in dentists, physicians and dancers. In addition, the development of a chronic arthritis may lead to mood and sleep disturbance. Inability to hold a pen or tools, to kneel, stand for long periods or to use ladders may have profound social and economic consequences.

Drug History

A record of the previous treatment must be sought. Statins are known to produce arthralgia and myopathy. Hydralazine, penicellamine and quinidine are likely to induce drug-induced lupus. Diuretics, salicylate, alcohol may precipitate gout.

Personal History

History of smoking, alcoholism.

EXAMINATION OF LOCOMOTOR SYSTEM

1. General physical examination
2. Examination of joints

1. General Physical Examination (GPE)

The examination begins with the observation of the patient entering the room

☞ *Observe for any abnormalities of gait and posture while patient is walking or ask him/her to walk.*

- The patient may be asked to stand and walk, even when it is obvious that this may not be possible. This will give an idea about the help the patient requires from others or from sticks, crutches, etc.
- **Painful gait (antalgic gait, Fig. 10.1).** It is jerky asymmetric gait with less time spent on weight bearing on painful leg or foot on the ground; with more severe pain the whole limb is held flexed and the foot is placed delicately on the ground for very short periods. The patient requires support to walk.
- **Painless gait.** In a painless gait, the normal smooth rhythm is disturbed either because of a short limb, a deformed or stiff joint or weak muscles. The effect of muscle weakness will depend on the site and degree of muscle pathology.
- **Trendelenburg gait.** Unilateral weakness of hip abductors produces pelvis drop on the opposite side while walking and during stance phase on affected side (standing).
- **Waddling gait.** Bilateral Trendelenburg gait (paralysis of glutei muscles) is waddling gait.

☞ *Observe for any difficulty in undressing, getting out of the chair and getting on to the examination couch*

- This will assess the disability.

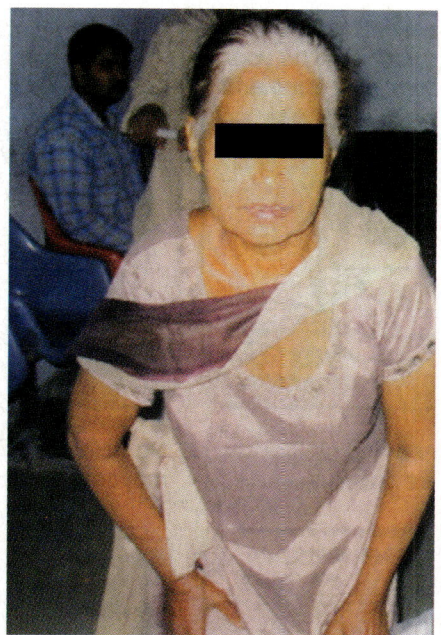

Fig. 10.1: Painful (antalgic) gait. Note that patient adopts a flexed posture, places both hands on the legs which are placed delicately on the ground due to pain.

☞ *Look at the muscles for wasting*

- The muscle wasting could either be due to *a primary* muscle disease, e.g. polymyositis, myopathy or *secondary* to a painful joint (disuse. Suddack's atrophy).

☞ *Look at bony structures for alteration in outline and shape or swelling*

- Fractures, tumours, infections and cysts can lead to alteration in shape/outline and swelling.

☞ *Look for any deformity*

- Deformities indicate disc disease or deforming arthritis (RA, OA).

☞ **Eyes.** *Examine the eyes for any abnormality*

Abnormality	Disease associated
Redness (conjunctivitis, iritis, episcleritis)	Rheumatoid arthritis, reactive arthritis, spondylarthritis,
Dryness of eyes (sicca syndrome)	Sjögren's syndrome
Blue sclera with multiple fractures	Osteogenesis imperfecta
Disturbance of vision	Giant cell arteritis
Blindness and deafness	Paget's disease

Physical Signs, Symptoms, Diagnosis and Differential Diagnosis

☞ **Mucous membrane.** *Look at mucous membrane for any abnormality*

Abnormality	Disease associated
• Buccal ulcers	SLE, Reiter's syndrome, Behçet's syndrome
• Anaemia (pallor), pancytopenia (necrotic ulcers)	Still's disease, rheumatoid arthritis, SLE

☞ **Skin.** *Inspect the skin for any lesion*

Lesion	Disease associated
• Nodules (subcutaneous swellings)	Amyloidosis, sarcoidosis, SLE
• Nodes on bony prominence	Osteoarthritis
• Petechiae	SLE, ITP
• Palpable purpura	Vasculitis
• Dry scaly lesion of psoriasis	Psoriatic arthropathy
• Erythema nodosum (painful, tender, oral, hard and red swelling on front of legs)	Sarcoidosis, reactive arthritis
• Haemorrhagic pustules	Gonococcal arthritis
• Rash (butterfly on face)	SLE, dermatomyositis
• Photosensitivity (sun-sensitivity rash)	SLE
• Raynaud's phenomenon	SLE, systemic sclerosis
• Livedo reticularis	Antiphospholipid syndrome

☞ **Hair.** *Look at hair for loss*

Hair loss	Disease associated
• Alopecia	SLE

☞ **Nails.** *Examine the nails for any abnormality*

Abnormality	Disease associated
• Clubbing of fingernails	Hypertrophic osteoarthropathy
• Nails pitting	Psoriatic arthritis (Fig. 10.2)
• Splinter haemorrhages, nail fold vasculitis	Vasculitis, SLE, and polyarteritis nodosa

☞ *Examine fingers and hands for any abnormality*

Abnormality	Disease associated
• Dactylitis, cutaneous infarct, gangrene	Vasculitis, rheumatoid arthritis, SLE
• Sclerodactyly (tight skin over the phalanges)	Scleroderma
• Broad stout, stubby fingers	Acromegaly, pseudohypoparathyroidism
• Pseudoclubbing	Hyperparathyroidism
• Arachnodactyly (see Fig. 1.19)	Marfan's syndrome

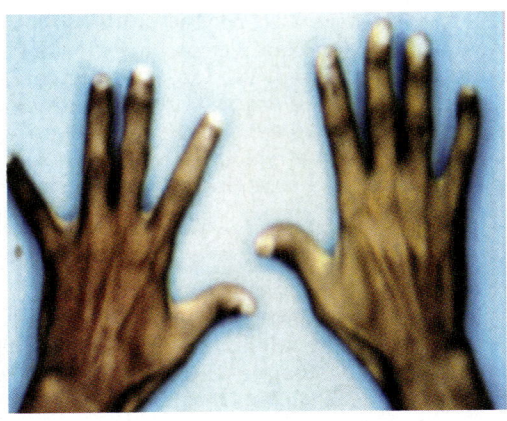

Fig. 10.2: Psoriatic arthritis involving PID and DIP joints with nail changes (pitting of the nails).

☞ *Examine neck, axillae, groin for any swelling*

Swelling(s)	Disease associated
Lymphadenopathy	RA, Felty's syndrome, sarcoidosis, tuberculosis

☞ *Examine the extremities for ulcer, deformity, etc.*

I. Lower extremities

Abnormality	Disease associated
• Leg ulcers (venous, arterial)	Rheumatoid arthritis, sickle cell anaemia, vasculitis, Felty's syndrome
• Varicose veins	Trauma, fracture
• Deformities	Trauma, RA, OA
• Flat foot	Congenital abnormality, wasting of muscles of sole
• Pes cavus (clawfoot) (see Fig. 1.22)	Polio, neuropathy, spina bifida
• Gouty tophi	Tophaceous gout
• Talipes equinus varus	Cogenital abnormality
• Neuropathic ulcer (see Fig. 1.23)	Neuropathy, tabes, diabetes, syringomyelia
• Large feet	Acromegaly
• Hammer toe	RA, trauma, wasting of small muscles of foot

II. Upper extremities

☞ *Look at hands (both front and back) for size, shape and any other abnormality.*

Abnormality	Significance/disease associated
• Large hands and palms	• Marfan's syndrome Gigantism

Contd.

Examination of Musculoskeletal and Locomotor System

Contd.

- Short hands (trident hands) with divergent fingers like spokes
- Spade like hands
- Wrist drop
- Ulnar deviation of hand
- Square hands
- Clawhand (*main engriffe*)
- Prayer's hand (*see* Fig. 1.21)

- Achondroplasia

- Acromegaly
- Radial nerve palsy, neuropathy
- Rheumatoid arthritis (RA)
- Nodular osteoarthritis (OA)
- Paralysis of interossei and lumbricals
- Diabetic cheiroarthropathy

Box 10.3: Subcutaneous Nodules

Type	Site
Gouty tophi (Fig. 10.4) seen in gout	Helix of the ear, overlying the joint or in finger pulps
Rheumatoid nodules in rheumatoid arthritis (Fig. 10.5)	Firm, non-tender nodules present at pressure points or frictional sites such as bony prominences
Nodules in SLE	Tendons of the hand
Rheumatic nodules in rheumatic fever	Present over the tendons on extensor surfaces of forearm, legs
Xanthomatous deposits in hypercholesterolaemia	Xanthomas may be present over joints, tendons, etc.

☞ *Look at the fingers for any abnormality/deformity*

Deformity	Rheumatic condition
• Arachnodactyly (long slender fingers see Fig.1.19)	• Marfan's syndrome
• Sclerodactyly (see Fig. 1.16B)	• Scleroderma

☞ *Look at the hands for any swelling*

Swelling	Rheumatic condition
• Heberden's nodes (hard bony nodules on dorsum of distal interphalangeal joints, Fig. 10.3)	• Nodular osteoarthritis
• Bouchard's nodes (hard nodules on dorsum of proximal interphalangeal joints, Fig. 10.3)	• Osteoarthritis (nodular)
• Rheumatoid nodules (firm painless subcutaneous nodules (Fig. 10.5)	• Rheumatoid arthritis

☞ Palpate for subcutaneous nodules by running the finger/thumb over the bony prominences or between thumb and finger if present in soft tissue.

The various subcutaneous nodules and their site for palpation are given in Box 10.3.

☞ **Measurement of muscle wasting.** Wasting of the muscle due to joint disease can be assessed by measurement with a tape at similar points of legs/thighs/arm/forearm, etc.

Muscle wasting in the joint disease is either disuse atrophy or due to disease process, i.e. infection or inflammation.

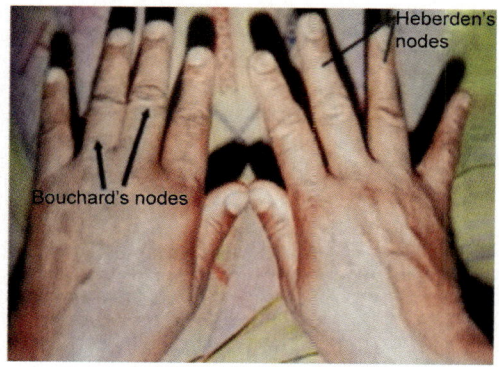

Fig. 10.3: Nodular osteoarthritis. Note the prominent involvement of distal interphalangeal joint with Heberden's nodes and proximal interphalangeal joints with Bouchard's nodes indicated by arrows in a patient with nodular osteoarthritis.

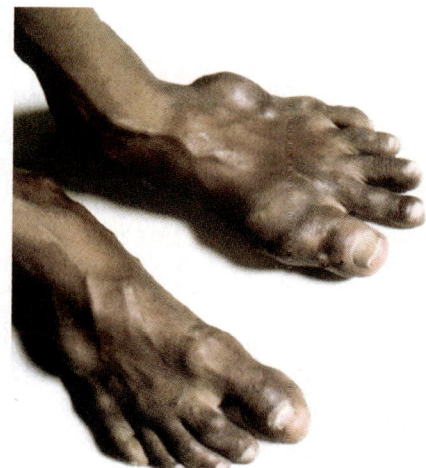

Fig. 10.4: Podagra. Acute gouty arthritis of first metacarpophalangeal joint of feet. (Note the swelling of the joints and tophi which were painful and tender.)

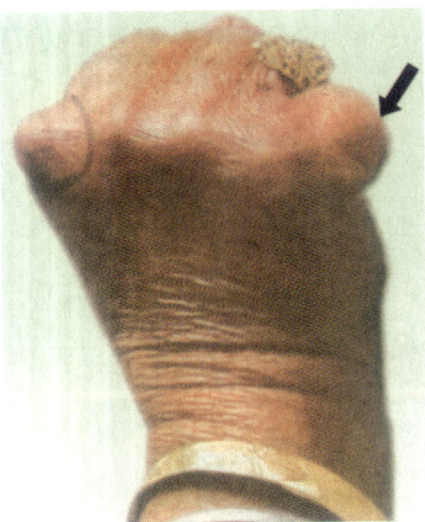

Fig. 10.5: Rheumatoid nodules. Note the cystic swellings.

EXAMINATION OF INDIVIDUAL JOINTS

The steps of examination include:
1. Inspection of the joint (look at the joint)
2. Palpation of bony landmarks and soft tissue structures (feel and palpate the joint).
3. Assessment of range of motion or the direction of joint movement (move the joint)
4. Special manoeuvres to test joint function

Inspection

You should look at the joint at rest as well as during movement.

Inspection at rest

☞ Note symmetry of involvement (Fig. 10.6). Is there asymmetric change in joints on both sides of the body or is the change only in one or two joints?

- Symmetric involvement of many joints especially of the extremities indicates rheumatoid arthritis (Fig. 10.6).
- Monoarthritis (involvement of one joint) indicates trauma, sepsis (Fig. 10.7), tuberculosis or gout as the cause.
- Asymmetric involvement of joints (pauciarthritis) is seen in reactive arthritis, psoriatic arthritis, Reiter's syndrome, ankylosing spondylitis.

☞ **Swelling**. Note any swelling of the joint or periarticular tissue.

Local oedema and redness is sometimes seen over the inflamed joint.

☞ **Measurement of range of movements.** Note the active and passive movements and their degree of motion.

Some joints such as the subtalar joint of foot which have limited movement can be tested passively. Relatively immobile joints (sternoclavicular, acromioclavicular, manubriosternal, costochondral and sacroiliac) have to be examined by palpation or stressing manoeuvres to evoke pain.

The *neutral zero method* of recording movement is recommended. All joints are considered to be in the neutral position when the body assumes classical anatomical position except joints of hands and feet.

In examining joints for range of movement, estimate the degree of limitation by comparing with the normal side. For accurate measurement, a goniometer (protractor) is used. Both active and passive movements should be assessed.

- Limitation of movements in a joint may be due to pain, muscle spasm, inflammation, increased thickness of the capsule; fibrous ankylosis, contractures, effusion into the joint, bony overgrowth, bony ankylosis, mechanical factors
- Hyperextensibility of joint occurs due to lax ligaments, e.g. Ehlers-Danlos syndrome, Charcot's joints (meniscal tear).

Remember painful active movements will give a poor estimate of true range of movement because of muscle spasm, hence other findings should be corroborated for diagnosis. Be gentle and careful during examination of painful joints.

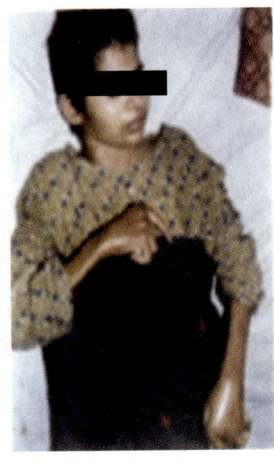

Fig. 10.6: Rheumatoid arthritis. Note bilateral symmetrical involvement of small joints of both hands, wrists, elbows and shoulders. There is associated deformities of the joints (deforming arthritis).

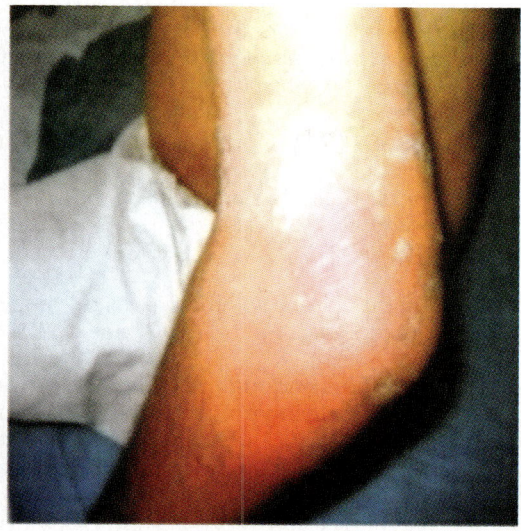

Fig. 10.7: Acute septic elbow.

- Joint swelling indicates synovitis (Fig. 10.8) or joint effusion.
- Periarticular swelling may be due to tendonitis, bursitis, muscle tear.
- Joint swelling may be due to bony enlargements or osteophytes.

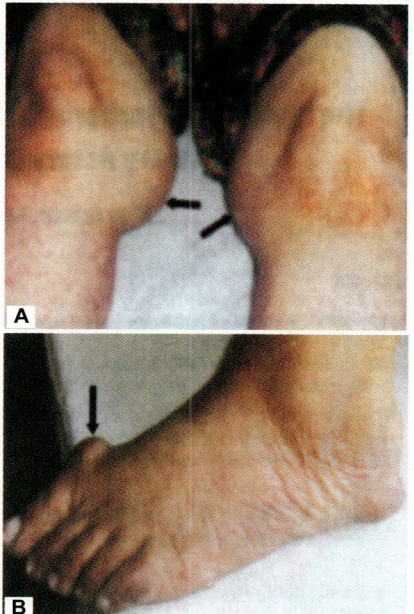

Figs 10.8A and B: Synovitis due to rheumatoid arthritis. (A) Note the boggy swellings (joint effusion) of both knees; (B) There is a rheumatoid nodule over the bony prominence of metatarsophalangeal joint of great toe (↓).

☞ Note any joint deformity or malalignment of bones. Look for any alterations in shape or outline or shortening of bone.

- **Dupuytren's contracture** (Fig. 10.9) is flexion contracture of the ring and little fingers.
- The term *valgus* is used to describe deviation of a limb distal to the joint away from midline, i.e. *Cubitus valgus* means carrying angle between the arm and forearm is decreased (<170°), *Cubitus varus* (carrying angle between arm and forearm increases), *genu valgus* means knock knee (knees are together but feet are apart) and *genu varus* to describe deviation towards the midline (bowed legs). *Coxa vara* means small angle between neck and shaft of femur.
- *Bowing of femur and tibia* is seen in Paget's disease of the bone.
- *Alteration in the shape of bones (bowing of legs)* occurs in rickets. Deformity of the chest in rickets (*rickety rosary*) is due to osteochondral enlargement.
- *Swan-neck, ulnar deviation of hand, Boutonnière and Z-shape deformities* are seen in rheumatoid arthritis (Fig. 10.10).

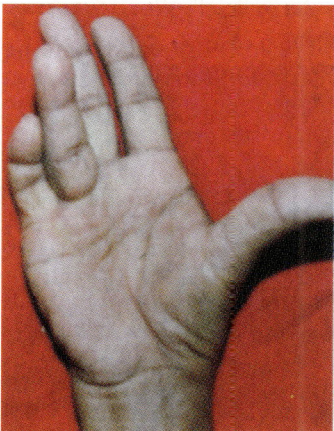

Fig. 10.9: Dupuytren's contracture of right hand.

☞ Note any muscle wasting around the joint(s). This is assessed by compa-ring the bulk of muscles on uninvolved side (joint).

- Muscle wasting around a joint occurs either due to disuse atrophy or by the disease process itself, for example, global wasting of the shoulder muscles may occur in glenohumeral arthritis called *disuse atrophy*.
- Arthritis or a splinted joint may cause disuse atrophy.

- Wasting of the small muscles of the hand may occur due to disease itself.
- Wasting of thenar muscle may be due to carpal tunnel syndrome (nerve entrapment in RA).

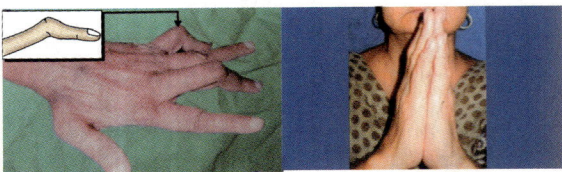

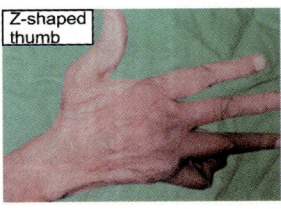

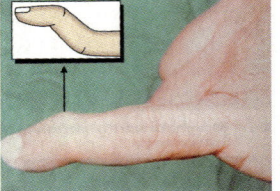

Fig. 10.10: Deformities of hand in deforming rheumatoid arthritis.

☞ Note the position or posture of the limb.

- Guarded posture—held in loose—pack position for capsulitis (adduction, internal rotation for shoulder).
- Mild flexion (10°) or neutral position is adopted for knee, elbow and wrist involvement

☞ Note any redness or erythema of the overlying skin

- Note any scar of previous surgery.
- Redness over a joint suggests septic or gouty arthritis or possibly rheumatoid arthritis.

☞ **Range of motion.** Ask the patient to perform joint movements. Note any limitation in range of motion or increased mobility (hypermobility) or joint instability from excessive mobility of the joint ligaments (ligamentous laxity).

Decreased range of movements (restricted movements) occur in arthritis, inflammation of periarticular tissue, fibrosis in or around a joint, or bony ankylosis (fixation).

Hypermobility of the joint is seen in Marfan's syndrome and Ehlers-Danlos syndrome, neuropathic joint (Charcot's joint). Pain on usage (stress pain) if occurs in all directions (universal) indicates synovitis while selective stress pain (one plane only) indicates periarticular lesion.

Note: Restriction of movements in one plane or direction indicates periarticular lesion; while restriction of all movements indicates joint problem.

Palpation (Feel and Move the Joint)

☞ *Palpate for the signs of inflammation of the joint, i.e. swelling, warmth, tenderness, etc.*

Swelling
i. Synovial membrane swelling gives real boggy or doughy feeling.

Palpable bogginess or doughiness of the synovial membrane indicates synovitis, which is often accompanied by effusion (Fig. 10.8A). Joint effusion from excess synovial fluid within joint space gives fluctuation test positive.
Swelling and tenderness over the tendon sheath or bursa indicate tendonitis or bursitis.

ii. Enlarged subcutaneous bursae may produce swelling over pressure areas (olecranon bursa at elbow).
iii. Localised swellings of long bones may be caused by infection (osteomyelitis), cysts or tumours or fracture.

Warmth. *Use the backs of your fingers to compare the warmth of the involved joint with its unaffected contralateral joint, or with nearby tissues if both joints are involved.*

Warmth indicates arthritis, tendinitis, bursitis, osteomyelitis.

Tenderness. *Elicit tenderness by applying firm pressure on the joint. Joint tenderness may be graded on the patient's response to firm pressure on the joint by holding it between finger and thumb as follows:*

Grade 1. The patient says the joint is tender
2. The patient winces due to pain
3. The patient winces and withdraws the affected part.
4. The patient does not allow the joint to be touched

N.B. Grade 4 tenderness occurs only in septic arthritis, crystal arthritis and rheumatic arthritis.

If tenderness is present, localise it as accurately as possible and determine whether it arises in the joint or in the neighbouring structures, e.g. in the supraspinatus or bicipital tendon rather than the shoulder joint.

☞ *Feel for the tendon sheath crepitus or joint crepitus.*

Tendon sheath crepitus is felt as a grating or creaking sensation when patient is asked to contract the muscle tendon involved. It is particularly common in tenosynovitis in the hand.

Joint crepitus is palpable crunching detected by feeling the joint with palm of one hand while it is moved passively with the other hand (Fig. 10.11). This may indicate osteoarthritis or loose bodies (cartilaginous fragments) in the joint space, but should be differentiated from nonspecific clicking of joints.

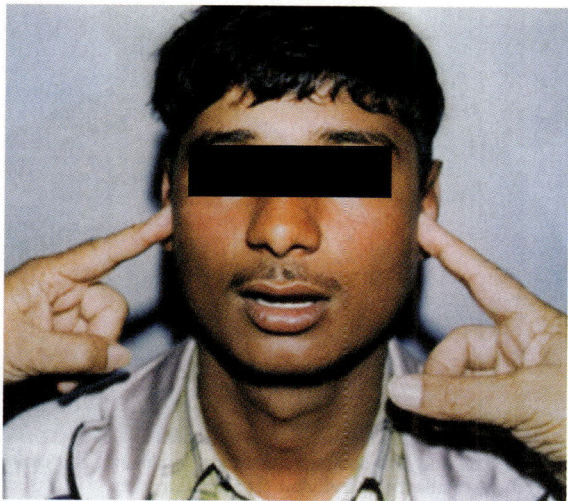

Fig. 10.12: Location and palpation of temporomandibular joint.

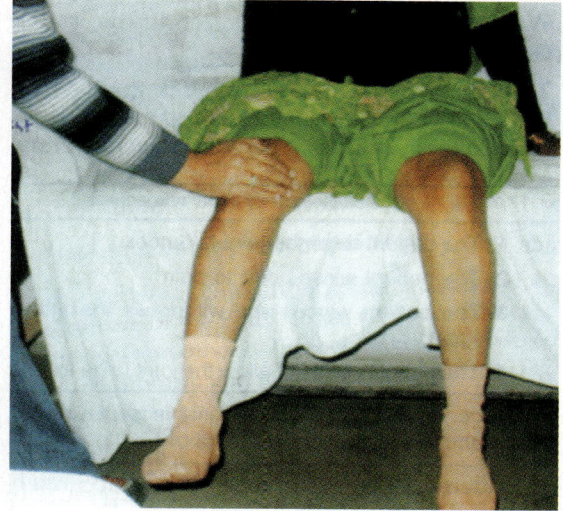

Fig. 10.11: Method of elicitation of joint crepitus.

TEMPOROMANDIBULAR JOINT

☞ **Inspection of the Joint.** *Inspect the joint for swelling or redness. Swelling may appear as a rounded bulge anterior to external auditory meatus.*

- Swelling, redness and restriction of movements indicate an inflamed joint.
- Swelling may also occur in subluxation or dislocation of the joint due to trauma or RA.

☞ **Palpation of the joint.** *Place the tips of your index fingers just in front of the tragus of each ear (Fig. 10.12) and ask the patient to open his or her mouth. The finger tips should drop into the joint space as the mouth opens. Check for the smooth range of movements and feel for crepitus.*

Snapping or clicking sound may be felt or heard in normal people.

Palpable crepitus or clicking may occur in poor occlusion, meniscal injury or synovial swelling due to trauma.

Range of movements. There are three types of movements at this joint;
  i. *Opening and closing of the jaw.* Ask the patient to demonstrate this movement.
  ii. *Prolusion and retraction of jaw.* This can be demonstrated by jutting the jaw forward and backwards. Ask the patient to follow you as you demonstrate the protusion and retraction of the jaw.
  iii. *Side to side or lateral movements.* Ask the patient to move the jaw from side to side.

- Normally as mouth is opened wide, three fingers, can be inserted between incisors.
- During normal protusion of the jaw, the bottom teeth can be placed in front of the upper teeth.

N.B. Any deviation from the normal indicates joint involvement.

THE SPINE

Applied Anatomy and Physiology

The vertebral column is a central bony structure of the body. It has two concavities; one of the cervical and other of lumbar spines, and two convexities, i.e. of thoracic and sacrococcygeal spines (Fig. 10.13A). These curves help to distribute upper body weight to the pelvis and lower limbs and also cushion the concussive effect of walking or running.

Important landmarks. Viewing from the behind, the important landmarks visible are depicted in Fig. 10.13B.

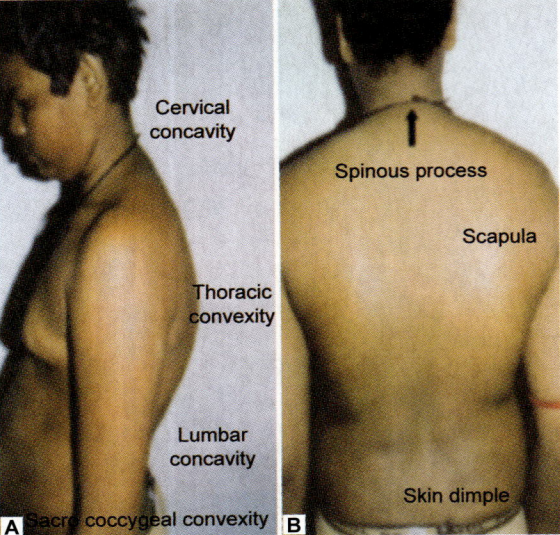

Figs 10.13A and B: Important anatomical landmarks and curves. (A) Patient's lateral view for various curves; (B) Patient's back for important landmarks
- spinous process of C_8–T_1 (↑) is prominent during forward bending
- Scapulae stand out prominantly
- Both shoulders are at same level.
- Skin dimples above the belt indicates posterior superior iliac spine. A line drawn above the posterior superior iliac spine crosses the spine of L4. A lumbar puncture is done just above this line.

Bony structures. The vertebral column has 24 vertebrae stacked on the sacrum and coccyx. A typical vertebra consists of:
1. *The spinous process projecting* in the midline posteriorly and transverse processes standing out at the junction of the pedicle and the lamina.
2. *Two articular processes* on each side of the vertebra, one facing up and another facing down at the junction of the pedicles and lamina. These are articular facets for joint articulations.
3. The vertebral canal is a large central space through which spinal cord passes. The smaller foramina is called *intervertebral foramina* formed by the inferior and superior articular processes of adjacent vertebrae, create a space for exit of the spinal nerve roots; and in the cervical vertebrae, the transverse foramen is for the vertebral artery.

The proximity of the spinal cord and spinal nerve roots to the vertebral bodies and to the intervertebral discs makes them vulnerable to compression by disc herniation, trauma and impingement from degenerative changes in the vertebrae.

Joints. The spinal column has slightly movable cartilaginous joints between the vertebral bodies as already described in the beginning.

A. Cervical Spine

Symptoms
i. **Neck pain** and difficulty in turning the head. Pain may be referred to the arm due to nerve root irritation at different sites at different level of involvement as follows:

1. Upper cervical spine affecting atlantoaxial joint	Pain radiating to occiput (C_2 root distribution).
2. Mid-cervical spine	Pain radiating into the interscapular region or into arms, often associated with local tenderness.
3. Lower cervical spine (C_6–C_7)	Widely referred pain into the interscapular region or into radial fingers and thumb.
4. C_8 involvement	Pain on the ulnar side of forearm and into ring and little fingers

Causes: Cervical rib, cervical spondylosis, Pancoast's tumour, angina, hiatus hernia, diffuse oesophageal spasm.

ii. **Neck stiffness:** It occurs due to muscle spasm due to cervical spine trauma or fracture or muscle injury.

iii. **Paraesthesias:** The patient may also report paraesthesias.

iv. **Neck movements**
- Nodding of the head occurs at atlanto-occipital joint (C_1)
- *Rotational neck movements* occur mainly at atlantoaxial joint (C_1 – C_2)
- The *flexion* (sternomastoid, scalene, paravertebral muscles), the *extension* (splenius capitis, trapezius, small neck muscles) and *lateral bending* (scalene and small intrinsic neck muscles) occur at the mid-cervical (C_3–C_5) level.

B. Thoracic Spine

Thoracic spines maintain a kyphosis throughout life. Movements in the thoracic spine are mainly rotational with little flexion, extension and lateral bending.

Symptoms
i. *Localised spinal pain or pain radiating round the chest wall*, mimicking cardiac or pleural disease.

- The **causes** of pain are tumour, trauma, infection (Pott's disease), ankylosing spondylitis, osteoporosis, degenerative disc disease, aortic aneurysm
  ii. *Progressive stooping and loss of height.* The patient with osteoporosis may complain of becoming progressively stooped (*Dowager hump*) with loss of height but without neurological features.
  iii. *Symptoms and signs of spinal cord compression*, e.g. paraplegia, sensory loss and loss of bowel and bladder control.

C. Lumbar Spine

The lumbar spine maintain lordosis which may be lost in ankylosing spondylitis and disc protusion. The main landmarks in lumbar region of vertebral column are the spinous process of L4/L5, which are level with the pelvic brim and the *"dimple of Venus"* which lie over the sacroiliac joint.

Symptoms

Backache and low back pain (read it at the end under brief synopsis of rheumatological diseases).

EXAMINATION OF THE SPINAL COLUMN

Patient should stand in erect posture in natural standing position—with feet together and arms hanging at the sides. The head should be in midline in the same plane as sacrum, and the shoulders and pelvis should be in the same plane.

Inspection

Posture
☞ Observe the posture, position of both neck and trunk when patient is entering the room.
☞ Assess the patient for erect position of the head, smooth, coordinated neck movements.
☞ Expose the patient's back for complete inspection.

- *Neck stiffness* indicates arthritis, muscle strain
- *Torticollis* (wry neck) indicates sternomastoid spasm or contracture
- *Cock-Robin position* indicates lateral flexion of neck due to erosion of atlas in rheumatoid arthritis.

Curvatures
☞ Inspect the patient from the side for spinal curvatures. Note any abnormal curvature of the spinal column whether as a whole or of part of it. The abnormal curvature may be in an anterior, posterior or lateral direction. The abnormal curvatures are:

- **Lordosis.** Anterior curvature is termed *lordosis*. There are normal lordotic curves in cervical and lumbar regions. Loss of lordosis occurs in acute disc prolapse.
- **Kyphosis.** Posterior curvature is termed *kyphosis* (Fig. 10.14). The thoracic spine exhibits a slight kyphosis normally, which increases with age. *Gibbus* is a localised angular deformity caused by fracture, Pott's disease (spinal tuberculosis) or by secondaries in the spines.

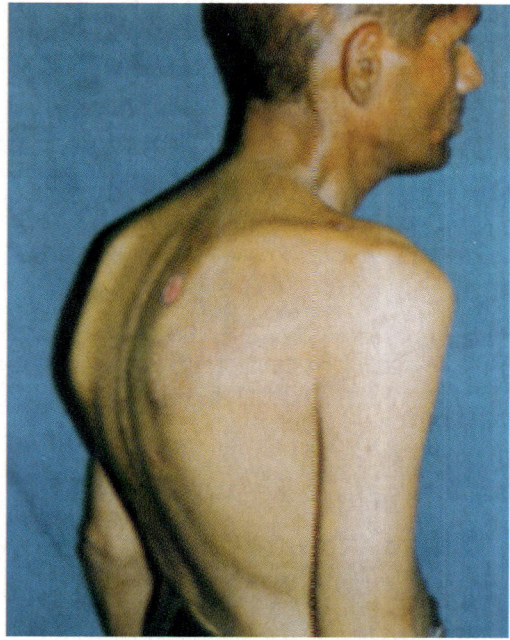

Fig. 10.14: Kyphosis.

- The *abnormalities of landmarks*, i.e. shoulder, ilias crests and skin creases below the buttocks are:
  1. Unequal shoulder heights are seen in scoliosis.
  2. Unequal lengths of iliac chests indicate hip or knee disease.
  3. Birthmarks postwine stain, hairy patches and lipoma commonly overlie spina bifida.
- **Scoliosis:** Scoliosis means lateral curvature of the spine and may be towards either side. It is associated with rotation of the bodies of the vertebrae.

In scoliosis bending of the patient due to acute disc protrusion is as follows;
- If protrusion is lateral to nerve root—patient bends away from lesion.
- If protrusion is medial to to nerve root—patient bends towards lesion.

When scoliosis is due to unequal leg lengths, it disappears on sitting because the buttocks then come at same level. Scoliosis secondary to skeletal anomalies shows a 'rib-hump' in spinal flexion combined due to rotation. Combined Kyphosis and scoliosis is often called *kyphoscoliosis* (Fig. 10.15) which is an idiopathic spinal deformity beginning in adolescence.

Palpation

☞ *In sitting or standing position, palpate the spinal processes of each vertebra by rolling the thumb with pressure over them and to note any tenderness.*

Tenderness suggests fracture or disc prolapse, infection or arthritis

☞ *In the lumbar region, check for any vertebral "step-off" (one spinous process seems either unusually prominent or recessed in relation to one above it). Identify any tenderness.*

Step-off occurs in spondylolisthesis, in which forward slippage of one vertebra may compress the spinal cord. Vertebral tenderness is suspicious for fracture or infection.

☞ *Palpate for tenderness over the sacroiliac joint, over and above the dimple overlying the posterior superior iliac spine.*

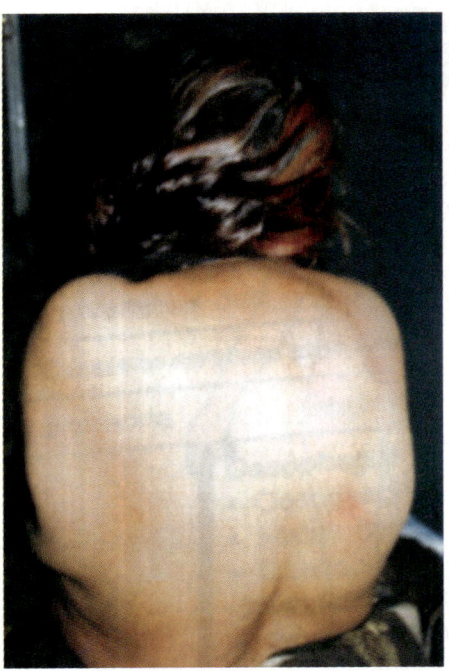

Fig. 10.15: Kyphoscoliosis.

For sacroiliac tenderness ask the patient to lie prone on a firm surface and apply firm pressure with palm of the hand over the sacrum.

Or

With the patient supine, fully flex the hip and knee and with firm pressure, abduct the thigh to stress the ipsilateral sacroiliac joint.

Pain arising from the sacroiliac joints may radiate into buttocks and posterior aspect of the thighs, but, unlike sciatica, does not go beyond knee. There is no reliable test to elicit tenderness of sacroiliac joint because both false positive and false negative results are common. In case of inflammation of sacroiliac joint, stressing of the buttocks to reproduce pain may be useful.

☞ *Tenderness: Elicit tenderness over spines*
  i. Use light percussion with the fist or tendon hammer to elicit spinal tenderness.

Pain on percussion of spines may arise from osteoporosis, infection or malignancy

☞ *Palpate the paravertebral muscles for tenderness and spasm. Muscles in spasm feel firm and knotted.*

Spasms occur in disc protrusion, myositis, prolonged abnormal posture and anxiety.

☞ *Elicit sciatic tenderness in sciatic notch*
  • With the hip flexed and patient lying on the opposite side, palpate the sciatic nerve between greater trochanter and the ischial tuberosity as it leaves the pelvis, i.e. in sciatic notch.

Sciatic nerve roots compression (L_4, L_5, S_1, S_2 and S_3) suggests a herniated disc or mass lesion irritating the nerve roots.

RAPID NEUROLOGICAL CHECK UP

☞ *Perform a detailed neurological check up noting any deficit in the limbs.*
  • Neurological deficit can occur due to compression of nerve root(s) or the spinal cord or the both.

TESTING OF SPINAL MOVEMENTS

☞ *Test the active and passive movements at various joints and note their range to identify any limitation or hypermobility.*

A. Testing of Cervical Movements

Flexion—Ask the patient to touch chin to chest.
Extension—Ask the patient to look up at the ceiling
Rotation—Ask the patient to turn the head to each side, looking directly over the shoulder
Lateral bending—Ask the patient to tilt the head sideways and try to touch the shoulder with the ear without raising the shoulder.

- Note any pain or paraesthesias in the arm reproduced by neck movement, suggesting nerve root involvement.

Warning: In patients with rheumatoid arthritis involving atlantoaxial joint or in patients with cervical injury, never try to elicit range of motion of the neck. Take the help of investigations such as X-rays for diagnosis.

B. Testing of Thoracic and Lumbar Spine Movements

The lumbar spines can flex, extend and bend laterally. The movements are tested as follows;

Flexion. Ask the patient to touch the toes without bending at the knees. *Note the smoothness, symmetry* and *range of movement* and the *lumbar curve.* As flexion proceeds, the lumbar concavity should flatten out.

Persistence of lumbar lordosis suggests muscle spasm or ankylosing spondylitis (Fig. 10.16C).

Measurement of Flexion of Spine (Schober's Test)

To measure the degree of flexion, first mark the spine at lumbosacral junction, then mark 10 cm above and 5 cm below this point (Fig. 10.16A) in standing position. Ask the patient to bend forwards as far as possible. A 4 cm increase between the two upper marks (10 cm mark + 4 cm) is normally seen (Fig. 10.16B). The distance between two lower marks remains same, i.e. 5 cm.

Extension: Place your hand on posterior superior iliac spine (Fig. 10.17A). Ask the patient to bend backward as far as possible.

Rotation: Stabilize the pelvis by placing one hand on the patient's hip and the other on the opposite shoulder. Now rotate the trunk by pushing the shoulder anteriorly and then pulling the hip posteriorly (Fig. 10.17B). Repeat the manoeuvre on the opposite side.

Lateral bending: Support the patient at the pelvis and at the shoulder, ask the patient to bend sideways as far as possible (Fig. 10.17C).

Decreased spinal movements occur in osteoarthritis, ankylosing spondylitis and other painful musculoskeletal conditions.

Tests for Degenerative Disc Disease

Tests for Nerve Root Compression in Prolapsed Disc

Prolapse of intervertebral disc is common at L_4/L_5 or L_5/S_1 level producing compression of the L_5 and

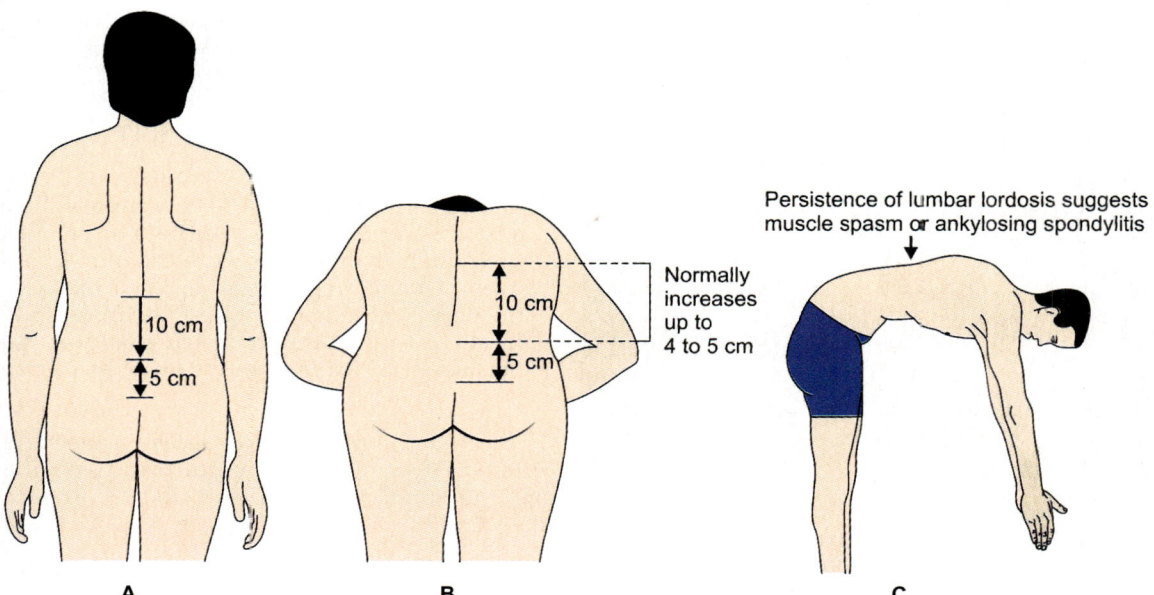

Figs 10.16A to C: Schober's test, measuring forward bending (flexion) of spine.

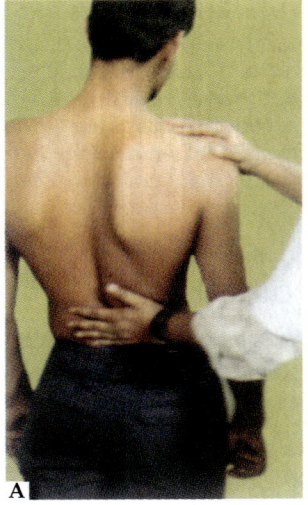
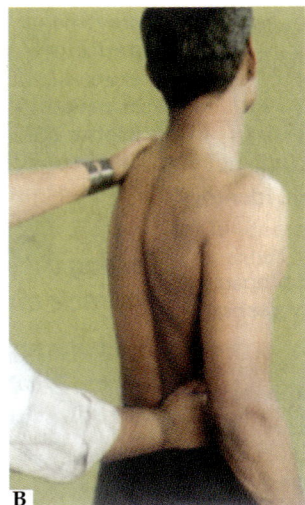
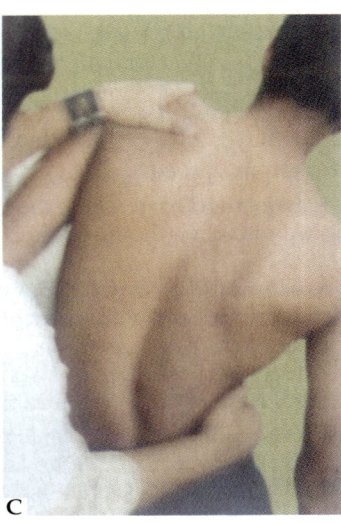

Figs 10.17A to C: Testing for the throacic and lumbar spine.

S_1 nerve roots respectively. *Straight-leg raising test* is used to stretch these roots.

Straight Leg Raising Test and Bragaard Test (Fig. 10.18)
- Make the patient lying supine and both legs extended.
- With knee extended, raise the leg on unaffected side by lifting the heel with one hand while preventing knee flexion with the other. Note the range of movement (normal up to 90° possible).
- Now repeat this manoeuvre on the affected side directing the patient to report as soon as pain is felt. Ask the patient to localise the pain or paraesthesia felt.
- When this limit is reached, augment the stretching of nerve roots by dorsiflexing the ankle (Bragaard test).
- Tests are said to be positive if pain occurs at <70° flexion of hip

Lassegue's Sign
- Perform the straight leg raising test as described in Fig. 10.18. When limit is reached, flex the knee to reduce the tension on sciatic nerve roots.
- Now further flex the hip.
- Now gently extend the knee until pain is reproduced once again, i.e. Lassegue's sign.

Bowstring Sign (Fig. 10.19)
- The posterior tibial nerve is now stretched like a bowstring across the popliteal fossa. Firm pressure is then applied with the thumb, first over the hamstring nearest the knee, then over the nerve in the middle of popliteal fossa and finally over the other hamstring tendon. Ask the patient which manoeuvre exacerbated pain (Fig. 10.19).

The test (sign) is positive if the second manoeuvre (pressure over middle of popliteal fossa) is painful and the resultant pain radiates from the knee to the back

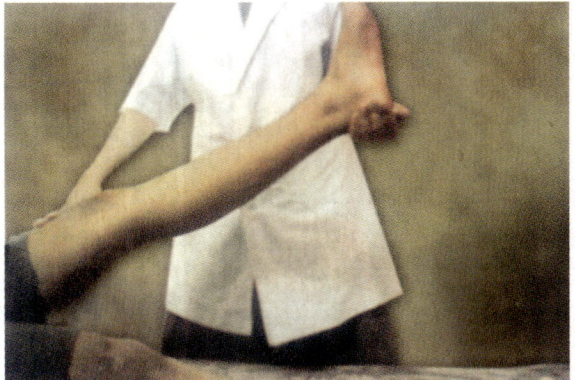

Fig. 10.18: Stretch tests for sciatic roots. *Straight leg raising test:* Normally about 90° of flexion at the hip is possible (varies from 70° to 120°) without producing pain. When the root is stretched over a prolapsed disc, the straight leg raising will be restricted before 70° flexion due to pain which will be felt in the lumbar region, not just in the leg.

Flip test (Fig. 10.20)
It is used to distinguish between sciatic nerve root irritation from malingering.

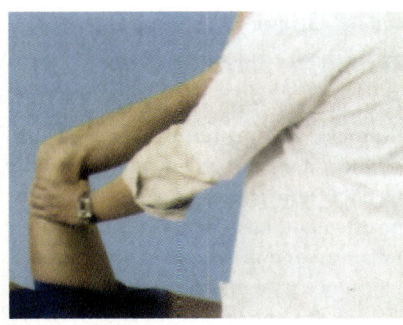

Fig. 10.19: Bowstring sign. Pressure over centre of popliteal fossa stretches posterior tibial nerve like a "bowstringing" across the fossa causing pain locally and radiation into back.

- The patient is made to sit on the edge of couch with the hips and knees flexed to 90°. Test the knee reflexes (Fig. 10.20A).
- Now extend the knee to an extent to elicit the ankle jerk (Fig. 10.20B).
- If there is sciatic root irritation, then patient will flip backwards to relieve tension on the nerve roots (Fig. 10.20B).
- In the absence of nerve root irritation (malingering), the patient's attention distracted to the ankle jerk, may allow full extension of the knee, i.e. to 90° (Fig. 10.20C).

Femoral Nerve Stretch Test (Figs 10.21A and B)

- Make the patient to lie prone, in case of flexion deformity of the hip to lie on the unaffected side.
- Flex the knee slowly, while asking the patient to report the onset of pain. If pain does not occur in the thigh or back, gently extend the hip with the knees remaining flexed (Fig. 10.21B).

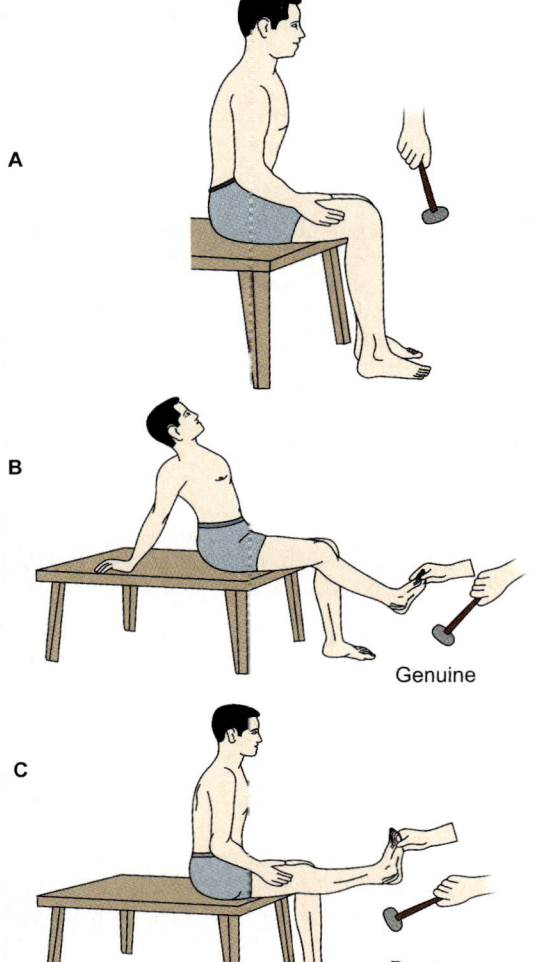

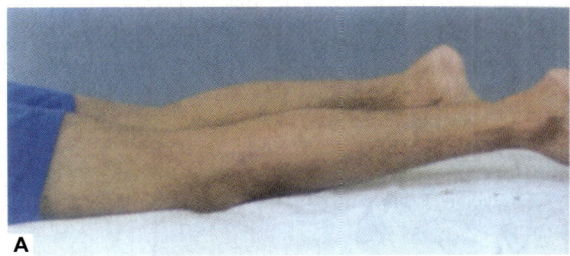

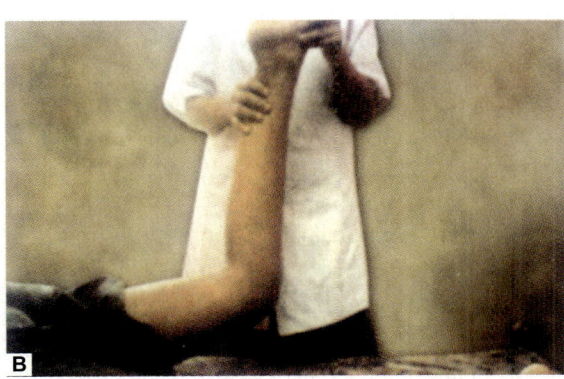

Figs 10.21A and B: Femoral nerve stretch test. (A) Patient lies prone and is free from pain because femoral roots are slack; (B) When femoral roots are tightened by flexion of the knee, pain may be felt in the back. If still no pain, femoral roots are further stretched by extension of the hip.

UPPER LIMB JOINTS

The Shoulder Joint

The shoulder joint (glenohumeral) is a ball and socket joint. It has a wide range of movements.

Figs 10.20A to C: Flip test. In the "flip" test, when attention is diverted to the tendon reflexes, the genuine patient will not permit full extension of the leg.

The rotator cuff muscles [SITS muscles—supraspinatus (S), infraspinatus (I), teres minor (T) and subscapularis (S)] surround the glenohumeral joint and are inserted into a fibrous capsule lining the joint and take part in the movements of joints. The movements at shoulder joint are:

1. Flexion 180°
2. Extension 60°
3. Abduction 180°
4. Adduction 50°
5. Rotation (external as well as internal up to 90°)

Examination of the Shoulder

If there is history of shoulder pain ask the patient to point to the painful area.

- Rotator cuff injury (tendinitis, tears, degeneration, tendon rupture) produces pain at lateral aspect of shoulder.
- Subacromial bursitis (calcific bursitis, arthritis) and capsulitis (frozen shoulder) produce pain at the top of shoulder.
- Head of humerus (tumour deposit, osteonecrosis, fracture/dislocation) and bicipital tendinitis produce pain at anterior shoulder.
- Joints—synovitis, osteoarthritis, dislocation, produce pain anteriorly and posteriorly.

Inspection

☞ *Inspect and compare the shoulder girdle from the front, scapulae and related muscles from behind. Note any muscle wasting, soft tissue swelling or difference in bony contour on the two sides.*

- Muscle atrophy suggests to a lesion in cervical nerves or periarthritis
- In scoliosis, there is elevation of one shoulder facing towards convexity.
- The shoulder contour gets flattened in its dislocation (i.e. in anterior dislocation, the lateral aspect is flattened while in posterior dislocation, the anterior aspect is flattened).

☞ *Look for swelling of the joint capsule anteriorly or a bulge in the acromial bursa under deltoid muscle.*

A significant amount of fluid may collect in the synovial cavity producing outpouching of bursa.

☞ *Survey the entire upper extremity for colour change, skin alteration or abnormal positioning.*

☞ *Stand behind the patient and observe the overall range of movements by asking the patient to place the hands at the base of the neck with elbow pointing sideways.*

☞ *Next ask the patient to put the arms down and to reach behind the back in-between the shoulder blades.*

☞ *Proceed further only if pain, swelling or limitation of movements is present.*

Palpation

Testing for range of movements at shoulder

The neutral position is with the arm to the side, elbow flexed to 90° with forearm pointing forwards. Because the scapula is mobile, true shoulder (glenohumeral) movement can be assessed only when the examiner immobilises the scapula between the thumb and the finger on the posterior chest wall.

☞ *Test the following movements at shoulder*

- Flexion and extension (Fig. 10.22)
- Abduction and adduction (Fig. 10.22)
- Rotation (external and internal) in neutral position (Fig. 10.22)
- Elevation

In clinical practice, internal rotation can best be compared by recording the height reached by each thumb up the back (*internal rotation and adduction*). This is tested by "asking the patient to scratch the back" or undo the bra strap (*Apley test*, Fig. 10.23). Similarly external rotation can be tested by asking the patient to place both hands behind the neck with elbows out to the side (tests external rotation and adduction Fig. 10.23, *Apley test*).

- Note any pain during the range of movement. In supraspinatus tendinitis (rotator cuff), a full passive range of movement is found, but there is a painful arc on abduction, with pain exacerbated on resisted abduction (Fig. 10.22).

Testing for the rotator cuff injury

☞ *Test the SITS muscles (Fig. 10.24)*

THE ELBOW JOINT

The elbow helps to position the hand in space and stabilises the lever action of the forearm. The joint is formed by the *humerus* and two bones of the forearm, the *radius* and the *ulna*. The three bony prominences, at the elbow are; *two epicondyles* (medial and lateral) of the humerus and tip of the *olecranon* which forms an equilateral triangle. The *subcutaneous bursa* overlying the olecranon is visible and palpable only when inflamed. The movements and the muscles involved are:

1. *Flexion* is carried out by biceps and brachioradialis

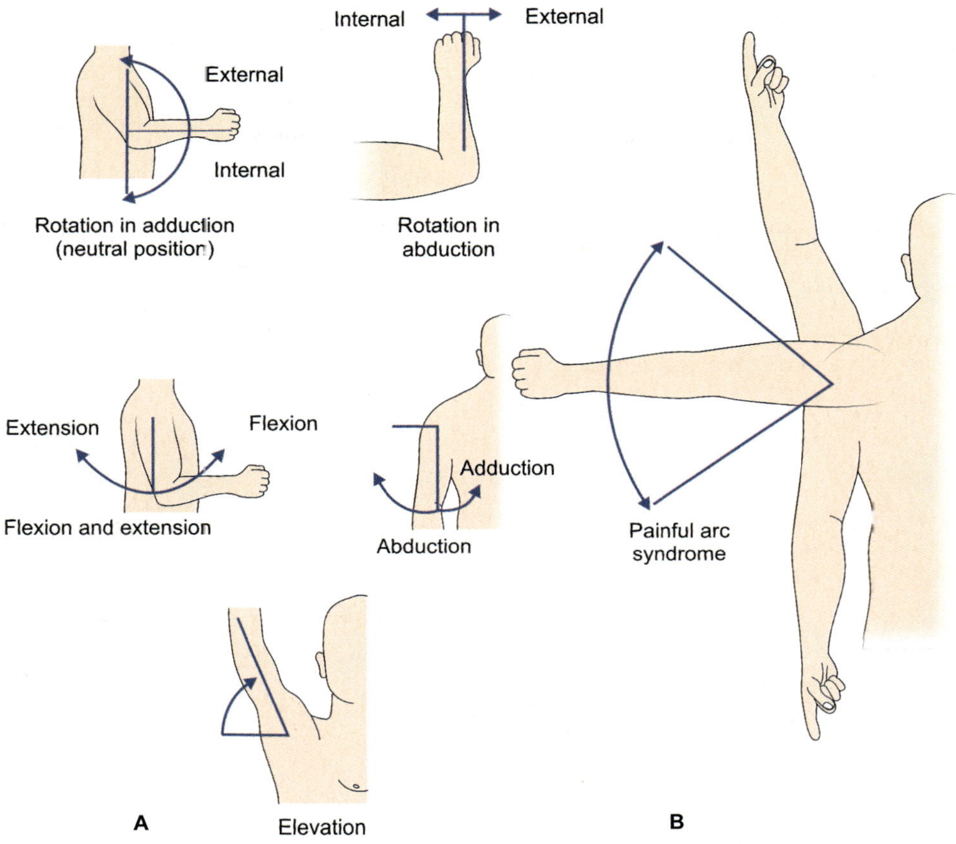

Figs 10.22A and B: Movements at the shoulder. **A.** The movements are tested against resistance. Stand in front of the patient and test the range of following movements at shoulder by asking the patient to:
 i. Move the forearm forwards (flexion) and backwards (extension)
 ii. Abduction and adduction. Raise the arm to shoulder level 90° against resistance with palms facing down. Now keeping the arm abducted bring it back to the side of chest (adduction)
 iii. Elevation. Raise the arms to 0° vertical position above the head with palms facing each other. This tests initial 60° movement
 iv. Rotation: Keep the arm by the side of the chest (adduction), rotate the forearm outwards (external rotation) and inwards (internal rotation). This is rotation in adduction.

B. Painful arc syndrome: Inability to perform these movements results in painful arc syndrome which is due to involvement of soft tissue around shoulder such as bursitis, capsulitis, rotator cuff tears or sprains or tendinitis.

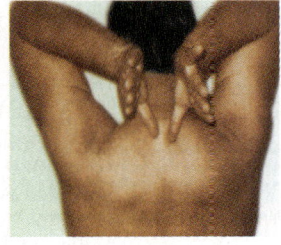

Fig. 10.23: Apley from above. Functional test of the infraspinatus and teres minor, that is, external rotation. Here the findings are quite normal. Internal rotation can be tested by asking the patient to scratch the back

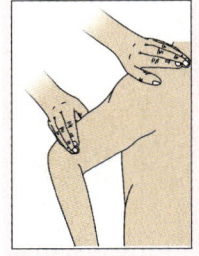

Fig. 10.24: Testing for rotator cuff injury.

SITS (*supraspinatus, infraspinatus, teres minor* and *subscapsularis*) muscle insert anteriorly at the shoulder, hence, palpate them on the greater tuberosity of the humerus with the patient's arm hanging by the side.

These muscles can also be tested (Fig. 10.24) by passively extending the shoulder by lifting the elbow posteriorly. This manoeuvre brings the rotator cuff on to the acromion. Palpate these muscles at the greater tuberosity of the humerus.

Tenderness over SITS muscles indicate sprains, tears or tendon rupture of the rotator cuff.

Drop-arm sign (ask the patient to abduct the arm fully up to 90° and then lower slowly) if positive (inability to hold the arm abduced at shoulder lines) indicates "*rotator cuff tear*".

2. *Extension* is done by triceps
3. *Pronator* teres does the *pronation*.
4. *Supination* is done by supinator

Examination of Elbow Joint

Inspection and Palpation

☞ *Support the patient's forearm with your opposite hand and flex the elbow to about 70. Inspect the contours of the elbow. Note any nodule or swelling.*

The causes of swollen elbow are arthritis, olecranon bursitis, epicondylitis and rheumatoid nodules.

☞ *Palpate the olecranon process and press on the epicondyles for tenderness. Note any displacement of olecranon.*

Medial (*golfer's elbow*) and lateral (*tennis elbow*, Fig. 10.25) epicondylitis are the common causes of pain and tenderness of elbow.

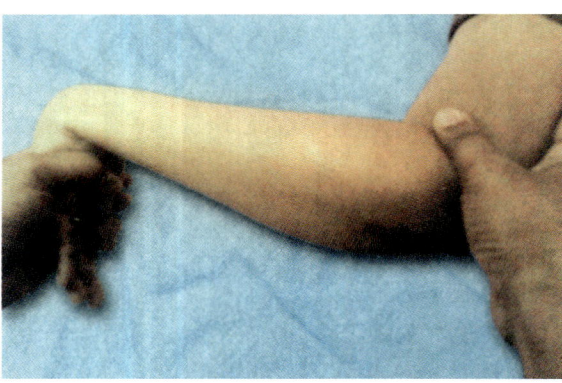

Fig. 10.25: Pain aggravation on dorsiflexion against resistance.

☞ *Palpate the groove between epicondyles and the olecranon, noting any swelling or tenderness.*

The synovium is most commonly accessible in this region if there is synovitis (normally neither synovium nor bursa is palpable). The ulnar nerve can also be palpated posteriorly between the olecranon process and the medial epicondyle.

Testing for Movements at Elbow Joint

The neutral position is with the forearm in extension. The following movements are tested:

☞ *Flexion and extension (Fig. 10.26):* To test these movements ask the patient to bend (flex) and straighten (extend) elbow.

☞ *Supination and pronation (Fig. 10.27).* With the patient sitting with an arm by the side and elbows flexed to minimize shoulder movement, ask the patient to supinate (turn up the palm) and pronate (turn down the palm).

THE JOINTS OF WRIST AND HANDS

The wrist joints include the *radiocarpal*, the distal *radioulnar joint* and *intercarpal joints*. On the dorsum of the wrist, there is groove of the radiocarpal joint.

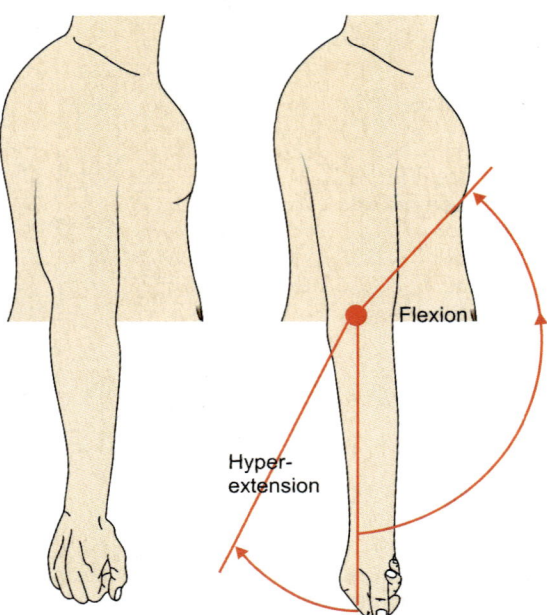

Fig. 10.26: Movements at elbow (e.g. flexion, hyperextension).

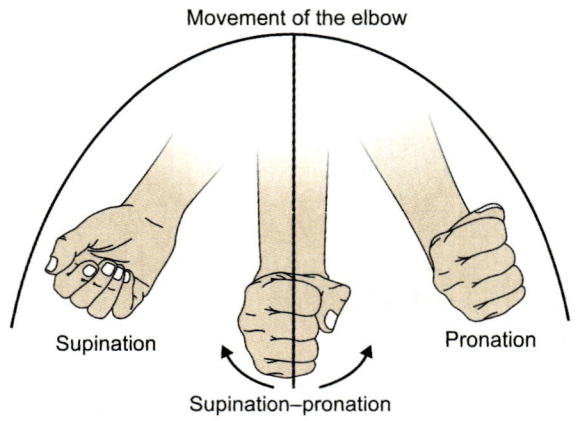

Fig. 10.27: Movements of the forearm/elbow (supination and pronation).

The joints of the hands include *metacarpophalangeal joints* (MCPs), the *proximal interphalangeal joints* (PIPs) and *the distal interphalangeal joints* (DIPs). Flex the hand and you will find the groove marking the MCP joint of each finger. It is distal to the knuckles and is best felt on either side of the extensor tendon on dorsal aspect of hand.

The movements at the wrist are *flexion* and *extension* (dorsiflexion), *deviation* (ulnar and radial) of the hand (Fig. 10.28).

The *pronation* and *supination* of the wrist result from respective muscle contraction in the forearm (already discussed).

Soft tissue structures important in the wrist and the hand are:

1. *Flexor retinaculum.* It is a transverse ligament across the wrist that holds the structures at wrist in place. The median nerve passes underneath it and provides sensation to the palm and the palmar surface of three and half fingers (*thumb, the index, middle and inner half of ring fingers*). It also supplies muscles of flexion, abduction and apposition of the thumb.
2. *Carpal tunnel.* It is a canal or tunnel beneath the flexor retinaculum, contains the sheath and flexor tendons of the forearm muscles and the median nerve.

Examination of Wrist Joints

Inspection

☞ Observe the position of the hands in motion to see if the movements are smooth and natural.

The movements are tested in neutral position, i.e. hand in line with the forearm and palm down (Fig. 10.28A).

Flexion. Ask the patient to flex the wrist against gravity, then against resistance (Fig. 10.28B).

Extension. Ask the patient to extend the wrist (dorsiflex) against gravity, then against graded resistance.

Ulnar and radial deviation. With palms down, ask the patient to move wrist laterally and medially (Fig. 10.28C).

☞ Inspect the hands and wrists (palm and dorsum) carefully for any swelling over the joints.

Diffuse swelling of hand(s) and wrist(s) is seen in arthritis and acute infection.
Localised swelling or ganglia arise from cystic enlargement.

☞ Look specifically for skin and nail changes, muscle wasting, joint deformity (ulnar or radial deviation).

The abnormalities of the hand associated with rheumatic diseases are rheumatic nodules, rheumatoid nodules, rheumatoid hands in RA (ulnar deviation of the hand).

☞ Observe contours of the palm, namely the thenar and hypothenar eminences.

Thenar atrophy indicates median nerve compression. Hypothenar atrophy indicates ulnar nerve compression (palsy).

☞ Note any thickening of the flexor tendons or flexion contractures in the finger.

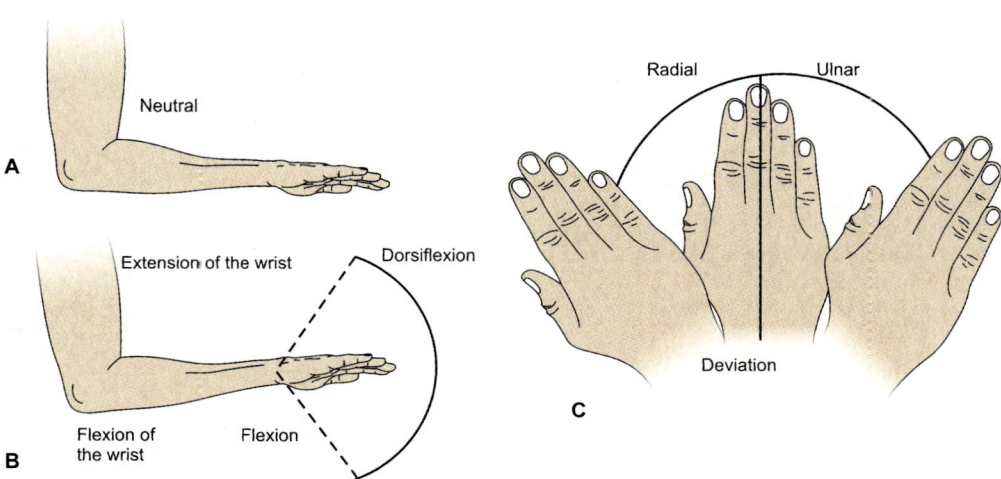

Figs 10.28A to C: Movements of the wrist.

Flexion contractures of 3rd, 4th and 5th fingers or Dupuytren's contractures (Fig. 10.9) arise from thickening of the palmar fascia.

Palpation

☞ *Palpate the wrist joint with your thumbs on the dorsum of the wrist and fingers beneath it (Fig. 10.29).*

Tenderness over distal radius occurs in *Colles' fracture*. Any tenderness or bony step-off indicates fracture.

Swelling and tenderness of joints indicate rheumatoid arthritis if bilateral or gonococcal infection if unilateral arthritis.

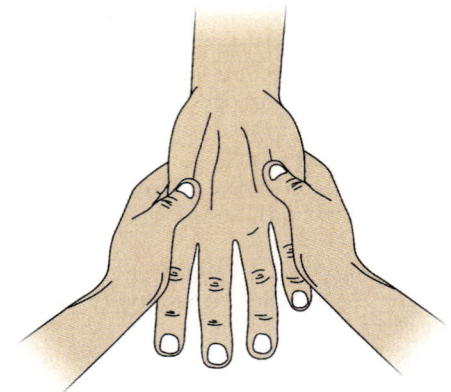

Fig. 10.30: To palpate and elicit tenderness at each metacarpophalangeal joint.

☞ Palpate the flexor tendons and tendon sheaths inserted on the thumb and fingers with your index finger for any *swelling* or *tenderness*.

Swelling and tenderness along the tendons indicate tenosynovitis.

Testing of the Movements

1. At wrist joint: They have already been described (Fig. 10.28).

2. At the finger joints: The movements are tested in relation to neutral position. The neutral position is with the fingers in extension.

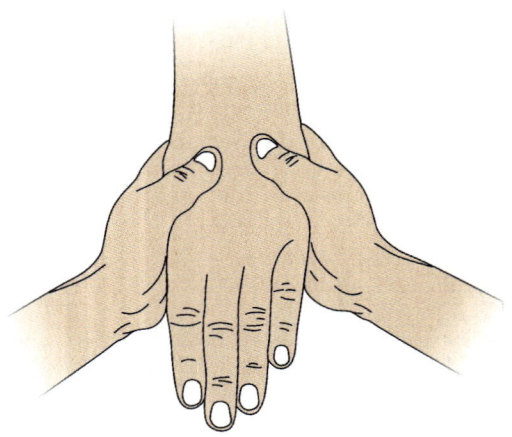

Fig. 10.29: Palpation of wrist joint.

☞ *Palpate the anatomical snuff box (a hollowed depression just distal to radial styloid process).*

Tenderness over snuff box suggests a scaphoid fracture.

☞ Compress the MCP joints by squeezing the hand from each side between the thumb and fingers (is equivalent to shaking hands). Alternatively use your thumb to palpate each MCP on each side of knuckles as your index finger feels the head of the metacarpal in the palm (Fig. 10.30). Note any swelling or tenderness.

Shaking hands are painful in synovitis of MCP

☞ Palpate the PIP joints between your thumb and index finger. *Note for swelling or enlargement or tenderness.* Using the same technique, examine DIP joints.

☞ *Flexion and extension* can be tested by asking the patients to make a tight fist with each hand, thumb across the knuckles, and then extend and spread the fingers. The fingers should open and close smoothly and easily. Test flexion and extension of MCP, PIP and DIP joints against gravity and against resistance (Fig. 10.31).

☞ *Abduction and adduction.* Ask the patient to spread the fingers apart (abduction) and back together (adduction). *Check for smooth coordinated movements.*

3. At the thumb (Fig. 10.32): Movements are tested in relation to neutral position (thumb along the side of index fingers and extended). The movements tested are:

☞ *Flexion and extension.* Ask the patient to touch the base of little finger with the thumb (flexion) and then to move the thumb back across the palm and away from the fingers to test extension (Fig. 10.32C).

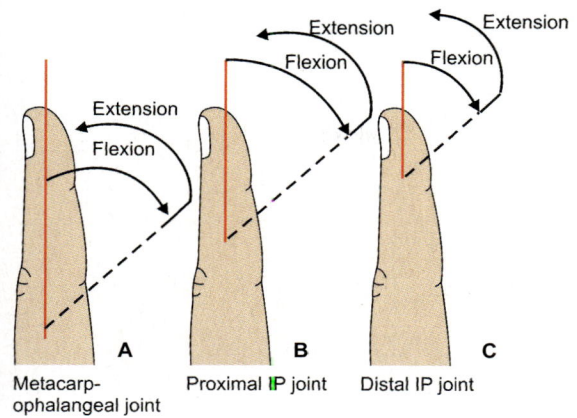

Figs 10.31A to C: Movement of the fingers. The movements are tested against gravity and against resistance.

- *Abduction and adduction.* Ask the patient to place the fingers and thumb in neutral position with the palm up, now ask the patient to move the thumb anteriorly away from the palm (abduction Fig. 10.32B) and then back to same position (adduction).
- *Apposition.* Ask the patient to touch the thumb to each of the other fingertips (Fig. 10.32C).

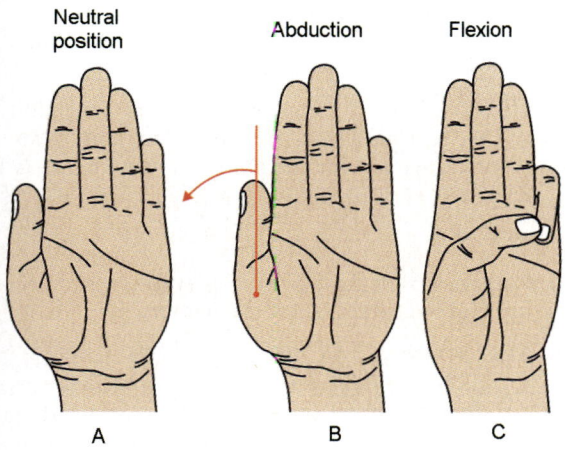

Figs 10.32A to C: Movements of the thumbs. (A) Neutral, (B) Abduction and adduction, (C) Flexion and extension and apposition

Assessment of Hand Function

- *Fine pinch.* Ask the patient to perform the pinch grip (between the thumb and index finger).

It may be decreased in scaphoid fracture.

- *Hand grip.* Assess the grip strength by asking the patient to grip two or three fingers of the examiner's hands. If the movements of the joints are not full, then patient will not be able to grip the fingers tightly.

Test for Sensations

- At the end, *test the sensation in the fingers.* Test median, ulnar and radial nerve sensation in the hand as discussed in nervous system examination.

Pain and numbness and objective loss of sensations on the ventral surface of first three and half fingers but not the palm along with weakness of abduction of the thumb indicates carpal tunnel syndrome which is confirmed by the tests described below.

Tests for Carpal Tunnel Syndrome

- *Thumb abduction test.* To test the abductor pollicis, ask the patient to raise the thumb perpendicular to the palm against resistance applied on the distal phalanx.

Patient is not able to abduct the thumb in carpal tunnel syndrome.

- *Tinel's sign (Fig. 10.33A).* Percuss lightly with your finger at the spot on the carpal tunnel. Tingling or electric sensations in the distribution of the median nerve constitute positive test and confirms the diagnosis of carpal tunnel syndrome.
- *Phalen's manoeuvre.* The manoeuvre is performed to compress the median nerve in the tunnel. The test is performed by asking the patient to press the back of the both hands (Fig. 10.33B) together at right angle. The appearance of numbness or tingling within a minute over the distribution of median nerve (palmar surface of lateral three and half fingers) indicates that the sign is positive, suggesting carpal tunnel syndrome.

LOWER LIMB JOINTS

The Hip Joint

The hip joint—a synovial joint is deeply embedded in the pelvis. The stability of joint is due to fitting of the head of the femur into the *acetabulum*, its strong fibrous capsule and powerful muscles, i.e. *flexors* (e.g. mainly *iliopsoas*), extensors (mainly *gluteus maximus*) adductor and abductor (*gluteus medium* and *minimus*).

The three principal bursae at the hip are: *Iliopsoas, trochanteric* and *ischiogluteal*.

Important Landmarks

On the anterior aspect of the hip, identify the iliac crest as the rim of pelvis at the level of LI. Follow

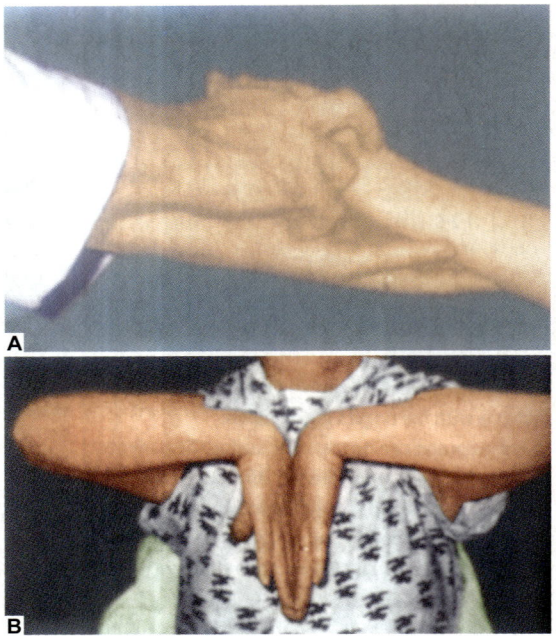

Figs 10.33A and B: Tests for carpal tunnel syndrome. (A) Tinel's sign; (B) Phalen's manoeuvre.

the downward curve to locate anterior superior iliac spine.

On the posterior aspect, the posterior superior iliac supine lies directly under the dimple just above the buttocks.

Symptoms of Hip Disease

1. *Hip pain:* It may be felt in the groin, anterior thigh or knee. The pain is worst during activity and walking, may be distressing at night.
2. *Stiffness:* The stiffness results in limitation of movements especially flexion and causing difficulty in putting on socks or shoes or cutting the toe nails. There may be difficulty getting in and out of the bath or sitting on a low chair.

Examination of Hip Joint

Inspection

☞ Inspect the hip while standing and observe the gait while walking. *Note any abnormality of gait.*
☞ Observe the patient from behind for *scoliosis* and *pelvic tilt* which may conceal a hip deformity or true shortening of one leg (Fig. 10.34). *If pelvic tilt occurs, measure the leg lengths.*
☞ Inspect the front and back surface of the hip for any *muscle wasting or bruising.*

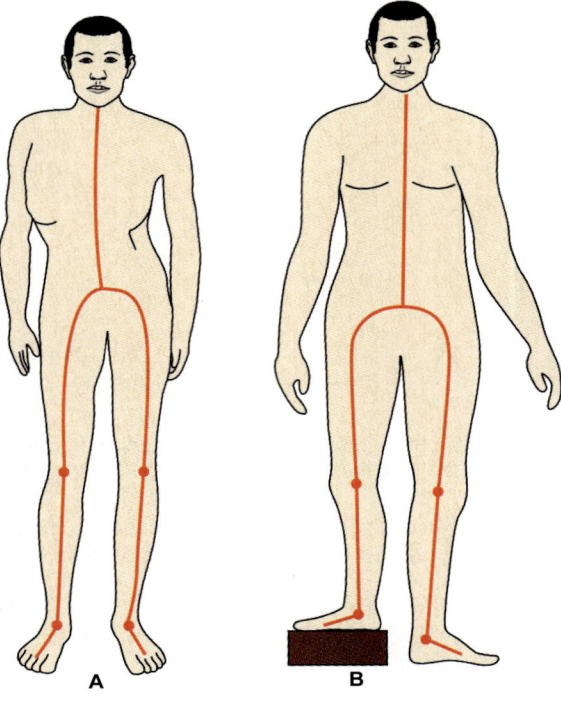

Figs 10.34A and B: Effect of true shortening right leg on posture. (A) Pelvic tilt and scoliosis; (B) Pelvic tilt and scoliosis are fully corrected by providing a shoe base.

Testing for Stability of the Hip (Trendelenburg's test)

☞ Ask the patient to stand first on one leg and then on the other, and observe any change in pelvic tilt on the non-weight bearing side (Fig. 10.35).

Palpation

☞ Palpate for local *tenderness* over the front of the hip and over the greater trochanter.
☞ Measurement of 'true' and 'apparent' shortening
  • For measurement of apparent shortening place the legs parallel with the patient lying supine. The length of the leg is measured from a fixed point, i.e. xiphisternum or umbilicus to the tip of medial malleolus on each side, provided there is no true shortening of one leg.

Apparent shortening is due to tilting of the pelvis, indicates adduction deformity of hip

  • For *true shortening*, measure the distance from anterior superior iliac supine to medial malleolus and compare it with the other side. Any difference is termed *'true'* shortening.

Examination of Musculoskeletal and Locomotor System

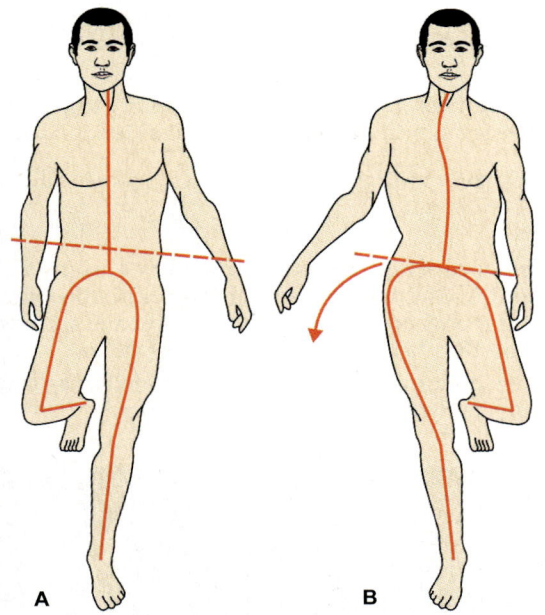

Figs 10.35A and B: Trendelenburg's test for testing the gluteal muscles.
A. Powerful gluteal muscles maintain the position normally on standing on one leg, i.e. the left leg in the figure;
B. Weakness of gluteal muscles on right side causes pelvic tilt on standing on the right leg.

True shortening results either from the disease of hip joint, i.e. dislocation of neck of the femur or fracture. There may be unilateral painless limp. Bilateral dislocation of hip produces lordosis, prominent buttock and abdomen with waddling gait.

Testing of Movements

The following movements are tested in neutral position (i.e. hip in extension, and patella pointing forwards).

☞ *Flexion.* With one hand on the iliac crest in a patient lying supine, use the other hand to flex each hip and note the range of flexion (0–120°).

☞ *Extension.* Try to stabilise the pelvis with one hand while the patient is lying in a lateral position. Attempt to extend the hip backwards by the other hand.

☞ *Abduction (Fig. 10.36A).* Stabilise the pelvis by grasping the opposite iliac crest with one hand. With the other hand grasp the ankle and abduct the extended leg (variable minimum 45°) until you feel the iliac spine move. This movement marks the limit of hip abduction.

Restricted hip abduction is common in osteo-arthritis.

☞ *Adduction (Fig. 10.36A).* With the patient supine, stabilise the pelvis, hold one ankle and move the leg medially across the body and over the opposite extremity.

☞ *Rotation (Fig. 10.36B).* Flex the leg to 90° at hip and knee, stabilise the thigh with one hand, hold the ankle with the other, and swing the lower leg medially for external rotation at the hip and laterally for internal rotation.

Rotation movements are restricted in hip arthritis.

THE KNEE JOINT

Knee joint is formed between the *femur*, the *tibia* and the *patella* (knee cap) with three articular surfaces. The medial and lateral epicondyles stand out as bony prominences on the medial and lateral aspects of the joint.

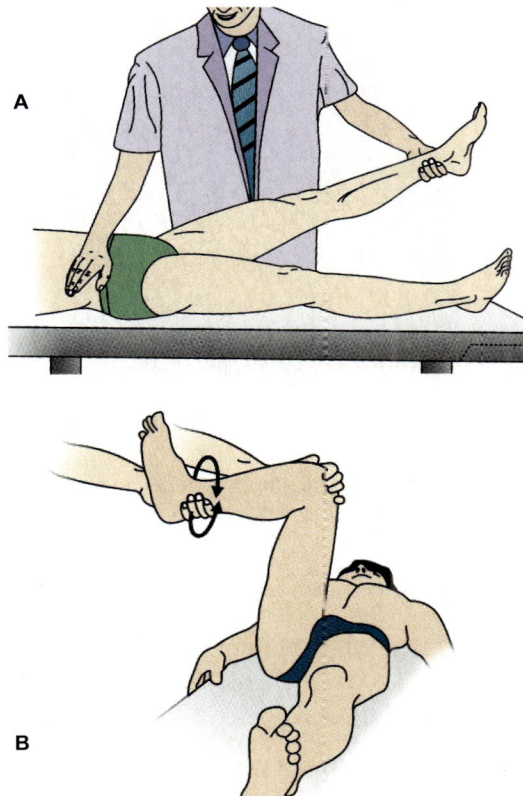

Figs 10.36A and B: Movements of the hip joint. (A) Testing the abduction and adduction of hip; (B) External (medial) and internal (lateral) rotation of the hip.

Examination of the Knee Joint

Inspection

☞ *Observe the gait for a smooth, rhythmic movements as the patient enters the room.*

The knee should be extended at heel strike and flexed at all other stages of swing and stance.

Stumbling or pushing the knee into extension with the hand during heel strike suggests quadriceps weakness.

☞ With the patient standing, note the presence of *bow legs (genu varum)* and knock-knees *(genu valgum, Fig. 10.37).*

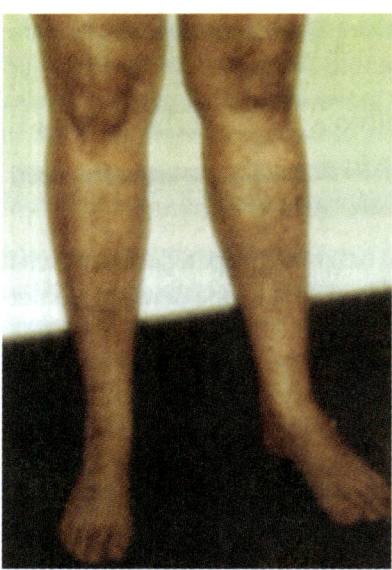

Fig. 10.37: Genu valgus or valgum.

☞ With the patient supine, inspect the limb alignment and note any *deformity, bony contour, erythema or swelling.*

A large effusion is seen as 'horseshoe' swelling just above the patella.
A synovial swelling in popliteal fossa indicates Baker's cyst.

☞ Look for *muscle wasting.*

The quadriceps rapidly wastes in disease of the knee joint.

Palpation

☞ With the knee flexed, palpate the joint line to elicit tenderness.

☞ Palpate the *ligaments, tendons and borders of menisci for any tenderness.*

Tenderness over the tendon or inability to extend the leg suggest quadricep's (patellar) tendon tear.

☞ *Perform patellar tap test (Fig. 10.38) if knee effusion is suspected.*

Presence of fluid can be confirmed by pushing the fluid from the suprapatellar bursa into the joint. On tapping on patella, it hits the femur and springs back, the phenomenon is called patellar tap.
If the amount of fluid is small, the patellar tap can only be elicited in the standing position.

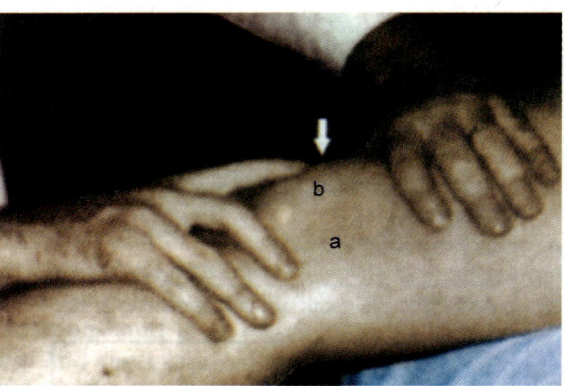

Fig. 10.38: Examination for knee effusion. Put the leg at knee in extension and parallel to floor. (a) Site of potential bulge of an effusion—posterior to patella, over joint line; (b) Application of pressure on patella to attempt ballottement (ballottement is positive in joint effusion).

☞ If quadriceps wasting is suspected, record and compare the muscle girth at a selected level above the patella (say 10 cm) in both thighs.

The difference between the muscle girth at thighs indicates quadriceps wasting on the side where it is decreased.

Testing the Movements of the Knee Joint

The principal movements of the knee are

☞ *Flexion and Extension (Fig. 10.39)*

Ask the patient to flex and extend the knee while sitting.

or

Knee flexion and extension can also be assessed by asking the patient to squat and stand up to provide support if needed to maintain balance.

Examination of Musculoskeletal and Locomotor System

☞ *Rotation.* To check internal and external rotation, ask the patient to rotate the foot medially and laterally.

Testing for Achilles Tendon

☞ Palpate the **tendon Achilles** from about the lower third of the calf to its insertion on the calcaneus. *Note any tenderness or swelling.*

Tenderness and swelling occurs in ruptured Achilles tendon or tendinitis
Tenderness of Achilles tendon at its insertion on calcaneous (enthesopathy) is common in ankylosing spondylitis and Reiter's syndrome.

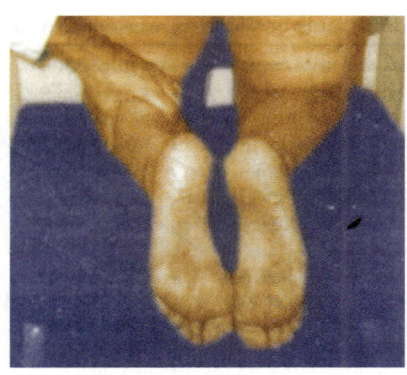

Fig. 10.40: Thompson's test. Squeeze the gastrocnemius muscle to assess the integrity of the Achilles tendon. Here foot is plantar flexed separate flexed with the test and thus is normal.

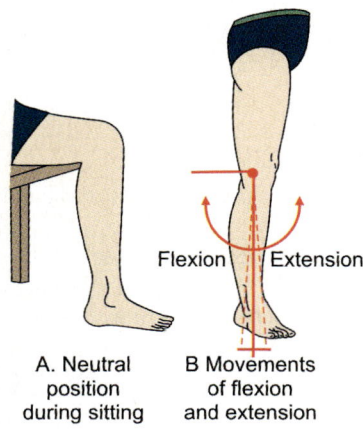

A. Neutral position during sitting
B. Movements of flexion and extension

Figs 10.39A and B: Movements of the knee joint. The movements are tested against gravity and against resistance. (A) Neutral position on sitting; (B) Flexion and extension.

☞ To test the integrity of the *Achilles tendon, perform Thompson's test* by asking the patient to kneel on a chair. Squeeze the calf and watch for plantar flexion at the ankle (Fig. 10.40).

Absence of plantar-flexion is a positive test, indicates rupture of Achilles tendon. Patients on steroid therapy are prone to this rupture.

THE ANKLE AND THE FOOT JOINTS

The ankle is a hinge and a weight-bearing joint between the *tibia*, the *fibula* and the *talus*. The three bony landmarks at the ankle are: the *medial malleolus* the *lateral malleolus* and *calcaneus*—the heel.

The ankle and foot are sites of sprain and bony injury in sports persons

Examination of the Ankle and Foot Joints

Inspection

☞ Inspect all surfaces of the ankles and feet, noting any *deformities, nodules* or *swellings* and any *calluses* or *corns*. Note the conditions of the *nails* and *skin*.

- *Talipes* (club foot) is usually a congenital deformity of foot.
- *Talipes equinus*. Patient walks on the foot due to extension of the foot.
- *Talipes valgus* is a condition in which the heel is turned outwards.
- *Talipes varus* is a condition in which the heel is turned inwards.

Palpation

☞ With your thumbs, palpate the anterior aspect of each ankle joint, and elicit any *tenderness* (Fig. 10.41).

- Arthritis of ankle causes diffuse pain and tenderness.

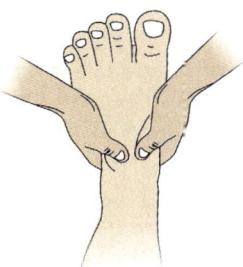

Fig. 10.41: To elicit tenderness at ankle joint in arthritis.

🖝 Feel the Achilles tendon for *nodules* and *tenderness*.

- Achilles tendinitis may produce painful swelling behind the ankle which worsens on walking or pressure from the footwear.
- In sub-Achilles bursitis, pain is similar to tendinitis (as discussed above) but the swelling bulges out on either side of the Achilles tendon.

🖝 Palpate the heel especially the posterior and inferior calcaneus, and the plantar fascia for *tenderness*.

- Tenderness under the heel at the insertion of plantar fascia occurs in calcaneous spur and plantar fasciitis.

🖝 Palpate the metatarsophalangeal joints for tenderness. Compress the forefoot between the thumb and fingers (Fig. 10.42). Exert pressure just proximal to the head of the 1st and 5th metatarsals.

Metatarsalgia occurs in trauma, arthritis and vascular insufficiency.
The cause of pain and tenderness in the foot are:
1. Plantar fascitis, synovitis involving MTP joints
2. Calcaneus fracture or stress fracture of metatarsal.
3. Arthritis, tenosynovitis, bursitis.
4. Plantar nerve neuroma (Morton's neuroma)

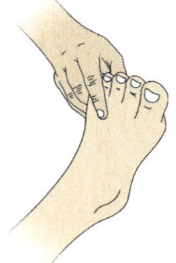

Fig. 10.43: To elicit tenderness on metatarsals.

Testing of Movements of Ankle

The movements that occur at the ankle include *flexion* and *extension* at the ankle joint and *inversion* and *eversion of the foot* at subtalar and transverse talar joints.

🖝 **Dorsiflexion and plantar flexion** (Fig. 10.44). Ask the patient to move the foot upwards (dorsiflexion) and downwards (plantar flexion) against gravity and resistance.

🖝 **Inversion and eversion.** Stabilise the ankle with one hand, grasp the heel with the other, and invert

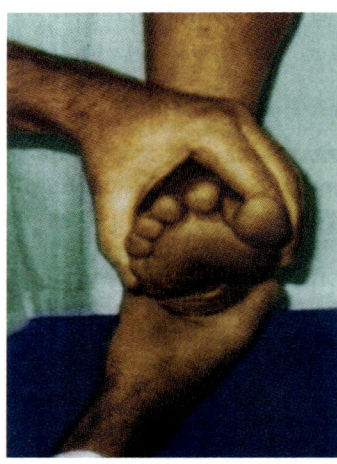

Fig. 10.42: Transverse arch squeeze test, to elicit the tenderness on metatarsophalangeal joint. Examiner squeezes the forefoot to accentuate the transverse arch. Pain from metatarsalgia or Morton's neuroma will increase on the plantar and dorsal aspects, respectively.

Tenderness on metatarsals is an early sign of rheumatoid arthritis. Pain and tenderness of first metatarsophalangeal joint is seen in acute gouty arthritis:

🖝 *Palpate the heads of 5 metatarsals and the grooves between them with your thumb and index finger for tenderness (Fig. 10.43). Place your thumb on dorsum of the foot and your index finger on the plantar surface.*

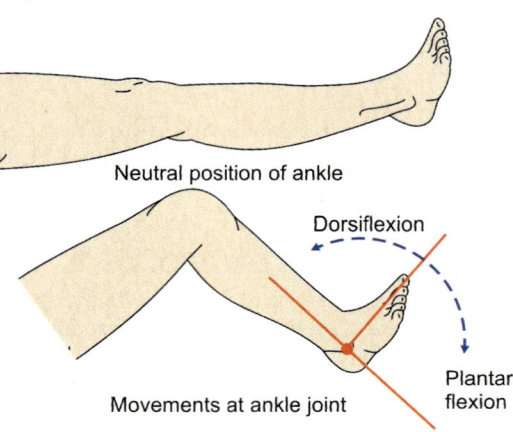

Fig. 10.44: Movements at the ankle joint. These movements are tested against gravity and against resistance.

and evert the foot (Fig. 10.45). These movements occur at tibiotarsal joints.

☞ **Metatarsophalangeal and interphalangeal.** Flexion and extension are illustrated in Fig. 10.46.

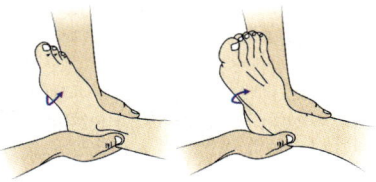

Fig. 10.45: Movements at tibiotarsal joint, i.e. inversion and eversion

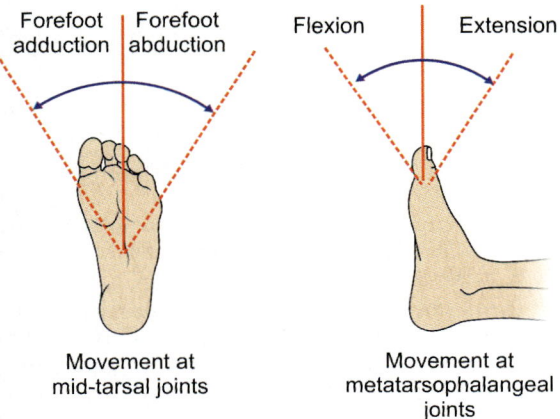

Fig. 10.46: Movements at metatarsal and metatarsophalangeal joints.

Hyperextensibility of Joints (Fig. 10.47)

It occurs in Ehlers-Danlos syndrome. The method of hyperextensibility is demonstrated in Fig. 10.47.

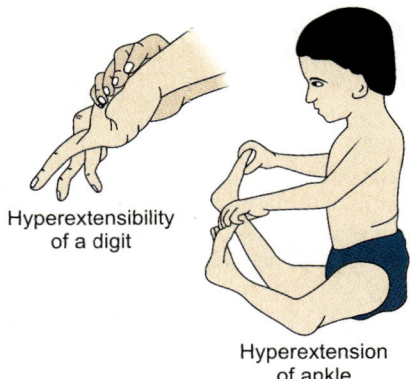

Fig. 10.47: Test for hyperextensibility of the digits in Ehlers-Danlos syndrome (diagram).

BRIEF SYNOPSIS OF RHEUMATOLOGICAL DISORDERS

DIFFERENTIAL DIAGNOSIS OF ARTHRITIS

The causes of monoarthritis (acute and chronic) and polyarthritis are tabulated (Table 10.3).

TABLE 10.3: Differential Diagnosis of Arthritic Syndromes

Acute monoarticular arthritis	*Chronic monoarticular arthritis*	*Polyarticular arthritis*
• Infective (gonococcal, non-gonococcal, i.e. *Staph.aureus* streptococcal, Gram-negative)	• Tubercular	• Rheumatoid arthritis
	• Syphilis	• SLE
	• Fungal	• Acute rheumatic fever
	• Brucellosis	• Reactive arthritis (Reiter's syndrome)
	• Perthes disease	
	• Osteoarthritis	
• Fracture		
• Hemathrosis (haemophilia)		
• Crystal induced		• Sarcoidosis
• Foreign body		• Vasculitis
• Osteoarthritis		• Bacterial endocarditis
• Ischaemic necrosis		
• Monoarticular RA		• Serum sickness
• Henoch-Schönlein purpura		• Drug-induced

Rheumatic Arthritis

- Affects children and adolescents.
- Starts as monoarthritis but becomes polyarthritis.
- Flitting type of joint pain involving mainly large joints, but small joints may also be involved.
- *John's other criteria,* i.e. chorea, carditis, erythema marginatum, subcutaneous nodules, etc may be present in small proportions of cases.
- It is usually, a non-deforming arthritis but occasionally recurrent rheumatic arthritis can lead to chronic *jaccoud arthritis*. In this arthritis, ulnar deviation of hand is a characteristic deformity.

Gouty Arthritis

- Occurs in middle aged males
- Attacks occur suddenly in early hours of the morning with excruciating pain in one of the big toes usually the left.
- Recurrent attacks are common.
- It is mostly a monoarthritis usually involving the first metatarsophalangeal joints called *podagra*.
- Attacks are precipitated by surgical trauma, diet excess in purine, alcohol, starvation, dehydration sepsis and diuretics.

- During attack, the joint is red, warm, swollen and tender.
- Recurrent attacks lead to chronic tophaceous gout (gouty tophi), uric acid stones and nephropathy.
- Diagnosis is confirmed by high urate levels during an acute attack.

Septic Arthritis

It can be *gonococcal* Or *nongonococcal* (*Staph.aureus, streptococcal* or *Gram-negative*) monoarthritis (hip, shoulder, knee), sometimes polyarthritis.
- Common in immunocomprised individuals. Damaged and prosthetic joints are predisposed to it.
- The joint involved is red, warm and swollen with limited mobility. There is fever with chills and rigors.
- Leucocytosis, X-ray and synovial fluid examination are diagnostic.

Tubercular Arthritis

- It occurs uncommonly. It occurs in extrapulmonary tuberculosis (10%).
- It is chronic granulomatous monoarthritis.
- It occurs commonly in debilitated children. In adults, alcohol dependence, diabetes and HIV predispose to it.
- It predominantly involves a large weight-bearing joint, i.e. hip or knee.
- It is characterised by insidious onset of pain swelling and restricted movments.
- Systemic manifestations, i.e. anorexia, night sweats, malaise occur in 50% cases.
- X-ray and synovial fluid examination are diagnostic.

PSEUDOGOUT (CALCIUM PYROPHOSPHATE DEHYDRATE—CPPD CRYSTAL DISEASE)

- This occurs in old people (>60 years) both in men and women.
- Acute atttack occurs due to crystal induced synovitis leading to pain and swelling of the joint(s) involved. Joints (knee, shoulder, elbow, ankle) are commonly involved than smaller joints.
- The attacks occur at irregular intervals.
- There may be deposition of CPPD crystals in articular cartilage and periarticular tissue called *chondrocalcinosis*.
- The **diagnosis** is confirmed by demonstration of calcium pyrophosphate crystals in the synovial fluid.

ACUTE CALCIFIC PERIARTHRITIS (HYDROXYAPATITE DEPOSITION DISEASE)

- It occurs in middle age (around 40 yrs) both in males and females.
- It may be *acute, subacute* or *chronic arthritis* characterised by pain and swelling of the joint involved (knee, shoulder, hip, etc.). Joint(s) is red and swollen.
- The characteristic feature is dystrophic calcification in which there is deposition of hydroxyapatite crystals in periarticular tissue leading to its destruction.

RHEUMATOID ARTHRITIS (RA)

- Occur in adolescents and adults of both sexes.
- Asymmetric deforming polyarthritis.
- Slow onset chronic polyarthritis with pain, morning stiffness and swelling of joints.
- Both small joints (common) and large joints (uncommon) are involved in all age groups.
- Systemic features, i.e. anaemia, weight loss and fever can occur.
- The characteristic signs of chronic arthritis are *deformities* (*swan-neck, Boutonniére deformity, ulnar deviation of hands*).
- *Extra-articular manifestations* include rheumatoid nodules, entrapment neuropathy (*carpal tunnel syndrome*), scleritis, diffuse fibrosing alveolitis, pleural and/or pericardial effusion, amyloidosis of kidneys and vasculitis.
- The **diagnosis** is based on clinical features, presence of rheumatoid factor (seropositive arthritis), anti-CCP antibodies and radiological studies.
- The 2010 ACR/EULAR classsification criteria for rheumatoid arthritis is depicted in Table 10.4.

TABLE 10.4: The 2010 ACR/EULAR Diagnostic Criteria for Rheumatoid Arthritis

	Points
1. Joint involvement	
• 1 large joint	0
• 2–10 large joints	1
• 1–3 small joints	2
• 4–10 small joints	3
• > 10 joints (at least one small joint)	5
II. Serology	
• RF/CCP negative	0
• RF or CCP positive at low titre <3 times upper limit of normals	2
• RF or CCP positive at higher titre >3 times of upper normal limits	3

Contd.

Contd.

III. Duration of synovitis	
• < 6 weeks	0
• 6 weeks or longer	1
IV. Acute phase reactants	
• Normal ESR/CRP	0
• Abnormal ESR/CRP	1

Diagnosis is based on presence of 10 or more points

SERONEGATIVE ARTHRITIS (HLA B-27 SPONDYLOARTHRITIS)

The seronegative polyarthritis is a group of disorders characterised by involvement of sacroiliac joints, peripheral inflammatory arthropathy and by absence of rheumatoid factor (RF). There is strong association towards family aggregation and **HLA B-27** positively. The disorders included are:

1. **Ankylosing spondylitis (AS).** It is a disease of adolescents (2nd and 3rd decades) with men three times more affected than women. The disease primarily involves the axial skeleton, peripheral joints and extra-articular structures. The disease has strong predilection to family aggregation and HLA B-27 positivity. Due to involvement of axial joints, back motion and chest expansion is limited. Hip pain and tenderness (sacroilitis) can be elicited by direct pressure. The **Schober test** which measures the flexion of lumbar spine is useful test for diagnosis.

2. **Reiter's syndrome.** It is characterised initially by a triad of arthritis, uretheritis and conjunctivitis. Later on rash, oral ulcers or balanitis may appear.

3. **Psoriatic arthropathy.** It occurs in 5–40% patients with psoriasis. It is characterised by distal polyarthritis involving small joints of hands and feet. It is chronic inflammatory condition, usually benign.

4. **Enteropathic arthritis.** It is non-deforming arthritis involving larger joint in patients with inflammatory bowel disease (ulcerative colitis, Crohn's disease, Whipple disease). Flare up of the disease are known, occur in the early course of the disease, usually affects knees and ankles. Attacks are self limiting without joint damage.

DEGENERATIVE ARTHRITIS (OSTEOARTHRITIS)

It is a degenerative arthritis involving the cartilage of joints. It occurs in old age due to wear and tear of the joints. It may be *primary* (idiopathic) or *secondary* due to some cause. It may be *localised* (involving one or two joints) or *generalised* (3 or more joints involved).

OA is characterised by gradual development of joint pain, stiffness, swelling and immobility (limitation of movements) of the joints. Swelling is caused by synovitis with effusion or by bony osteophytes. Crepitus may be heard over the joint involved. Bony enlargement with osteophytes formation lead to bony deformity.

The generalised OA involving three or more joints is dominated by *Heberden's* nodes at distal interphalanged joints and *Bouchard's nodes* at proximal interphalanged joints and predominates in women and has familial transmission.

COSTOCHONDRITIS

Tietze's syndrome. It is costochondritis involving the middle age and both sexes equally. It is characterized by pain and swelling of second and 3rd costochondral joints near the sternum.

LOW BACK PAIN

Sciatica. It is characterised by low back pain that radiates along the sciatic nerve. It occurs due to irratation of sciatic nerve roots anywhere in the canal, intervertebral foramina, in pelvis or buttocks. The **causes** include prolapse of intervertebral disc, spinal tumour, degenerative disease of the spine or spondylolisthesis. *Straight leg raising test* is positive. There will be sensory or motor deficit with absent or depressed ankle jerk.

Lumbar spondylosis. This is common disorder of old age and causes chronic or recurrent low back and leg pain. The spinal roots involved are L_4–L_5 and L_5–S_1. This is due to degeneration of nucleous pulposus and annulus fibrosus.

The lower back pain radiates downwards along the nerve roots involved. Sneezing, coughing or movements aggravates the pain of prolapsed disc.

The radicular pain, dermatomal sensory disturbance (paraesthesias, hyper or hypoanaesthesia) and adminished or absent deep tendon jerks are specific to the roots involved. It can be a unilateral or a bilateral disease.

1. *Lumbar disc prolapse (10.48): Acute low back pain in young* associated with bending or lifting weight is characteristic of acute lumbar disc protusion. Sudden movement and coughing will increase it. In addition, there may be compression of nerve roots (*cauda equina syndrome*). If sacral nerve roots are involved, there may be loss of sphincter control and perianal sensations. These acute episodes may be superimposed on previous disc degeneration.

Acute back pain in middle and old age may be due to osteoporotic fracture and is not associated with neurological symptoms. This type of pain is increased by spinal flexion but is relieved on lying down.

2. *Infective pain* associated with malaise, weight loss, night sweats, usually indicate tuberculosis

Physical Signs, Symptoms, Diagnosis and Differential Diagnosis

(Pott's disease) or pyogenic infection of the spine. The patient feels difficulty in moving the spine. The infection may involve intervertebral disc (caries), adjacent vertebrae, and at times it may tract into psoas muscle (*psoas cold abscess*) presenting as a swelling in the groin or may lead to painful flexed hip.

Diagnosis: The diagnosis is made on clinical features and limited movement of lumbar spines i.e. *flexion, extension, lateral flexion* and *rotation* and exclusion of the hip disease by FABERE test (Fig. 10.49).

The confirmation of the diagnosis is done by radiology and MRI/CT scanning.

FABERE TEST (Fig. 10.49)

This test helps to confirm or exclude hip disease as a cause of low back pain. The manoeuvre causes locking of the hip joint.

Method

For the FABERE (Flexion, Abduction, External Rotation) test, have the patient lying supine. Passively flex, abduct, and externally rotate the lower extremity at the hip so that the lateral malleolus touches the contralateral patella. Then apply downward force on the ipsilateral knee (Fig. 10.49). Repeat on the contralateral side for control.

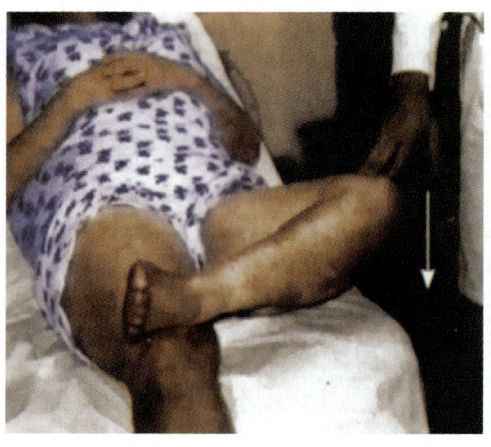

Fig. 10.49: FABERE test. Patient lies supine with passive flexion, abduction, external rotation of the lower extremity. Here the left leg is being assessed. Downward force on the ipsilateral knee is applied. Excellent test to assess the function of the hip status, helps to confirm and exclude the disease of the hip.

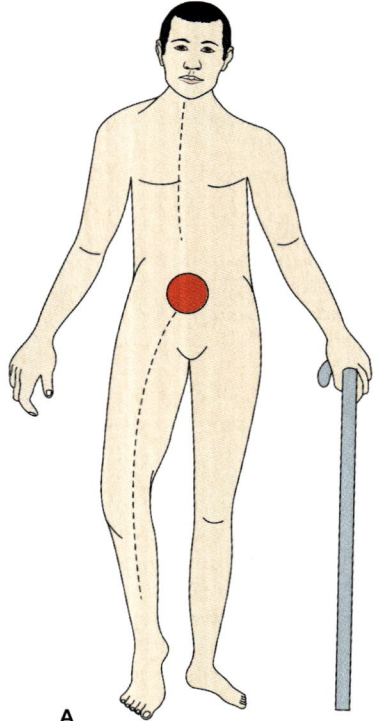
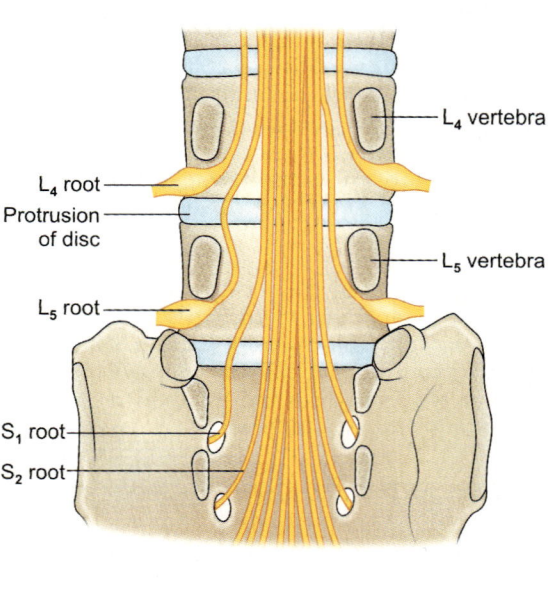

Figs 10.48A and B: Compression of lumbosacral nerve roots by herniation of disc. (A) Clinical presentation with site and radiation of pain to the leg (diagram). There is compensatory scoliosis; (B) Common site of prolapse of the disc (diagram).

During the manoeure, if pain occurs, it indicates lower back pain due to radicular involvement, disc disease or ankylosing spondylitis not hip joint disease (as hip joint is locked)

SYSTEMIC LUPUS ERYTHEMATOSUS (SLE)

It is an immune-mediated multisystemic connective tissue disorders in which autoantibodies raised against the cell components cause injury to the connective tissue/collagen tissue and blood vessels, hence also called *collagen vascular disorder*.

The cause remains unknown, but hereditary, complement deficiency, drugs, infections and disordered immunity play some role in its pathogenesis.

It is characterised by:
- *General features*, e.g. fever, fatigue, myalgia, malaise, tiredness.
- *Polyarthritis* involving the small joints causing painful tender joints and morning stiffness.
- A *butterfly rash* over the malar area (cheeks) is common.
- *Serositis* (pleuritis, pericarditis, effusion in pleural and pericardial cavities), *fibrosing alveolitis* can occur.
- *Proteinuria* due to lupus nephritis occur in two-thirds cases. *Nephrotic syndrome* can also occur.
- *Anaemia, thrombocytopenia, pancytopenia,* and *splenomegaly* (*Felty's syndrome*) occurs in children.
- Depression, seizures, psychosis
- Conjunctivitis, episcleritis, optic neuritis
- Vasculitis of the finger's tips, Raynaud's phenomenon, urticaria, livedo reticularis.
- Nausea, vomiting, diarrhoea, intestinal pseudo-obstruction

Diagnosis is made on the clinical features and confirmed by presence of autoantibodies (*ANA*, *anti-Smith*).

Differential Diagnosis

Being a multisystemic disorders, it comes into differential diagnosis of:
1. Polyarthritis (small joints arthritis)
2. Nephrotic syndrome
3. Vasculitic syndrome
4. Photosensitive rash.

ANTIPHOSPHOLIPID SYNDROME

This syndrome occurs in small number of cases of SLE, is characterised by vascular (venous) thrombosis, abortions and presence of antiphospholipids antibodies (lupus anticoagulants and anti-cardiolipin). Other causes of this syndrome are:
1. Other autoimmune disorders
2. Infections (viral, bacterial, treponemal)
3. Malignancies
4. Hematological disorders
5. Systemic diseases, i.e. pernicious anaemia, diabetes, and dialysed patients.

SCLERODERMA (SYSTEMIC SCLEROSIS)

It is a multisystemic disorder of connective tissue of unknown aetiology characterised by
 i. *Raynaud's phenomenon*—spastic tricolour skin phenomenon.
 ii. *Sclerodactyly* (thickening of skin over fingers and toes)
 iii. Asymmetric polyarthritis involving small joints causing pain, swelling and stiffness of fingers.
 iv. Hypomotility of gut and gastro-oesophageal reflux.
 v. Intestinal fibrosis of the lung leading to cor-pulmonale.
 vi. Pericarditis (with or without effusion) heart failure, arrhythmias.
 vii. Proteinuria and progressive renal insufficiency.
 viii. Dry eyes (Sjögren syndrome)

Diagnosis is suspected on clinical features and confirmed by investigations (*antinuclear antibodies, radiology* and *skin biopsy*).

POLYMYALGIA RHEUMATICA

It is a condition characterised by muscle stiffness (shoulder and pelvic girdle muscles) and joint pains. It is more common in elderly female. **Symptoms** (headache and joint pains) are worst in the morning and last for minutes to hours. Fever, tiredness, weight loss and sweating are common accompaniments.

Diagnosis is made on clincial symptoms, palpable temporal artery, raised ESR and CRP and temporal artery biopsy.

HENOCH-SCHÖNLEIN PURPURA

It is a form of vasculitis induced by type III hypersensitivity reaction. It involves children and adolescents, usually follows upper respiratory infection or food and drug allergy.

It is characterised by purpuric spots (arms, legs, buttocks), abdominal colic, polyarthritis and haematuria.

Diagnosis is confirmed by renal biopy.

MARFAN'S SYNDROME

It is an inherited disorder of collagen/connective tissue transmitted by autosomal dominant trait characterised by:
  i. *Musculoskeletal features,* i.e. long and thin extremities, arachnodactyly (long slender fingers), tall stature (the length of lower segment is more than upper segment, arm span exceeds the height), thumb protrusion sign (positive).
  ii. *Ectopia lentis* (dislocation of lens)
  iii. *Dilatation of the root of aorta or aortic aneurysm.*

Diagnosis is suspected on clinical features and confirmed by positive family history and two of the three clinical manifestations, i.e. skeletal, ocular and cardiovascular.

EHLERS-DANLOS SYNDROME

It is a genetically inherited disorder of connective tissue characterised by *hyperelasticity of the skin, hypermobility of the joints* and *fraglity of the tissue* and *blood vessels* resulting in easy bruisability and bleeding tendency.

Skin is hyperextensible like rubber (*rubber man syndrome*), gaping wounds, pepper-like thin scars, gum bleeding following dental extraction and recurrent haemoptysis are other common manifestations.

The joint manifestations include laxity and hypermobility of joints (Fig. 10.46) with recurrent haemarthroses, congenital talipes equinovarus, dislocation of hips, etc.

OSTEOGENESIS IMPERFECTA

It comprises heterogenous group of rare inherited disorder of collagen tissue characterised by:
1. Reduction in bone mass, brittle bone leading to multiple fractures in childhood.
2. Blue sclera, dental abnormalities (dentiogenesis imperfecta)
3. Progressive hearing loss
4. Positive family history.

FIBROMYALGIA

Fibromyalgia is a common soft tissue rheumatism characterised by pain, stiffness, paraesthesia, non-restorative sleep, easy fatigueability and widely distributed bilateral symmetrical tender 16 points (two occipital, two cervical, two trapezius, two superaspinatus, two at second rib, two lateral epicondyles, two gluteal, two greater trochanter and two over knees)
- It affects middle and old aged females (50 yrs of age)
- Patient complains of pain and stiffness of trunk, hip, shoulder girdles or low back pain radiating to buttocks or pain and stiffness of neck and shoulder.

Diagnosis is made on the history and physical examination demonstrating 11 tender points out of 18 described and exclusion of other rheumatic disorders.

Unit XI

Dermatological Disorders

- Symptoms of Dermatological Disorders
- History
- General Physical Examination
- Examination of Skin Lesion
- Brief Synopsis of Skin Disorders

SYMPTOMS OF SKIN DISORDERS

PRURITUS

Skin itching is called *pruritus*. The **causes** are:

1. **Common skin disorders**
   - Scabies (Fig. 11.1)
   - Atopic eczema, allergic contact dermatitis (Fig. 11.2)
   - Candidiasis, herpes zoster
   - Urticaria
   - Insect bites (e.g. flea, bed bug)

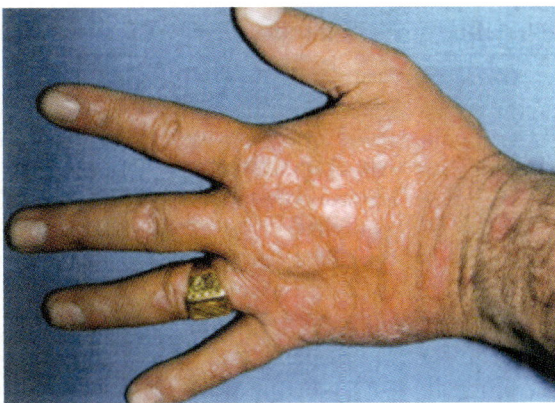

Fig. 11.2: Allergic contact dermatitis.

2. **Systemic diseases** with or without skin involvement
   a. *Metabolic diseases*
      - Hypothyroidism, carcinoid syndrome
   b. *Neoplastic diseases*
      - Chronic lymphatic leukaemia (CLL)
      - Lymphomas and other carcinomas
   c. *Haematological disease*
      - Polycythaemia vera
   d. *Renal failure*
      - Uraemia
   e. *Liver diseases*
      - Cholestasis particularly primary biliary cirrhosis
   f. *Miscellaneous*
      - Senile, psychogenic
      - Drug-induced

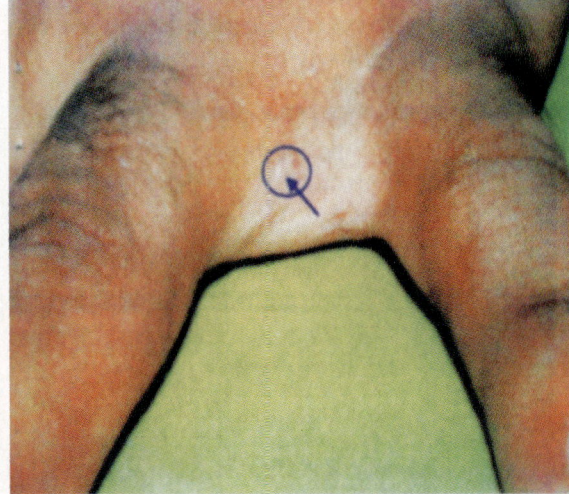

Fig. 11.1: Scabies. Note the burrow caused by the mite in the interdigital region.

Physical Signs, Symptoms, Diagnosis and Differential Diagnosis

Symptom Analysis

Ask about the following

Q. **When does it occur? Is it worst at night?**
- Itching due to scabies is worst at night.

Q. **History of insect bite.**
- Wasp and inset stings can lead to itching.

Q. **History of allergy or intake of a drug.**
- Drug allergy/anaphylaxis can produce pruritis.

Q. **Ask about metabolic disease of (hypothyroidism, carconoid), leukaemias, obstructive jaundice, uraemia and bronchial asthma.**
- Read systemic diseases causing pruritus.

Q. **History of pain abdomen or worm expulsion.**
- Worm infestations can lead to pruritis in children and adolescents.

RASHES

These are eruptions occuring over the skin or mucous membrane and may be associated with fever. The rashes may be **macular, papular, vesicular, pustular** or **haemorrhagic**. Fevers associated with rash are called *exanthematous fevers*. If rashes occur in the mucous membrane, they are called *enanthems*. The distribution of the rashes and time of their appearances are characteristic, i.e.

Day of skin rash	Exanthematous fever
Ist day of fever	Chickenpox
Second day	Scarlet fever
Third day	Smallpox (eradicated)
Fourth day	Measles
Fifth day	Typhus
Sixth day	Typhoid

Make enquiries about the rash

Q. **Is it macular, papular, vesicular, pustular or haemorrhagic?**

Q. **Day of onset of rash.**

Q. **Is rash associated with fever?**

Q. **Does rash itch?**

Q. **Ask about associated symptoms.**

ABNORMAL SKIN COLOURATION

- Ask about any pigmentation (localised or generalised) or depigmentation.
- Pigmentation, i.e. localised (freckles), generalised
- Depigmentation (loss of pigment), e.g. vitiligo, albinism.

SUBCUTANEOUS NODULES/SWELLINGS

Q. **Ask about any nodules (swelling over the skin)**
- Neurofibromatosis, xanthomas, etc. produce subcutaneous nodules.

SKIN INFECTIONS

Q. **Ask about skin lesion with fever, toxaemia.**
- Boil, carbuncle, herpes (simplex, zoster), tuberculosis are common skin infections.

DISFIGUREMENT

Acne, leprosy

Q. **Ask about itchy skin lesion.**

Q. **History of depigmentated patches.**

Q. **Are there any anaesthetic lesion?**

Q. **History of disfigurement.**

WEEPING SKIN LESION (ECZEMA)

Q. **Do the skin lesions exude fluid?**
- Eczema and pemphigus (rupture of bullae) lesions can exude fluid.

FLUID FILLED VESICLES/BLISTERS

Q. **History of burn, drug, etc.**
- Pemphigus is characterised by fluid-filled blisters.

TROPHIC ULCERATION

Q. **Ask about trophic ulcer.**
- Prolonged hospitalisation, e.g. surgery, fracture, etc. can produce trophic ulcer at pressure points.

Q. **History of neurological deficit, i.e. hemiplegia, paraplegia, etc.**
- Neurological diseases can lead to trophic changes.

Q. **History of skin or systemic disease.**
- Leprosy can lead to trophic ulcers.
- Diabetes, peripheral neuropathies due to any cause can lead to trophic ulceration.

HISTORY

Present History

A complete history should be taken with special emphasis on the following points:

1. **Symptoms associated with lesions**, e.g. itching, pain, burning or numbness. Ask

about these symptoms as they form clues to clinical diagnosis. Itching is the most common dermatological symptom. In some diseases, i.e. scabies, it is particularly worst at night. The causes of itching have been listed in the beginning (read pruritus). Some skin disorders are not itchy (e.g. rash of secondary syphilis, xanthomas). Loss of sensation is prominent in leprosy.

2. **Evaluation of the lesions/symptoms**

   Ask about the skin lesion/symptom and analyse its characteristics
   - Site of involvement
   - Duration of lesions
   - Manner in which the lesion progressed or spread
   - Associated aggravating or relieving factors
   - Period of resolution or improvement in chronic cases
   - *Rash/Rashes:* Ask about the rash, if present, ask about its time of appearance and its distribution. Ask about peeling of skin (erythroderma).
   - *Ask about any subcutaneous swellings,* i.e. neurofibroma, xanthomas, cysticercosis, sarcoidosis, rheumatic nodules, gouty tophi, etc.
   - *Pigmentation.* Ask about only pigmentation, whether localised or generalised.
   - *Hair:* Ask about loss of hair (alopecia)
   - *Ask about history of loss of sensation and amputation if done,* for leprosy.
   - *Fluid filled vesicles.* Ask about fluid filled vesicles for pemphigus which ruptures and produce denuded surface.
   - *History of surgery, prolonged bed rest/recumbency* for bedsores.

In our country self-applied remedies often cause irritant contact dermatitis.

- *Enquire about certain systemic symptoms (Table 11.1) for disorders likely to produce skin eruptions* (read the causes of pruritus in the beginning).
- Ask about associated systemic symptoms, e.g. cough, sore throat, joint pain, dyspnoea, fever for infection and autoimmune condition, malaise, arthralgia (e.g. psoriatic arthropathy) and pemphigus (Table 11.1).

Past History
- Ask about past history of such a disease or past history of drug intake.
- A history of same condition in the past may be a clue to the diagnosis (e.g. *recurrent herpes simplex, fixed drug eruptions*).

Family History

Family history is relevant in atopic skin conditions, psoriasis, genetic disorders such as icthyosis (Fig. 11.3), infections (e.g. impetigo and dermatophyte infections) and infestations (e.g. scabies, pediculosis). A history of the same genital condition in the sexual partner may be obtained in the conditions like *genital candidiasis* and other *sexually transmitted diseases*.

Personal History
- Ask about place of work, hobbies or recreational activities, use of cosmetics and ornaments, and sexual exposure.
- Ask in details about the medicines taken already and medicines being taken or being applied locally.

- Work contacts may produce irritant or allergic contact dermatitis.

TABLE 11.1 : Skin Lesions Clue to Systemic Disorders, their Analysis

Skin eruptions	Associated systemic diseases	Enquire about
1. Erythema nodosum (refer to Fig. 11.27)	Sarcoidosis, tuberculosis, post-streptococcal infections, connective tissue disorders, drugs	Cough and expectoration • Dyspnoea • Sore throat • Joint pains • Drugs
2. Pyoderma gangrenosum (Fig. 11.4)	Ulcerative colitis, rheumatoid arthritis	Rectal bleeding and joint pains
3. Dermatitis herpetiformis (Fig. 11.5)	Gluten-induced enteropathy	Family history and change in bowel habits
4. Generalised purpura	Idiopathic thrombocytopenic purpura, dengue and other blood disorders	Family history, haematuria, fever and weight loss
5. Dermatitis artefacta	Personality disorders	Stresses or anxieties

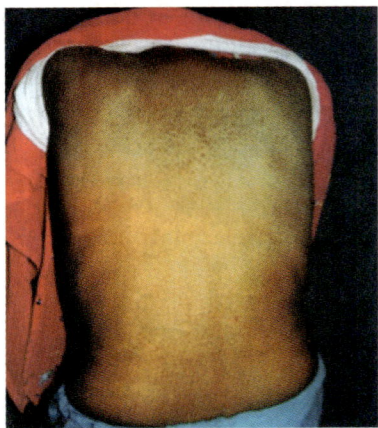

Fig. 11.3: Icthyosis: Note the dry scaly lesions of the skin on the back.

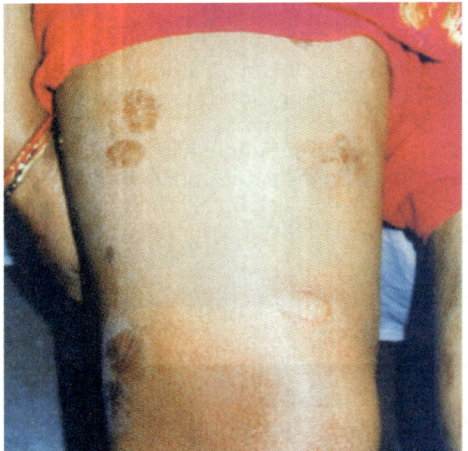

Fig. 11.4: Healed lesions of pyoderma gangrenosum.

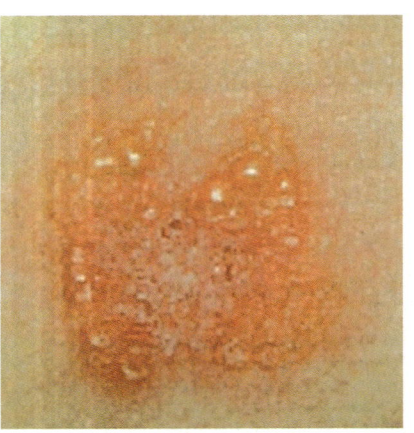

Fig. 11.5: Dermatitis herpetiformis.

- Ornaments and cosmetics are incriminated in contact dermatitis
- Sexual exposure is important for diagnosis of sexually transmitted diseases, HIV.
- History of photosensitivity in photodermatitis.

EXAMINATION

Sequence of Examination
- Ask the patient to remove any dressing, wigs or make up
- Before inspecting any rash or lesion, inspect the colour of the skin and nails.
- Examine the skin as a whole for state or condition, colouration, swelling/ulcer/blisters/scabs.

I. GENERAL EXAMINATION

☞ *Examine the skin for moistness, greesiness, loose or tight skin, elasticity, atrophy or hypertrophy.*

1. Moistness

It is due to sweating. Sweating may be decreased (*anhidrosis*) or increased (*hyperhidrosis*).

Decreased sweating (dry skin) may be seen or felt in dehydration, hypothyroidism, avitaminosis A, scleroderma, xeroderma, icthyosis, old age anasarca and due to anticholinergic drugs. Patchy decreased sweating occurs in autonomic neuropathy (diabetes, leprosy).

Increased sweating (moist skin) is common during defervescence in fevers (malaria, pneumonia, septicaemia), acute MI, rheumatic fever, thyrotoxicosis, tuberculosis (night sweats), acromegaly, nervousness, phaeochromocytomas, carcinoid syndrome, hot weather or excessive humidity (heat exhaustion).

Localised sweating over the one side of face is noted in trigeminal neuralgia, histamine headache gustatory hyperhidrosis in neurological disease, asthenia, nervousness, Raynaud's disease, debility and thyrotoxicosis.

Abnormal form of sweating, i.e. coloured (yellow) sweating is noted in severe Jaundice, urinous sweating in uraemia, bloody sweating in haemorrhagic disease. **A cold and clammy skin** (sweating with coldness) is noted in shock, MI generalised peritonitis and severe pain.

2. Loose/Thin/Thick/ Wrinkled Skin

The *loose skin* hanging in folds may be found in old age, progeria (premature senility), loss of fluid from oedematous skin, enuchoidism (hypogonadism), dehydration (pinched up fold of skin), pseudoxanthoma elasticum (a rare inherited disease).

Tense or tight skin (the skin cannot be lifted by pinching) is found over the areas of inflammation, oedema, cellulitis, scleroderma, morphoea.

Hyperelastic skin (skin can be stretched to some extent) is found in *Ehlers-Danlos syndrome* (a congenital connective tissue disorder). In this disorder the skin is fragile and heals with cigarette paper scars.

Thick and hypertrophied skin. It occurs in acromegaly, cretinism, myxoedema, *avitaminosis A and C*, elephantiasis, xeroderma, icthyosis, neurofibromatosis, leprosy (leonine face), manual workers, maid servants (hypertrophied palms).

Thinness and atrophy of skin. It is common in old age (senile atrophy), trophic changes during prolonged immobilisation, oedematous skin, malnutrition, wasting diseases, insulin therapy and idiopathic atrophy. The atrophy is best demonstrated by pinching a fold of the inelastic skin on the dorsum of hand.

Skin Colour

☞ *Look for any abnormal skin colouration*

The normal skin colour varies depending on lifestyle, light exposure as well as constitutional and ethnic factors.

Pallor denotes paleness; can be transient due to haemorrhage or shock and intense emotional upset, or in patients with atopy—an inherited susceptibility to develop hay fever, asthma and eczema. It must be remembered that pallor does not mean yellowness or jaundice. A pale skin is also seen in hypopituitarism and hypogonadism (*Kallmann's syndrome*). The abnormal colouration of skin is depicted in Box 11.1.

Abnormal redness (erythema) of skin may be due to:
- Cherry-red colour in carbon monoxide poisoning
- Overheating (Fig. 11.6)
- Extreme exertion
- Sunburn or photosensitivity
- Erythroderma (e.g. exfoliative dermatitis) in which majority of the skin surface is red, could be due to skin conditions, drugs (Fig. 11.7)
- In febrile illness
- Inflammatory skin disease
- Exanthematous skin disease

Box 11.1 Abnormal Skin Colouration

Colour	Disorder/state
Shallow brownish discolouration	Uraemia
Bluish tinge or colouration	Cyanosis produced by abnormal haemoglobin (sulph or methaemoglobin). It has been discussed under CVS and respiratory system examination
Pink colouration	Carbon monoxide poisoning
Yellow colouration	Mepacrine, jaundice (discussed under examination of abdomen)
Red colouration	Clofazimine, rash
State grey colouration of exposed parts	Phenothiazines

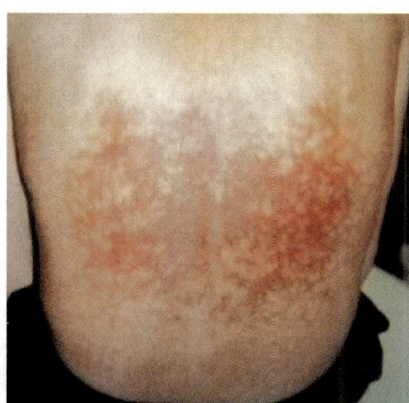

Fig. 11.6: Erythema ab igne on the back due to hot water bottle.

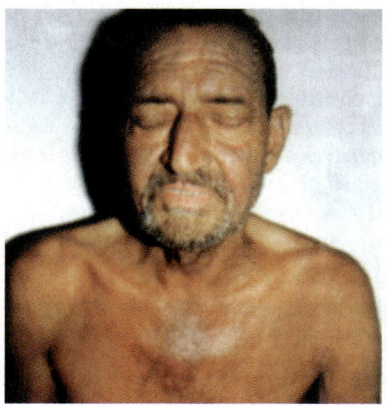

Fig. 11.7: Erythroderma (exfoliative dermatitis) induced by a drug. Note the diffuse erythema and exfoliation of skin.

- Local redness may be due to telangiectasia or disseminated intravascular coagulation and purpura.

Cyanosis refers to bluish discolouration of skin, produced by presence of reduced haemoglobin >5 g either locally, as in impaired peripheral circulation, or generally, when oxygenation of the blood is defective. The presence of abnormal haemoglobin such as methaemoglobin (i.e. due to aniline dyes, dapsone, primaquine, phenazopyrine, etc.) or sulphaemoglobin may lead to cyanosis. Carboxyhaemoglobin in carbon monoxide poisoning leads to cherry-red colour of the skin and cyanosis, called *red cyanosis*.

Cyanosis may be central, peripheral, mixed, differential and local. Local cyanosis could be due to Raynaud's disease, scleroderma, peripheral arterial and venous occlusion, thrombophlebitis, varicose veins.

Jaundice refers to yellow colouration of the skin and mucous membrane of conjunctivae due to increased serum bilirubin >2.5 mg%. The *lemon yellow colouration of skin* may be seen in haemolytic anaemia while *deep yellow to orange or yellowish-green colouration* is seen in obstructive jaundice. *Orange-yellow colouration* to the skin may be due to carotenaemia from which jaundice has to be differentiated by examining the conjunctivae which are also orange-yellow in jaundice but not in carotenaemia.

Loss or Excess of Skin Pigmentation

Loss of normal pigmentation (melanin) in the skin is usually congenital, called *albinism* (Fig. 11.8); if it is localised, it is called *piebaldism*. Patches of white and dark pigmented skin is seen *in vitiligo*.

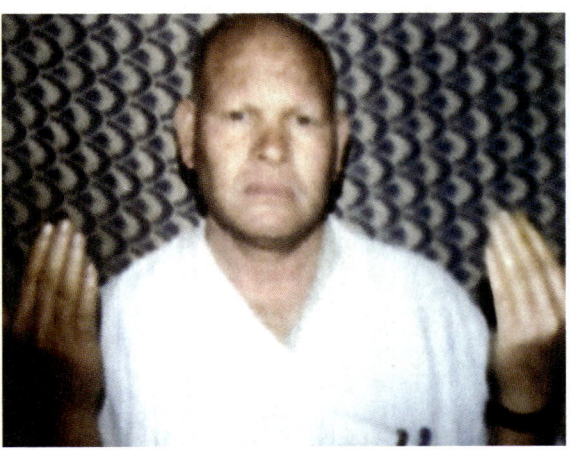

Fig. 11.8: Albinism. There is congenital widespread loss of pigment. Note the heterochromia (loss of pigment in the iris).

Hyperpigmentation refers to excess of pigmentation of the skin which could be either drug induced (Box 11.2) or haemosiderosis, carotenaemia (bronze pigmentation) and chronic arsenic poisoning. Brown pigmentation may be *localised* or *generalised*. *Erythema ab igne* a reticular pattern of pigmentation of legs is seen in women who habitually sit near the fire, can be seen on the back (Fig. 10.6) or belly with use of hot-water bottle. The causes of pigmentation are given in Box 11.3.

Box 11.2 Drug-induced Pigmentation

Drug	Pigmentation
Amiodarone (class III anti-arrhythmic)	Slate-grey, seen on exposed parts
Arsenic	Diffuse bronze with superimposed rain drop depigmentation
Bleomycin and busulfan	Brown pigmentation
Chloroquine	Blue-grey pigmentation on exposed parts
Mepacrine	Yellow
Clofazimine	Red
Minocycline	Slate-grey, seen on scars, temples, shins and sclera
Phenothiazines, psoralens	Slate-grey on exposed parts

Box 11.3 Causes of Pigmentation

- Loss of normal colour / pigment — Vitiligo, albinism (total absence, Fig. 11.8)
- Brown pigmentation of skin, mucous membrane and creases of the palm and scars — Addison's disease (see Fig. 9.18) or hypopituitarism, idiopathic
- Blotchy pigmentation of the face, "melasma or chloasma" — Pregnancy, postpartum
- Pallor of skin and mucous membrane — Anaemia
- Black pigmentation of skin — Haemochromatosis, kala-azar
- Pink, plethoric complexion of skin — Polycythaemia, alcoholism, Cushing's syndrome

☞ Examine the skin for pigmentation (localised or generalised) or depigmentation.

A. Localised Brown Pigmentation

Localised pigmentation may be seen in pellagra and in scars of various kinds. It can be idiopathic. The localised brown hyperpigmentation are:

Dermatological Disorders

1. **Chloasma**: A mask-like pigmentation of face associated with brown pigmentation of nipples and of linea alba. It is seen in pregnant women and women taking oral contraceptives.
2. **Melasma:** It is similar to chloasma, is seen in Asian and African males.
3. **Brown-coloured naevoid lesion:** It is light brown discolouration of skin over trunk, buttocks, and thighs seen in Albright's syndrome.
4. **Café au lait spots (Fig. 11.9):** They are brown patches (localised lesions) seen in neurofibromatosis (more than 5 spots of >1.5 cm² area are diagnostic).

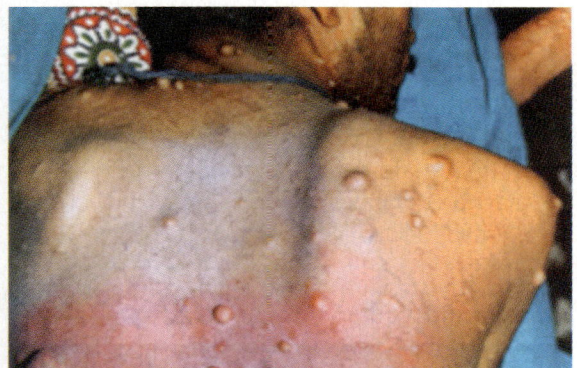

Fig. 11.9: Neurofibromatosis. Note the multiple small swellings on the skin with diffuse pigmentation and *café au lait* lesions.

5. **Freckles or (ephelides):** They are sharply defined light-brown macules seen on face or exposed sites in fair-skinned persons or are seen in xeroderma pigmentosum.

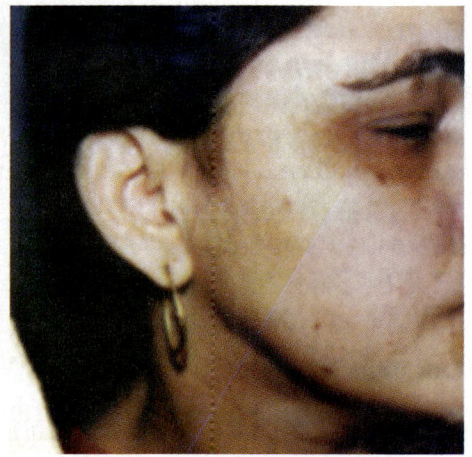

Fig. 11.10: Congenital melanocytic naevi over the face.

6. **Lentigines:** These are macules larger than freckles, are seen on palms, soles and genitalia. Solar lentigines are seen over sun-exposed area.
7. **Post inflammatory hyperpigmentation:** It occurs following eczema and dermatophytosis, drug eruptions, lichen planus.
8. **Congenital melanocytic naevi:** They can occur on any part of the body (Fig. 11.10).
9. **Acanthosis nigricans:** A circumscribed thickening and hyperpigmentation of skin giving a typical texture in axillae, neck, genitalia, groin. It may be hereditary, due to endocrine disorders (insulin resistance syndrome) and could be due to malignancy.

B. Generalised Hyperpigmentation

Diffuse/generalised hyperpigmentation over sun-exposed areas commonly occurs due to exposure to sunlight. Diffuse pigmentation is classically seen in Addison's disease over sun-exposed areas, flexures, bony prominences, mucosal surfaces, mucocutaneous junctions, nipples, palmar creases, genitalia. Previously pigmented lesion or scars also become darker. *The causes of generalised brown hyperpigmentation* are:

1. **Endocrinal diseases,** e.g. Addison's disease, pituitary tumour, Cushing syndrome, Nelson's syndrome, acromegaly.
2. **Collagen vascular diseases,** e.g. SLE, dermatomyositis.
3. **Drugs and metals,** e.g. heavy metals, cancer chemotherapy.
4. **Debilitating diseases,** e.g. HIV infection, kala azar, malaria, tuberculosis, advanced malignancies, megaloblastic anaemia, alcoholism, hepatic failure, biliary cirrhosis, chronic renal failure.
5. **Metabolic diseases,** e.g. haemochromatosis, porphyria.
6. **Neurofibromatosis (Fig. 11.9).**

Swelling/Nodule/Ulcer

☞ *Look for any swelling(s) or ulcer on the skin*
- Neurofibromatosis (Fig. 11.9), xanthomas (tuboeruptive), lipomas, fibromas, sarcoidosis cysticercosis, malignancy produce cutaneous or subcutaneous swelling(s).
- Rodent ulcer, bedsores, diabetic foot ulcer, basal cell carcinoma, scrofuloderma are common causes of skin ulcer.

☞ *Look for any bleeding into the skin, i.e. purpura, bruises, ecchymosis, haematoma, etc.*
- Bleeding occurs into the skin in bleeding disorders and disorders of capillary fragility,

while bleeding into deeper tissue resulting in haematoma is due to coagulation disorders (haemophilia, liver disease, anticoagulant therapy).

Note: Haemorrhagic skin lesion unlike that of erythema cannnot be obiterated by digital pressure. They are pink or red in colour. They tend to change in colour and disappears unlike capillary naevi and skin pigmentation.

Site of Involvement

☞ Look for specific sites for involvement, i.e. scalp, eyelids, face, lips, extremities, axillae and genitalia.

Special sites or areas of predilection are:
- Photodermatosis involves sun-exposed areas and spares shielded areas.
- Atopic dermatitis in children frequently involves the antecubital and popliteal fossae, e.g. flexor surfaces.

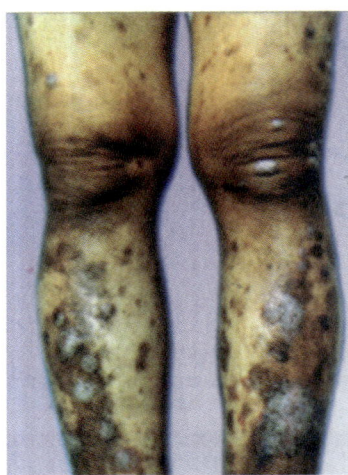

Fig. 11.11: Psoriasis. Note the dry scaly pruritic lesions over the extensor surface of the legs.

- Psoriasis involves the extensor surfaces of legs (Fig. 11.11), joints (elbow, knee) scalp, natal cleft and nails.
- Cutaneous candidiasis produces maceration of the skin in body folds especially in the obese, induces erosion and intertrigo. In infants, napkin may encourage Candida infection.
- Seborrhoeic dermatitis is seen in areas where there is high density of sebaceous glands, i.e. scalp, forehead, eyebrows, nasolabial folds, presternal areas, etc.
- Acne involves cheek (Fig. 11.12), forehead, shoulder and back

Specific sites of involvement are:
1. **Scalp:** Seborrhoeic dermatitis, lichen planus, alopecia, psoriasis.
2. **Eyelids:** Atopic dermatitis, contact dermatitis (cosmetics), angioedema, dermatomyositis, xanthelasma, basal cell carcinoma.
3. **Face:** Acne (Fig. 11.12), atopic dermatitis, butterfly rash (rosacea, erysipelas, lupus pernio, SLE, erythema infectiosum), naevi, freckles, basal and squamous cell carcinomas.
4. **Lips:** Herpes labialis, dermatitis (atopic, contact) angular stomatitis, angio-oedema, urticaria, impetigo, erythema multiforme, squamous cell carcinoma.
5. **Hands:** Dermatitis, psoriasis, fungal infections, erythema multiforme, photodermatoses, scabies, warts, vasculitic skin lesions.
6. **Feet:** Dermatitis, psoriasis, fungal infection, vasculitis, corns, callosities, pitted keratolysis.
7. **Axillae:** Psoriasis, contact dermatitis, acanthosis nigricans, boils, erythrasma, scrofuloderma.
8. **Genitals:** Psoriasis, lichan planus (penis), lichen simplex (scrotum, vulva), fixed drug eruptions, sexually transmitted diseases/genital warts, balanitis, squamous cell carcinoma (penis, vulva).

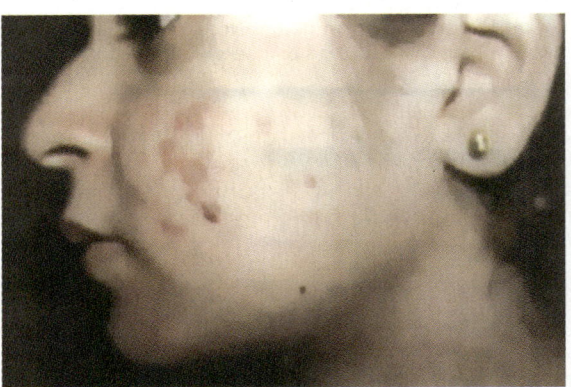

Fig. 11.12: Acne vulgaris—a chronic skin condition manifesting as comedomes or black heads due to blockage of pilosebaceous glands commonly involves the face, chest and back where sebaceous glands are present in abundance. The condition occurs commonly in adolescent males and females.

II. EXAMINATION OF SKIN LESION

A. Distribution of the Lesion

Skin disorders are generalised, localised or regional. Recognition of the characteristic distribution facilitates the diagnosis greatly by narrowing down the diagnostic possibilities.

☞ Inspect the distribution of the lesion, e.g. symmetrical or asymmetrical, centripetal or centrifugal, etc. Note the following points:

1. Is the lesion/rash localised, universal, symmetrical?
2. Does the lesion/rash follow an anatomical (dermatomal) pattern or central/peripheral distribution?
3. Does it affect special sites (flexor or extensor areas)?
4. Are areas/regions of predilection for some skin disorder involved?
5. Are there other clues to the diagnosis at distant sites?
6. Are there any incidental findings, e.g. genitalia involved?

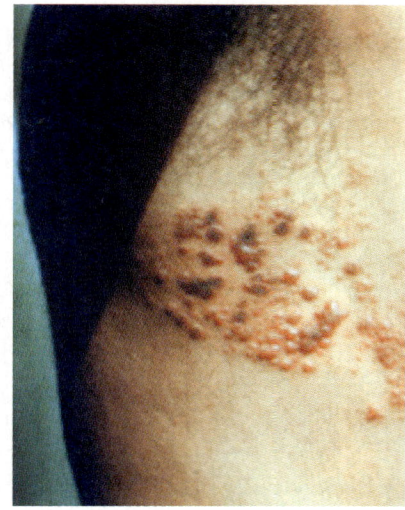

Fig. 11.13: Herpes zoster infection. Note the distribution of skin lesion along the dermatome.

Universal, Symmetric vs Asymmetric Lesion

- *Localised distribution* of lesion is seen in contact dermatitis, e.g. necklace, ear-rings, lipstick dermatitis.
- *Universal* and *symmetrical eruptions* favour the systemic or constitutional cause.
- *Asymmetrical eruptions* spreading from a single focus favour fungal, bacterial or viral infections. They occur in cooks, hair dressers, barbars who hold the tool in dominating hand while handling irritant material in the other.

Anatomical Pattern of Central vs Peripheral Distributions

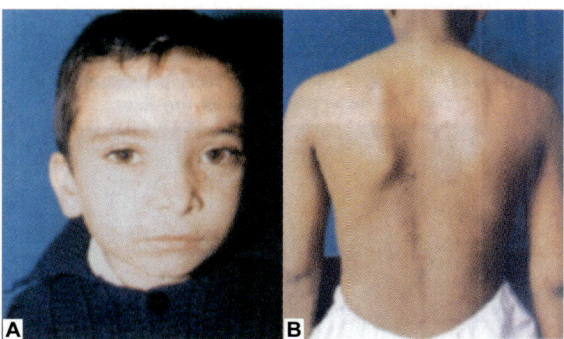

Figs 11.14A and B: Chickenpox. Note the centripetal distribution of the skin eruptins in two brothers. (A) Lesions over the face; (B) Lesions over the back. Simultaneous infection in two brothers indicates direct transmission of infection.

- *Dermatomal distribution* (Fig. 11.13) of the rash favours the diagnosis of herpes zoster infection. Some common diseases such as chickenpox (Fig. 11.14) and pityriasis are *centripetal in distribution*; while erythema nodosum, erythema multiforme and smallpox are *centrifugal (peripheral) in distribution*.
- *Ringworm* involves groin (tinea cruris), hands (tinea unguium) (Fig. 11.15), feet (tinea pedis), scalp (tinea capitis) and beard (tinea barbae).
- Swelling around the eyelids without redness indicates acute nephritic or nephrotic syndrome or trichinosis; whereas irritation around eyes indicates contact dermatitis.

B. Morphology of Skin Lesions

Skin lesions are said to be *primary* when they arise *de novo* as the first manifestation of skin disorder.

Secondary lesions: Secondary lesions arise from the changes in the primary lesions. They trace the

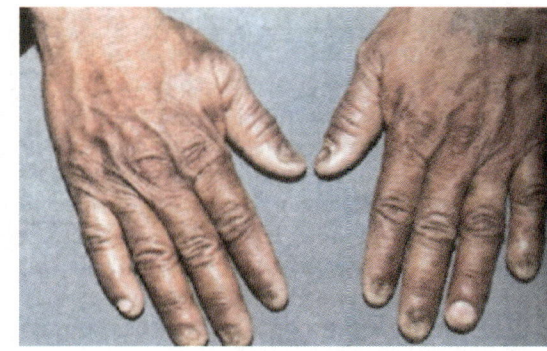

Fig. 11.15: Tinea unguium (fungal infection of hands). Note the thickening and discolouration of nail plates. Oncholysis is frequent.

evolutionary course of the primary into secondary lesions and are thus helpful to the clinical diagnosis. After the distribution of the lesion, the morphology of the lesion should be defined. Most lesions (primary as well as secondary) have special names (Table 11.2) which should be used to describe the skin lesion. Sometimes early primary lesion may be obscured by scratch marks, crusting and ulceration, therefore, these must be sought and when found, inspected closely.

☞ Note the morphology of the lesion using a lens if necessary. Palpate the lesion. Note whether lesion is smooth or rough, dry or moist and is there any sweating?

☞ Note the configuration/shape (a tumour or ulcer) and arrangement of the lesion

☞ Examine the lesion using uniform bright light and the part of patient undressed according to the spread of the lesion. Note the following points:
1. What are their shapes?
2. What are their sizes?
3. What is their colour?
4. What are the characteristics of their margins and surfaces?

The lesion should be described as per terminology used (Table 11.2).

C. Colour of Skin Lesion

☞ Examine the skin colour

Most skin lesions vary in colour, i.e.

- Violaceous scaly discrete flat-topped papules are seen in lichen planus
- Yellow coloured hue or tubercles are seen in xanthomatosis (Fig. 11.16).
- Depigmented or reddened anaesthetic skin lesions are seen in leprosy (Hansen's disease, Fig. 11.17). The lesions are located in the skin that is normally cooler than body temperature.
- A pink heliotrophic rash over the cheeks is seen in dermatomyositis and SLE.
- Ash-leaf depigmented (Shagreen patch) lesion on the trunk and adenoma sebaceum on the face indicate tuberous sclerosis (Fig. 11.18).

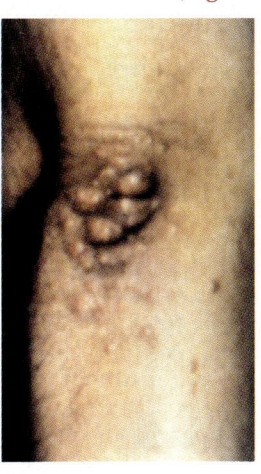

Fig. 11.16: Tuboeruptive xanthomata on the elbow of a patient with dyslipidemia.

TABLE 11.2: Terminology Used in Skin Lesions

Skin lesion	Description	Diseases in which they are present
I. Primary lesions		
Papule	A circumscribed, raised solid area of skin, less than 0.5 cm in diameter An elevated area of skin greater than 2 cm in diameter, can result from coalescence of papules	Moles, small neoplasms, lichen chronicus simplex, secondary syphilis, dermatomyositis called Gottron's papules
Macule	A flat circumscribed area of altered colour or texture	Chloasma, freckles, vitiligo, syphilis, von Recklinghausen disease
Vesicle	A small circumscribed fluid filled skin lesin (<0.5 cm in diameter)	Eczema, chickenpox, herpes (simplex, zoster) drug eruptions
Bulla	A large vesicle (>0.5 cm in diameter) or fluid filled blister is generic term used both for vesicles or bulla	Fungal, bacterial (staphylococcal scalded skin syndrome), herpes, erythema multiforme, bullous pemphigoid, pemphigus, SLE, epidermolysis bullosa, porphyria cutanea tarda, drug reactions (toxic epidermal necrolysis)
Pustule	A pus-containing blister, large collection of pus area is called furuncle	Rosacea, pustular psoriasis, adverse drug reaction, Reiter disease, bacterial superinfection of skin lesions

Contd.

Contd.

Skin lesion	Description	Diseases in which they are present
Abscess	Collection of pus in a cavity, more than 1 cm in diameter	Bacterial infections of skin by pus forming organisms
Wheal (urticaria)	A transient elevated reddened area associated with scratching and dermal swelling	Physical urticaria (solar, dermatographism, cholinergic)
Angioedema (Fig. 11.19)	A diffuse swelling or oedema that extends into the subcutaneous tissue (Fig. 11.19)	Vasculitis, hepatitis B and C infection, serum sickness, hereditary angioedema
Nodule	A raised solid skin mass >0.5 cm in diameter	Read the causes of skin and subcutaneous nodules already described
Petechiae	Small pin-head size (<3 mm in diameter) macules containing blood. It occurs due to extravasation of blood into the skin	Causes of petechiae, purpura, ecchymosis and haematoma are same such as: • Trauma • Fixed drug eruptions • Blood dyscrasias • Endocarditis • Henoch-Schönlein purpura
Purpura	Extravasation of blood into skin producing a large macule or papule that does not blanch on pressure	
Ecchymosis	A large petechiae (>3 mm) is called ecchymosis	
Haematoma	A localised collection of blood producing a swelling	
Burrow	A linear or curved tract (particularly caused by a burrowing scabie mite)	It is a characteristic lesion in scabies, guinea-worm, filaria
Comedome (the black head)	A plug of keratin and sebum wedged in a dilated pilosebaceous orifice	Acne
Telangiectasia	Dilatation of small cutaneous blood vessels that blanch on pressure	It is seen in nevus telangiectasia, Louis-Barr syndrome (ataxia-telangiectasia), Fabry disease, xeroderma pigmentosum, hereditary haemorrhagic telangiectasia

II. Secondary lesions

Skin lesion	Description	Diseases in which they are present
Scales	Dried flakes of dead skin arising from the horny layer	The scaly lesions are present in tinea versicolor, pityriasis rosea, psoriasis and seborrhoeic dermatitis
Crust and scabs	Dried exudate (blood or fluid) on the skin looking like a scale	They are formed in oozing eczema, bullous dermatosis, abrasions, pyodermas and burns
Erosion	A denuded area of skin with loss of epidermis	They occur in traumatic skin lesion
Ulcer	A denuded area of skin with loss of epidermis and a part of dermis	They are seen after trauma, in tuberculosis, granulomatous diseases, dermal leishmaniasis and as rodent ulcer
Excoriation	Linear marks or erosions produced by scratching	It occurs in all pruritic dermatosis
Fissure	A slit in the skin	Acanthosis nigricans
Sinus	A channel or cavity that permits the discharge of fluid or pus	Scrofuloderma
Scar	The healed area of the skin in which normal skin has been permanently replaced by fibrous tissue	It is seen following healing of deeper skin lesion
Keloid scar	Excessive scar formation	It is seen on healing of deeper burns
Atrophy	Thinning of the skin	It occurs in leprosy, syphilis, scleroderma, senile skin and congenital or hereditary dysplastic processes
Striae	A streak-like linear, atrophic pink or white skin lesion caused by a change in connective supporting tissue	They occur in Cushing's syndrome (pink), pregnancy (white) and following ascites

Physical Signs, Symptoms, Diagnosis and Differential Diagnosis

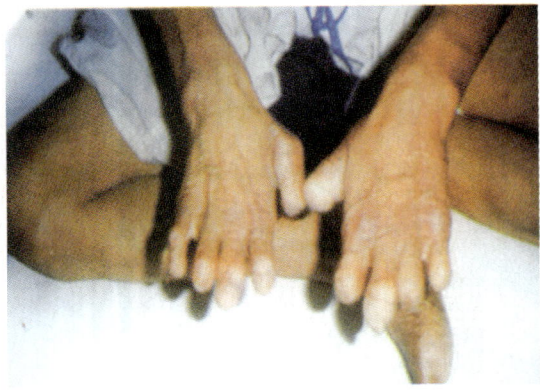

Fig. 11.17: Hansen's disease (leprosy).

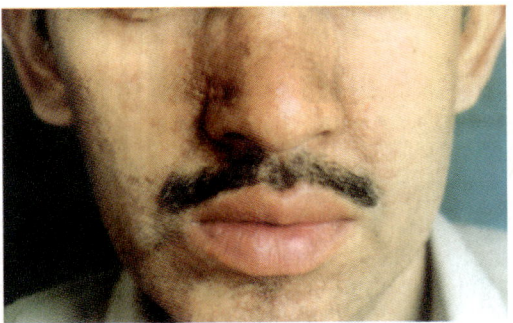

Fig. 11.18: Tuberous sclerosis, i.e. adenoma sebaceum over the face.

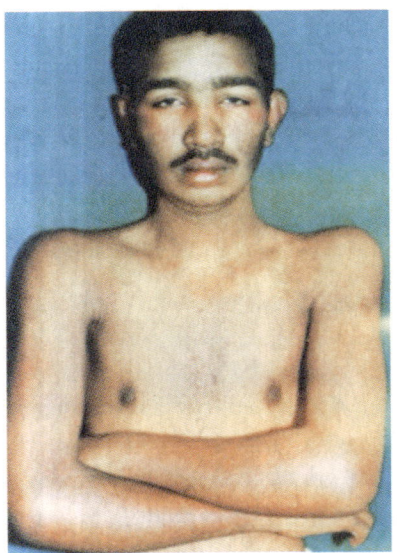

Fig. 11.19: Angioedema. Note the diffuse swelling over the body due to oedema of subcutaneous tissue including face and lips.

- Portwine stain (a tumour consisting of dilated capillary vessels) may be associated with *Sturge-Weber syndrome* (Fig. 11.20). *A salmon-coloured patch due to capillary plexus may be seen as capillary naevus (naevus flammeus).*
- Cavernous haemangioma (Strawberry naevus—Fig. 11.21), de Morgan's spots are cherry-angiomas.

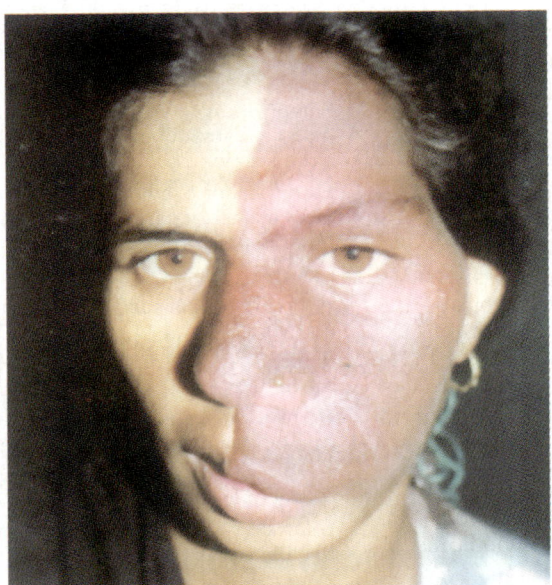

Fig. 11.20: Sturge-Weber syndrome. Note portwine stain (capillary haemangioma) of left side of face.

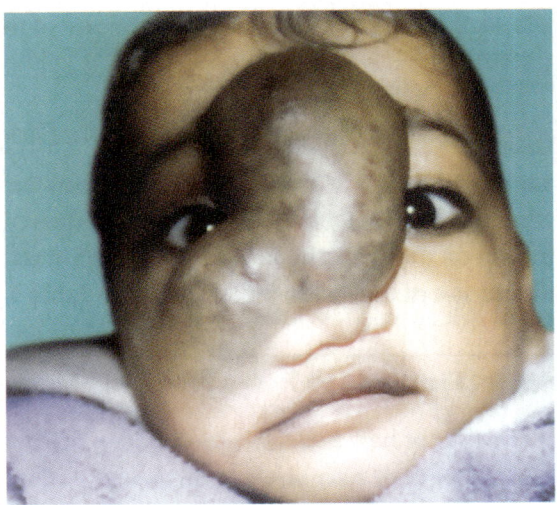

Fig. 11.21: Cavernous haemangioma (strawberry naevus) in a child. Note the well demarcated round, lobulated growth on the face at the base of the nose and obstructing both the eyes.

Palpation

I. Interventional Physical Examination

Palpation (feeling of the skin) is specially important to assess the quality of scale, thickness of the lesion, texture, teethering and temperature. Simple squeezing will identify the characteristic teethering and epidermal dimpling over dermatofibroma, scratching will reveal dermatographic wheals and rubbing will provoke erythema in mastocytosis while picking or removing the crust may reveal underlying pus.

II. Examine other Areas for Physical Signs

Individual features may suggest a diagnosis hence, search other features of the disease to support the diagnosis, for example, scaly plaques suggest psoriasis, therefore, examine other areas, i.e. nails for psoriatic pits and oncholysis. Similarly, presence of discrete purplish leison (lichen planus) search mouth for striae.

EXAMINATION OF NAILS

Examine the nail for change in shape, colour, ridges, pits, thickening or hypertrophy, infection of nail bed (paronychia), nail bed infarcts, tumour (warts) and nail bed pulsations.

☞ Look for the shape and colour of the nails.
- Abnormal shapes are:
  - *Koilonychia* (spoon nails). It is characteristic shape of the nails in iron deficiency anaemia but can also be seen due to nail trauma in manual labourer and rickshaw pullers, in thyrotoxicosis, syphilis, porphyria, ischaemic heart disease
  - *Platynychia* (flat nails) is also seen in hereditary iron deficiency.
  - *Clubbing of the fingers* (read it in Unit on CVS and respiratory systems examination)

☞ Look for ridges/lines/thickening or hypertrophy/pits/ infection and any other abnormality.
- The important changes in the nails and their associated conditions are described in Table 11.3.

☞ Look for nodules/tumours of the nails
- Warts around the finger nails may occur in nail biters
- Subungual fibroma (warty swellings) may be seen in tuberous sclerosis

- Glomus tumour (neurovascular glomus bodies). Sometimes may be seen through the nail as small dark spot.

Abnormal Colouration of Nails (Box 11.4)

Box 11.4	Change in the Nail Colour as a Clue to Diagnosis
Nail colour	Diagnosis
White nails or Terry's nails (leuconychia, Fig. 11.22)	Hypoalbuminaemia, chronic liver disease, other wasting diseases, congenital
Pale	Anaemia, shock
Orange or lemon yellow	Carotenaemia, mepacrine toxicity
Yellow	Jaundice, tetracyclines, and lymphodema
Bluish	Cyanosis, side effect of an cyanides
Red	Palmar erythema carbon monoxide poisoning, polycythaemia, embolic lesions of subacute bacterial endocarditis, vasculitis
Black (melanin)	Addison's disease, Peutz-Jeghers syndrome, hemochromatosis, side effect of cytotoxic drugs
Green	Pseudomonas infection (paronychia)
Petechiae, purpura, ecchymosis	Bleeding or coagulation disorders
Rash	Disease or drug-induced

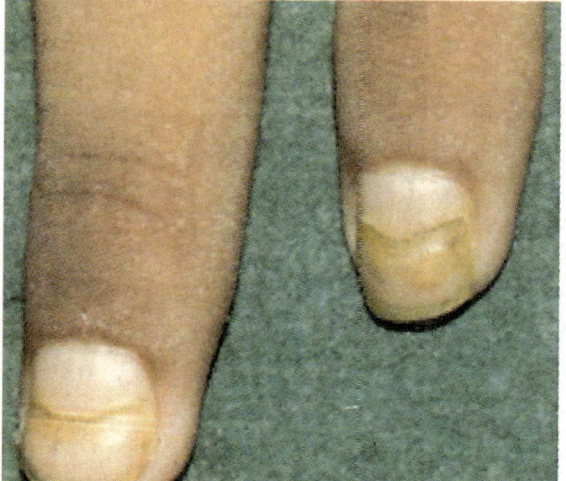

Fig. 11.22: Terry's nails (white nails) in a patient with cirrhosis of liver. Note the transverse lines across the nails.

TABLE 11.3: Important Changes in the Nails

Change	Association
Bitten nails (thimbling of nails)	Personality disorder
Splinter haemorrhages (haemorrhagic streaks under the nails)	Minor trauma, systemic vasculitis, SABE, trichinosis, rheumatic fever, cryoglobinaemia
Pitting of nails	Psoriasis, eczema
Onycholysis (rat bitten nail). It is detachment of nails from their bed	Trauma, hyper- and hypothyroidism psoriasis, lichen planus, ringworm infection
Brittle nails	Peripheral vascular disease, iron deficiency, use of nail varnish or cuticle remover
Transverse ridging	Acute illness, Zn deficiency
White line (transverse across the nails, i.e. Mee's line)	Arsenic poisoning, high fever, Hogdkin's disease, palmar keratosis
Absent nail	Nail-patella syndrome
Fungal infection (thickening, crumbling and discoloration) (Fig. 11.23)	Candidiasis, ringworm
Red half-moons (red lunula)	Congestive heart failure
Blue half-moons (blue lunula)	CuSO₄ poisoning, Wilson's disease
'Half and half nails (see proximal half resembles ground glass, while distal half is pink or reddish brown)	Chronic renal failure (CRF) disappears after successful renal transplantation and after dialysis

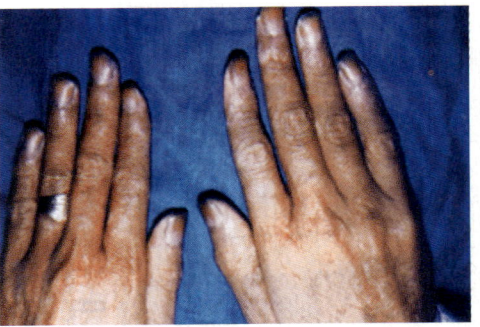

Fig. 11.23: Fungal infection of the skin.

EXAMINATION OF HAIR

1. Hair Loss

☞ *Inspect the pattern of hair loss. Visually inspect the pattern on the patient's head, face, axillae, body and pubic area.*

- Patchy hair loss of head suggests tinea capitis, alopecia areata, trichotillomania
- Temporal and occipital hair loss (male *baldness pattern*) suggest androgenic alopecia.
- Complete loss of head hair suggest alopecia totalis.
- Complete loss of all body hair indicates alopecia universalis.

2. Hirsutism (excessive hair growth)

☞ *Look for excessive body hair*

- Male type of excessive hair growth over face in female is either genetic, idiopathic or due to adrogenaemia
- Secondary hirsutism occurs in Cushing's syndrome, adrenogenital syndrome, adrenal hyperplasia, polycystic ovarian syndrome (*Stein-Leventhal syndrome*), ovarian tumour, steriods and ACTH therapy. These patients need full endocrine assessment.

BRIEF SYNOPSIS OF COMMON SKIN DISORDERS

SCABIES (THE ITCH)

Scabies is a common contagious pruritic condition involving the skin of an individual sensitised to the female mite *Sarcoptes scabei* or its products.

Mode of transmission. The disease is usually contracted by close personal contact or by sharing of contaminated towels, bed-linens and clothings. Holding the hand is less common mode of spread because warmth is necessary for the mite to remain mobile. The condition is common among children, mentally subnormal and immunocompromised individuals. Overcrowding, poor personal hygiene and poverty are predisposing factors.

Clinical Features

The patient complains of pruritus and skin lesions. The pathognomonic lesions are *burrows* which appear as slightly elevated, brownish, tortuous lines or dots. The site of burrows include finger-webs (*refer to* Fig. 11.1), wrists, elbows, ankles, breasts and genitalia. The face and scalp are usually spared. The point of entry of the mite in the burrow is denoted by a tiny vesicle at one end that contains the mite. The mite can be removed at the end of a needle or the burrow.

CARBUNCLES

A carbuncle is a deep infection of many contiguous hair follicles by *Staph. aureus*, is characterised by intense inflammatory changes in the surrounding and underlying connective tissues. Rupture through multiple sites on the surface gives the typical *sieve-like appearance*. Sometimes, the entire core of the lesion is shed off leaving a *deep ulcer with purulent floor*. Common sites are the nape of neck, the shoulders, hips or thighs. They occur in old persons, patients of diabetes and malnutrition.

IMPETIGO CONTAGIOSA

It is a contagious superficial pyogenic infection of the skin (Fig. 11.24). It is of two types:
1. **Nonbullous impetigo** occurs in pre-school going or young school-age children and is due to infection caused by *Staph. aureus* or *Group A streptococci* or both.
   The initial lesion is a thin walled vesicle which ruptures and exudes serum that dries up and form crusts. The crusts even finally separate to leave erythema and hypopigmentation.
2. **Bullous impetigo** is encountered in newborn, is caused by *Staph. aureus*.
   In *bullous impetigo*, the vesicles do not rupture but enlarge to form bullae up to 2–3 cm in diameter which can persist for 2–3 days. Lesions are commonly seen on the face but can occur on any part of the body. The ruptured bullae lead to crusts formation.

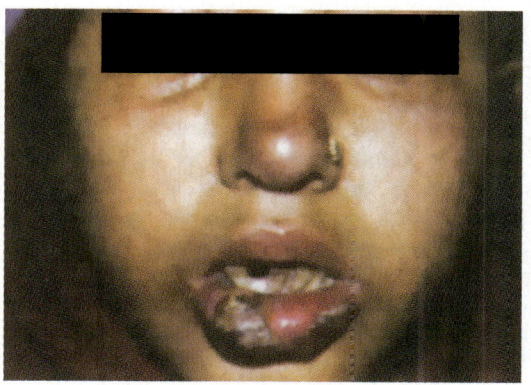

Fig. 11.25: Herpes labialis.

lead to 'S crum pox'; while damage to skin over a finger may produce *whitlow* especially in nursing mother.

Type II causes genital infection, i.e., *vulvovaginitis* (produces burning sensation), *dysuria* and *lymphadenopathy*. Extragenital infection of the thigh or buttockes may cause myalgia and dysesthesia of the affected skin.

The clinical features and complications of herpes simplex are given in Box 11.5.

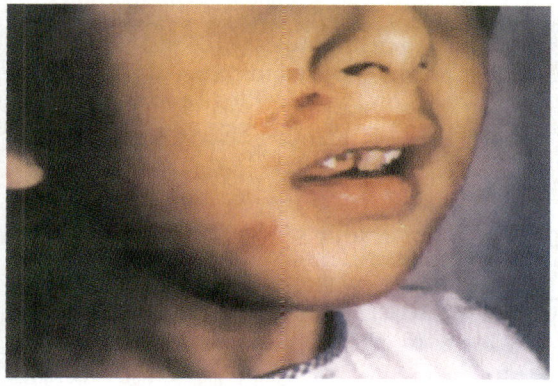

Fig. 11.24: Impetigo contagiosa.

HERPES SIMPLEX

There are two types of herpes simplex infections—HSV types I and II.

Clinical Features

Primary herpes infection by HSV-I may cause asymptomatic gingivostomatitis in children but in others there may be symptoms such as stomatitis associated with buccal ulceration (Fig. 11.25), marked local lymphadenopathy and systemic features. Trauma to skin may introduce virus and

Box 11.5: Clinical Features of Herpes Simplex

Type I
- Herpes labialis (Fig. 11.25) (cold sores)
- Keratoconjunctivitis
- Finger infections (whitlows)
- Encephalitis
- Primary gingivostomatitis
- Genital infection (vulvovaginitis in females)
- Erythema multiforme involving lips, face and mucous membrane

Type II
- Genital infection
- Neonatal infection (acquired during delivery)

VARICELLA-ZOSTER VIRUS (VZV) INFECTION

The disease affects patients of middle age or old age. Pain, tingling and dysaesthesia may precede the appearance of skin lesion. It produces vesicles, papules and bullous lesion throughout the dermatome (*refer* to Fig. 11.13). Secondary infection or postherpetic neuralgia may follow an attack of shingles (zoster infection). Postherpetic trigeminal neuralgia can occur and may lead to infection of eye.

URTICARIA

It is a common reaction pattern to foods (nuts, shellfish) and food additive, drugs (salicylates, indomethacin), and more rarely to an underlying systemic disease.

All types of urticaria are due to release of mediators (*histamine*, *serotonin* and *other kinins*) which cause increased permeabililty and accumulation of fluid into extravascular space. The urticaria may be *immunological* (atopy, food allergy, drug allergy, dermatographism, angioedema, serum sickness, blood transfusion reactions) or *non-immunological* (drugs, i.e. opiates, salicylates, NSAIDs, antibiotics, contrast media).

Non-immunological physical urticaria is precipitated by heat, cold, sweating, pressure, sun exposure, etc. *Acute urticaria* is widespread and lasts for a few days may be a manifestation of type I allergic reaction, even associated with serum sickness like reaction, hence, history often reveals a clear-cut cause, i.e. particular food or drug. *Chronic urticaria* is arbitrarily defined as disease lasting for more than 6 weeks.

Urticarial eruptions (Fig. 11.26) are itchy wheals, sometimes accompanied by deeper and more diffuse swelling (angioedema) of eyes or lips, but genital swelling is less common. Lesions begin as erythematous macules that evolve into pink oedematous wheals with a surrounding flare. The number and size of wheals is variable. The wheals are evanescent lesions that seldom present longer than 12–24 hours.

The urticaria may be associated with systemic features, e.g. headache, fever, arthralgia, syncope, nausea, vomiting and pain in abdomen. The most serious complications of acute urticaria are:
 i. *anaphylactic shock* characterised by pallor, sweating, hypotension and collapse bronchospasm.
 ii. *angioedema* (refer to Fig. 11.19).

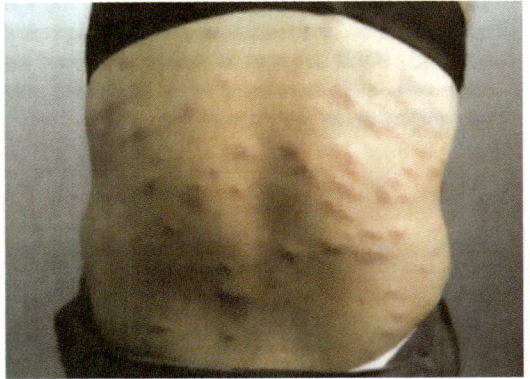

Fig. 11.26: Chronic urticaria: Note the pink oedematous wheals with surrounding flare (wheal and flare lesion).

ERYTHEMA NODOSUM (*refer to* Table 11.1)

This reaction is vasculitis involving the deeper dermis and subcutaneous fat producing painful nodules or plaques (Fig. 11.27) on the skin of thighs and arms. It may be provoked by *unknown factor*, *drugs* (penicilline, sulpha, oral contraceptive) and *systemic diseases* (sarcoidosis), *inflammatory bowel disease* and *infections* (bacterial, viral, fungal).

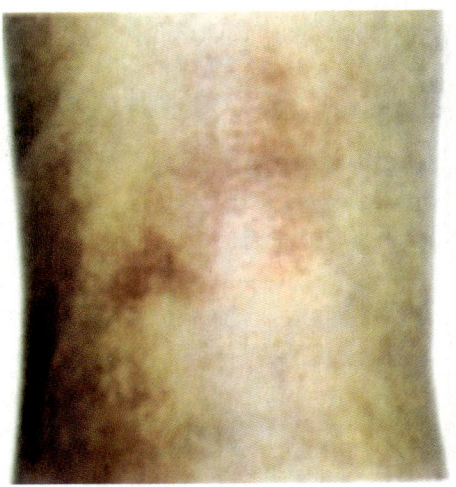

Fig. 11.27: Erythema nodosum.

Painful palpable nodules or plaques up to 5 cm in diameter, dusky blue-red in colour appear in crops over 2 weeks on the lower legs and thighs. They slowly fade to leave bruising and staining of the skin. Malaise, fever and joint pain (arthralgia) are common.

STEVENS-JOHNSON SYNDROME

It is an immune-mediated severe bullous reaction pattern due to varied aetiological factors, i.e.
 i. Herpes simplex infection (usually type I) provokes recurrent attacks
 ii. Mycoplasma
 iii. Bacterial infections, e.g. streptococci, vaccinia, tuberculosis
 iv. Drugs, e.g. sulphonamides, sulphonylureas (chlorpropamide), barbiturates, NSAIDs (ibuprofen, piroxicam) and anticonvulsants (phenytoin).

"*Stevens-Johnson sydrome*" is common in children, adolescents and adults. It is characterised by prodromal symptoms (malaise, fever), severe erythematous or bullous lesions involving skin and mucous membranes and palate. Bullae rupture cause erosions, ulceration and bleeding. The lips are covered by characteristic massive haemorrhagic crusts (Fig. 11.28).

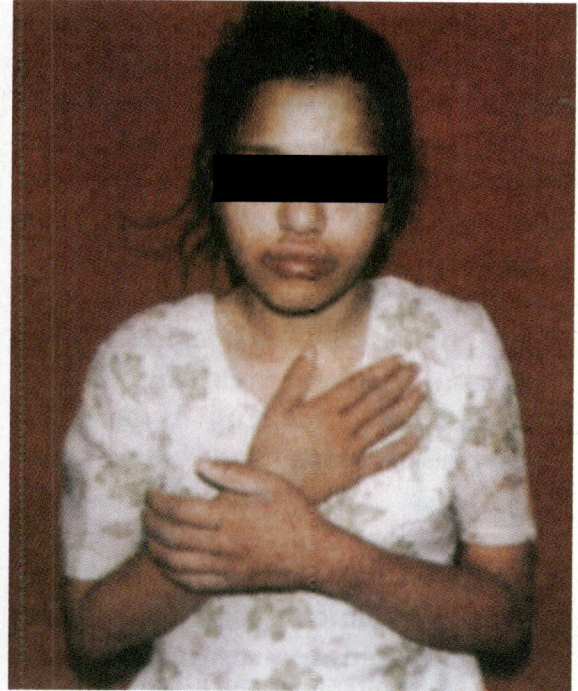

Fig. 11.28: Stevens-Johnson syndrome due to ibuprofen.

Eye changes include conjunctivitis, corneal ulceration, uveitis or panophthalmitis. Genital lesions are frequent. Marked constitutional symptoms such as fever may accompany skin lesion. Lung and renal involvement may occur.

NEUROFIBROMATOSIS (VON RECKLINGHAUSEN'S DISEASE)

The characteristic cutaneous features are scattered, light brown (*café au lait spots*) macules and flesh-coloured smooth polypoidal swelling, i.e. neurofibromas (*refer to* Fig. 11.9). *Molluscum fibrosum* (skin tags) are sessile, pink-coloured tumours widely distributed over the trunk. *Plexiform neuromas* are uncommon and tend to follow the course of a nerve, usually on the face, neck or trunk. Oral lesions are uncommon. Small circular pigmented hamartomas of iris (*Lisch nodules*) appear in early childhood.

More than 5 café au lait spots suggest the diagnosis of neurofibromatosis.

PSORIASIS

It is a chronic noninfectious, inflammatory skin disease characterised by erythematous silvery white plaques over the extensor surface of knees (*refer to* Fig. 11.11) and elbow as well as on the scalp. It is common in adult age. The course is unpredictable with exacerbations and remissions.

Genetic and immune abnormality, trauma (*Koebner phenomenon*), emotional disturbance, infections, drugs and HIV infection act as predisposing or precipitating factors.

Simple plaque psoriasis produces salmon-pink silvery white plaques which on scrapping reveals a glistening membrane and on removal reveals, small bleeding spots (*Auspitz's sign* is positive). It involves exterior surface of elbows, back, scalp, flexures palms and soles and nails.

Pustular psoriasis (localised and generalised) is characterised by pustules, there may be associated fever.

Guttate psoriasis: It is common in children and young adults, characterised by crops of small rain drop like shiny scales on the trunk and extremities. This may precede an upper respiratory infection.

Exfoliative or erythrodermic psoriasis. The skin is red and scaly over the trunk and extremities. Itching and burning are troublesome.

Complication. Psoriatic polyarthritis.

ACNE VULGARIS

It is a skin disease of teenagers characterised by blockage of pilosebaceaus ducts of sebaceous glands of face, chest and back. It involves both sexes. Peak incidence is between 16 and 20 years.

It occurs due to increased sebum production, abnormalities of microbial flora, hyperkeratinisation, inflammation of the duct and hyperandrogenism. It can be familial.

Skin Lesions

Comedones both open (*black heads*) and closed (*white heads*) due to plugging of pilosebaceous orifice and accretion of sebum and keratin in deeper layers are characteristic lesions. Inflammatory papules, nodules and cyst formation follow these lesions leading to scarring and disfigurement.

Site of the Lesion

Face (*refer to* Fig. 11.12), shoulder, upper chest front and back and chin (violin players called *Fiddler's neck*) are sites of involvement. Increased local trauma and premenstrual tension may cause exacerbation.

Variants

1. Acne neonatorum (infantile)
2. Acne conglobate

3. Acne fulminans
4. Acne excorice
5. Occupational acne
6. Drug induced acne
7. Acne due to virilisation or adrenal hyperplasia.

ALOPECIA AREATA

It is a common condition of idiopathic nature, characterised by well-defined patches of baldness usually on the scalp. *Alopecia totalis* describes complete loss of scalp hair and *alopecia universalis* refers to complete loss of all hair on the body.

There is often a personal or family history of atopy. Alopecia areata is associated with Down's sydrome and other autoimmune disorders such as thyrotoxicosis, Addison's disease, Hashimoto's thyroiditis and pernicious anaemia.

This occurs in both sexes and all races, and is usually seen in young adults or children. Only 25% cases are seen over the age of 40 years.

Skin Lesions

Patches of hair loss (baldness) can occur on any part of the body, e.g. beard, eyebrows but the scalp area is frequently involved (Fig. 11.29). Asymptomatic hair loss is first noticed by the relative or barber or hair dresser. Patches tend to regrow over the course of several months within the scalp margin in adults.

Children with atopy may develop loss of all scalp hair (*alopecia totalis*). Alopecia totalis is less common among adults.

Loss of hair from all body sites (*alopecia universalis*) may occur by extension from other sites.

Pathognomonic signs of Alopecia Areata

Broken off hairs of 3–4 mm long which taper off towards scalp (*exclamation-mark hair*) are pathognomonic of active disease.

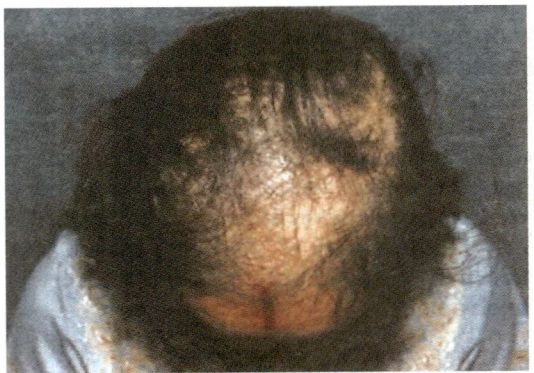

Fig. 11.29: Alopecia areata: Note the patchy loss of scalp hair in a young female.

LUPUS VULGARIS

Immunity acquired during primary tubercular infection protects the individual for several years, hence, after a long latent period reinfection may occur. Depending upon the level of immuity, skin necrosis may be mild (*lupus vulgaris*), moderate (*tuberculosis verrucosa cutis*) or extensive (*sacrofuloderma*) or widespread and extensive (*tuberculosis orificialis*).

Lupus vulagaris is the most common cutaneous tuberculosis producing varied manifestations. Although face is the commonest site of involvement in the West, in India the buttocks, thighs, legs and upper extremities are commonly affected. Erythema, scaling and scarring plaques are seen. In severe cases, cutaneous tissue appear **'gnawed'**, hence, the term lupus' (meaning 'wolf'). Lupus vulgaris represents high level of immunity, hence, skin lesion (necrosis) is mild. The cutaneous lesion show granuloma formation with central caseation.

SCROFULODERMA

This type of tuberculosis of the skin is an extension of infection into the skin from an underlying focus, usually the lymph node (Fig. 11.30) and occasionally from the underlying tuberculosis of bone or joint. It commonly follows cervical or axillary lymphadenopathy where the underlying lymph nodes enlarge and overlying skin gets infected, breaks down to form discharging sinuses. The ulcers are soft with undermined edges and heal by linear cord-like scars.

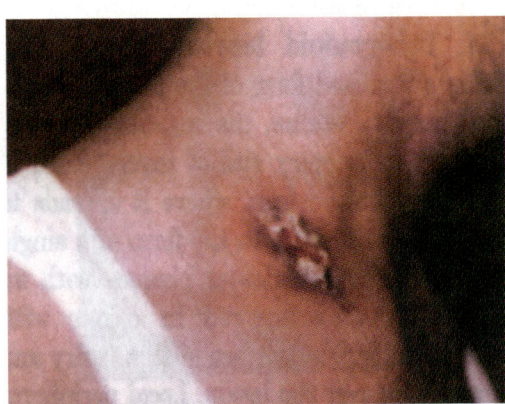

Fig. 11.30: Scrofuloderma commonly follows rupture of tubercular lymphadentis. Note the sinus and pigmentation around it.

LEPROSY

Leprosy is not a skin disorder but a systemic disorder, where skin involvement forms an important and distinct spectrum. Leprosy (*Hansen's disease*) caused by *M. leprosy* is classified depending on the immune status of an individual into *tuberculoid*, *borderline* and *lepromatous*.

The skin lesions occur in two main polar types of leprosy, e.g. *tuberculoid* and *lepromatous*.
1. **Tuberculoid leprosy** (Fig. 11.31B): Being a localised form of the disease due to good immune status, the organism may be confined to primary site of involvement in the neural tissue from where it spreads to the skin. Lesions are in the form of a single or a couple of macules or plaques with an elevated rim, dusky red in colour with central pallor. The surface of skin is dry and anaesthetic over the lesion. Local peripheral nerves may be enlarged and thickened. Biopsy shows tuberculoid granuloma with no bacilli.
2. **Lepromatous leprosy.** Immunity is lacking and presenting symptoms usually pertain to systemic involvement especially respiratory system, e.g. nasal congestion, cough, etc. The skin lesions are in the form of plaques, nodules, macules and papules which are erythematous and multiple and have no loss of sensation. With untreated disease, the facial skin become thicker giving the individual a "*leonine face*' (Fig. 11.31A). Involvement of nerves due to increasing damage may lead to '*clawhand*', *wrists drop* and *footdrop*. Loss of sensation leads to trophic changes and autonomic disturbances. Involvement of bone and digits give rise to their resorption (*loss of digits*) and muscle wasting. Loss of a part/parts is common, therefore, these patients prefer to become beggars.

FIXED DRUG ERUPTIONS (Fig. 11.32)

The pathogenesis of this type of reaction is unknown. Most of the drug reactions are immunlogically mediated either by hypersensitivity type I reaction (penicillin induced) or by immune complex or by photoallergic reactions. The face, hands and genitalia are commonly involved. Bright red, sometimes pruritic or even blistered plaques or annular lesions are seen. There is associated burning and discomfort. The lesions are fixed in site and appear within hours of offending drug administration. They will occur at exactly the same sites if the drug is given again at another time. Postinflammation is a characteristic feature. Phenolphthalein (a laxative), NSAIDs (Fig. 11.32) tetracyclines, phenacetin, sulphonamide, salicylates and oral contraceptives pill are known to cause them.

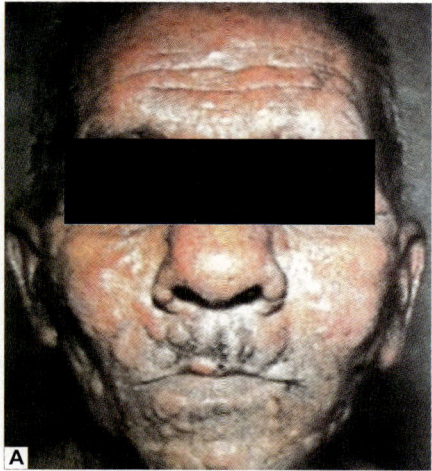

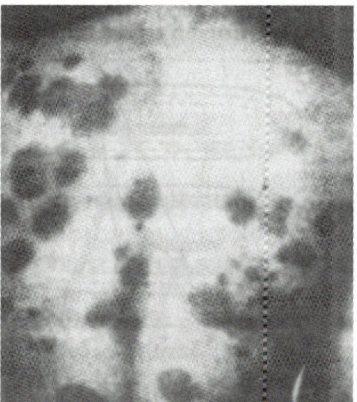

Fig. 11.32: Fixed drug eruption due to NSAIDs.

PEMPHIGUS

Pemphigus is an autoimmune bullous disorders of skin and mucous membranes, characterised by intraepidermal blisters formation.

Pemphigus can be divided into two groups:
1. **Pemphigus vulgaris** (Fig. 11.33): Blisters occur in deeper epidermis.
2. **Pemphigus foliaceus.** It is superfacial form of pemphigus.

Pemphigus vulgaris: Patients are usually between ages of 40 and 60 years and 90% have HLA-DR_4 linkage. It is common in India.

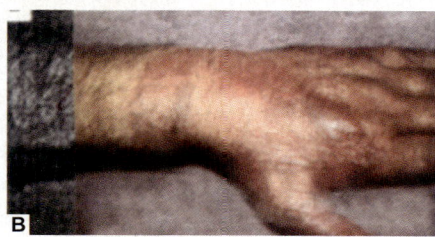

Figs 11.31A and B: Leprosy. (A) Leonine facies in lepromatous leprosy. Note the papulonodular lesions with thickening of skin; (B) Note the macular illdefined anaesthetic lesion in tuberculoid leprosy.

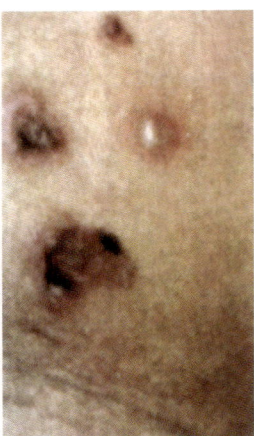

Fig. 11.33: Pemphigus vulgaris. Note the blisters, erosions and crusted lesions.

In majority of patients, lesions may be confined to mucosal surfaces; 50% cases have initial involvement of mouth with bright red painful erosive lesions with denuded mucosa. In a few patients, this may be the only site of involvement.

Most commonly, the primary skin lesion is a flaccid blister, occurring anywhere on the normal skin. Such lesions (blisters) soon rupture to leave behind moist eroded lesions which have a tendency to spread. The characteristic sign, e.g. *Nikolsky's sign* of the disease is elicited by applying lateral pressure on normal looking skin at the periphery of active lesion, results in the formation of new bulla or if applied to the pre-existing bulla results in the spread of bulla (*bulla spread sign*). When large areas of the skin are eroded, fluid loss and catabolic changes may produce severe metabolic disturbance. Secondary bacterial infection of denuded skin is common.

Pemiphigus foliaceus: The primary lesions are flaccid blisters which are scaly and crusted erosions. The lesions are localised to face, scalp, chest and upper back. The lesions may spread and lead exfoliative erythroderma. Mucous membranes are infrequently involved. Heat and sun exposure may exacerbate the symptoms.

The diagnosis is confirmed by the (i) cytological examination of blister fluid and by; (ii) direct immunofluorescent staining of a skin sample obtained from the edge of a fresh blister.

ATOPIC DERMATITIS/ECZEMA

Atopic dermatitis is chronic pruritic skin disorder of unknown aetiology associated with personal or family history of atopy and a typical distribution and morphology. Itching is severe, distressing, and there is tendency for lichenification and frequently raised levels of IgE.

The disorder is genetically predisposed and risk of transmission is 60% if both parents are affected. The *predisposing factors* are:
- Dietary products, e.g. milk, egg, etc.
- Heat humidity, dryness of skin
- Contact with wollen clothes.

Skin Lesions

The cardinal skin lesion of atopic dermatitis is itch and scarching that produces rash and not the rash that itches. Atopic eczema usually begins before the age of 6 months but, paradoxically seldom presents during neonatal period. The rash remits spontaneously in two-thirds of children before the age of 10 years. The distribution of rash in adults is on the face, trunk and extremities. The **diagnosis** is made by presence of pruritus, morphology and distribution of the lesion (face, trunk, extremites), relapsing or chronic dermatitis and positive family history, cheilitis, conjunctivitis, wool or food intolerance with sweating, high IgE level, type I hypersensitivity, white dermographism (*Hanifin and Rajka's diagnostic criteria*).

SEBORRHOEIC ECZEMA (DERMATITIS)

It is chronic skin disease involving typical areas of skin which are rich in sebaceous glands. Its cause remains unknown but a yeast like fungus *Malassezia furfur* appears to be a perpetuating factor. The condition runs in families but the precise mode of inheritance is not known, *Pityriasis capitis* (dandruff) is probably the mild form of seborrhoeic dermatitis.

Skin Lesion

It can occur in infancy during first 2 months of life with lesions on the scalp (*cradle cap*) and trunk. It is rare in childhood but becomes common during middle age (18–40 years) and old age.

The three common patterns involving seborrhoeic dermatitis are:
1. Scalp, ears, face and eyebrows
2. Interscapular (Fig. 11.34) and presternal areas of skin.
3. Flexures of axillae, umbilicus, breasts and groin.

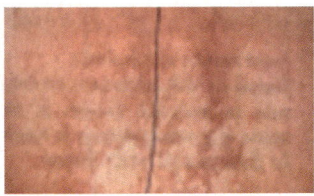

Fig. 11.34: Seborrhoeic dermatitis. Note the erythematous plaques with greasy scales in the interscapular region.

Unit XII

Vitals and the Unconscious Patient

- Symptoms
- History
- General Physical Examination
- Systemic Examination
- Brief Synopsis of Different Comas

SYMPTOMS

Unconsciousness or Coma

Definition: Coma or unconsciousness is defined as persistent loss of consciousness in which the subject lies with eyes closed and shows no response to external stimulus. In deep coma the corneal, pupillary, pharyngeal reflexes and the tendon and plantar reflexes are absent. With lesser degree of coma (precoma), pupillary reflexes, reflex ocular movements and other brain stem reflexes are preserved and there may or may not be rigidity of the limbs and extensor plantar response.

Alteration in Consciousness

The term **'stupor'** refers to state of disturbed consciousness when an individual responds only to the vigorous painful stimuli by groaning, opening the eyes or with irregular respiration.

Drowsiness. It is a sleepy state from which patient can be aroused by external stimulus and can remain alert for some time.

Confusion. It is a state of reduced mental clarity. Disorientation with hypoactive presentation has been called *"acute confusion"* or *"torpor"*.

Delirium. It is a state of agitation (high arousal) in which there is confusion and often hallucinations.

Coma-like States

Coma is characterized by complete unarousability. Several other syndromes also render the patients unresponsive are described because of their special importance as follows:

1. **Vegetative state:** This is awake coma in which the eyes remain open giving the appearance of wakefulness but patient is unresponsive. There is an absolute absence of response to commands and an inability to communicate. There may be yawning, grunting and random movements of limbs and head. There are accompanying signs of extensive bilateral cortical damage, i.e. Babinski signs, decerebrate or decorticate limb posturing and absent response to visual stimuli. Autonomic nervous system functions are preserved. The vegetative state results from global damage to the cerebral cortex most often following cardiac arrest or head injury.

2. **Akinetic mutism:** It is state of partial or full awakefulness (awake coma) in which patient lies immobile with eyes open and is unable to talk. It results from hydrocephalus, mass in the region of third ventricle, bilateral frontal lobe lesions.

   Abulia. It is milder form of akinetic mutism with same significance. Person will have change in behaviour with decreased rate and complexity of language and speech.

3. **Locked-in-state:** It is a state of pseudocoma in which patient appears to be unconscious, immobile and unresponsive but can open and move the eyes on command. Often these patients communicate with movements of eyes, a form of *'sign language'*. These individuals are thus *"locked in, or imprisoned within their own bodies"*. It results from pontine infarction or haemorrhage due to basilar artery occlusion.

4. **Coma vigil (vigilant coma):** It is a state of disturbed consciousness with muttering. In this state, person is vigilant but unresponsive. It is observed

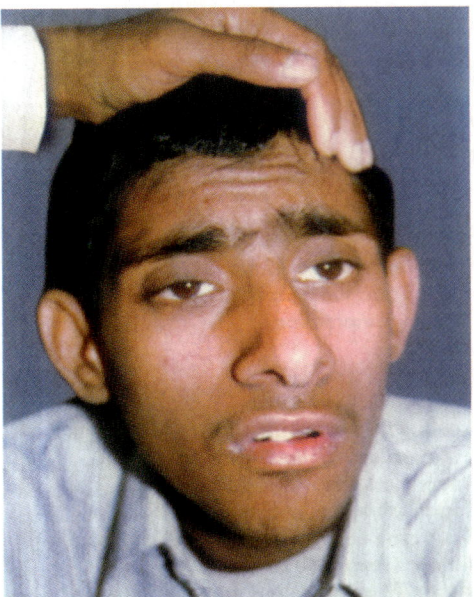

Fig. 12.1: Catatonia. A patient with hypomobile face and vacant look. He appears to be distressed and makes no responsive movements.

in infectious fevers such as typhoid, dengue or pneumonia.
5. **Catatonia (Fig. 12.1):** It is hypomobile syndrome associated with major psychosis. In its typical form, the patients appear awake with eyes open but make no voluntary or responsive movements, although they blink spontaneously and may not appear distressed. The characteristic feature is that the limbs maintain their posture when lifted or moved by the examiner.
6. **Hysterical pseudocoma:** It indicates voluntary attempt to appear comatosed. Patients resist to examination. Eyelid opening is actively resisted. Blinking occurs to visual threat when the lids are held open. The eyes moves concomitantly with head rotation. All these signs negate brain damage.

Causes of Coma

A normal level of consciousness is maintained by activation of the cerebral hemispheres by brain stem reticular activating system (RAS). Hence, coma occurs either due to extensive bilateral damage to celebral hemisphere or cerebral oedema or brain stem compression or damage. The causes of coma are:

I. **Brain stem and cerebellar lesions, e.g.** cerebellar infarction, tumour, haemorrhage, trauma, infections (e.g. encephalitis, brain abscess, meningitis).

II. **Lesions of cerebral hemisphere with oedema, with or without brain stem compression,** e.g. infarction, haemorrhage, encephalitis, meningitis, tumour, status epilepticus, cerebral malaria, trauma (subdural, extradural), hydrocephalus, hypertensive encephalopathy

III. **Metabolic abnormalities, e.g.** diabetic ketoacidosis, respiratory failure, hepatic failure, adrenal crisis, renal failure, hypopituitarism, cardiac failure, hypothyroidism, hyponatraemia (severe), hypoxia, hypokalaemia, hyper- and hypocalcaemia, vitamin deficiencies (e.g. B_1, nicotinic acid, B_{12}).

IV. **Drugs and physical agents causing cerebral dysfunction, e.g.** anaesthetic agents, drug overdose and alcohol ingestion. Hyper- and hypothermia.

V. **Psychogenic, e.g.** hysteria.

Head injury, epilepsy, poisoning, hypo- or hyperglycaemia, cerebral embolism and SAH are common causes in young age; While CVA, intracranial infection, head injury, cardiac arrhythmias, hypo- or hyperglycaemia are common in old age.

ASSESSMENT OF A PATIENT WITH COMA

An account of events preceding coma are most infirmative, hence, must be obtained directly from the friends or relatives and supplemented by any other information from the third personnel/ambulance personnel/eye witness, etc. It is imperative to know when the patient was last seen alert and conscious because the possible diagnosis is influenced by the onset of coma.

HISTORY

Present History

In many cases, the cause of coma is immediately evident (e.g. trauma, cardiac arrest or known drug ingestion); while in others information have to be gathered from third party regarding the:

i. **Onset of coma:** The cerebrovascular episodes, drug abuse or intoxication, hypoglycaemia, a life-threatening infection (septicaemia) or postictal condition cause sudden onset of coma; whereas coma associated with diabetic ketoacidosis, chronic renal failure (uraemia) or hepatic encephalopathy develops insidiously.

ii. **Details of preceding neurological symptoms:**
   - A history of headache preceding coma indicates intracranial space occupying lesion.
   - Seizures whether focal or generalised indicate intracranial tumour, brain abscess, encephalitis or brain haemorrhage.

- Dizziness, diplopia occurring before coma indicate transient vascular episodes such as cerebral vasospasm.
- A history of trauma with concussion followed later by fluctuating consciousness, confusion, stupor and coma indicates subdural haematoma.
- A history of trauma followed by a brief lucid interval before lapsing into coma suggests extradural haemorrhage.

iii. **Use of medications, illicit drugs or alcohol.** Patients with drug-induced coma may be known or identified by neighbours, family, medical attendants or the ambulance driver or recovery of drug containers or wrapper or alcohol from their homes by the attendant.

iv. **A history of depression or suicidal tendencies** must be taken into account of unexplained coma.

v. **A thorough search of the patient** may reveal hospital outpatient attendance card, unfilled prescriptions, drugs or even syringes. *Diabetics or hypertensives or epileptics* often carry some form of identification either in their clothing (pocket) or as a wrist band or necklace.

Past History

History of liver, kidney, lung, heart disease (arrhythmias) or other medical illnesses such as *diabetes, hypothyroidism, Addison's disease* must be sought. Hypoglycaemia is characterised by stupor or coma with signs of sympathetic overactivity (pallor, sweating, tachycardia, seizures) and patient can be aroused easily by I.V. 25% glucose in case of doubt of diabetic vs hypoglycaemic coma before blood or urine sample is taken for examination.

Family History

- Heart disease (cardiomyopathies)
- Stroke
- Hyperlipidaemia

Personal History

- Ask about occupation, habits (smoking, alcoholism)

EXAMINATION

General Physical Examination (GPE)

Proper diagnosis of a case of coma depends on the recognition and interpretation of certain clinical signs such as brain stem reflexes, proper use of diagnostic tests. It is a common practice that acute respiratory and cardiovascular problems should be attended to on priority basis than neurological examination. Therefore, vital signs must be maintained such as clear airway, intubation and oxygenation (Fig. 12.2), pulse, BP before subjecting the patient to further evaluation. The immediate basic assessment will guide series of investigations and immediate resuscitative measures (Table 12.1).

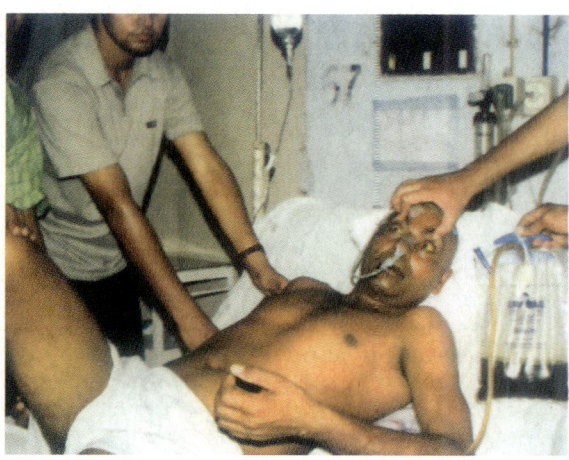

Fig. 12.2: Hepatic coma. Presence of jaundice and dark-coloured urine in presence of unconsciouness indicate hepatic coma. Ammoniacal smell from the breath present.

TABLE 12.1: Immediate Assessment of Coma and Remedial Measures

Assess	Check	Remedy
1. Is the airway patent?	Blood gases	Intubate and give O_2 (Fig. 12.2)
2. Is the patient convulsive?	EEG/blood glucose	I.V. glucose, O_2 and diazepam
3. Are there signs of head or face injury?	CT scan	Neurological examination
4. Is the neck fractured?	X-ray	Splint neck
5. Is there major haemorrhage?	Pulse, BP	Maintain BP and circulation
6. Is there an evidence of diabetes mellitus?	Blood/urine sugar	Give glucose if hypoglycaemia, otherwise treat appropriately
7. Is there an evidence of drug overdosage or misuse such as needle pricks?	Pupils and respiration	Naloxone or other appropriate antidote

General Observations

☞ *Note the general appearance, nourishment, dress and cleanliness.*

Severe emaciation with altered consciousness, suggest disseminated tuberculosis, HIV infection

malignancy, diabetes, Wernicke-Korsakoff psychosis.
- Shabby dress and uncleanliness indicate psychiatric disorder.

☞ Note for any evidence of trauma or exposure. Note any marks of injection or superficial thrombophlebitis.

- Signs of external trauma may be associated with fractures and intracranial bleeding.
- Marks of injections or thrombophlebitis indicate drug abuse/overdose.

☞ Look at face for pallor or signs of shock, injury and asymmetry

- Marks of injury or head injury indicate it to be cause of coma (concussion, contusion and laceration).
- Pallor and shock indicate blood loss (internal or external) if trauma is suspected. It may indicate fluid loss in a patient with diarrhoea and vomiting.
- A symmetry of face indicates CVA as the cause of coma.

☞ **Skin.** *Examine for: Colour (cyanosis, jaundice, purpura, rashes, pigmentation); texture (coarse, dry in hypothyroidism) and presence of infection sites (diabetics, drug), warmth, temperature, haemorrhagic spots*

- Cyanosis indicates type 2 respiratory failure
- Jaundice indicates hepatic coma
- Bleeding spots indicate blood dyscrasias
- Coarse and dry skin suggest myxoedematous coma
- Warmth or high temperature suggest hyperthermia, and coldness indicates hypothermia as the cause of coma.

☞ **Smell.** Alcohol and ketones may be smelt. In hepatic failure (ammonical odour) and uraemia (smell of urine), a distinct smell is present (Table 12.2).

☞ Always look for the important diagnostic clues (Table 12.2) so as to reach proper diagnosis.

☞ Look for state of hydration

The state of hydration is assessed by:
i. *Skin elasticity or turgor:* It is demonstrated by pinching up a fold of skin and then released. It remains as a ridge and subsides slowly if skin elasticity is lost otherwise it returns immediately to its normal position.

Loss of elasticity is not true index of hydration as it is lost in old age and due to loss of collagen in the skin.

TABLE 12.2: Clinical Clues to the Cause of Coma

Finding	Diagnostic clues
Haemorrogic spots	Purpura, bleeding diathesis
Smell of breath	Diabetic ketoacidosis, uraemia, alcohol, hepatic encephalopathy, aluminium phosphide poisoning
Seizure	Meningitis, encephalitis, cerebral malaria, brain haemorrhage, status epilepticus
Pyrexia	Septicaemia, meningitis, encephalitis, thyroid crisis, vasculitis
Jaundice	Hepatic coma (Fig. 12.2)
Perspiration	Anxiety, phaeochromocytoma, thyrotoxic crisis
Bradycardia	Stokes-Adams, myxoedema coma, OP poisoning, raised ICP, hypothermia, obstructive jaundice
Tachycardia	Hyperthyroidism, shock, CHF, infections
Hypotension	Shock, Addisonian crisis, AMI, drug intoxication, internal haemorrhage
Hypertension	Hypertensive encephalopathy, raised ICP (intracranial pressure), subarachnoid haemorrhage
Tachypnoea	Diabetic coma, metabolic acidosis, infection (pneumonia), respiratory failure
Rapid, shallow breathing	Alcohol intoxication, acidosis, diabetes
Dilated pupils	Autonomic hyperactivity
Papilloedema	Hypertensive encephalopathy, brain tumour, subarachnoid haemorrhage
Neck rigidity	Meningitis, subarachnoid or intracerebral haemorrhage, meningoencephalitis, meningism (typhoid, malaria)
Tongue/cheek bite	Status epilepticus
Cardiomegaly	CHF, hypertensive heart disease, valvular heart disease
Arrhythmias	AMI, CHF, valvular heart disease
Pulmonary rales/crackles	Pulmonary oedema, CHF, pneumonia
Hepatomegaly	CHF, hepatic failure
Asymmetric deep tendon reflexes	CVA, subdural haematoma, mass lesion
Plantar extensor	Raised intracranial pressure, hypoglycaemia
Primitive reflexes present	Dementia, frontal lobe lesions

Vitals and the Unconscious Patient

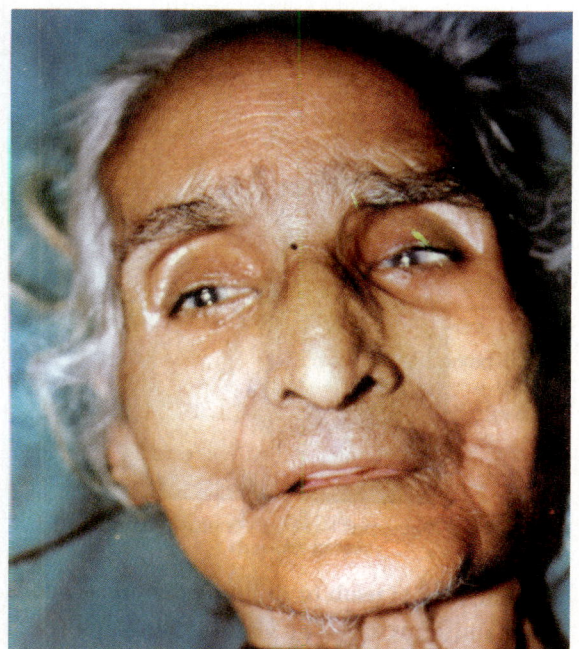

Fig. 12.3: A dehydrated patient. Note the sunken cheeks and eyeballs with dry tongue. Her systolic BP was <90 mm Hg. The skin was dry, wrinkled with loss of elasticity.

ii. *Intraocular tension*: In dehydration, the eyeballs are soft and shunken (Fig. 12.3) due to low intraocular pressure or tension.
iii. *Recording of BP*: Low blood pressure and postural drop in BP indicates dehydration and intravascular volume depletion due to fluid loss, i.e. diarrhoea, vomiting, burns, sweating, diabetes, diuretics, pancreatitis, etc.
iv. *Dry tongue and mouth:* A dry tongue and mouth may indicate dehydration but are commonly seen in smokers and mouth-breathers, hence, these signs may be deceptive.
v. *Jugular venous pulse and pressure (JVP):* The jugular venous pressure is low in volume depletion, hence veins are collapsed and not visible.

☞ *Examine ear and nose for bleeding*

- Bleeding from the ear occurs in fracture of middle cranial fossa (cranial trauma) or base of skull.
- Discolouration over the mastoid due to bruising (*Battle's sign*) suggests middle cranial fossa fracture.
- Bleeding from nose (epistaxis) with CSF rhinorrhoea indicates anterior cranial fossa injury.

The Vitals

1. The Pulse

☞ *Count the pulse rate, analyse its rhythm, character, volume and any other abnormality.*

- Count the pulse for at least 15 seconds if the rhythm and heart rate appear to be normal, multiply the reading by 4 to get the pulse rate or heart rate in beats/min (bpm). If the rate is too slow or too fast, then count the pulse for full one minute.
- The pulse should be analysed for *rate, rhythm, character, volume and presence or absence of radio-femoral delay*. When the rhythm is irregular, the heart rate should be counted by cardiac auscultation to know the *pulse deficit*. The pulse deficit (difference between heart rate and pulse rate) is because of non-conduction of weak cardiac beats to peripheral pulse.

> The rate of pulse varies from 60 to 90 bpm (average 72–75 bpm) during activity in a normal healthy individual. The rate is somewhat higher in children, and women, and is increased by standing, during eating and emotional stress.

Heart rate <60/min is called **bradycardia** and more than 100/min is called **tachycardia**. The causes of decreased and increased heart rate are given in Table 12.2.

Arrhythmias (atrial fibrillation, ventricular ectopics) are associated with embolic stroke followed by altered sensorium.

2. Blood Pressure

☞ *Measure BP in both the arms at least once*

- Blood pressure is measured using a sphygmomanometer cuff wrapped around the upper arm. The method of measurement and a checklist for measurement are discussed in CVS examination. It is important to use the correct size of the cuff. The length of inflatable bladder of the cuff should be 30–35 cm and width should be 12.5 cm (12–14 cm) for an average adult.

Blood pressure should be taken in both the arms at least once. Normally there may be difference of <10 mmHg in both the arms. Subsequent readings should be repeated on the arm with high pressure difference.

An internationally recognised JNC VIII classification which defines the normal and abnormal blood pressure is depicted in Box 12.1.

Extreme degree of hypertension (accelerated, malignant) is associated with hypertensive encephalopathy and subarachnoid haemorrhage

Box 12.1	JNC VIII Classification of hypertension	
Category	Systolic (mm Hg)	Diastolic (mm Hg)
Normal	<120	<80
Prehypertension	120–139	80–89
Stage 1 hypertension	140–150	90–99
Stage 2 hypertension	≥160	≥100

(Table 12.2). Hypotension with altered sensorium is observed in poisoning (alcohol, barbiturates), internal bleed, septic shock and myocardial infarction (cardiogenic shock).

3. Respiration

☞ *Count the respiratory rate and analyse its rhythm and pattern in unconscious patient*

- Count the respiratory rate for a full half minute and multiply it by 2 to get respiratory rate per minute. This should be counted when patient's attention is diverted elsewhere. For example, count the respiratory rate when you are counting the pulse rate.

Normal respiratory rate in adults is 14–18 breaths/min. Tachypnoea implies respiratory rate more than normal. Tachypnoea with altered sensorium indicates metabolic acidosis, diabetic ketoacidosis, CNS infections and respiratory failure (Table 12.2).

Pattern of Respiration

Respiration patterns though considered important in the coma diagnosis, but are of a little help in localisation of the lesion.

Hyperventilation (rapid breathing) indicates hypoxia, acidosis, poisoning, infection and may be psychogenic.
- Central neurogenic hyperventilation indicates lower midbrain/upper pontine lesion
- Apneustic breathing suggests lesion in lower pons.

Slow, shallow, regular breathing suggests metabolic or drug effect (opiates, barbiturates). The presence of cyanosis, activation of extrarespiratory muscles, flapping tremors, intercostal recession indicate type 2 respiratory failure (Fig. 12.4).

Rapid, deep (kussmaul) breathing suggests metabolic acidosis, diabetic ketoacidosis, uraemia, hepatic failure and pontine lesion.

Cheyne-Stokes breathing (hyperapnoea alternates apnoea) suggests bihemispherical damage or metabolic coma.

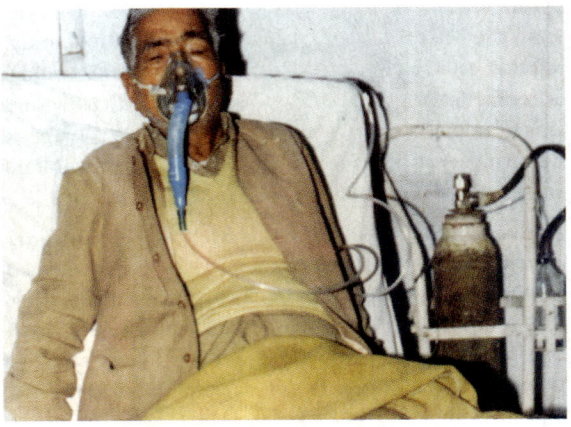

Fig. 12.4: Respiratory failure (type 2) with CO_2 narcosis. The patient had cyanosis, tachypnoea, tachycardia, flapping tremors. He is being shifted to respiratory intensive care unit (RICU).

Biot's breathing is also a periodic breathing seen in meningitis where there is sudden increase or decrease of respiration in paroxysms.

Agonal gasp (gasping respiration) is a terminal respiratory pattern, suggests bilateral lower brain stem lesion.

Sighing breathing is characterised by interruption of normal respiration by deep sighing breaths. It is seen during excitement and hysteria.

Temperature

The warmth of the skin felt with back of the hand over covered body part (neck, chest, abdomen) is a good indicator of fever, but an apparently normal temperature does not exclude hypothermia or hyperthermia.

☞ *Record the oral, rectal or axillary temperature in a patient with altered consciousness as the situation demands.*

Fever or pyrexia refers to an elevated body temperature (>37.2° or > 99°F) above the normal limits in an individual. The average oral temperature is usually quoted as 37.1°C (98.6°F). It may fluctuate considerably, i.e. in early morning, it may fall as low as 35.8°C (96°F) and in the evening it may rise to 37.2°C (99.0°F) called circadian rhythm. *Rectal temperature* is higher than oral temperature by an average of 0.4 to 0.5°C (0.7 to 0.9°F) approximately. In contrast, the axillary temperature is lower than oral temperature by approximately 1°C, hence, is considered less accurate than other two measurements.

Choice of site for recording

Most patients prefer oral to rectal temperatures. Oral temperature recording is not recommended in an unconscious patient or restless/violent patients as recordings may be less accurate and thermometer is likely to be broken. The sites of temperature recording in unconscious patient are axilla, groin (inguinal) and rectum (children).

High temperature. Rise in temperature in unconscious patient could be due to CNS infection (encephalitis, meningitis) or septicaemia, thyroid crisis, meningism (subarachnoid haemorrhage) or heat stroke).

Hyperthermia/hyperpyrexia: It refers to extreme elevation in temperature above 41°C (106°F). It could be due to heat stroke, heat exhaustion cerebral malaria, pontine haemorrhage, neuroleptic administration or malignant hyperpyrexia (an inherited abnormality).

Hypothermia: It refers to an abnormally low temperature below 35°C (95°F) rectally. Low-reading clinical thermometers are available and should be used when hypothermia is suspected. Temperatures as low as 27°C are not uncommon and core body temperatures below 20°C have been recorded in patients who subsequently survived. The **causes** of hypothermia with altered consciousness are:
1. Sudden or accidental exposure to low temperature environment.
2. Malnutrition, starvation
3. Myxoedema coma
4. Hepatic failure, diabetic ketoacidosis, hypoglycaemia, uraemia.
5. Head trauma, spinal cord injury
6. Drug-induced (barbiturates, opiates, *benzodiazepine*, phenothiazines, alcohol).

SYSTEMIC EXAMINATION

Neurological Examination

Level of Consciousness

An application of Glawgow Coma Scale not only provides a grading of coma by numerical scale but allows serial comparisons to be made for prognostic information particularly in coma due to trauma and poisoning (Box 12.2). This scale should be applied in each and every patient under observation and should be charted out from time to time by nursing or medical staff. If the patient is not arousable by conversation, calling the patient's first name, a sudden loud noise, then increasingly intense stimuli are used to determine the threshold for arousal and the optimal motor response of each side of the body. Tickling the nostrils with a cotton wisp is a modest stimulus to arousal—all but deeply stuporous or comatose patients will move the head away and rouse to some degree and may use the hand to remove the offending stimulus. Responses to noxious stimuli (squeezing the Achilles' tendon, sternal pressures, supraorbital pressure with thumb) should be appraised critically.

The fundamentals of neurological examination are:

☞ Assess the level of consciousness according to Glasgow Coma Scale (Box 12.2).
- It gives prognostic information in a comatosed patient, Serial observatinos are to be made.

☞ Look for the signs of head injury, e.g.
Local bruising
Penetrating wounds and fracture
Bleeding from nose, ear or other sites

Box 12.2 Glasgow Coma Scale

Scale	Score
Eye opening (E)	
• Spontaneous	4
• To loud voice	3
• To pain	2
• None	1
Best motor response (M)	
• Obeys	5
• Localises	4
• Abnormal flexion	3
• Extensor response	2
• None	1
Verbal response (V)	
• Oriented	5
• Confused, disoriented	4
• Inappropriate words	3
• Incomprehensible sounds	2
• None	1
Coma score (E + M + V)	
• Minimum	3
• Maximum	15

Note: Patients with head trauma scoring 3 or 4 have an 85% chance of death or vegetative state; while scores above 11 indicate only 5–10% chance of death or vegetative state and 85% chance of moderate disability or good recovery. Intermediate scores have intermediate prognosis.

- Scalp oedema and haematoma (local swelling) can easily be palpated while *"battle sign"* (bleeding/bruising of skin behind pinna) "suggest basal skull fracture. Similarly bleeding from the ear is a sign of trauma and fracture.

- Purpura and neck stiffness indicate meningococcal septicaemia and meningitis.

Abnormal Posturing

☞ *See the limbs for posture, tone and movement. The patient's posture should be observed first without intervention.*

- **Decorticate rigidity or posturing** describes stereotyped arm and leg movements either occurring spontaneously or induced by sensory stimulation. It is characterised by flexion of elbows and wrists and arms supination against the rigid body; suggests bilateral cerebral damage above the midbrain (i.e. internal capsule/cerebral hemisphere).
- **Decerebrate rigidity** (Fig. 12.5) **or posturing** describes extension and adduction of elbows and wrists with pronation; suggests corticospinal damage in the midbrain or caudal to diencephalon. It occurs due to hemispheric mass compressing the midbrain or posterior fossa/cereberal lesion, or hypoxic or hepatic/toxic encephalopathy.
- *Arms extension with flaccid legs or leg flexion* have been associated with low pontine lesions.
- *Total flaccidity* of all the four limbs and hypotonia indicate the involvement of pontomedullary junction.

- *Multifocal myoclonus* is almost always an indication of a metabolic disorder (e.g. uraemia, anoxic encephalopathy, drug intoxication).
- *Bilateral asterixis (flapping tremors)* is a certain sign of metabolic encephalopathy, respiratory failure (Fig. 12.4) or drug intoxication.
- *Rigidity and opisthotonous* position indicates either strychnine poisoning or tetanus (Fig. 12.6).

Note: Acute lesions of any type frequently cause limb extension regardless of location, and almost all extensor posturing become flexion as the time passes, so posturing alone cannot be utilised to pinpoint the anatomical site of the lesion.

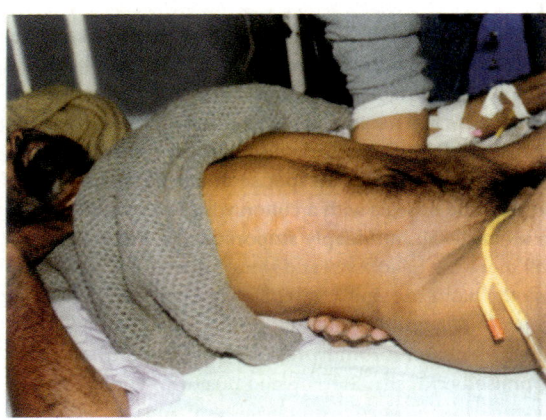

Fig. 12.6: Unconscious patient presenting with abdominal rigidity, trismus and provoked muscle spasms. He appears to be a case of tetanus. The arching of the back is demonstrated by putting the hand behind the back.

Neck Rigidity

☞ *Elicit neck stiffness by gently flexing the neck.*

- Neck stiffness is protective mechanism, indicates meningeal irritation either due to blood in CSF or infection. It may disappear in deep coma.

Causes of coma with neck rigidity

- Subarachnoid haemorrhage
- Meningitis, e.g. bacterial (Fig. 12.7), viral, fungal, etc.
- Encephalitis
- Intracranial bleed
- Posterior cranial fossa lesion (e.g. tumour, haemorrhage)
- Cerebral malaria

Pupillary Size and Reaction

☞ *Examine the size, equality and inequality of pupils and their reaction to light*

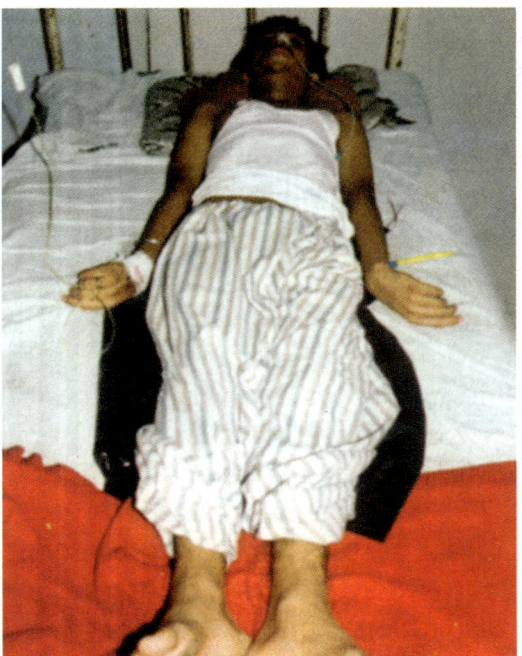

Fig. 12.5: Decerebrate rigidity in a patient with coma due to encephalitis.

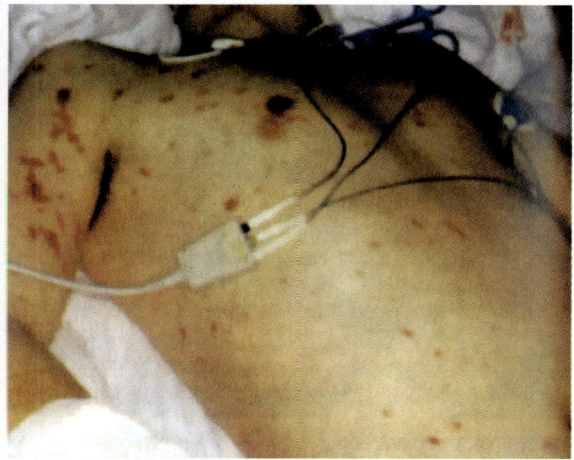

Fig. 12.7: Meningococcal meningitis. The patient had meningococcal rash over the trunk and extremities with neck rigidity.

- It provide valuable information regarding the site of lesion in an unconscious patient (Fig. 12.8).

1. The small pupils (1 to 2.5 mm) that react to light indicate metabolic encephalopathy or bilateral cortical lesions (hydrocephalus or thalamic haemorrhage).

   With early midbrain lesion, the pupils become mid-dilated and non-reactive to light. As the damage to the midbrain increases, the pupils become dilated and fixed. The ciliospinal reflex is also lost at this stage. The use of mydriatic eye drops by a previous examiner, self-administration by a patient or direct ocular trauma may cause misleading pupillary enlargement.

2. Very small pinpoint (<1 mm) pupils with reaction to light characterize narcotic or barbiturate poisoning. In bilateral pontine lesions (haemorrhage) pupils are small pinpoint but unreactive to light (Fig. 12.8A). The response to naloxone and the presence of reflex eye movements distinguishes the two.

3. Unilateral 3rd nerve palsy (Fig. 12.8B) causes unilateral pupillary enlargement (<6 mm) which could be due to ipsilateral lesion (mass lesion of midbrain) or due to contralateral compression of 3rd nerve in midbrain against the opposite tentorial margin (*contrecoup effect*).

4. Unilateral small pupil of a Horner's syndrome (Fig. 12.8C) is detected by failure of the pupil to enlarge in the dark, is seen in cerebral haemorrhage that affects the thalamus (sympathetic system).

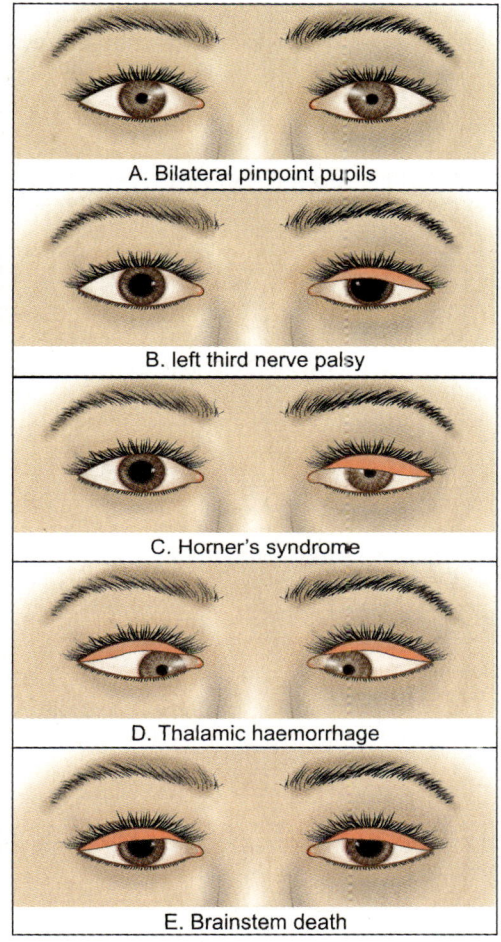

Figs 12.8A to E: Various pupillary abnormalities.
A. Bilateral pinpoint pupils occur in opiate and hypnotic poisoning, pontine haemorrhage and brain stem lesions.
B. Left third nerve palsy (ptosis, mydriasis, absent light reflex) occurs in midbrain lesion cavernous sinus thrombosis.
C. Left side Horner's syndrome (ptosis, meiosis, anhidrosis, enophthalmos, loss of ciliospinal reflex) occurs due to cervical or brain stem sympathetic involvement.
D. Thalamic haemorrhage produces deviation of eyes towards the nose and pupils are small, later become large and unreactive.
E. Brain death with fixed, dilated, unreactive pupils with eyes closure.

Ocular Fundus Examination

☞ *Examine the fundus by ophthalmoscope*

The fundoscopic examination can detect subarachnoid haemorrhage (subhyaloid haemorrhages), hypertensive encephalopathy (exudates, haemorrhage, vessel crossing changes, papilloedema) and increased intracranial pressure (papilloedema) as a cause of unconsciousness.

Eye Movements

☞ Examine them as these are cornerstones of physical diagnosis in coma because they allow a large portion of the brain stem to be analysed (Fig. 12.9).

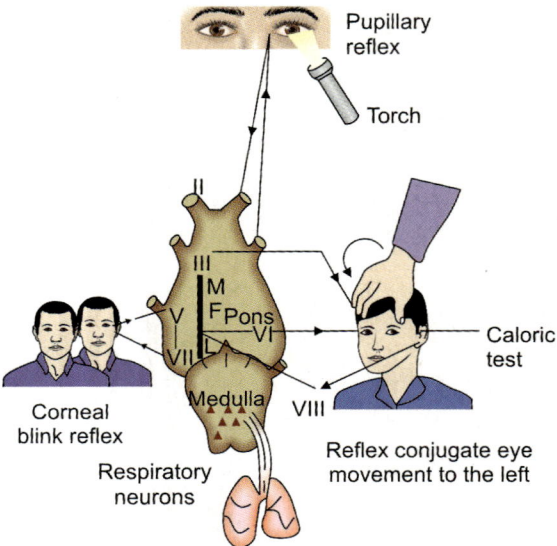

Fig. 12.9: Brain stem reflexes in coma examination (read the text).

- The eyes are first observed by elevating the lids and noting the resting position and spontaneous movements of the globes.
- Horizontal divergence of the eyes at rest is normally observed in coma.
- An adducted eye at rest indicates lateral rectus palsy due to 6th nerve in the pons; and when bilateral, it is often a sign of raised intracranial tension (*false localising sign*).
- An abducted eye with pupillary dilatation indicates 3rd nerve palsy in the midbrain.
- Skew deviation, i.e. vertical separation of the eyes (ocular axes), sometimes with elevation of one eye and depression of the other results from pontine or cerebellar lesions.
- Spontaneous ocular movements may be observed in structural lesions in the posterior fossa.
- Conjugate horizontal ocular deviation at rest indicates damage to the pons on the side of paralysis of gaze or frontal lobe lesion on the opposite side (Fig. 12.10).

Brain stem Reflexes

☞ *Oculocephalic reflex (doll's eye movements)*

The oculocephalic reflexes depend on the integrity of the ocular motor nuclei and their interconnecting tracts that extend from the midbrain to the pons and medulla. Rotate the patient's head from side to side and observe the movments of the eyes. In coma with intact brain stem, there is conjugate movements of the eyes in a direction opposite to the head movement. This is normal phenomenon. Failure of movements to one side not the other indicates unilateral gaze palsy due to brain stem lesion; while bilateral brain stem lesion leads to loss of eyes movements in any direction.

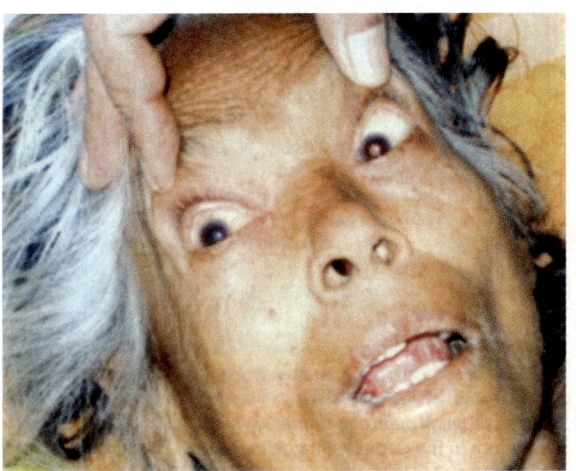

Fig. 12.10: Spontaneous conjugate horizontal ocular deviation in an unconscious patient at rest indicates either pontine or frontal lobe lesion (read the text).

- On vertical or horizontal rotation of the head, the conjugate deviation of the eyes (evoked doll's eye movements) to the opposite side, signifies the intact brain stem and implies that the coma originates from damage to cerebral hemisphere. The opposite—absence of doll's eye movements signifies damage within the brain stem but can be produced infrequently by profound overdoses of certain drugs.
- Spontaneous conjugate horizontal deviation in a comatosed patient indicates pontine damage on the same side or frontal lobe damage on opposite side.

Warning: Oculocephalic reflex test must not be attempted if there is a little doubt about trauma to the cervical spine.

☞ *Observe for spontaneous or induced nystagmus.*

Oculovestibular reflex (caloric test): It tests the integrity of pathway from labyrinth in the ear to the midbrain via medial longitudinal fasciculus (Fig. 12.9) which connects the 6th and 8th cranial nerves to contralateral 3rd nerve. This test is useful when doll's eye movements cannot be elicited for example deep coma.

The test is performed by irrigating the external auditory canal with cold water in order to produce convection currents in the labyrinth. After a brief period, there is deviation of both eyes to the irrigated side and nystagmus occurs to the opposite side. *Nystagmus* is the response to be seen in this test, therefore, medical students can remember the acronym (COWS—cold water opposite, warm water same) which will remind them the direction of nystagmus to cold and warm water. The absence of nystagmus despite conjugate deviation of the eyes indicate hemispherical lesions.

- In conscious patient, there is nystagmus with slow phase towards irrigated ear (brain stem) and fast phase in opposite direction.
- In comatosed patient with intact brain stem there is tonic conjugate movements of the eyes towards the stimulated side.
- The loss of conjugate deviation indicates brain stem damage.

☞ *Test the corneal reflex (blink reflex)*

Corneal blink reflex (corneal reflex) tests the integrity of pontine pathways between 5th and 7th cranial nerves which form the afferent and efferent pathway of this reflex respectively. The loss of corneal reflex indicate brain stem damage. CNS depressants diminish or eliminate the corneal responses.

Other Abnormal Ocular Movements

☞ *Look for other abnormal ocular movements, i.e. bobbing, dipping, oscillations, abnormal deviation, etc.*

- **Ocular bobbing** describes a brisk downward and slow upwards movements of the eyes, indicates cerebellar tumour or haemorrhage.
- **Ocular dipping** describes a slower downward and faster upward movements of the eyes, denotes anoxic damage to the cerebral cortex.
- **Rapid ocular oscillations** may occur especially after poisoning with tricyclic antidepressants.
- **Rapid conjugate lateral movements** should suggest focal motor seizure originating in contralateral frontal lobe.

- In thalamic infarct, the **eyes are pushed downwards and medially** as if patient is looking at his/her own nose (Fig. 12.8D)
- **Oculogyric crisis** (tonic deviation of eyeballs upwards or to one side for minutes to hours) is seen in encephalitis lethargica or Japanese B. encephalitis (it is a rare phenomenon now (Fig. 12.11).

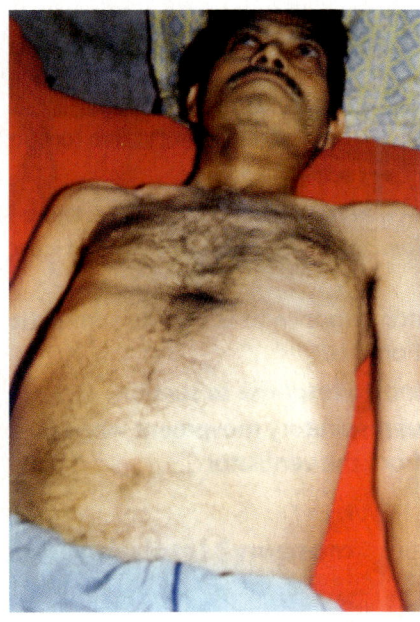

Fig. 12.11: Oculogyric crisis. Note the tonic deviation of eyeballs upwards, occurs intermittently in a patient with encephalitis (idiopathic encephalitis) is rarely seen now-a-days

Motor Responses

☞ *Elicit tone, posture and tendon jerks on both sides to detect unilateral or bilateral paralysis.*

Presence of focal signs or unilateral paralysis indicates focal structural damage to the brain (hemiplegia); while bilateral absence indicate metabolic or drug—induced coma (non neurologic coma).

The **causes** of non-neurological coma are:
1. Hyper or hypoglycaemic coma.
2. Metabolic coma, i.e. renal failure, hepatic failure, respiratory failure.
3. Endocrinal causes, e.g. myxoedema coma, pituitary apoplexy.
4. Electrolyte disturbance
5. Physical coma, i.e. heat stroke, heat exhaustion, hypothermia
6. Drugs (CNS depressants) and poisons.

- The only evidence of paralysis may be abnormal flaccidity on the affected side. In case of hemiplegia in unconscious patient, the paralysed limb falls suddenly with a thud when both upper limbs are raised and then released suddenly.
- Facial asymmetry indicates 7th nerve palsy.
- Alteration of deep tendon jerks and plantar extensor response on the paralysed side indicate contralateral corticospinal involvement; but in deep coma, plantar reflexes lose their significance because they may become extensor on both the sides.
- Presence of primitive reflexes suggest encephaltic/encephalopathic lesion of brain

OTHER SYSTEMS EXAMINATION

- **Cardiovascular system (CVS) examination** for cardiomegaly, murmurs and carotid artery bruit.
- **Respiratory system examination,** e.g. crackles/rales or abnormal breath sounds for any underlying respiratory disorder.
- **Abdominal examination** for any mass, signs of hepatic or renal insufficiency, ascites, rigidity, etc.

BRAIN DEATH TESTING

The widespread utility of mechanical ventilation has improved survival of patients with severe brain damage. The clinical diagnosis of brain death is now an inevitable aspect of practice in intensive care units on patients receiving ventilatory support.

Prior to testing for brain death, it is necessary to confirm that the cause of the irreversible brain damage has been established (e.g. intracranial bleed, encephalitis) and reversible causes (hypothermia, drug intoxication and metabolic defects) have been excluded. The diagnosis of brain death depends on fulfilling a set of preconditions, all of which must be present, and then apply a series of clinical tests (Table 12.3). The brain death tests should be performed by two experienced physicians either together or separately. The tests are then repeated after an interval of 6–24 hrs before labelling *"brain death"*.

BRIEF SYNOPSIS OF DIFFERENT COMAS

METABOLIC VERSUS NEUROLOCIAL COMA
(Table 12.4)

HEPATIC COMA

It may be *acute* (occuring with 8 weeks of hepatic illness) or *chronic* (disease with 6 month duration).

TABLE 12.3: Diagnosis of Brain Death and its Testing

I. Preconditions for brain death

1. Deeply comatosed patient
2. Exclusion of reversible causes of coma;-
   - There must be no suspicion that coma is due to depressant drugs, e.g. narcotics, hypnotics, tranquillisers.
   - No evidence of hypothermia (rectal temp. >35°C)
   - No profound abnormality of electrolytes and acid-base disturbance
   - No metabolic or endocrinal cause of coma
3. Establish the cause for severe irreversible brain damage. There should be no doubt that patient is suffering from irreversible brain damage (intracranial haemmorhage, encephalitis and others causes)

II. Brain death tests (all brain stem reflexes are absent)

- The pupils are fixed, dilated, and unreactive to light
- The corneal reflexes are absent
- The vestibulo-ocular reflexes are absent, i.e. there is no eye movement following an injection of 20 ml of ice-cold water into ear in turn.
- There is no motor response to adequate stimulation within cranial nerve distribution
- No gag reflex and no response to suction
- No spontaneous respiratory movement when the patient is disconnected from the ventilator

Causes

Acute hepatic coma	Chronic hepatic encephalopathy
1. Acute viral hepatitis of all types (except hepatitis A), drugs and poisons	1. Chronic hepatitis B, C and non A–non B
2. Pregnancy with hepatitis	2. Alcoholic cirrhosis Postnecrotic/post-hepatitic/cryptogenic cirrhosis and Biliary cirrhosis, Cardiac cirhosis
3. Autoimmune hepatitis	3. Wilson's disease, Budd-Chiari syndrome
4. Wilson's disease, Budd-Chiari syndrome	4. Drug and toxin induced
5. Reye's syndrome in children	5. Hemochromatosis
6. Shock, hyperthermia or hypothermia	6. Veno occlusive disease
	7. Nonalcoholic fatty liver disease

Symptoms and Signs

1. **Cerebral features**; i.e. poor alertness, disturbed concentration, behavioural changes, drowsiness, confusion, disorientation, disturbed sleep pattern, slurred speech, constructional apraxia convulsions and coma.
2. **Jaundice** (moderate to severe)
3. **Fetor hepaticus** (an ammonical breath odour).
4. **Flapping tremors**
5. **Liver dullness:** The liver span is reduced in acute coma.
6. **Bleeding diathesis** (purpura, ecchymosis, GI bleed)
7. **Signs of portal hypertension** (ascites, oedema, splenomegaly) are present in chronic hepatic encephalopathy not in acute coma.
8. **Neurological manifestations.** There may be cerebral oedema but neurological signs can occur in chronic hepatic encephalopathy.
9. **Hepatorenal syndrome** is rare occurs in chronic hepatic encephalopathy but not in acute coma.

Diagnosis: Diagnosis is suggested by jaundice and other clinical features, confirmed by LFT, ultrasound, serum ammonia levels and abnormal EEG.

Differential Diagnosis

All the conditions causing metabolic coma come into its differential diagnosis (read metabolic coma Table 12.4).

DIABETIC KETOACIDOSIS (DKA) OR DIABETIC COMA

It develops in type 1 diabetic patients under following situations:

I. Undetected or undiagnosed type 1 diabetes.
II. Patients of type 1 diabetes on treatment with insulin may miss the dose or develop it under stress or following an infection or some other precipitating factor.

Clinical Features (Table 12.5)

- History of polyuria, polydipsia and polyphagia. There is history of weight loss
- Unconscous or semiconscious patient.
- Frequent vomiting with abdominal pain.
- Signs of dehydration, air hunger, Kussmaul breathing and hypotension are characteristics signs.
- There may be fever and leucocytosis.
- Tendon jerks are diminished and plantars are normal.

TABLE 12.4: Clinical Features of Two Important Comas

Feature	Neurological coma	Metabolic coma
1. State of consciousness	Coma usually with agitation	Silent coma (no agitation or resistance)
2. History of trauma	May be present. There may be signs of injury, e.g. bruising, bleeding	No history or evidence of trauma
3. Focal neurological deficit/neck stiffness	Present	Absent
4. Brain stem reflexes	Doll's head ocular movements are lost on one side or both sides	Doll's head eye movements are preserved usually except in deep metabolic coma. They are always preserved in drug-induced coma
5. Physical signs	Neck stiffness, plegia/paresis of limb(s), seizures, abnormal posture and reflexes, and signs of raised intracranial pressure (headache vomiting, papilloedema) indicate neurological disorders as the cause	Hyperpyrexia, abnormal smell, air hunger flapping tremors indicate metabolic disorder as the cause
6. Breathing	Deep, sturtorous	Slow and shallow
7. Pupils	Unequal pupils or unilateral pupillary involvement indicates neurological disorder	Bilateral small pupils occur in drug induced (opiate, barbiturates and other drugs) coma
8. Ocular fundi	Abnormal	Normal
9. Common cause	Meningitis, encephalitis, subarachnoid or intracerebral haemorrhage, status epilepticus, brain tumour and infarction	Hypo- or hyperglycaemia, uraemia, liver cell failure, hypothermia, heat stroke or heat exhaustion respiratory failure, drug overdosage, endocrinal and electrolyte imbalance

- Acetone smell.
- Thin lean built, emaciated.

Diagnosis is suspected in young patient of type I diabetes on insulin who has either omitted insulin or took too little insulin following infection or stress. Confirmation is done by high blood glucose level and ketonemia.

Differential Diagnosis

It has to be differentiated with other coma in diabetes, i.e. hyperosmolar nonkenotic diabetic coma (Table 12.5).

HYPEROSMOLAR NONKETOTIC DIABETIC COMA (TABLE 12.5)

This is common in type 2 diabetes patients. It is precipitated by some factor, e.g. procedures, drugs, infection. The clinical hallmark of the syndrome is *hyperglycaemia, hyperosmolality* and *dehydration* without ketoacidosis (no ketone or minimal ketone).

TABLE 12.5: Differentiating Features of Two Types of Coma in Diabetes

	Hyperosmolar nonketotic coma	*Diabetic ketotic coma*
Body constitution	Obese	Thin, lean
Occurrence presentations	Type 2 diabetes present with complications	Type 1 diabetes polyuria, polydipsia and polyphasia
Precipitating factors	Procedure, drugs, documented infection, etc.	Too much food with no or a little insulin or infection
Serum Na⁺	135–155 mEq/L	150 mEq
Blood glucose	Usually >600 mg%	Usually <600 mg%
Osmolarity	Usually <340 mosm/kg	>340 mOsm/kg
Ketosis	Absent or minimal	Present
Insulin	Small dose required (insulin independent)	Large dose required (insulin dependent)
Fluids	Half normal saline (0.45% NaCl)	Normal saline
Mortality	Higher	High

Diagnosis. It is suspected in every patient of coma with type 2 diabetes. Diagnosis is confirmed by very high level of blood glucose (>600 mg%) high osmolarity (>340 mOsm/kg and high sodium (>150 mEq).

RESPIRATORY FAILURE

Failure of the respiratory system to maintain normal partial pressure of O_2 and CO_2 in the blood is called *respiratory failure*. For all practical purposes, PaO_2 less than 60 mmHg or $PaCO_2$ more than 50 mmHg indicates respiratory failure. It may be *acute* (acute alteration in blood gases) or *chronic* (slow alteration of blood gases).

Causes (Table 12.6)

TABLE 12.6: Causes of Respiratory Failure

Acute respiratory failure	*Chronic respiratory failure*
1. Acute asthma	1. An inhaled foreign body
2. Interstitial lung disease or fibrosis	2. Status asthmaticus
3. Pulmonary embolism	3. COPD and its acute exacerbation
4. Pulmonary oedema (acute LHF)	4. Multiple ribs fracture
5. Adult respiratory distress syndrome (ARDS)	5. CNS depressants, poisoning
6. Pneumothorax	6. Idiopathic hypoventilation syndrome
7. Pneumonia, infections	7. Pickwickian syndrome
8. Environmental pollutants	
9. Sedatives or narcotics	
10. Retention of sputum	

Symptoms

The clinical symptoms irrespective of its type incltude cough, sputum, haemoptysis dyspnoea, hypercapnoea, disturbed consciousness (Fig. 12.4).

Physical Signs

- Increased respiratory rate, cyanosis, disturbed consciousness
- Flapping tremors (CO_2-induced narcosis)
- Crackles and rales on both sides of the chest
- Physical signs of basic respiratory disease

Diagnosis is suspected on clinical findings and confirmed by blood gas analysis.

HYPOGLYCAEMIA

It is defined as 'fall in blood glucose concentration below lower limit of normal. Severe hypoglycaemia refers to fall in blood glucose concentration below 40 mg% (2.2 mmol/L), may lead to coma. Spontaneous hypoglycaemia is classified traditionally into: (i) *Postprandial or reactive* which occurs only in response to meals and (ii) *fasting* which occurs after few hours of fasting. Fasting hypoglycaemia usually occurs in the presence of disease, while postprandial hypoglycaemia occurs in the absence of a recognisable disease. Hypoglycaemia in diabetes may be *episodic* or *continuous* for some period. Hypoglycaemia in diabetes is mostly induced by treatment either by insulin or by oral hypoglycaemics.

Causes

I. **Postprancial hypoglycaemia**
   - Alimentary (dumping syndrome following gastric surgery)
   - Insulin or OHA induced
   - Galactossaemia
   - Hereditary fructose intolerance

II. **Fasting hypoglycaemia**
   - Common cause is insulinoma or insulin like growth factor produced by non-pancreatic tumour or administration of large dose of insulin or OHA.

Precipitating Factors

- Other drugs, e.g. pentamidine, quinine, salicylates.
- Hypopituitarism, Addison's disease, hypoglucagonemia
- Liver diseases, e.g. hepatitis and cirrhosis
- Pancreatitis
- Renal failure
- Congenital enzymatic deficiency, e.g. glucose-6-phosphatase
- Miscellaneous, e.g. malnutrition, pregnancy

Clinical Features

The symptoms and signs are:

CVS	: Palpitation, tachycardia, anxiety, cardiac arrhythmias.
CNS	: Tremors, confusion, headache, tiredness, difficulty in concentration, incoordination, slurred speech, drowsiness, convulsions, coma.
GI tract	: Nausea, vomiting
Skin	: Sweating, hypothermia

Diagnosis is confirmed by *Whipple triad*, i.e.
1. Symptoms and signs of hypoglycaemia.
2. Low blood sugar usually less than 40 mg/dl
3. Reversal of symptoms and signs with administration of IV glucose.

Differential Diagnosis

The hypoglycaemic coma is to be differentiated from hyperglycaemic coma (Table 10.7).

POISONING INDUCED COMA

Any substance which produces adverse reactions/effects in a living organism is called **poison**. Acute poisoning is the most common cause of non-traumatic coma in young persons (<35 years of age). Hospital-based data suggests that about 10% of all coma admissions are due to poisoning.

Poisoning may be *suicidal* (self, intentional) or *accidental* and *homocidal*.

Although accurate history is an important clinical weapon for diagnosis, but at times, is difficult to obtain from patients who are confused or obtuneded and information obtained from the relatives and friends may not be dependable.

TABLE 12.7: Comparison of Clinical Features of Hypoglycaemic and Diabetic Coma

	Hypoglycaemic coma	*Diabetic coma*
History	Regular dose of insulin and no food	Too little or no insulin with food
Precipitating factor	Severe unaccustomed exercise	Untreated/hidden infection
Symptoms	No vomit/occasional vomit	Frequent vomiting with abdominal pain
Physical signs	• Skin and tongue moist	• They are dry due to dehydration
	• Pulse is bounding	• Weak/feeble pulse
	• Normal breathing	• Rapid shallow breathing (Kussmaul)
	• No air hunger	• Air hunger present
	• No abnormal smell of breath	• Smell of acetone
	• Tendon reflexes brisk	• Diminished
	• Plantars are extensor	• Plantars are normal (flexor)
Urine	No glucose/ketone	Glucose and ketone bodies are present
Blood	Low blood glucose	High blood glucose
	Bicarbonate level and pH normal	Low bicarbonate and pH

Poisoning is likely to be missed if it is not suspected. The suspicious circumstances include:
1. Unexplained coma in a previously healthy person.
2. A history of underlying psychiatric illness such as depression.
3. Financial loss, marital dispute, personal rivalary/Jealousy
4. Coma following ingestion of food, drink or medication. The onset of illness in industrial workers or occupational workers may indicate chemical poisoning.
5. Patients falling ill immediately after landing from a foreign country or after arrest for criminal activity should be suspected of having illicit drug concealed in body cavity or the GI tract.

Clinical Features

Before proceeding for detailed examination, ensure A, B, C of cardiopulmonary resuscitation. Proceed to examine the patient as follows:
1. *Level of consciousness by Glasgow Coma Scale.*
2. *Look for respiratory effort, cyanosis, presence or absence of cough and gap reflex.*

- Respiratory rate is decreased in OP and benzodiazepine poisoning while it is increased in salicylate poisoning. Acidotic breathing occurs in methanol, ethanol, ethylene glycol
- Cyanosis occurs due to poisoning by CNS depressants and methaemoglobinemia and salicylates poisoning

3. *Record pulse and BP*
   - Heart rate is slow in poisoning by OP compound and opiates, antidepressants, increased in halogenated hydrocarbons, tricyclic antidepressants.

- Hypertension occurs in poisoning due to cocaine, amphetamines, MAO inhibitors.
- Hypotension occurs due to poisoning by antidepressants, cyanide, arsenic, CO and aluminum phosphide.

4. *Note the size of pupil and reaction.*
   - Pupils are constricted in poisoning by OP compounds, opiates, carbamates, barbiturates and phenothiazines.
   - Pupils are dilated due to poisoning by atropine, LSD, nicotine, amphetamines and tricyclic antidepressants.
5. *Look for needle marks/pricks for opiate poisoning*

6. *Measure the temperature* (low reading rectal thermometer)

- Body temperature may be high in atropine and anticholinergic poisoning, ectasy and cocaine intoxication. Temperature is low in CNS depressants poisoning.

7. *Look at the all orific for drug packets (cocaine)*
8. *Look for the odour of the breath, vomitus, colour of the nails and urine*

- Alcoholic smell (ethyl alcohol), pungent smell (aluminium phosphide poisoning).
- Colour of nails for cyanosis in CNS depresents poisoning

The nature of poisoning will be revealed after investigations and toxological screening.

HEAT STROKE (HYPERTHERMIA)

Definition: It is defied as hyperpyrexia due to complete breakdown of thermoregulatory mechanism with failure of sweating. It occurs when the core or rectal temperature rises to or above 41°C. Above 42°C, hypothalamic control of temperature is lost.

Precipitating factors. They are:
1. **Environmental,** e.g. high temperature, high humidity ($\geq 75°C$) and lack of wind
2. **Endogenous,** e.g. deficient perspiration, obesity, alcoholism and debility.
3. **Exogenous,** e.g. improper clothing, dehydration, heavy exercise, febrile illness and drugs e.g. anticholinergics and phenothiazines.

Clinical Features (read Table 12.8)

Diagnosis is confirmed by clinical features and high temperature.

HEAT EXHAUSTION

Definition: It is exhaustion of the body due to hyperthermia. It occurs in acclimatised persons following heavy or vigorous exercise. It occurs in troops landed in hot climates. It is the result of either water depletion or both salt and water depletion resulting in sweating and dehydration.

Clinical Features

Both heat stroke and heat exhaustion are hyperpyrexia induced disorders with clinical features discribed in Table 12.8.

Diagnosis: It is suspected on clinical grounds and presence of high temperature. *Presence of sweating differentiates it from heat stroke.*

TABLE 12.8: Clinical Symptoms and Signs of Heat Stroke and Heat Exhaustion

Heat Stroke	Heat Exhaustion
• Onset acute or insidious	• Onset acute or insidious
• Nausea, vomiting, dizziness, vertigo and thirst	• Increasing thirst, giddiness, fatigue, muscle weakness and syncope
• Sweating present	• Sweating absent
• Sensorium impaired, seizures, drowsiness and coma supervene	• Mental confusion, judgement impaired
• Signs of dehydration present without sweating	• Signs of dehydration with sweating skin
• Skin is dry and flushed	• Skin is wet
• Tempetature is >41°C	• Temperature is usually < 41°C
• Cyanosis, jaundice and petechiae are marked features	• Neurological signs, e.g. paraesthesias, movement incordination, cerebellar signs and hallucinations are marked features
• **Person is hot and dry**	• **Person is hot and wet**

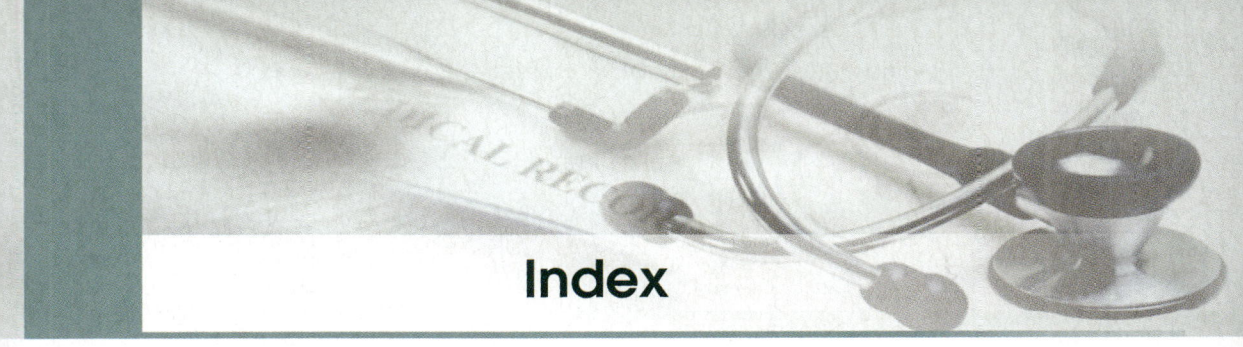

Index

A chronic recurrent or episodic headache 154
A Kayser-Fleischer ring 8
A lithotripsy scar 136
Abdominal
  breathing 42
  distension/swelling 264
  girth measurement 288
  reflexes 219
  wall oedema (parietal oedema) 26
Abdominojugular reflux test/manoeuvre 83
Abnormal
  colouration of nails 419
  deposits on the retina 167
  gaits 226
  posturing 434
  redness 411
  respiratory patterns 41
  skin colouration 408
Abnormalities of
  chest 41
  lips 9
  penis 139
  sensations 242
Abscess 313
Acanthosis nigricans 351, 352, 413
Accessory (XI) nerves 199
Accommodation reaction 164
Acne vulgaris 414, 423
Acrocephaly 5
Acrocyanosis 24, 121
Acromegaly 363
Acute:
  abdomen 304
  arterial ischaemia 115
  diarrhoea 263
  erosive 299
  lymphadenitis 339
  nephritic syndrome 147
  renal failure 146
  rheumatic activity 111
  severe asthma 62
  severe dyspnoea 62
Addison's disease 364
Adiadochokinesis 223
Adrenal tumours 356

Adson's test 118
Adult polycystic kidney disease 148
Adventitious/added sounds 54, 95
Aegophony 54
Aerophagia (air swallowing) 259
Agranulocytosis 324
Air conduction 195
Akinetic mutism 427
Albinism 412
Allen's test 117
Allodynia 236
Alopecia areata 424
Alport syndrome 129
Amaurosis 179
Amaurosis fugax 120
Amenorrhoea 348
Anaemia 79, 321
Anaesthesia 236
Anal reflex 221
Analgesia 236
Angioedema 418
Anhidrosis 370
Ankle and the foot joints 399
Ankle
  clonus 218
  jerk 217
  oedema 25
Anorexia nervosa 260
Anosmia 176
Anus 293
Anus, rectum and prostate 292
Aortic and other pulsations 286
Apex beat 89, 90
Aphthous ulceration 10, 272
Aplastic anaemia 343
Apneustic breathing 432
Appearance 1
Appetite 259
Arachnodactyly 21, 22
Areas of auscultation 94
Areflexia 218
Arterial
  bruit 97, 101, 291
  pulse 83
Arteritis 115
Arthralgia 111
Artrial fibrillation 359
Ascites 290, 307
Assessment of a patient with coma 428
Astasia-abasia 227

Asteriaxis 290
Asymptomatic
  bacteriuria 148
  urinary abnormalities 148
Ataxia 196, 248
Athetosis 230
Atopic dermatitis/eczema 426
Atrial fibrillation 85
Attrition of
  teeth 11
  teeth and recession of gums 11
Audible ejection clicks 95
Audiometry 195
Auditory acquity 195
Autoantibodies 405
Autonomic nervous system (ANS) 243

Babinski's response 220
Back of abdomen 292
Balanoposthitis 149
Barium meal study 301
Barrel-shaped chest 42
Basal
  cell carcinoma 413
  ganglia (extrapyramidal lesion) 246
Biceps (C5–C6) 215
Bicipital tendon 382
Bilateral XII nerve palsy 202
Bilirubin 308
Bitot's spots 7
Bitten nails 420
Bleeding 327
  gums 332
  per rectum/hematochezia 261
Blood
  disorders 337
  loss 321
  pressure (BP) 87
BMI 3, 78
Bone
  conduction 195
  pain 372
Bouchard's nodes 379
Boutonnière deformity 382
Bovine cough with hoarseness 32
Bowing of legs 137, 381
Bowstring sign 388

445

Brachycephaly 5
Bradycardia 430
Brain death testing 438
Brain stem
　　evoked potentials 195
　　reflexes 436
Breast
　　cysts 319
　　diseases 319
　　lump 313
Breath sounds 52
Brief synopsis of different
　　comas 438
Broca's area 173
Bronchial
　　asthma 62
　　breath sound 53
Bronchiectasis 59
Bronchogenic carcinoma 65
Bronchophony 54
Bronchopleural fistula 68
Brudzinski's sign 234
Bruisability 365
Bruising 328
Buerger's disease 120
Bulbar palsy 202
Bulbocavernous reflex 221
Bulimia nervosa 260
Bursa 372

Café au lait spots 413
Calculating ability 172
Caloric test 198
Candidiasis 407
Capillary pulsations 85
Caput medusae 275
Carbuncles 420
Carcinoma of
　　breast 319
　　tongue 13
Cardiac dyspnoea 61
Cardiovascular system 71
Carotid pulsations 81, 83
Carpal tunnel syndrome 243
Cataract (lens opacity) 8
Catatonia 428
Cauda equina syndrome 403
Causes 248
Causes of
　　abdomen pain 258
　　anaemia 321
　　coma 428
　　trigeminal nerve palsy 190
Cavernous
　　haemangioma 418
　　sinus thrombosis 186
Central
　　chest discomfort/heavi-ness 35
　　cyanosis 78
　　or retrosternal chest pain 35
　　vein occlusion 169
Cerebellar 225

Cerebral
　　haemorrhage 251
　　thrombosis 251
Cerebrovascular accidents 251
Cervical spine 384
Chancre 140
Chancroid 139, 140
Cheiroarthropathy 351
Chest
　　examination 41
　　expansion 45
　　pain (cardiac) 71
　　pain (pleuritic) 35, 66
Chickenpox 415
Chilblain 24
Chloasma 413
Cholelithiasis 282
Chorea 228
　　gravidarum 229
Chronic
　　arterial disease 115
　　cholecystitis 282
　　diarrhoea 263
　　leg ulceration 125
　　lymphocytic leukaemia
　　　(CLL) 340
　　myeloid leukaemia (CML) 341
　　obstructive pulmonary
　　　disease (COPD) 63
　　pernio syndrome 121
　　renal failure 147
　　tophaceous gout 402
Chvostek's sign 354
Cirrhosis of liver　a 290
Classification 99
Cleft lip/hare lip 9
Cleft palate 14
Clonus 208, 217
Clubbing of the fingers 38
Clue to systemic disorders, their
　　analysis 409
Cochlear functions 195
Cognitive functions 170
Coin test 57
Colorectal cancer 303
Colour vision 177
Coma vigil 427
Common
　　abnormalities 285
　　skin disorders 420
　　symptoms 153
　　urinary symptoms 127
Condition of arterial wall 85
Congenital adrenal hyperplasia 365
Conjugate gaze palsy 184
Conjunctiva 7
Conjunctival haemorrhage 7
Consciousness 170, 427
Consecutive (glucomatous) 167
Constipation 263
Constructional ability 172
Co-ordination and gait 222

Cornea 7
Corneal
　　arcus 7
　　opacities 7
　　reflex (blink reflex) 437
　　reflex 189
　　ulcer 8
Cortical (postcentral gyrus) 236
Corticospinal tracts 203
Cough 31
Coughreflex 200
Courvoisier's sign 282
Crackles or rales or crepitations 56
Cranial nerves 176, 247
Craniotabes 5
Creases of the palm 322
Cremasteric reflex (Lr–L2) 220
Crigler-Najjar 308
　　syndrome 269
　　type 2 308
Crohn's disease 302
Cryptorchidism 356
Cusco's speculum used to display 146
Cushing syndrome 363
Cutaneous candidiasis 414
Cyanosis 38, 78
Cystocoele 145

D'accoucheur hand 21
D'accoucheur hand or obstetric
　　hand 355
Dacrocystitis 6
Dactylitis 22
Daivympie's sign (lid retraction) 360
Dark-coloured urine 309
Deafness 198
Decerebrate rigidity 434
Decorticate rigidity 434
Deep
　　palpation 278
　　pressure pain 241
　　vein thrombosis (DVT) 122
Defaecation 221
Deformities of fingers 22
Deformity of the chest 42
Deltoid reflex 216
Delusions 171
Dental caries 10
Dermatitis herpetiformis 409
Dermatological disorders 407
Dexamethasone suppression test 364
Diabetes
　　insipidus 348
　　mellitus 368
Diabetic
　　coma 439
　　dermopathy 351
　　foot 24, 351
　　nephropathy 370
　　neuropathy 369
　　retinopathy 169
　　stiff hands 351

Index

Diagnosis of respiratory disorders 60
Diarrhoea 262
Differential cyanosis 79
Differential diagnosis 143
    of arthritis 401
    of masses in different areas of abdomen 295
Differential signs of congenital heart diseases 112
Dilated superficial veins 275
Dinner-fork deformity 229
Diplopia 6
Discolouration of urine 270
Disorders of
    ocular movements 184
    speech 173
Displacement of apex beat 90
Disseminated intravascular coagulation (DIC) 338
Distant vision 178
Distended neck veins 38
Disuse atrophy 381
Divarication of recti 276
Does it radiate to any site/direction? 258
Dolicocephaly 5
Doll's eye movement 197, 436
Donovanosis 140
Dowager hump 385
Down syndrome 20
Dribbling of urine 130
Drop-arm sign 391
Dry skin 410
Dumb-bell shape chest 42
Dupuytren's contracture 311, 381
Dysarthria 175
Dysdiadochokinesis 223
Dyskinesia 232
Dysphagia 31
Dysphasia or aphasia 173
Dysphonia 176, 199
Dysphonia (hoarseness) 31
Dyspnoea 34
Dyspnoea, orthopnoea and paroxysmal nocturnal dyspnoea 72
Dystonia 230
Dysuria 131

Ear 8
Ecchymosis 327
Ecchymotic patches 329
Edinger-Westphal nucleus 181
Effect of respiration on JVP 82
Electronystagmography 196
Empyema thoracis 66
Encephalocoele 5
Endocrinal disorders 347
Enlarged kidney(s) 286
Enophthalmos 183
Enthesopathy 399
Epididymis 142
Epilepsies 252

Episodic weakness 160
Epistaxis 29, 327
Erythema
    marginatum 111
    nodosum 422
Erythroderma (exfoliative dermatitis) 411
Erythromelalgia 24
Examination of
    abdomen 273
    abdominal lump/mass 294
    breasts and axillae 313
    cardiovascular system 89
    female genitalia 143
    gait 226
    groin and genitalia 138
    nails 419
    respiratory system 36
    skin lesion 414
    thyroid gland 353
Excessive use of the tendon 374
Exophthalmos (proptosis) 182, 359
Expansile pulsations in epigastrium 276
Exteroceptive (superficial) sensation 239
Eye movements 436

Fabere test 404
Facial
    asymmetry 156
    dyskinesia 232
    expression 1
    nerve paralysis 192
    pain 155, 191
    puffiness 131
    weakness 194
Factors II, V, VIII, IX, X, XI, XII 344
Fasciculations and fibrillations 231
Fascinante or short shuffling gait 226
Fatigue/tiredness 267
Fatty abdomen 276
Features of two common types of joint disease 373
Femoral
    hernia 139, 292
    nerve stretch test 389
Fever or pyrexia 432
Fibroadenoma 313, 319
Field of vision 177
Fifth (trigeminal) cranial nerve 187
Finger flexion 215
Finger to finger test 223
Finger-nose test 223
Fingers
    as clue to diagnosis 21
    for deformities 21
First (ophthalmic) division 188
Fissuring 12
Fixed drug eruptions 425
Flapping (asterixis) 228
Flapping tremors 273

Flatulence 265
Flatus 264
Flexor retinaculum 393
Flip test 388, 389
Fluctuation test 143
Fluid thrill 289
Foetus 264
Foot joints 399
Forced expiratory time 58
Fourth (trochlear) nerve palsy 184
Fovea 167
Freckles 413
Frenulum linguae 15
Frenulum of tongue 13
Fundus 167
Funnel chest (Cobbler's chest, pectus excavatum) 42
Fur (coating) 12
Furunculosis 40

Gag reflex 200
Gait apraxia 227
Galactorrhoea 314, 348
Gall bladder 281
Gall bladder mass/palpable gall bladder 281
Gasserian ganglion 188
Gastritis 299
Gastro-oesophageal reflux disease 300
Gaze palsy 185
General
    observations 429
    physical examination (GPE) 429
Generalised
    distended abdomen 276
    lymphadenopathy 19
    oedema 26
    purpura 409
Genu valgus 398
Geographic tongue 12
Gibbus 385
Gigantism 363
Gilbert 308
Gilbert's syndrome 269
Gingivitis 11
Girth of abdomen 278
Glabellar tap reflexes 210
Glasgow Coma Scale 433
Global aphasia 174
Glossitis 332
Glossopharyngeal neuralgia 199
Goitre 357
Gonococcal urethritis 141
Gouty arthritis 379
Gouty tophi 379
Gower's sign 206
Gradenigo's syndrome 185
Grading of goitre 353
Grasp reflex 210
Grasping and avoiding reflexes 210
Graves' disease 354, 359, 361

Groin 292
Group of muscles 209
Guarding 279
Gum 11
Gum hypertrophy 11
Gynaecomastia 315

Haemarthrosis 328
Haematuria 129
Haemoglobinuria 270
Haemolytic anaemia 343
Haemophilia a 339
Haemostasis 327
Hair loss 420
Half and half nails 137
Halitosis 266
Hallucinations 171
Hand deformities 374
Handgrip 209
Hands 20
    for any swelling 379
Hashimoto's
    disease 358
    thyroiditis 358, 363
Head movements 5
Headache 153
Heart sounds 94
Heartburn and acid reflux 262
Heat
    exhaustion 442
    intolerance 348
    stroke 442
Heberden's nodes 379
Hematemesis 261
Hemiballismus 'ballism' 230
Hemifacial spasms 194, 233
Henoch-Schönlein purpura 405
Hepatic coma 438
Hepatobiliary systems 257
Hepatomegaly 305
Hepatosplenomegaly in
    haematology 330
Herpangina 41
Herpes
    labialis 421
    simplex 421
    zoster infection 415
Hiccup 266
Hip pain 396
Hirsutism 348, 420
History of coma 428
Hoarseness 199
Hoffmann's sign 215
Homan's sign. 123
Horner's syndrome 183
Horseshoe kidney 285
Hutchinson's teeth 11
Hydatid thrill/sign 290
Hydration, state of 4
Hyperacusis 192
Hyperaesthesia 236
Hyperalgesia 236, 240

Hyperelastic skin 411
Hyperextensibility of joints 401
Hyperkeratosis of palms 20
Hyperpathia 236
Hyperpigmentation 413
Hyper-reflexia 218
Hyper-resonance 50
Hypertension 88
Hypertensive retinopathy 169
Hyperthermia/hyperpyrexia 433
Hypertonia 207
Hypertrichosis 364
Hyperventilation 137
Hypoaesthesia 236
Hypoalgesia 240
Hypoglossal (XII) nerve 201
Hypogonadism 368
Hypogonadotrophic hypo-
    gonadism 368
Hypoparathyroidism 367
Hypothermia 433
Hypothyroidism 362
Hypotonia 207
Hysterical gait 227

Icthyosis 410
Idiopathic (Bell) palsy 192
Ileocaecal mass 298
Impetigo contagiosa 421
Impotence 348
In vitiligo 412
Inability to maintain posture 229
Incisional ventral hernia 277
Increased sweating
    (hyperhidrosis) 347
Infantalism 3
Infarction 186
Inguinal hernia 292
Inguinal lymph nodes 292
Insight 172
Inspection of thyroid 353
Intelligence 172
Intercostal recession 43
Intermittent claudication 116
Internal jugular pulsations 81
Internuclear ophthalmoplegia 185, 187
Intra-abdominal 294
Intraocular tension 431
Inversion and eversion 401
Involuntary movements 154, 227
Iris 8
Iritis 163
Iron deficiency anaemia 344
Irregularly irregular pulse 85
Ischaemic attacks 250
Ishihara's test plates 179

Jacksonian epilepsy
    (focal epilepsy) 252
Janeway lesions 113
Jaundice 7, 268, 272, 308
Jaw jerk 189, 216, 249

Joint
    crepitus 383
    of muscle 371
    pain 372
    position sense (JPS) 240
Jones diagnostic revised criteria for
    rheumatic fever 111
Judgement 172
Jugular venous pulse and pressure
    (JVP) 79

Kallmann's syndrome 411
Kaposi's sarcoma 14
Kayser-Fleischer ring 7, 8
Keratoconjunctivitis 8
Keratomalacia 8
Kernig's sign 234
Kidneys 285
Klebsiella rhinoscleromatis 40
Knee
    clonus 217
    jerk 216
    joint 397
Knee-heel test (the heel-shin test 224
Knee-heel test 224
Knocked knees 137
Knock-knees 398
Koilonychia 419
Koplik's spots 14
Kussmaul's sign 82
Kyphoscoliosis 386
Kyphosis 385

Labia majora 144
Labrinthine disease 196
Lacunar infarct (small vessel infarct)
    251
Large purpuric spots 333
Lassegue's sign 388
Lens 8
Lentigines 413
Leprosy 424
Leucocytosis 324
Leucoerythroblastic anaemia 325
Leuconychia 419
Leucopenia and neutropenia 323
Leukaemias 325
Leukaemoid reaction 324, 325
Leukoplakia of the tongue 12, 271
Levator palpebral superioris muscles
    (lps) 181
Lhermitte's sign 236
Lichen planus 13
Lid lag 360
Limb girdle myopathy 206
Linea nigra 275
Lipodystrophy or lipoatrophy 351
Lips 9
Livedo reticularis 121
Liver 280
Liver dullness 287
Lizard/reptile tongue 13

Index

Ileopsoas abscess 298
Lock jaw or trismus 232
Locked-in-state 427
Locomotor system 371
Loin pain/renal pain/ureteric pain 127
Lordosis 385
Loss of
    libido 370
    vision 169
Low back pain 403
Lower cranial nerves IX, X, XI and XII 202
Lower limb
    ischaemia 116
    joints 395
Lower motor
    neuron 194
    neuron lesion 246
Lumbar spine 385
Lump in the neck (lymphadenopathy) 31
Lung
    abscess 61
    sounds 56
Lupus
    pernio 9
    vulgaris 424
Lymph nodes 18, 19
    examination of 333
Lymphadenopathy 339
Lymphocytosis 325
Lymphoedema of the breast 314

Macrocephaly 4, 5, 16
Macroglossia 12, 350
Macrosomia 16
Macular
    degeneration 167
    region 167
    sparing 177
Malar flush 79
Maldon teeth 10
Male genitalia 139
Mammary souffle 101
Marasmus 3
Mass in epigastrium 296
Mass in or over the abdominal wall 296
Mass in the hypogastrium 298
Measles 14
Measurement of ankle/brachial pressure index (ABPI) 119
Measurement of JVP 82
Mediastinal compression/mediastinal mass/superior vena cava syndrome 69
Megaloblastic anaemia 345
Meibomian gland 6
Melanocytic naevi 413
Melasma 413
Membranous 147

Memory 172
Meningeal irritation 233
Meningococcal meningitis 435
Mental status 170
Meralgia prosthetica 243
Metallic (prosthetic) sounds 95
Method of
    auscultation 51
    examination 82
Microalbuminuria 370
Microcephaly 4
Micturition 222
Midsystolic clicks 95
Migraine 153
Milking sign (waxing and waning of the grip) 229
Minora 144
Mirizzi's syndrome 282
Mixed cyanosis 79
Moebius sign 361
Mongoloid face 16
Monoarthritis 402
Monoarticular arthritis 401
Mononeuritis 242
Mons pubis 144
Mood or emotional state 170
Morphology of skin lesions 415
Motor
    function 247
    responses 437
    system examination 203
Mouth thrush 272
Movements
    at the shoulder 391
    of ankle 400
    of the chest (expansion of the chest) 42
Mucosa 13
Murmurs 97
Murphy sign 281
Muscle
    cramp 233
    spasm 232
    strength and power 209
    weakness 204
Muscular dystrophies/myopathies 249
Myalgia 161
Myasthenia gravis 206, 254
Myasthenic 204
Myelodysplastic syndromes 330, 341
Myelofibrosis 342
Myeloid metaplasia 342
Myelomatosis 326
Myoclonus 230
Myoglobinuria 270
Myokymia 232
Myopathies 204
Myotonia 208, 249
Myotonic jerks 219

Nail dysplasia 137
Nails 22

Nasal
    discharge/running nose 29
    obstruction 29
    pain 30
    regurgitation of fluids 199
    septum 39
Nasopharynx 170
Nausea and vomiting 260
Neck stiffness 17, 170, 234
Necrobiosis lipoidica diabeticorum 352
Nephrolithiasis 148
Nephrotic syndrome 147
Nerve lesion 242
Nervous system 153
Neurofibromatosis (von Recklinghausen's disease) 413, 423
Neuropathic joint (Charcot joint) 25
Neuropathic ulcer 378
Night 'bone' pain 371
Nipple
    discharge 314
    inversion 314
Nocturia 77
Normal areas of resonance and dullness on chest 46
Normal fundus 166
Normal palpable structures in the abdomen 273
Normal traube's area on left side 48
Nose 9
Numbness 161, 235
Nystagmus 157, 196

Obesity 3
Occlusion of central artery of retina 169
Occlusive arterial disease 115
Ocular fundus 166
Ocular pain 6
Oculocephalic reflex 195, 436
Oculogyric crisis 437
Oculovestibular reflex (caloric test) 437
Oculovestibular reflex 195
Odour/smell 4
Odynophagia 31, 257
Oedema 25, 77
    of the lids (periorbital oedema) 6
    of the lids 6
Olfactory (first) cranial nerve 176
Oligoarticular 376
Oliguria/anuria 128
On slit-lamp examination 8
Opacification of cornea 7
Opening snap (os) 95
Ophthalmopathy 359
Ophthalmoplegia 187
Ophthalmoscope 166, 435
Opisthotonus 233
Optic (second) cranial nerve 176
Optic atrophy 167
Optic neuritis 168
Oral lesions 13

Orientation to time, place, person 172
Orthopnoea and PND (paroxysmal nocturnal dyspnoea) 34
Orthostatic (postural) hypotension 88
Osler-Weber-Rendu disease 328
Osteoarthritis 403
Otitis externa 169
Outer most point of the cardiac impulse felt 91
Oxycephaly 4

Pain (joint pain) 371
Pain abdomen 257
Pain due to tendon involvement 371
Painful (antalgic) gait 377
Painful finger tips 79
Palatal reflex 221
Pallor 322
Palmar erythema and janeway lesion 79
Palmomental reflex 210
Palpation (digital examination) 293
Palpation 277
    for sinus tenderness 40
    of trachea 44
    of various pulses 84
    of wrist joint. 394
Palpebral fissure is wide 6
Palpitation 75
Pancytopenia 330
Panhypopituitarism 364
Papanicolaou (pap) smears 146
Papillae 12
Papilloedema 167, 168
Paraesthesias and dysaesthesias 236
Paraphasias 174
Paraphimosis 141
Parasternal heave 91
Paratonic rigidity (gegenhalten phenomenon) 208
Paronychia 419
Pattern of respiration 432
Peau d' orange of the breast 315
Pectoral reflex 216
Pelvic abscess 299
Pelvic inflammatory disease (PID) 151
Pemphigus 425
Pendular
    jerks 219, 229
    knee jerks 224
Penis 139
Percussion 46
    of Traube's semilunar space 291
Pericardial
    knock (rub) 97
    rub 92
Pericarditis 73, 114
Perimetery 180
Peripheral cyanosis 78
Peripheral sensory system (spinal cord) 234
Peripheral vascular system 115

Peristaltic sounds 291
Periumbilical mass 296
Pes cavus 23, 378
Petechiae 419
Phalen's manoeuvre 395, 396
Phimosis 140
Photodermatitis 410
Pigeon chest 42
Pitting oedema 26
Pituitary dwarfism 3
Plantar reflex 220
Platybasia (basilar invagination) 5
Platynychia 419
Pleural effusion 66
Pleural fluid aspiration 66
Pleural rub 55, 56, 57
Pleuropericardial rub 57
Pneumonic consolidation 59
Polyarticular 376
    arthritis 401
Polycythaemia 338
Polydactyly 21
Polyneuropathies 252
Polyp 40
Polyuria 128
Polyuria and polydipsia 347
Porphyria 270, 413
Portal hypertension 309
Portwine stain 418
Posterior
    columns 235, 238
    roots 234
Postinfective polyneuropathy 253
Postpolio paralysis 207
Post-tussive suction 57
Post-zoster neuralgia 191
Practical classification of headache 153
Prayer's hand 21
Precocious puberty 348
Precordium 89
Prepuce 140
Pressure sores 25
Pretibial myxoedema 361
Profile for coagulation disorders 344
Prognathism 15, 364
Prolactin secreting pituitary tumour 315
Pronator sign 229
Proprioceptive sensations 240
Protein energy malnutrition 3
Pruritus (itching) 269
Pruritus 407
Pseudobulbar palsy 203
Pseudocoma 428
Pseudohypertrophy of calf muscles 206
Pseudoptosis 184
Psoas cold abscess 404
Psoriasis 414, 423
Psoriatic arthritis 378
Psychogenic 267
Psychogenic vertigo 157
Pudal's sign 289
Pulmonary
    collapse 65
    dyspnoea 61
    embolism 64
Pulse deficit 84
Pulsus
    alternans 86
    bigeminus or trigeminus 86
    paradoxus 86
Pupillary
    abnormalities 163
    reactions to light 163
    size and reaction 434
Pupils 163
Pupils are fixed, dilated, and unreactive to light 438
Purpura 327, 419
Purpuric spots 333
Pursed-lip breathing 37
Pursuit gaze movements 185
Purulent urethritis (gonorrhoea) 150
Pyoderma gangrenosum 409
Pyorrhoea 11
Pyramidal tracts 203

Quinsy 15

Radiating 72
Radiculopathy 244
Radiofemoral delay 85
Raised intracranial
    pressure 168
    tension 247
Rapid tapping gait 227
Rashes 408
Raynaud's phenomenon 120, 121
Rebound phenomenon 224
Recession of intercostal spaces 43
Red pin test 179
Redness of eyelids 6
Referred pain 257
Reflex
    eye movements 197
    rigidity 208
Reflexes 210
Regional lymphadenopathy 18
Reinforcement or Jendrassik's manoeuvre 217
Reiter's syndrome 403
Renal masses 356
Renal tubular defects 148
Renin-angiotensin system 26
Reptile tongue 229
Respiration 432
Respiratory rate and rhythm 41
Rest pain 371
Reticular activating system (RAS) 428
Retinal
    atrophy 167
    haemorrhages 168
    vein occlusion 169
Retinitis pigmentosa 167
Retroversion of the uterus 151